Nursing
elderly
people

To all our 'old people', and their friends,
who are the recipients of our care

Nursing elderly people

Sally J. Redfern BSc PhD RGN

Senior Lecturer, Department of Nursing Studies
King's College (KQC), University of London, London

Foreword by
Dorothy E. Baker BSc PhD RGN SCM
Senior Lecturer in Nursing,
University of Manchester

Churchill Livingstone

EDINBURGH LONDON MELBOURNE AND NEW YORK 1986

CHURCHILL LIVINGSTONE
Medical Division of Longman Group Limited

Distributed in the United States of America by Churchill
Livingstone Inc., 1560 Broadway, New York, N.Y. 10036,
and by associated companies, branches and
representatives throughout the world.

First published 1986

ISBN 0-443-03084-7

British Library Cataloguing in Publication Data
Nursing elderly people.
  1. Geriatric nursing
  I. Redfern, Sally J.
  610. 73'65   RC954

Library of Congress Cataloging in Publication Data
Main entry under title:
Nursing elderly people.
  Includes index.
  1. Geriatric nursing.   I. Redfern, Sally J.
[DNLM: 1. Geriatric Nursing. WY 152 N974603]
RC954.N886   1986   610.73'65   85–16676

Produced by Longman Singapore Publishers (Pte) Ltd.
Printed in Singapore

Foreword

It would be unusual if nurses when asked of their work 'whose side are you on?' did not answer 'the side of the patient, of course.' And this answer would come not only from clinical nurses, since our nursing leaders also are much exercised about 'accountability', 'quality assurance', 'the nurse as the patients' advocate'. Elderly people tend not to be amongst the most privileged of patients, but we must assume that the generalised concern for 'the patient' does not exclude them.

If we are indeed on the side of the elderly patient, acting as her or his advocate, we will immediately recognise the complexity and delicacy of our work, and the depth of knowledge and understanding necessary for it. In this volume Sally Redfern and her fellow contributors have made a major contribution to that knowledge and understanding. They alert us to make the necessary meticulous assessment of each nursing situation, and, in co-operation with the patient, to construct an appropriate care plan.

In ideal circumstances the next steps—acting on the plan and evaluating its effectiveness—would proceed without obstacle. In practice, the necessary resources of time, competent assistance and equipment are not always available, and the plan, even if formulated, often cannot be carried out. Short cuts are taken, 'getting through the work' becomes the norm, and wider aims, such as helping the

patient to become independent, are abandoned. There may even be pressures which result in the nurse suspending the rules which govern the normal civilities between adults. Through no fault of her own, the nurse finds herself involved in a standard of care which in no way reflects her ideals as 'the patient's advocate'. What now of 'quality assurance'?

A positive response to inadequate resources, arising from thoughts inspired by this book, might perhaps be considered. Rather than 'coping' and 'muddling through' in the time-honoured manner, the nurse might record those items on the care plan which she has not been able to carry out, and the consequences for the patient. This information could be passed to the nurse managers, thus providing them with valuable data to support their claims for resources, as well as assisting them in their endeavours to remain in close contact with what Stacey describes as 'the clinical coal face'. These insights could, in appropriate circumstances, be shared with the members of the Health Authority and the Community Health Council, to their great benefit.

Were such a practice adopted widely by nurses working with elderly patients, the precepts of this excellent book could both illuminate and ultimately change nursing practice. In any case, the book provides a stimulus for nurses to eliminate the gulf between the succession of fine sounding slogans about nursing and the reality of life on the ward or in the home of the frail and sick. The outcome may both bring comfort to the elderly and pose a challenge for those in highest authority, and for the nurse in between there is no escape from the question 'whose side are you on?'

Manchester, 1986   D. E. B.

Preface

Our attempt has been to combine the expertise of many people concerned with care of elderly people (nurses, social scientists, doctors and other specialists) into a comprehensive nursing textbook. We cover social, psychological and physiological aspects of ageing, the common nursing problems of elderly people, and provision of health care. Our approach is a warm-blooded, humanitarian one in which old people are seen as a precious 'commodity' who have wisdom and other positive contributions to make to society. This book will have been successful if it encourages its readers to value the old people they care for and to promote opportunities for well-being and psychological growth rather than helplessness and deterioration in their old age.

The intention has been to produce a text which is not overly parochial and which can cross cultural and geographical boundaries. The material on the organisation of health care and provision of services, however (especially Part 3 and Part 4), necessarily emphasises a British perspective, although much of it is appropriate to other western industrial countries.

We hope the book will be a key text for nurses specialising in the care of elderly people, which would include post-basic course students. In addition, since many student nurses will care for old people when they are qualified, either by choice or otherwise, this book should provide them with useful reference material. A truly comprehensive nursing textbook for the elderly might encourage more student nurses to choose to specialise in this field, particularly if they use the book during their basic training. The readership might also include doctors joining departments of geriatric medicine and other members of the health care team, all of whom require some knowledge of nursing and the nurse's role. Above all, our aim is that the book will appeal to the socially aware nurse of post-industrial societies in which social problems such as ageing populations, mass unemployment and increased leisure time are of major concern, and in which ageism will take its place, along with sexism and racism, as an acknowledged discrimination issue.

The illustration on the cover of this book was chosen to reflect a positive view of old age. It shows two white-haired women who could be friends, engaged in a challenging activity not traditionally regarded as female. The activity is self-initiated, there are no health care workers in sight, and it could be located in a hospital or community setting. The exclusion of men from the picture is not deliberate, but it does illustrate the fact that most old people are women. This reason alone would dictate departure from convention and the use of the female gender throughout this book when referring to old people in the singular.

The book contains four parts. In *Part 1*, the focus is on what it means to be old and the changes which may occur as a result of ageing.

Although the term 'aged' is used as a category to describe old people, it is inappropriate because 'ageing' and 'aged' are time-dependent concepts. A child 'ages' over time but is not classified as aged. Lumping all old people into a homogeneous, rigid category, although convenient, denies recognition of their individual differences. It also increases the risk of their being classified as a low status minority. This occurs with other groups, such as 'the disabled'. It is usual to distinguish between functional and chronological age, especially with reference to child development; we talk, for example, of the 'mental age' of a child. Similarly, not all old people are functionally, physiologically, psychologically and socially at the same point at the same age. The use of classifications such as 'retirement age' encourages misleading categorisation. In practice the outcome is that 'old age' is often negatively regarded as a period of non-productivity and illness, when it can be, and often is, a time of positive experience, health and optimism, especially as a result of the technological, material and social advances in our society. In Chapter 1, Malcolm Johnson explores these ideas. The attitude held by society tends to demean old people and reflects the destructive stereotyping of ageism, not dissimilar to that experienced by women and black people. Problems of frailty do occur, but they vary according to people's life experiences, to variations in exposure.

In Chapter 2, Sally Robbins continues the discussion on the fallacy of ageist stereotyping. Some of the psychological theories of ageing are described as are the effects of changes in role and the impact of life events. The research evidence on changes in cognitive processes (intelligence, learning, memory, perception, etc.) which result from growing older does not always support the assumption of inevitable decline. People adjust to being old in different ways, and adjustment is a healthy lifetime process not confined to old age. Health care demands and health care itself would alter substantially if in both preventive and reactive medicine greater account were taken of old people's individuality.

Some of the physiological theories of ageing are summarised by Gerry Bennett in Chapter 3. He describes the physiological changes which occur with age and emphasises the importance of distinguishing between changes which occur as a result of age alone and those which accompany diseases common in old people.

Part 2 contains 18 chapters and has a clinical emphasis, covering the nursing problems commonly experienced by old people. It takes a client-centred individualised approach and acceptance of the 'nursing process' is explicit in most of the chapters.

Communication and sensory deficit are central to Chapters 4, 5 and 6. In Chapter 4, Jill Macleod Clark explains the principal components of communication. She focuses on the nurse's role in assessing and meeting the needs of elderly patients with communication difficulties in general, but particularly those with speech impairment following a stroke. In Chapter 5, Katia Gilhome Herbst reminds us that to be old and deaf constitutes a double stigma as well as double handicap, and deafness is often associated with 'daftness' (incorrectly) and with depression (correctly). The prevalence of deafness is much higher than is generally believed and most old people have some hearing loss. Nurses have an important role in assessment of hearing loss, in improving communication with deaf old people, and in helping them take advantage of personal and environmental hearing aids. Bob Greenhalgh, in Chapter 6, notes that most people who are partially sighted or totally blind are elderly. He discusses assessment of visual ability, the factors which influence sight, and the nurse's contribution to the rehabilitation of old people with impaired sight.

Chapters 7 to 16 attend to essential human needs and functions which often present difficulties in old age. In Chapter 7, Amanda Stokes-Roberts discusses the importance to old people of maintaining their earlier activities and interests, and the factors which influence an old person's ability to keep occupied. Amanda identifies what can be done to keep old people in the environment of their choice and to enhance their well-being in institutions.

Mobility is the subject of Chapter 8, and Lynn Batehup and Amanda Squires discuss the prevalence of immobility of old people and the factors which affect their mobility. The specific mobility problems of people with certain pathologies (Parkinson's disease, hemiplegia, arthritis, amputation, falls) are described, and guidance is given on their management. The relative merits of stroke units on recovery of patients compared with conventional care are discussed. The subject of mobility continues in Chapter 9 on care of the foot. Foot problems tend to be given low priority, yet they cause so much pain and incapacity for old people and are relatively easy to prevent and to treat. Mike Hobday discusses the common problems and their management. There is much nurses can do to relieve an overstretched chiropody service.

Difficulty in breathing also limits mobility. In Chapter 10, Angela Heslop covers cardio-vascular and respiratory fitness of old people, and the nursing management of people with breathing difficulties. Keeping fit with regular exercise is advocated for younger people. The right kind of exercise is equally important for old people, both in good and in poor health.

It is tempting, particularly for those living alone or with mobility problems, to eat unwisely. Sue Thomas, in Chapter 11, describes the risk factors which affect the nutritional status of old people, the preva-lence of malnutrition, and the nutritional problems which occur. She gives guidance on how to help old people to eat properly and outlines the nutritional services available in the United Kingdom.

Old people find it embarrassing to talk about their bodily functions, particularly problems of elimination, and the prevalence of urinary incontinence is probably higher than that published. In Chapter 12, Christine Norton describes elimination needs and the assessment and management of people with defaecation and micturition difficulties. She discusses the controversy surrounding the emergence of the incontinence adviser into a

nursing climate in which all nurses might regard themselves as specialists.

Deaths of old people from hypothermia frequently make headlines, and the recog-nition and management of hypothermia occu-pies a major part of Chapter 13. Michael Green urges that nurses and doctors should be vig-ilant for abnormally low and high body temperatures in old people, should be aware of those in the population at risk, and should become politically active in an effort to improve the financial and social circumstances of this vulnerable group.

With increasing numbers surviving into very old age, many more immobile old people are at risk from pressure sores. The prevention and management of pressure sores forms a major part of Sally Redfern's discussion in Chapter 14. As with incontinence, manage-ment of people with, or at risk of developing, pressure sores requires a multi-disciplinary team approach, but these are areas in which nurses can take the lead.

Chapter 15 covers sleep and rest. We all need adequate sleep, yet the function of sleep continues to be debated. Morva Fordham discusses sleep patterns of old people compared with young, and the effects of different patterns on daytime behaviour. She describes the multiple causes of sleep prob-lems of old people and emphasises the nurse's role in assessing and managing these problems.

In Chapter 16, Christine Webb returns to the subject of stereotyping and prejudice, and discusses the widespread myth that old people, particularly women, are asexual. Sexual expression tends to be discouraged, particularly in institutions and for old people with disabilities. Nurses are in an ideal position to act as advocates in helping old people fulfil their need for self-respect, companionship, love and intimacy. Like sexuality, pain is a personal and private ex-perience. In Chapter 17, Susan Gollop outlines the effect of ageing on the experience of pain. She focuses on the assessment of pain and the various ways in which the nurse can intervene in caring for an old person in pain.

Chapters 18 and 19 refer to the elderly

mentally frail. Although dementia is common in the very old, it is not, as is often thought, synonymous with ageing, a point made clear by Julia Brooking in Chapter 18. Julia also clarifies the difference between dementia and confusion, and provides an optimistic approach to treatment and care of these frail old people. She goes on in Chapter 19 to discuss another common problem for old people, depression, and highlights its social, biological and psychological antecedents. Suicide and other so-called 'functional' disorders of old people are discussed briefly, and the approaches to care which are most helpful are identified. This should be useful material for nurses without specialised psychiatric training.

Old people consume nearly a third of the National Health Service drugs budget and this proportion is likely to increase. In Chapter 20, Jill David discusses both the value and the hazards of drug use for old people. Nurses have a crucial role in teaching patients about their drugs, in monitoring progress and reporting side-effects, and in preparing patients (or relatives) to administer their own drugs safely when discharged from hospital.

Part 2 ends with Chapter 21 by Jo Hockley on death and dying. She discusses the causes of death in the elderly and where people die. 'Natural' deaths seem to be much less common today, perhaps because few occur at home. Useful guidance is given on the management of problems often experienced by people who are dying, including care of relatives. Following this is a discussion of the merits of hospice care and a comment on euthanasia. The chapter ends with a poem written by a 90-year-old patient just before her death, which carries a message for all nurses— to ensure that patients do not die alone.

Part 3 examines the provision of care for elderly people and focuses mainly on a British perspective. Helen Evers' Chapter 22 is essential reading if we are to understand the organisation of care for old people in this country. She outlines some of the characteristics of the elderly population and describes the historical development of health service provision, noting that needs and services seldom match

well. Helen draws on research into the organisation of nursing and highlights the perennial problems of this low status specialty, particularly those of long-term care. The arguments are strongly made for nurse-led long-term care units without the clinical atmosphere of the hospital, where old people who require little medical attention can live in a homely, personalised environment, and where the links with community nursing are strengthened. Long-term care is the focus of Chapter 23 in which Barbara Wade refers to research carried out with old people living in long-term geriatric wards and residential and private nursing homes. The impression which emerges is one of inflexibility by the authorities and little choice for old people. Barbara advocates a 'supportive model' of care which would be appropriate to all settings and would give old people and their relatives the choice and freedom they seek.

Psychiatric care for elderly people has developed as a specialty more recently than geriatrics, and there is a serious shortfall of psychogeriatricians and specialist nurses. In Chapter 24, Julia Brooking identifies the facilities required for the elderly mentally frail, facilities which are not available for most of these old people. It is their families who are left with the major burden of care.

Virtually all hospital nurses care for old people, but, in Chapter 25, Pauline Fielding focuses on the variety of organisation and facilities provided in geriatric units, and specifies the basic requirements of such units. Comprehensive assessment of an old person's level of independence is an essential prerequisite for successful nursing intervention, and planning for the patient's discharge from hospital should begin soon after admission. The important role that nurses working in geriatric units have is emphasised, in protecting the patients from the negative effects of an impersonal and institutionalised environment.

Although integration of hospital and community services for old people is an attractive proposition, separation of these services is the reality today. In Chapter 26, Fiona Ross describes the complexity and challenge for the nurse caring for old people at home, and she describes the organisation of primary health care and social service provision in this country. She argues for development of the district nurse as the key worker for old people in the primary care team, responsible for preventive as well as therapeutic nursing. This would leave the health visitor free to continue to focus on child care.

In Chapter 27, Alison While describes the surveillance and health promotion and maintenance functions of health visitors, and agrees that, apart from the few who specialise in care of old people, most health visitors give priority to child care. She regards the health visitor as essential in maintaining the wellbeing of old people at home, and believes that rather than extending the role of the district nurse as advocated by Fiona Ross, health visitors should expand their clientèle to include all members of the family, i.e. old people as well as children. Alison While also gives us insight into the problems of growing old in inner-city areas, into the ageing experience of people from ethnic minorities, and into violence against old people.

In *Part 4*, Sally Redfern draws together issues raised in earlier chapters and discusses others relevant to the care of old people. The focus in Chapter 28 is the elderly person, in Chapter 29 it is the elderly patient or client, and in Chapter 30 it is the nurse's role and health care provision for old people. Chapter 28 refers to some of the earlier discussions on the impact of an ageing population; it highlights the experiences that women, men and people of different ethnic origin have in being old, victims of discrimination and dependent on inadequate services. More positively, some aspects of 'successful ageing' are discussed, together with ways in which nurses can help old people to stay healthy.

Some of the major issues concerning the quality of living and of dying for the frail old person who needs short-term hospital care or continuing support are discussed in Chapter 29. We focus on communication with elderly patients or clients, on the organisation of nursing in different institutional settings, and

on surgery for old people. Striking a balance between allowing old people the rights to which any individual is entitled and avoiding unnecessary risk is a continuing theme, and is perhaps the key to high quality nursing. The theme continues in the discussion on the quality of dying in which the focus is the patient's right to refuse treatment, informed consent, and the care of dying people.

In discussion of the nurse's role, in Chapter 30, the main concerns are the debate about independent nurse practitioners and nurse education. An attempt has been made to give an overview of health care provision and to make recommendations for the future. In the final section we identify some of those areas in nursing elderly people which would benefit from further research. Nurses who examine their own practices, who continue to learn about nursing old people and who investigate nursing issues themselves, will ensure that the quality of nursing will improve and, with it, the quality of life for old people.

I am grateful to Dorothy Baker for writing the Foreword. She is a specialist and teacher on the nursing of elderly people, and an advocate for the elderly in her work as a member of a local Health Authority. Her research on the organisation of nursing in geriatric wards is well known to the profession.

This book would not have been written without each contributor's commitment and patience. Many waited a long time between sending me their chapters and the final appearance in print. I am indebted to Churchill Livingstone, particularly to Ellen Green who put the idea to me in the first place, and to Sally Morris and Dinah Bagshaw who nursed me through all the stages of production. Specific thanks go to Pat Shipley who gave me much of her time in discussion of my ideas and her skill at constructive criticism, to Pam Coles, Joyce Hine, Doreen Newman and Christine Terrey for their high quality typing of this manuscript, and to Beryl Bailey for her indexing skills.

London, 1986   S. J. R.

Contributors

Lynn Batehup BSc RGN DipN
Clinical Teacher, St George's Hospital and Department of Nursing Studies, King's College (KQC), University of London, London

Gerald C. J. Bennett MB BCh MRCP
Consultant in Geriatric Medicine, The London Hospital, Whitechapel, London

Julia I. Brooking BSc RMN RGN DipN Cert Ed RNT
Lecturer in Psychiatric Nursing, Department of Nursing Studies, King's College (KQC), University of London, London

Jill A. David BSc MSc RGN HV MIBiol
Director of Nursing Research, Royal Marsden Hospital, London

Helen K. Evers BSc MSc PhD
Senior Research Fellow, Department of Social Medicine, University of Birmingham, Birmingham

Pauline Fielding BSc PhD RGN
Director of Clinical Nursing Research, Bloomsbury District Health Authority, The Middlesex Hospital, London

Morva Fordham BSc MSc RGN SCM RNT
Lecturer, Department of Nursing Studies, King's College (KQC), University of London, London

Katia Gilhome Herbst MA PhD
Projects Officer, The Mental Health Foundation, London

Michael F. Green MA MB BChir FRCP
Consultant Physician in Geriatric Medicine, States of Guernsey, Channel Islands

Robert Greenhalgh BA CQSW
Honorary Chairman of the Partially Sighted Society, Principal of Training, South Regional Association for the Blind

Susan M. Gollop BSN MSN RGN RNT
Senior Lecturer, Nursing Studies, North East Surrey College of Technology, Surrey

Angela Heslop DipN RGN RCNT
Clinical Teacher in Continuing Nurse Education, Bloomsbury Health Authority. Research Fellow, Department of Medicine, Charing Cross Hospital, London

Mike C. Hobday BA MChS
Head of Chelsea School of Chiropody, London

Jo Hockley RGN SCM
Symptom Control and Support Sister, St Bartholomew's Hospital. Sister at St Christopher's Hospital, London

Malcolm L. Johnson
Professor of Health and Social Welfare, The Open University, Milton Keynes, Bucks.

Jill Macleod Clark PhD BSc RGN
Lecturer, Department of Nursing Studies, King's College (KQC), University of London, London

Christine Norton MA RGN
Formerly Incontinence Adviser, Bloomsbury Health Authority, London

Sally J. Redfern BSc PhD RGN
Senior Lecturer, Department of Nursing Studies, King's College, (KQC), University of London, London

Sally E. Robbins BSc MPhil
Senior Clinical Psychologist, Psychology Department, Maidstone Health Authority

Fiona M. Ross BSc RGN NDNCert
Queen's Institute Lecturer in Community Nursing, Department of Nursing Studies, King's College (KQC), University of London, London

Amanda Squires MCSP SRP
Superintendent Physiotherapist, Dulwich Hospital North, Camberwell Health District, London. Part-time tutor, Degree Course for the Remedial Professions, Polytechnic of Central London

Amanda Stokes-Roberts DipCOT, SROT
Head Occupational Therapist, Bolingbroke Hospital, London

Sue Thomas SRD DipHE
Formerly Dietitian to the Geriatric Unit, St James' Hospital, Balham, London

Barbara E. Wade RGN BEd PhD
Director, Daphne Heald Research and Development Unit, The Royal College of Nursing, London

Christine Webb BA MSc PhD RGN RSCN RNT
Principal Lecturer in Nursing, Bristol Polytechnic

Alison E. While BSc MSc PhD RGN HVcert
Lecturer, Department of Nursing Studies, King's College (KQC), University of London, London

Contents

PART ONE

Ageing and old age

1

M. L. Johnson

The meaning of old age

The process of ageing is classically depicted as one of constant and inexorable decline after reaching a peak of bodily function and efficiency around the end of the second decade of life. Moreover, the later years of life are conventionally seen as ones where pathologies of mind, body and social relationships take place. Indeed the period known as old age has been seen, until very recently, as one of withdrawal from the mainstream of life due to infirmity.

Elaborating on traditional presentations of ageing as an inexorable process of decline, modern medical science has created a pathology model of ageing which indicates declining function in all bodily systems. Also reflecting accounts in literature, history, biblical sources and folk lore, psychologists and psychiatrists have produced a body of data which they claim follows a decremental pattern. The advance of chronological age is said to produce a consistent erosion of capacity for memory, cognition, learning and creativity. In terms of psychological health later life is associated with widespread confusional states, dementia and depression of epidemic proportions. Social scientists have made their own contributions to the prevailing picture, by focusing on the poverty of retired people, their high consumption of health and social services, their 'burdensome' claim on social security budgets. Research has focused largely on the negative impact of retirement and its consequences for conjugal relationships, levels of morale and isolation from former social networks.

This chapter will attempt to reconcile this sombre picture of the ageing process with some recent trends both in research and in the patterns of behaviour to be observed amongst the increasingly large numbers of people who are active in later life. In doing this we will give some attention to the life histories of individuals and the value of biographical analysis in gaining a more authentic picture of the social processes of ageing. It will also be necessary to look briefly at the constraints which limit the opportunities for elderly people to fulfil their potential—thus helping to reinforce the negative stereotypes of old age.

THE BIOLOGY OF AGEING

Later chapters (particularly Chapter 3) deal in detail with the physical changes which accompany ageing processes. For present purposes it is necessary only to indicate what the biological and clinical sciences have to say about the human body throughout the lifespan.

Accumulated evidence points fairly unequivocally to the declining efficiency of most bodily systems with age. Once biological maturity has been reached—between the ages of 15 and 25 years—the degenerative processes begin. In the early stages the reductions in function are small, but continue over time in an increasing and cumulative fashion. Rates of age-related degeneration vary considerably. Moreover, the onset of decline occurs at different points in the life-path for different parts of the body. Within individuals, the variance from statistical norms will be influenced by genetic inheritance, lifestyle and factors such as obesity, diet, exercise and medical history.

This brief sketch of biological decline is indicative of the overall position. It offers a picture of the human body as an organism which increases in stature and efficiency during the first two decades of life, reaching

its peak around the middle of the third decade. From that point the speed of decline is variable but inevitable. Amongst the intervening factors which can influence and even arrest the pace of advancing physical inefficiency are two broad categories of action. The first concerns the behaviour of individuals—their diet and general lifestyle. The second is the increasing capacity of medical science to treat, ameliorate or cure those conditions which speed up the ageing process or lead to premature death. With increased capacity to manipulate these variables it has been possible to increase dramatically the numbers of people, in developed societies, who live a full lifespan.

Yet, whilst biology conveys an uncompromising message of degeneration and medicine a complementary one of increasing illness associated with age, there is a cross-current of evidence of a more positive kind. Its effect is to offer the prospect of a less pathological mode of growing old which allows continuity of life experience and a wide range of activity. The debate about how far modifications of personal conduct combined with good medical care can create supernormal life expectancy and how far it can lead to a healthier existence is now in full flow. After decades of negative findings and decrementalism, there has arisen an antithetical concept of ageing with more positive connotations. Perhaps best encapsulated in the vigorously optimistic pages of Fries and Crapo's (1981) volume *Vitality and Ageing: Implications of the Rectangular Curve*, the dialogue now offers ageing as both an inexorable decline and as a process capable of considerable manipulation. The new debate claims that what have been previously considered as normal processes of ageing can be considerably slowed down. Indeed the image of the rectangular curve is offered as one which reflects the impact of better health so that the major maladies of adulthood are compressed into a relatively short space of time immediately prior to death. The survival curve will become rectangular rather than one of linear decline, after an early peak.

The argument the book seeks to advance is that the present upper limit for human longevity, of about 115 years, is unlikely to be extended in the foreseeable future, but that progress in health and welfare will delay the onset of the most damaging ailments of later life. It is contended that most of the disabling conditions of old age are self-inflicted (through alcohol, tobacco, poor diet, lack of exercise, etc.), or occur as a result of the way society is organised in that it may cause ill health (environmental pollution of various kinds) and fail to provide adequate health and welfare services. A remedy for these causes of illness lies in health education, political action and more positive personal behaviour. Were this approach to be adopted, the authors predict a general raising of health standards. Consequently, the chronic illnesses of insidious onset (cancers, rheumatism, degeneration of the heart and so on) will reach an acute stage later in life and concentrate themselves in a short period of perhaps three years prior to death. Thus the downward curve of survival would become more like a rectangle (Fig. 1.1).

Whilst the extension of life and health debate is being conducted in a somewhat value-laden manner, there is a growing body of scientific evidence for the more optimistic view which needs to be unravelled. Within governmental thinking, pressured by rising demand for medical services and the desire to reduce public spending, the focus of this new trend is on the behaviour of individuals. Smoking, diet, exercise, early medical consultation, prophylactic medication and changes in lifestyle are all the subject of health education programmes. The individual is seen to be responsible for his or her own health state and responsible for reducing claims on health resources. In parallel, there is another view (to which we return later, Townsend 1981) which rejects the emphasis on personal conduct and urges changes at a different level, that is, in patterns of work, transport and social organisation—social and political solutions which will make life safer for all.

RESEARCH ON OLD AGE

Studies of ageing and old age (gerontology) are no longer rare, as might have been claimed confidently as little as 20 years ago. But in the intervening period the growth of geriatric medicine, the expansion of academic and policy related research, along with changes in the demographic structure, have

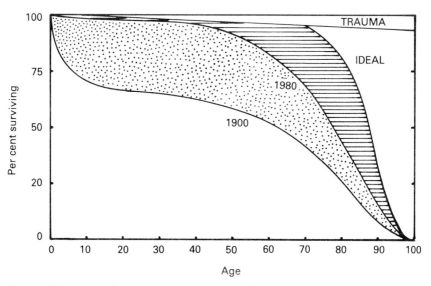

Fig. 1.1   The rectangular curve. *Source: Fries and Crapo 1981.*

made later life more important and better understood. Having said this, it is essential to recognise that gerontology is still very youthful as a field of study. Much material has been gained through recent research which has aided our social and medical understanding of old age; but it remains largely confined to studies of the maladies which come with age.

CONTRIBUTION TO THE PATHOLOGY MODEL

The history of British research into old age over the past 100 years tends—as do contemporary studies—to be linked to the resolution of problems connected with the rising proportion of elderly people in the population and their absolute numbers. In 1881 people over the current retirement ages in England and Wales (65 for men and 60 for women) formed little more than 5 per cent of the population. By the turn of the century it had risen to more than 6 per cent. At the last published census in 1981 it had advanced strikingly to 17 per cent, with the greatest expansion taking place in the 75 plus age groups.* A century ago, the great concerns brought to public attention by the growing school of social surveying reformers, were with poverty, illnesses and institutional care of the aged. These culminated in the report of the Royal Commission on the Poor Law (1905–09), which laid down a blueprint for the welfare state, and more immediately led to the introduction of old age pensions.

During the next half century the interests put so firmly on the political agenda by the researches of Charles Booth (1902), Seebohm Rowntree (1901), Beatrice Webb (1926) and Bowley and Burnett Hurst (1912) remained fixed. As founders of the social survey method, they each contributed powerfully effective descriptions of the nature and extent of poverty, ill health and social breakdown.

* The figures given here are for people over retirement ages, i.e. 60 for women and 65 for men. Sometimes statistics are given for those *over 65 only*. This is the case in Helen Evers' Chapter 22.

Their detailed statistical accounts provided evidence of a kind which circumscribed the everyday conditions of the artisan classes, including older people. Between them these pioneers had uncovered areas of ignorance so vast and forms of need so fundamental that few of their successors reached out beyond the territory they had defined. As a result, it became a commonplace that old age for those from all but the most privileged classes was characterised by physical illness, poor nutrition, inadequate housing and fear of the pauper's death. Thus, whilst important basic scientific research proceeded slowly on the biological bases of ageing, the greatest efforts of medical research were to do with ill health both physical and mental. (Handbooks which attempt to provide syntheses of existing work tend to be a sound guide to the pattern and distribution of existing research. In gerontology such a series of handbooks was published, under the general editorship of James Birren (Binstock and Shanas 1976, Birren and Schaie 1977, Finch and Hayflick 1977). In 1981 a new series edited by Carl Eisdorfer, *Annual Reviews of Gerontology and Geriatrics*, appeared. The foci of attention remain in the clinical management and pathologies of later life; and the same is true of the leading *Journal of Gerontology*.)

This small, but consistently growing body of knowledge, provided a basis for Sheldon (1948) to complete his important study of old people in Wolverhampton early after the Second World War. In the resulting book he was able to provide a taxonomy of the sicknesses which were attributed to old age and to suggest ways in which these could be medically managed. Significantly, the studies which followed have been developments of specialist areas of his broad-ranging studies. Incontinence, falls, strokes, dementia, confusion and depression remain high in the profile of medical research.

Social scientists in Britain have always been fewer in number in the gerontological field, despite their work having had enormous impact both on the public consciousness and politically. They too have been preoccupied with the causes and consequences of poorer physical health and social deprivations which appear to follow retirement from work. After the major policy reforming studies at the turn of the century there was a lull in activity. The interwar years produced a very modest literature about the effects of retirement, but it has failed to leave any permanent mark.

The resurgence of interest in social welfare provision occasioned by the Second World War and the wartime planning for a welfare state served to refocus attention on old age. Beveridge's pension plan revived the debates of the first decade of the century, about the quality of life after retirement (Macintyre 1977). Income, health and housing resumed their position at the head of the agenda—an agenda which has survived almost intact to the present day. But as empirical studies of life circumstances of old people began, they soon developed specialist orientations (Cole 1962, Townsend 1962, Brockington and Lempert 1966, Tunstall 1966). Apart from Peter Townsend's *The Family Life of Old People* (1957) there have been few notable studies which look at the subject in the round. In particular, research of a social and medical kind alike, gave pride of place to studies of 'need'. As a result the enormous output of research which has been produced since the early 1950s has provided a highly detailed account of the structural characteristics of the retired population, the illnesses which are likely to afflict them, the sources of their income, the quality of their housing, their occupancy of hospital beds and consumption of general practitioner (family doctor) services, their need for social support services at home, the changes in family support which have necessitated increased public provision and the quality of institutional care. More recent work has turned to the effectiveness of social policy provision to meet the needs of elderly people, particularly as the rising (and ageing) of this sector of the population became apparent. Studies of geriatric care, old people's Homes and the whole range of domiciliary services, both statutory and voluntary, became increasingly common.

The pathology model of ageing can, of course, be extended too far, for studies within what is here called 'normal ageing' do exist. Psychologists, although equally afflicted by the desire to depict old age as a deviance from the arbitrary norms of early adulthood, have nonetheless done much to identify the general characteristics of retired populations. Yet until very recently their explanations of normal cognitive functioning, personality integration, memory retention and learning skills have served to reinforce the image of old age as a period of chronic decline. These studies have formed the main stream of 'human growth and development' studies which map the whole life as a series of age related stages. Until the upsurge of 'lifespan' studies in the United States, influenced by the work of Goulet and Baltes (1970), Nesselroade and Reese (1973) and Baltes and Schaie (1973), the last stages of any publication or taught course on human development, presented a picture of expected (and therefore normal) decline on all major parameters. Only in the past few years has this orthodoxy been firmly challenged, drawing strength from a close scrutiny of prior assumptions and inappropriate methodologies (Taub 1980). Thus, for example, it is now claimed that the view of decrements in memory function with age are in some measure due to the inappropriate nature of the tests (coming as they do from an earlier culture, old people find them meaningless) and the failure to recognise that as people grow into middle age and beyond they sift information more carefully and store only the essential, rather than whole chunks of undigested material (Labouvie Vief 1982).

LIFE-HISTORY APPROACHES

Equally there are shifts of interest to be observed across the social sciences. As the editor of an international and multidisciplinary journal, *Ageing and Society*, I receive and read over 100 articles a year, submitted for publication. The bulk remain in the mould outlined, but increasingly there is an awareness of the need to theorise, to examine the political economy of old age and to view old age as a particular product of a life lived (Taylor and Ford 1981, Townsend 1981, Walker 1981, Estes 1982).

It would be possible to further document and classify the output of age related research, but this would be as lengthy as it is unnecessary. Convincing evidence of the pathology orientation of studies in old age can be readily found in the series of annual publications produced by the Centre for Policy on Ageing (formerly National Corporation for the Care of Old People), entitled *Old Age: A Register of Social Research*. This annual compendium contains details of all the serious work being undertaken in the field. Each year an analysis is produced by Hedley Taylor of the main subject areas and the percentage of projects under each heading. The volume for 1979/80 identified 165 studies under 40 headings. Of the headings themselves, only three could be said to be of a non-problem centred kind, and contributing 8% to the total. Typical headings are labelled: rehabilitation, sheltered housing, information needs, mental disorder, residential care, etc.

Too much emphasis on these features of the body of research on ageing could lead to a misunderstanding of the purpose of drawing attention to them. There is no implication that this work is in any important sense bad, only that it is providing us with a distorted picture of later life which lacks congruence with my own studies and experience of work with older people. It has led both policy makers and the world at large to see old age as synonymous with sickness, poverty and mental decrepitude. The fact that these conditions do occur amongst the older members of our society is neither to be denied nor ignored. What is important, however, and a central proposition of this chapter, is to recognise that much of what professional observers and helpers see as pathological and problematic is not seen in that way by older people themselves.

For some years now I have been involved in both theoretical writing and empirical studies

of social ageing, as well as in social policy issues in old age. Throughout this period I have been anxious to encourage researchers and analysts to take more account of how elderly people see and value their own lives, in particular in the context of their life-histories. In other places I have written at length about the relationship between life experience and the experience of old age. Inevitably, former lifestyle and practices are powerful and formative factors, not only in the material conditions of life in retirement, but also in the way it is perceived and interpreted. All too little account is taken of these factors in determining what society will do for its older members. Indeed I frequently use a metaphor which compares the social and medical pathologists with spectators in the arena at the end of a marathon race who see the runners enter for the last lap tired and bruised. They see their task as attending to relieving the weariness and the pain of the runners without ever asking how the race was run or what plans they may have for further racing.

The importance of biography*

To suggest that by collecting biographical accounts of people's lives we will see a more dynamic and authentic picture is not to say that it solves all problems or that it has no drawbacks. Among the drawbacks are the ways researchers deal with personal stories and explanations of events which may be subject to poor recall, partial interpretation and internal contradiction. Such accounts are said not to be 'objective' or 'scientific'. But biographical studies of ageing do not take every statement from the teller as factually true. The student of biographies is concerned with the *meaning* of social events as seen through the eye of the self-observer. Like all observers, his or her view will be selective and subject to interpretation. This is obvious from any biography or autobiography you may read. But this very selection tells us much about the

* Parts of this section are taken from Johnson (1979).

way individuals see themselves. In the case of older people it is possible to see the present as a product of the past even when interpretations they might put on particular events are suspect or facts are open to correction. For what emerges is a distillation of their view of themselves and what has happened to them, which has survived through life and will provide the basis for the future. It is the basis of their self-esteem and self-image.

Robert Butler (1963), whose book on old age in America won a Pulitzer Prize, has written of the significance of what he calls the life review. He argues that reminiscence is an integral part of human psychological health and an aspect which increases with age (and the amount of life to review). We have a constant need to reconstruct our self-images and personal histories in the light of recent and current happenings (Strauss 1959, 1977). Thus personal biographies are possessions which we all have and which we tend to keep in good repair, incorporating new material all the time. They provide the framework for so much decision making. This is evident in the way people—especially older people—tell and retell stories about those parts of their lives which, in retrospect, were most important to them. For my own father, the Second World War and his six years as a gunner in Britain and Europe undoubtedly provided a high spot. The events and relationships of that period had a profound effect on his life.

Those who 'take' biographies from others always have a theme or themes which they want to pursue. As Stimson (1976) in explaining his biographical approach to drug users said:

> The successful in this world provide us with suitable biographical accounts of their success. For some the success is explained as personal endeavour in a free society, for example the rags to riches career of a working-class boy who makes it to company director. For others, especially women, personal beauty is the way out of the slum. Yet other biographies show the early development of talent—the pop star whose parents always knew he would be successful by the way he handled his toy guitar as a child. (Stimson 1976, p 1).

By taking a particular dimension of life such as work, sport, love life, etc., it is always essential to examine the developments (or career) of the chosen theme and the way in which it interacts with other continuing careers like marriage, relations with children and involvements in other major activities. A person's biography can be seen as the product of a number of separate but related careers moving along side by side and influencing each other, sometimes minimally, sometimes dramatically. The path—or career—of their health is an important influence on everyone's life.

It is in the very process of unfolding a biography that relationships can be most fruitfully observed. For there you see the whole and continuing nature of, say, the marital relationship or the employer/employee relationship. It is the history which gives meaning to the major events which may not otherwise come to notice. In the setting of later life such histories are vitally important. They provide the explanations which are needed when crises occur and professionals are deciding the future.

If the argument so far has been clear, it will be apparent that by seeing relations and relationships as continuing processes within personal histories, we can see both the satisfactory and the problematic features of old age more clearly. Much of the literature in geriatrics, nursing, social work and other caring professions dealing with older people concerns itself with externally defined pathology. For example, the presence of severe chronic bronchitis, or persistent post-bereavement depression leading to self-neglect, can be seen as objectively observed states which require professional intervention. These crises are often 'life events' which may be misunderstood and misinterpreted if the processes which preceded them are not examined.

Robert Butler, who uses the biographical approach as a method in psychiatry, writes:

> I have used the concept of the life review in my psychotherapeutic work with older persons. Life review therapy includes the taking of an extensive autobiography from the older person. . . . Use of

family albums, scrapbooks and other memorabilia
. . . evoke crucial memories, responses and
understanding in patients. . . . Such life-review
therapy can be conducted in a variety of settings
from senior centers to nursing homes. Even
relatively untrained persons can function as
therapists by becoming "listeners" as older
people recount their lives. (Butler 1975, p 413).

Clearly, a great depth of understanding is
not always required. But when a serious situation is perceived by the helper which might
lead to radical changes in lifestyle for the older
person (e.g. hospitalisation or transfer to an
old people's Home), then biographical knowledge becomes important. If helping means
assisting others to achieve their own objectives (insofar as circumstances allow) then
these objectives need to be uncovered. Unfortunately, they are rarely lying on the surface
and are often not articulated in response to
direct questions of the 'Tell me what you want
. . .' sort. My own experience is that the interviewer needs to be clear about the objectives
of the inverview and to be armed with key
questions which will stimulate the right sort of
reminiscence. Roy Fairchild (1977) talks about
these questions as 'openers' and 'hookers'.

As Maggie Kuhn the leader of the American
Gray Panthers movement, says:

> Old people ought to have a sense of history. They
> must be encouraged to review their own history,
> valuing their origins and past experiences. If we
> could stimulate life review, we could see what we
> have lived through and the ways in which we
> have coped and survived (Kuhn 1977, p 30).

Just as many younger people are unclear
about where they are going and what they
want from life, so too with some older people.
But experience of life-history interviewing
shows that the process of exploration draws
attention to the important features of that life
and almost automatically raises questions
about how those lost elements might be
reconstructed (however imperfectly) in the
changed circumstances of later life. For
example, for many retired women who had no
paid employment, the most satisfying part of
their lives was when their children were at
home. It may be that no acceptable substitute
is available to meet that latent need, but if we

were more concerned with meeting individual
needs than dispensing the resources we have
available (home helps, meals-on-wheels, old
people's clubs, etc.) more solutions might
emerge, like the new fostering schemes
whereby a family takes in an older person for
a short time and provides a substitute and
sympathetic family life.

Whilst manuals and textbooks are readily
available to explain the taking of a medical
history, diagnostic interviews or on casework
method, there are few guides to biographical
interviews. The ground rules are simple to
understand though less easy to carry out. First,
establish a clear interest in the interviewee for
his or her own sake. Second, approach the
interview without introducing the subject of
the person's 'problem'. Third, express a real
interest in her (or his) life and what (s)he sees
as its major themes and events. By listening
hard and talking only as much as is needed to
move the story on, the account will unfold and
the 'problem' will fuse into a context which will
give it meaning and possibly suggest some
solutions. Paul Thompson's excellent book
The Voice of the Past (1978) provides a helpful
interview guide. Ken Plummer has more
recently provided a detailed manual in his
Documents of Life (1983). At a simpler level
Help the Aged's *Recall* (1981) pack is also
valuable.

It is no longer necessary to defend the
biographical approach as a technique. Its roots
can be found, as Rosenmayr (1981) has
reminded us, in the European tradition of
sociology and exemplified in such classic
studies as *The Polish Peasant* (Thomas and
Znaniecki 1927). In the literature of psychology
the processes of life development go back to
Freud and Jung, taking a specific biographical
form in the work of Erikson (1950). More
recently, there is evidence of its impressive
application in studies of middle age by
Neugarten (1968) and Valliant (1977), amongst
others. At the same time there has been
increasing sociological attention to life-
histories, particularly in relation to ageing and
old age. In America Glen Elder's (1974) retro-
spective accounts in *Children of the Great*

Depression and Tamara Hareven's (1981) recent volume are testimony to the confident and increasingly sophisticated analysis of whole or partial biographies. In France Anne-Marie Guillemard's (1972) study of retirement has been followed by others in this form, the latest to be reported being Gaullier's (1982) researches on the redundancy experience of men in their fifties. The most widely read life-history studies of recent years have been Dan Levinson's (1978) *The Season of a Man's Life* and the linked volume of more dramatically depicted accounts in Gail Sheehy's (1974) best selling book *Passages*. Their success has served to legitimise an approach which has had to struggle for respectability, despite its long and honourable history. This may explain the dearth of such studies in Britain, where the prevailing views about suitable methodologies for the study of ageing processes have favoured more structured survey-based approaches.

Cohorts, generations and history

The essential argument for viewing ageing throughout the lifespan as a continuous and ever-changing process, which takes different forms in each successive cohort, has already been made. But before going on to look at the practical issues which arise out of these shifting patterns we must give some attention to conceptual tools and the ways they are to be applied.

The notion of 'generation' as a description of biological and lineage relationships goes back into ancient history. It provides much of the organising framework of Jewish history as recorded in the Old Testament and was an equally well-developed set of relationships in classical Greece. It served then as a system of age-grading which made possible the allocation of roles, relationships, economic tasks and patterns of authority. In modern western societies the temporal aspects of generational differences have come to the fore. Social organisation no longer rests on lineage, nor does it indicate any universal attribute of authority or status. Indeed, as we have already

observed, the longer-lived generations are more likely to find themselves suffering from status deprivation than from celebration of their seniority. Within studies of ageing it has been common to avoid the wider applications of the term 'generation' and to confine attention to the social membership category which is formed by the different layers of family formation. In its looser usage, 'generation' can mean a group of individuals who share a common experience, such as 'the Second World War generation' or Glen Elder's collective term 'Children of the Great Depression'. Within the setting of this paper the pioneering work of Leonard Cain used the term in this way. In writing of 'the new generation of elderly people' he was referring to a demographic cohort rather than a sociobiological category. To avoid confusion, and because it appears to be a more valuable device, attention here will be confined to age cohorts.

A cohort is constituted by the coincidence of the birth of its members within a specified time period. This is not to say that a cohort is merely an age group in the manner commonly adopted when presenting population based data in tabular form. The routine analysis of data by dividing subjects into five or 10 year age groups is one of the principal practical reasons why we have neglected the historical dimension in social science and medical empirical research. It leads to the comparison of arbitrary age segments in a way which assumes that any differences are attributable to age. It is the unconsidered use of that practice which leads to the age labelling this Chapter is attempting to challenge.

What constitutes the organising experience of a cohort which will allow its proper segregation (for analytical purposes) from the rest of a given population is a matter of historical judgment. It is a judgment which acknowledges the unifying influence of social structure on the experience of individuals. There is no opportunity here to elaborate the long-standing debate about the duality of ego and community in the lives of individuals which has consumed social scientists for many decades. Readers are referred to an excellent summary by Philip Abrams (1982), who also provides in his volume *Historical Sociology a* most coherent argument for the combining of historical and sociological analysis.

Abrams' concern is with the refinement of 'sociological generation' and he employs that term, but his argument is one which can equally serve the more specific subset—the cohort. He draws attention to the way in which human history, or what is sometimes called the tide of events, acts as a powerful force in shaping people's lives. These forces are part of the 'structure' within which lives are lived. They are capable of creating such a distinctive set of common experiences (as in wartime) that those who have shared in them are bound together in their thinking and their actions, by the events they shared. Using this approach a sociological generation could include people drawn from a variety of age groups, and for this reason I choose to confine attention to age-based cohorts for use in relation to old age.

In considering the parameters of a cohort, it is essential to consider the pervading influences in the lives of those encompassed. Jane Synge (1981), in her study of Canadian family patterns of people born in the last decade of the nineteenth century and in the early part of the twentieth century, lays particular stress on the need to integrate personal and historical factors in family life, for a group which were born in a specific and transitional historical phase. She continues: 'In addition, data from these sources may also indicate whether characteristics that we currently associate with ageing may stem in part from the specific features of the early life experience of people now in their seventies and eighties.'

Similarly, Martin Kohli et al (1983), in reporting a study of flexible retirement in Germany, observed how the arrangement of life experiences into age stages imposed severe limitations on people who were forced to take early retirement. 'Historically, not only the chronological age at which the socially structured transitions in the life-course occur, has changed, but the character of the temporal organisation itself.' He goes on to identify factors relevant to his sample of early retirees,

which include 'the development of an age-graded school system, of other age-graded systems of public rights and duties, the transformation from a demographic pattern of random experience to a pattern of predictable lifespan and the narrowing of the age for the "normative" events of the family cycle and work career'.

Thus, in examining those who now fall into the groups called old, it is increasingly necessary to find demarcations of historical identity. My own markers in this process include the commencement of the First World War, the points at which universal education was extended, and—in relation to health and social welfare—the extent of adult working life completed before the full introduction of the welfare state in Britain (Phillipson 1982).

HEALTH, RETIREMENT AND WORK

In looking at those who are currently old, it is important not to treat the whole age span (say from 65 to 105) as forming a single group. Even more to the point we should not presume that each new group of elders will be like the last. New cohorts bring new experiences, strength and expectations.

In a book about her views on ageing, Maggie Kuhn (Hessel 1977), quotes a section from Alex Comfort's (1977) volume *A Good Age*, which summarises the position well:

> Unless we are old already, the next "old people" will be us. Whether we go along with the treatment meted out to those who are now old depends on how far society can sell us the bill of goods it sold them—and it depends more upon that than upon any research. No pill or regimen known, or likely, could transform the latter years of life as fully as could a change in our vision of age and a militancy in attaining that change (Comfort 1977, p 13–14).

Attention on 'the active elderly' usually focuses on the retention of physical and psychological fitness to lead a life in much the same way as younger people. It implies being ambulant, capable of walking distances, carrying purchases, negotiating busy roads and coping with public transport; essentially the retention of functional capacities in dealing with what are known as activities of daily living. Clearly this is one of the interpretations which must be taken into account, for the decline in physical health and strength is a seriously limiting factor of older people. But the severe onset of these conditions is being kept at bay until later in the lifespan, and this, combined with a less hostile environment, could release a more creative phase during retirement.

So, in addition to functional health, we need to examine two other forms of increased activity which coincide with and are stimulated by a greater healthiness. The first might be termed 'corporate consciousness and action', the second the 'recolonisation of eldership'.

Functional health in old age, it is well established, is highly correlated with previous lifestyle and status. Shanas and Maddox sum it up neatly when they say:

> In general the lower the socioeconomic position of an individual, the higher the prevalence of disease and the higher the age-specific death rate. These commonly observed associations between socioeconomic position, illness and life expectancy have a complex explanation. Indices of socioeconomic position usually include measurements of income, occupation and education. Such factors, singly or in combination, are reflected in different styles of life and differential access to, and use of, health resources. For instance, low income, a manual occupation and minimal education generally predict a high incidence of disease and elevated death rates in all industrialised countries (Shanas and Maddox 1976, p 602).

The implication of these relationships is that middle-class people are more likely to survive into old age, whereas artisans whose work has been particularly arduous or dangerous to health die at earlier ages. In general this picture is supported by official data on mortality, resulting in a situation whereby those who do survive into retirement can expect to live to age 80 and beyond. Population projections indicate that, from 1986 until the end of the century, those aged 85 years and over will increase in numbers constantly and dramatically to 60% above the current total. The consequences of more people living a full lifespan are mixed. They are expected to remain independent and living in the community for longer but in doing so will suffer the accumulated affects of chronic disease.

The detail of age-related health status is not an essential part of this chapter, but it has been necessary to lay the ground for our understanding of the extended period of physical and psychological well-being, sufficient to allow adequate social functioning. It can be simply but graphically illustrated by pointing to the rising average age of admission to old people's Homes. Ten years ago average admission age was in the lower seventies, with places being given on occasions to people still in their sixties. Now it is difficult for elderly people to gain admission to an old people's Home before their eightieth birthday.

As this group of 'old old' consolidates its position, changes in the social structure of the retired population as a whole will be taking place. There will be more people within it, at all ages, whose socioeconomic position is higher than that of previous cohorts; reflecting improvements in working conditions, the *embourgeoisement* (the growth of the middle classes) of mid-twentieth century Britain, with its better nutrition, housing and education. In sum, there will be more older people throughout the age ranges who have health sufficient to allow for full and active participation in society. These new cohorts will have experienced relative prosperity, support of the welfare state and the rise of consumerism. A new and more aggressive climate of expectation can be anticipated to replace the polite acquiescence and minimal expectations to which researchers and practitioners are currently accustomed. Cohort changes provide the key to many of the likely developments in the future. Life experience for groups of people of the same age group inevitably conditions their expectations and their responses to social and economic circumstances. Those who are currently over 70 years of age in Britain were born in an Edwardian era which marked the end of Britain's dominance of world trade, an era which led directly to the First World War. The interwar depression followed, being terminated by the 1939–45 war, which in turn brought several years of continuing hardship. Only in the 1950s, when this group of people were already moving towards the end of their working (employment) life, did prosperity of a pervasive kind emerge. This historical phase has therefore been one of privation followed by relative plenty, creating amongst those who are now old an understandable sense of comparative well-being.

Again drawing on my own recent life-history studies (Johnson 1982a) it is clear that relative deprivation is the linchpin of satisfaction or dissatisfaction in later life. For this generation their reference groups are principally themselves in the past and their own parents in retirement. Any objective assessment of living standards would give support to the view that Mark Abrams (1980) discovered, that the current cohort is comparatively well off and perceives itself as such. Yet for those who saw the welfare state constructed during their mid-life or earlier and particularly those who were young in the immediate post-war period, the comparison will have an increasingly negative effect. Current expectations of income in retirement are having to be radically revised, whilst projections about the costs of future financial support for the retired give little cause for optimism.

Frustration and unmet expectations may breed political reaction. In most of Europe there is a long way to go, but during the period under consideration in this paper, the strong likelihood is that successive cohorts will not only be more highly motivated to take action, but their higher skills will facilitate an organised lobby of a kind as yet unknown in Britain. Their demand for opportunities to carry out work in its various forms is likely to become more insistent.

CORPORATE CONSCIOUSNESS AND ACTION*

Corporate consciousness and action can reasonably be predicted, then, as the response of the increasingly articulate and socially

* The ideas in this section and the next were first reported in Johnson (1982).

skilful retired population. It will be a group which is less poor overall than its predecessors, as occupational pensions and home ownership supplement state support. Like its American counterpart it is likely to seek a better deal for retired people in everyday transactions where prejudice and commercial practice limit their opportunities. There are no immediate signs of a common consciousness emerging amongst older people in Britain. Certainly no political allegiance is observable yet. But there are signs of an increasing commercial recognition of retired people as a worthwhile market, especially in transport, holidays, domestic equipment and personal services. Banks, building societies, insurance companies, employers and the trade unions continue to exercise unremittingly ageist discrimination against retired people in a manner which may not be tolerated for much longer.

The American experience of increasing consciousness by elderly people of their common position arose out of their desire to challenge commercial interests and later to act as lobbyists in influencing government policy at state and federal level. Perhaps inevitably, those who became involved in organised activity to secure better treatment from those offering goods and services in the market-place were what Pratt (1976) in his book *The Gray Lobby* calls the 'slightly privileged'. In first pursuing preferential treatment amongst traders of all kinds, and then in the 1960s focusing more clearly on political influence, a number of influential national groups emerged. The largest and most durable of them are: The American Association of Retired Persons (AARP) and the National Retired Teachers Association (NRTA), which function in national affairs as one body; The National Council of Senior Citizens (NCSC), which was set up in the 1960s to campaign for Medicare, and then extended its interests, has a less middle-class membership than AARP; more cross-sectional in their membership and more campaigning in their approach than either of these are the Gray Panthers.

Together these mass-membership organisations (their combined membership is counted in millions) are able to act as foci for political reform within the United States and to influence state and federal policy directly. In recent years the US Senate passed legislation raising the compulsory retirement age for public employees to 70 years. Such a development is currently inconceivable in Britain because elderly people are not organised, nor do they appear to wish to be organised on their own behalf. But relative deprivation has proved to be the most powerful force for dissatisfaction in later life. It is likely to increase dramatically as those who expected a long and comfortable retirement find themselves in straitened circumstances because of inflation; also, governments may want to execute a backlash against retired people in favour of employed and unemployed younger people. Should these speculations come to pass, they could be the triggers for mass-membership organisations on the American model. If they do arise, these groups will undoubtedly seek re-entry into all the corners of social and economic life, to establish a respected place for old age.

RECOLONISATION OF ELDERSHIP

Recolonisation of eldership is an expression of this desire to re-enter the social world on equal or even positively discriminated terms. The phrase adopted here is not meant to denote the return to another golden age but takes eldership to mean recognition of and due respect for experience. At its core this 'recolonisation' is about self-respect and mutual respect across generations. It requires society to make a more generous place for old age; but one which also allows greater opportunity for intergenerational support and cross-generational exchange.

In his study of early retirement in France, Xavier Gaullier (1982) depicts the post-war period of policy on old age as having gone through three phases. The first period he saw as the transformation of old age into retirement. The second, in the 1960s, was characterised by the transformation of old age into

the third age (a period of leisure, autonomy and self-realisation). In the latest stage, dating in France from about 1976, he sees the policy for old age as having become a policy on unemployment. Rising unemployment has brought about earlier and earlier enforced retirement (down to age 50 years in some parts of the country). Gaullier writes:

> An individual is declared "old" by authorities responsible for employment and rejected definitively from the job market uniquely on account of his age, regardless of his state of health, his biological or psychological ageing. . . . There is no longer a promotion of a way of life but rather the payment of allowances to the unemployed. . . . For a long time old-age policy favoured the social insertion of the elderly, the new policy brutally excludes them from social life (Gaullier 1982).

These observations have a familiar ring not only in the British context, but in almost all the countries in Europe and North America, where economic recession has led uniformly to early retirement and redundancy, coupled with a reduction of services and monetary benefits. In this account the author attributes the crisis in old-age policy to weaknesses in the capitalist structure as well as to the political allegiance of governments to the 'working population'. Certainly, structural factors are pre-eminent in the situation. The restitution of France's third age conception is not likely to be achieved by individual effort. Yet a return to conceptions of society which provide open access to all its major arenas for older people is simply to restate a tenet of human rights.

Within the reconstructed forms of eldership, there will need to be provision for a great diversity of lifestyles. Thus the most important reforming function to be performed would be the systematic removal of constraints on personal decision making. So the agenda might well include the removal of paternalistic practices amongst health and social welfare practitioners, housing managers and so on, who presently take significant decisions for older people with little or no real consultation. It is, then, a restoration of the civil rights which have become so eroded, as Alison Norman (1980) has reminded us. Her discussion on the balance between rights and risk in referred to in some detail in Chapter 29.

AN AGEIST MODERN WORLD

A picture has been created in this chapter of old age which is viewed as an illness and regarded as unproductive. Whilst attention has been drawn to many positive aspects of later life, the prevalent image in developed societies is one of bodily decline and reduced ability to be socially useful. Associated with these beliefs goes an attitude of mind which demeans elderly people. In many respects it reflects the negative stereotyping of women and of black people which we now know as sexism and racism. Ageism is an equivalent term.

Whilst it would be foolish to pretend that growing old is a period of endless vitality and growing excitement, it is important to draw to the fore the neglected positive features of old age. The whole truth about it is not to be found in the pathology models of the professionals or of the traditional researchers. A more balanced view will recognise that the later stage of life will be very different for people with different social statuses and personal experiences. It will incorporate a respect for individual life-histories and their formative influence on the character of old age. At the same time it will acknowledge the way society can minimise or extend the opportunities and satisfactions of being an elder. Even the language it uses about those who are old will be more thoughtful—less ageist. Perhaps we should begin by abandoning the word 'geriatrics' as a term to describe people and retain it for its only proper use; as a title for the practice of medicine on older people.

REFERENCES

Abrams M 1980 Beyond three score years and ten. Age Concern, Mitcham
Abrams P 1982 Historical sociology. Open Books, Shepton Mallet Somerset

Age Concern 1976 Profiles of the elderly, Vols 1–8. Age Concern, Mitcham
Baltes P B, Shaie W (eds) 1973 Life-span developmental psychology: personality and socialization. Academic Press, New York
Birren J E, Schaie K W (eds) 1977 Handbook of the psychology of aging. Van Nostrand Reinhold, New York
Booth C 1902 Life and labour of the people of London. Macmillan, London
Bowley A L, Burnett Hurst A R 1912 Livelihood and poverty. London
Brockington F, Lempert S M 1966 The social needs of the over eighties. Manchester University Press
Brown E 1982 Older Americans' use of health maintenance organisations. Research on Aging 4 (June): 2
Butler R N 1963 The Life review: An interpretation of reminiscence in old age. Psychiatry 26:1
Butler R N 1975 Why survive? Being old in America. Harper and Row, New York
Cain L D 1964 Life course and social structure. In: Faris R E L (ed) Handbook of modern sociology. Rand McNally, Chicago
Cain L D 1967 Age status and generational phenomena: the new old people in contemporary America. Gerontologist 7
Cole D 1962 The economic circumstances of old people. Occasional Papers on Social Administration. Bell, London
Comfort A 1977 A good age. Mitchell Beazley, London
Eisdorfer C (ed) 1981 Annual review of gerontology and geriatrics. Springer, New York
Elder G 1974 Children of the Great Depression. University of Chicago Press, Chicago
Erikson E 1950 Childhood and society. Norton, New York
Estes C 1982 Dominant and competing paradigms in gerontology. Ageing and Society 2 (July): 2
Fairchild R 1977 Life story conversations: diversions in a ministry of evangelistic calling. United Presbyterian Program Area on Evangelism, New York
Finch C D, Hayflick L (eds) 1977 Handbook of the biology of aging. Van Nostrand Reinhold, New York
Fries J F, Crapo L M 1981 Vitality and aging: implications of the rectangular curve. W H Freeman, San Francisco
Gaullier X 1982 Economic crisis and old age—old age policies in France. Ageing and Society 2 (July): 2
Goulet L R, Baltes P B (eds) 1970 Life-span developmental psychology: research and theory. Academic Press, New York
Guillemard A M 1972 La retraite—une mort sociale. Mouton la Haye, Paris
Hareven T K (ed) 1981 Aging and the life course. Guildford Press, New York
Haug M 1979 Doctors and older patients. Journal of Gerontology 34 (November): 6
Help the Aged 1981 Recall: a reminiscence guide. Help the Aged, London
Hessel D (ed) 1977 Maggie Kuhn on ageing. Westminster Press, Philadelphia
Johnson M L 1976 That was your life: A biographical approach to later life. In: Munnichs J M A, van den Heuval W J A (eds) Dependency and interdependency in old age. Martinus Nijhoff, The Hague

Johnson M L 1979 An ageing population: relations and relationships. Open University Press, Milton Keynes

Johnson M L 1982 The implications of greater activity in later life. In: Fogarty M (ed) Retirement policy, the next fifty years. Heinemann, London

Johnson M L 1982a Ageing, needs and nutrition—a study of voluntary and statutory collaboration in community care for elderly people. Policy Studies Institute, London

Kohli M, et al 1983 The social construction of ageing through work. Ageing and Society 3 (March): 1

Labouvie-Vief G, Blanchard-Fields F 1982 Cognitive ageing and psychological growth. Ageing and Society 2 (July): 2

Levinson D 1978 The seasons of a man's life. Knopf, New York

Macintyre S 1977 Old age as a social problem, some notes on the British experience. In: Dingwall R, et al (eds) Health care and health knowledge. Croom Helm, London

Nesselroade J R, Reese H W (eds) 1973 Life-span developmental psychology: methodological issues. Academic Press, New York

Neugarten B (ed) 1968 Middle age and ageing: a reader. University of Chicago Press, Chicago

Norman A 1980 Rights and risk. Centre for Policy on Ageing, London

Office of the Population Censuses and Surveys 1979 Population projections 1977–2017. Series pp 2 No 9. HMSO, London

Phillipson C 1982 Capitalism and the construction of old age. Macmillan, London

Plummer K 1983 Documents of life. Allen and Unwin, London

Pratt H J 1976 The gray lobby. University of Chicago Press, Chicago

Report of the Royal Commission on the Poor Law (1905–9) 1909 HMSO, London

Rosenmayr L 1981 Age, lifespan and biography. Ageing and Society 1 (March): 1

Rowntree B S 1901 Poverty: A study of town life. Macmillan, London

Russell L B 1981 An ageing population and the use of medical care. Medical Care 19 (June): 6

Shanas E, Maddox G 1976 Aging health and the organisation of health resources. In: Binstock R H, Shanas E (eds) Handbook of aging and the social sciences. Van Nostrand Reinhold, New York

Sheehy G 1974 Passages: predictable crises of adult life. Dutton, New York

Sheldon J H 1948 Social medicine of old age. Oxford University Press, Oxford

Stimson G 1976 Biography and retrospection: some problems in the study of life histories. Unpublished paper presented to the British Sociological Association Annual Conference

Synge J 1981 Cohort analysis in the planning and interpretation of research using life histories. In: Bertaux D (ed) Biography and society. Sage, Beverley Hills

Taub H A 1980 Life-span education: A need for research with meaningful prose. Educational Gerontology 5

Taylor R, Ford G 1981 Lifestyle and ageing. Ageing and Society 1 (November): 3

Thomas W I, Znaniecki F 1927 The Polish peasant in Europe and America (2 vols). Over Publications, New York

Thompson P 1978 The voice of the past: oral history. Oxford University Press, Oxford

Townsend P 1957 The family life of old people. Routledge and Kegan Paul, London

Townsend P 1962 Last refuge. Routledge and Kegan Paul, London

Townsend P 1981 The structured dependency of the elderly. Ageing and Society 1 (March): 1

Tunstall J 1966 Old and alone. Routledge and Kegan Paul, London

Valliant G E 1977 Adaptation to life. Little Brown, Boston

Walker A 1981 Towards a political economy of old age. Ageing and Society 1 (March): 1

Webb B 1926 My apprenticeship. Longman Green, London

S. E. Robbins

2

The psychology of ageing

INTRODUCTION

Psychologists divide the human lifespan into stages which correspond roughly with chronology: babyhood and infancy, 0–2 years; childhood, 2–12 years; adolescence, 12–18 years; adulthood, 18–65 years; and old age, 65+ years. There is a strong tendency within developmental psychology to concentrate on the first two or three of these stages, breaking them down into tiny subsections and tracing minute changes in behaviour, whilst leaving the last two stages of adulthood and old age largely unexplored. Old age is thought to start at around 60 or 65. When we talk about ageing we are usually referrring to a process which involves people in this old age group. It is as though those of us who are under 65 are immune to the phenomenon of ageing. Alongside the lack of exploration of developmental stages in old age goes a tendency to make simple generalisations about 'the elderly', mostly of a gloomy and derogatory nature.

In recent years there has been some increase of interest in adult development. Levinson (1978) outlined the Seasons of a Man's Life from the novice phase in the early twenties through to the late adult transition in the early sixties, and Kubler-Ross (1975) outlines five stages of the dying process. However, to date we have no accepted way of dividing either adulthood or old age into developmental stages. A tentative classification for old age might include three stages;

the young active group, 65–75 years; the older retired group; and the aged survivors, 85+ years. In this chapter, through drawing on information from a wider group, I shall be concentrating mainly on those aged between about 65 and 85 years, our information on the 'aged survivors' being at present quite sparse.

Fundamental questions

There are three fundamental points to be examined:
1. Change. What psychological changes do we see as part of the ageing process?
2. Adjustment. How do people adjust to the changes involved in ageing?
3. Context. How do questions of psychological change and adjustment relate to the Health Service context?

We will examine each of these three questions in turn.

CHANGE

The question of changes which are related to the ageing process will be dealt with in two main sections, the first summarising the role changes which accompany old age and the second looking at changes in psychological functioning of the individual person.

Role change

Life events

The attainment of old age by a large proportion of the population is a relatively recent phenomenon. The current elderly population are often the first in their family to face the life events of later life. Some of these events are simply by products of living a long life, such as multiple bereavements; however, many others are dictated by contemporary cultural patterns. The attainment of 'retirement age', qualification for pensions and concessions, and, for many old people, changes in housing, are examples of culturally determined role changes in western industrialised countries in

the 1980s. Life events of this sort constitute stresses whatever the quality of the change (Gunderson and Rahe 1974) and both bereavement and retirement are clearly linked to subsequent illness and death (Murray Parkes 1975). The impact of the life event of retirement is aptly illustrated by a quote from Adela Irskine's chapter in *The Challenge of a Long Life* (Pincus 1981). 'It was as if the structure of my life had collapsed—almost like being hit by a physical blow . . . after the first fine careless rapture, the feeling: God! What have I done?' (p 143)

Effects of role changes

Western retirement encourages the shedding of responsibilities and the acceptance of a more dependent lifestyle. The lower social and economic status that ensues leads to a lowering of expectations of the elderly person and by the elderly person. The role changes of later life together with individual and social adjustments to them, can easily act in a cyclical manner, with burdens removed and progressively less expected of old folk until their value as contributors to society is both restricted and weakened. The negative effects that no longer being needed have on elderly people are emphasised by Lily Pincus (1981) in her examination of the challenge of a long life.

It is generally assumed that the sociological and physical signs of decline of the elderly are paralleled by a psychological deterioration. This view is consistently reinforced by the media, and when individuals are thus induced to say 'my mind is not as sharp as it was' or 'it's too much for me to think about at my age' we usually find ourselves nodding tacit agreement, albeit sympathetically. To be old is to accept the role of incompetent. We demonstrate this attitude whenever we unthinkingly help old folk without considering whether the person actually wants or needs special care.

The cultural stereotype

The cultural stereotype of old age in contemporary Britain commonly runs along these lines; great achievements occur relatively early in life, mostly in the teens, twenties and thirties, and the picture thereafter is one of steady decline. In old age we are expected to become either nice old ladies and charming old gentlemen, or awkward old biddies and dirty old men. The individual character is lost and devalued regardless of whether the positive or the negative stereotype is applied.

The cultural stereotype is not without factual support. Scientific advances have largely been made by young people. Marconi transmitted the first radio signals at 21 and Bell made the first telephone at the age of 29. Lehman (1953) looked at the achievements of great chemists in relation to chronological age and reported that their peak of productive output occurred between the ages of 30 and 34 years. Whatever the balance of evidence behind the expectation of decline and impairment in old age, the effect of the stereotype when internalised by elderly folk may well be that of a self-fulfilling prophecy. It is difficult to maintain motivation and concentration on psychological tasks when you and everyone else around you believes that all old people become mentally frail and demented, and so when someone asks you to do a test you do badly—just as everyone expected.

The experience of ageing

Current literature suggests that the actual experience of ageing can be quite different from the stereotype. Most adults feel younger than their chronological age anyway and this feeling increases with advancing age. Kastenbaum et al (1972) investigated the concepts of personal and interpersonal age with the help of 75 people aged between 20 and 69. They concluded that personal age, that is the age a person feels, is so distinct from chronological age that gross errors are likely to occur whenever the two are confused. Moreover, several recent descriptions of the process of ageing based on self reports suggest that the long accepted image of merciful retirement matching encroaching feebleness of mind and body may be far from

correct (Blythe 1979, Pincus 1981, Stott 1981). These authors emphasise in particular the great differences which exist between individual experiences of ageing. They suggest that enormous variability in the ageing process in inevitable considering the diversity of life experiences and personal circumstances which obtains in old age.

Individual change

This section will attempt a summary of the information currently available regarding the changes in individual psychology which occur with the ageing process. After outlining the experimental data in this area, the methodological questions which are raised by the data will be examined.

Experimental evidence

The research data on individual change during ageing are summarised under six headings—intelligence, learning and memory, problem solving, perception, sex differences and personality. (Table 2.1 summarises the evidence). During these summaries the terms cross-sectional and longitudinal will often be used to describe experiments. A cross-sectional study involves taking measures from different groups of subjects. In a longitudinal study the same subjects are tested repeatedly over time.

Intelligence. Most of our information on intelligence and ageing comes from studies using the Wechsler Adult Intelligence Scale (WAIS). Wechsler (1944) reported the findings from his standardisation of the WAIS as showing a peak in intellectual capacity in the mid to late twenties. The test was standardised on approximately 2000 men and women who ranged in age between 16 and over 75 years. A cross-sectional design was used. This result was similar to that found in the earlier standardisation studies for the Wechsler–Bellevue scale in which the highest scoring group was the early twenties. It was thought by many that this intellectual peak paralleled the acquisition of biological maturity and that the subsequent decline in intellectual capacity mirrored the

Table 2.1 Summary of experimental evidence of change in cognitive abilities

Studies suggestive of cognitive decline with ageing.	Studies suggestive of preservation of cognition with ageing
Wechsler (1944), Eisdorfer and Wilkie (1973) Blum et al (1972)*— Intelligence Cunningham et al (1975)— Fluid intelligence	Bayley and Oden (1955)*, Owens (1966),* Savage et al (1973)*— Intelligence Terman and Oden (1959)*—Concept mastery Gilbert (1973),* Green (1969)*—Verbal ability
Gilbert (1941)—Learning and memory Monge and Huttsch (1971)—Paired associate memory Eisdorfer et al (1963)— Serial learning Canestrari (1966)— Learning verbal associates Talland (1965)—Immediate memory under stress Craik (1968)—Supraspan memory Schonfield and Robertson (1966)—Free recall	Schonfield and Robertson (1966)—Recognition Memory Savage et al (1973)*— Verbal and perceptual motor learning Harwood and Naylor— Learning German
Young (1966), Heglin (1956)—Problem solving Bromley (1957)—Abstract thinking Goldfarb (1941)—Complex reaction time Rabbitt (1965, 1981)— Ignoring irrelevant information	Wetherick (1964), Smith (1967)—Problem solving

* Longitudinal studies.

physical decline seen in later life. Following the standardisation studies, the assumption of intellectual decline with age was built into the WAIS norms. Apart from its use in research work, the WAIS is by far the most popular test of intellectual ability in adults.

The WAIS is composed of two sets of subtests, one measuring verbal ability and one measuring performance, or spatial, ability. The effects of age on test score were particularly marked in four of the five performance subtests of the WAIS: block design, object assembly, digit symbol and picture arrangement. These subtests are all timed. These findings led Wechsler to classify the subtests into two categories as far as ageing effects were concerned. One group, known as 'hold' tests, showed little difference between the young and old subjects whilst the other group, known as 'don't hold' tests, were more poorly done by older subjects. The two categories both contain two verbal and two performance subtests. The two groups could be used to calculate a 'deterioration quotient'. For this, scores on the 'hold' tests were compared with scores on the 'don't hold' tests and the relationship interpreted in relation to that expected in a person of that age.

The discovery that certain tests showed more age effects than others has led some to draw a parallel with the idea of fluid and crystallised intelligence. This conceptualisation of intellectual ability is particularly linked with Cattell (1963). Fluid intelligence is thought to reflect a person's basic potential to acquire new ideas and adapt to new situations, and is thought to stem from qualities inherent in the central nervous system. By contrast, the term crystallised intelligence was used to denote learned intellectual skills based on cultural and environmental experience. It seems logical that tests which reflect accumulated experience might show little decrement with advanced age, and might even show an increasing score. The vocabulary subtest of the WAIS is often cited as a possible example of a test reflecting this crystallised intelligence. The tests which show more of an age effect might reflect a more ephemeral fluid ability which ebbs as ageing progresses. If fluid intelligence does indeed decline more rapidly than crystallised intelligence, one would expect correlations between measures of the two to be higher in young subjects than in old ones. Cunningham et al (1975) confirmed this in a cross-sectional comparison using the WAIS vocabulary subtest to measure crystallised intelligence and Raven's progressive matrices to measure fluid intelligence. So far, then, studies suggestive of some decline in intellect during ageing have been noted. Not all studies agree with this. In 1959 Terman and Oden reported on a follow-up study involving a large group of especially gifted people in their early forties. Their subjects consistently showed a higher score on the concept mastery test than when tested 12 years before. Bayley and Oden (1955) had also reported increasing levels of intellectual ability between the ages of 20 and 50. In another longitudinal study 96 men were tested using the army alpha test at the age of 50 again 11 years later. There were no significant differences between scores at the different ages. On retesting 31 years after the original there was a pattern of increasing ability (Owens 1966). Blum et al (1972) reported a decline after the mid sixties in their 20 year study. Savage et al (1973) studied a group of elderly people in Newcastle over a seven-year period. Many of those studied were over 75 years old. The group of primary interest here is those who lived in the community, of whom there were 190. Savage et al reported no change in the overall intelligence quotient (IQ). Performance IQ improved whilst verbal IQ declined a little, a pattern opposite to that reported by Wechsler. This study, however, cannot be seen as conclusive. Many subjects died during the seven-year period. Those who lived to be tested throughout may comprise a special 'survivor' group. However, further longitudinal studies do give some support to these findings. Both Gilbert (1973) and Green (1969) reported no decline in verbal abilities in advanced old age in selected groups. In a 10-year longitudinal study, Eisdorfer and Wilkie (1973) found a small statistically significant decline in abilities in their 60–70 years age group, and a slightly larger decline in the 70–80 years age group. Furthermore, they suggest that the changes are too tiny to be of any practical significance. Finally, Schaie and Strother (1968), using a mixed cross-sectional and longitudinal design, confirmed that purely cross-sectional data exaggerates age-related changes, except where speed is of prime importance. In conclusion then it seems that intellectual decline is not a universal and inevitable part of growing old.

Learning and memory. In an early study Gilbert (1941) demonstrated a decline in performance with age on a variety of tasks of learning and memory. A large body of the experimental literature since that time would support this.

The decrement found by Gilbert was particularly noticeable in a paired associate task, when a series of paired stimuli are to be remembered. Later studies suggest that the time period between pairs was particularly important. Older people did badly when there was little time to produce an answer (Monge and Hultsch 1971). This also seems to be true of serial learning tasks, in which a series of individual items is presented for memorisation (Eisdorfer et al 1963). There is some evidence that older people are more affected by established linguistic habits since they apparently find learning new associations for words of high associative strength particularly difficult (Canestrari 1966).

The term immediate memory refers to a memory mechanism which registers incoming information and keeps it for a few seconds. Immediate memory appears to be little affected by ageing according to the results of memory span experiments. Only under conditions of very high task difficulty, for instance when required both to respond in conditions of interference and to search and match incoming material with remembered items, does the immediate memory of elderly subjects appear less efficient than that of their juniors (Talland 1965).

When memory span is exceeded, that is when material is stored for more than a few seconds or when a great deal of material is presented, age effects are often found (Craik 1968). Much research in this area has concentrated on finding the locus of the age-related deficit, and it seems that in many instances the problem lies in the retrieval stage of memory. Schonfield and Robertson (1966) used a free recall task with five age groups from the twenties to sixties. Free recall means that subjects may remember material in any order once the information has been presented. There was a clear relationship between age and performance for the recall task, with the older subjects scoring poorly. However, when a recognition task was used, in which the correct answers were chosen from among distractors, the age factor had no effect.

As with the intelligence studies, not all the experimental evidence is indicative of age-related decline. A study of learning ability was included in Savage et al's (1973) longitudinal study in Newcastle. They used both a verbal and a perceptual motor test of learning and found no real evidence of declining ability. Similarly, experiments which focus on ability to retain newly learned information suggest that there is little or no age effect, particularly if the material is fully learned initially. Huppert (1982) quotes an Australian study by Harwood and Naylor to illustrate the potential learning capacity of the old. After 80 people aged 63–91 were given weekly German lessons for three months, more than half passed an exam which schoolchildren normally attempt after three years tuition. It is interesting to note that the elderly people themselves were amazed at their ability.

Problem solving. The expectation of poor problem-solving ability among old people is logical given that there are many tasks of this sort in intelligence tests, and of course much research suggests poorer intelligence test performance in old age. Young (1966) compared an 'old' 45–76 years age group with a 'young' 29–45 years age group on a complicated problem-solving task. She found not only that the older people performed less well than their juniors, but also that the two groups did not differ in measured intelligence. Conversly, Wetherick (1964) found that his most difficult problem-solving task was best solved by older people. He also suggested that they gained most from test experience, in terms of improving from problem to problem. Subjects were matched in overall intelligence. Later experiments suggest that, as well as intelligence, memory factors and the degree of abstractness of the task used can affect problem-solving performance. It may be that some reported age effects are due to these factors rather than an age-related deficit in problem-solving ability per se. The evidence we have to date suggests that elderly people are best able to solve problems when the information given is both concrete and personally relevant. It seems that older people more often use concrete methods to solve problems than abstract principles (Bromley 1957). This may well be linked to educational experience. Elderly people are also reported to adhere to tried and trusted methods rather than use new and more efficient problem-solving methods. If a series of problems is given, all solvable by the same method, and then a problem which could be solved using a more simple method is interpolated, it is often said that the older subject is more likely to stick to the inefficient method than is the young subject (Heglin 1956). However, it seems once again that other factors are also important. Smith (1967) produced different results in a very similar experiment and concluded that factors other than age were probably influencing the results. She felt that level of intelligence was probably the most important influence.

Perception. The stereotype of perception in the aged person is one of dulled senses— Shakespeare's 'sans eyes . . . sans everything'. In this short summary we will examine this point with particular reference to speed of response and the effect of irrelevant information.

A wide variety of experimental studies have reported a slower reaction time in elderly subjects than in younger people. This is often explained as being due to perceptual deficits. In fact, experiments focusing on perceptual sensitivity show only a minimal loss between average young and old people (Birren and Botwinick 1955). The slight differences found in simple reaction time are disproportionately increased as the task becomes more complex (Goldfarb 1941). It seems that it is the decision process and the associative aspects of the task which make for the disproportionate effect. This means that the phenomenon is one of central slowing rather than a peripheral effect (Birren and Botwinick 1955). Further investigation of this effect shows that the older person can react as quickly as the young in many instances but that when there is time to review the situation more the old people tend to respond more slowly. Much of the slowness appears to be a behavioural preference rather than a deficit per se.

A tendency to be adversely affected by irrelevant information is reported to be a perceptual concomitant of old age (Rabbitt 1965, 1981). Rabbitt feels that the elderly in general find it difficult to ignore irrelevant information, probably because they tend to process smaller 'chunks' of information at a time. He goes on to relate this to practical issues affecting old people, suggesting that they may find group conversations particularly difficult to follow and that they are disadvantaged in reading. Schonfield (1974) thinks there may be even greater practical effects. He suggests that roadside advertising may adversely effect the elderly car-driver, and that more effort should be made to shield old people from surplus information whenever a task requiring great concentration is in hand.

Sex differences. The differential survival rates of the sexes have been well documented and publicised, but it is more rare to find reliable reports of sex differences in psychological processes. For the purpose of this summary only a few specific examples of sex differences in ageing will be examined.

Britton and Britton (1972) reported that in women survival itself appeared related to personality characteristics. Women who were more involved, active and satisfied, lived longer than their less engaged colleagues. Personality and survival did not appear associated for men. Savage et al (1977) reported a variety of sex differences in personality in their Newcastle sample. The men scored more highly on 'ego strength', while the women were more tense, sensitive, insecure and overprotected. With regard to self-image, the women showed more conflict and contradiction between their basic identity, self-acceptance and behavioural functioning than did the men. Differential ageing patterns are suggested by a problem-solving experiment employing subjects of both sexes aged between 41 and 76 years (Young 1971). The younger subjects showed the customary pattern of males being superior to females on the task, but for subjects aged 60 or more, the pattern was reversed. Although this could be simply an artefact of the different generations involved the author speculated that the males showed more decline in ability with age than the females, and that this might be related to physiological changes, particularly in cerebral circulation.

Personality. Part of the popular stereotype of personality in old age is an expectation that the old will be self-opinionated, unwilling to change and possibly boring. As seen above in 'The cultural stereotype', grannies and grandpas are supposed to be benign and contented or irascible and depressed. To fit the culturally accepted mores one must lose drive and ambition with age and one's interest in sex must fade rapidly (see Chapter 16). In this section we will examine some studies of measurable personality characteristics and old age, both cross-sectional and longitudinal.

Schaie and Marquette (1972) reviewed the current literature on personality and ageing. Reported personality differences between old and young included increases with age in introversion and cautiousness, and decreases in need for achievement, heterosexuality, responsivity and psychopathology. However, many studies of the aged using personality assessment actually find a remarkable similarity in personality between the old and the younger age groups with whom they are compared. This, of course, says nothing about how introverted, cautious etc. they are.

Botwinick (1973) considers reports of increased cautiousness and rigidity in the aged to be of particular importance, and this is echoed throughout much of the literature. He cites a variety of evidence suggesting that elderly subjects are more likely to 'play safe' than their juniors, but it is evident that the increased cautiousness so often reported as an ageing effect is a far from unitary phenomenon. The same verbal label is employed for a great variety of personality characteristics displayed in many different experimental studies. Furthermore, there is clear evidence from Edwards and Vine (1963) that differences in a personality measure of cautiousness between age groups can be caused by differences in intellectual ability. Chown (1962) thinks the same is true of reported increases in 'rigidity' in old age. Intellectual factors can force people into dealing inadequately with complex situations whatever their basic personality. Once again experiments on 'rigidity' are very varied in nature though purporting to examine the same personality trait.

An American study of 87 men aged 55 to 84 years attempted to look at personality and adjustment before and after retirement and also to delineate personality types in the aged (Reichard et al 1962). The methods used included intensive interviews, ratings and psychological tests. The results suggested that a critical period of adjustment occurred shortly before retirement during which the men were agitated about the problems and implications of retirement. There was no one way of reacting to the problems presented. Reichard et al outlined five styles of personality found in their group: 'constructiveness' involving self-awareness, flexibility and general satisfaction, 'dependency' reflecting a passive and unambitious style of life, 'defensiveness' which involved being habit bound, compulsively active and emotionally overcontrolled, 'hostility' which is summarised as an aggressive and competitive style, and 'self hate', a strategy adopted by a few men, which was composed of a self-critical, depressed and pessimistic mode of living.

A more recent study included an analysis of personality in a larger investigation of memory and ageing (Botwinick and Storandt 1974). The experimenters felt that the subject group was a little better educated and of higher social class than the norm. They concluded that their group showed no relation between age and life satisfaction, and only a negligible link between sense of control over life and age. The female subjects also completed both a scale measuring depression and a general personality test. There was a slight tendency towards more depression in older subjects, but no age effects at all in the personality test.

As with the studies of intellectual ability, it is important to consider information gathered from longitudinal research as well as the cross-sectional data summarised above. In 1972 Britton and Britton reported the results of a nine-year study carried out in a village in Pennsylvania. They included a broad assessment of activity, health, attitudes, relationships, life satisfaction and conformity, and studied a group of 146 people aged 65 years and above. Most of those studied had sought and found continuity and consistency in their lives, but these were individual patterns showing both continuity and change in personality. The effects of external events were complex. It seemed that outside factors were filtered through the individual's personality system and had both indirect and at times multidirectional effects. Britton and Britton felt that on average the quality of personality adjustment declined, but that individuals separately showed patterns of improving personality adjustment as well as of declining.

An English longitudinal study by Savage et al (1977) sampled 82 subjects living in the community. They agreed with Botwinick and Storandt's (1974) cross-sectional survey in reporting no relation between life satisfaction and age. However, Savage et al are more unusual in reporting a number of other areas in which old people scored differently from the adult norms. On the general personality measure their subjects were more reticent, introspective, silent, reserved and detached than the norm. They showed cautiousness in their emotional expression, were shy, felt inferior, and were critical and uncompromising. There was also a higher level of emotional instability than was expected. An assessment of self-concept revealed the group were decisive and definite about themselves, and felt a strong sense of moral worth and of worth within their families. Although these subjects were rather defensive, their self-esteem was quite high and they were not particularly self-critical.

Methodological issues

The research summarised above gives some

evidence to the popular idea that ageing involves a psychological decline, and more especially an intellectual decline. In science, as in current affairs, there is a tendency to report the bad news and the spectacular differences rather than the intriguing similarities. Certainly a great deal of the experimental literature is of this sort.

Occasionally in the summary we have seen that a supposed 'ageing effect' is later explained by another factor. In order to have confidence in an experimental finding we need to be sure that the effect reported cannot be attributed to any other factor. Moreover, we have to feel that we can generalised from the particular experiment to elderly people at large, or at least to a reasonable subsection of them, if the information given by an experiment is to hold any practical importance. In many experiments on ageing there are flaws in the methodology which reduce our confidence in one or other of these points. We will examine these methodological points briefly in the two sections which follow.

Alternative influences on results. Many studies employ a cross-sectional method in which people of different ages are compared with each other on particular experimental variables. This is true of many of the early intelligence studies. When this method is used, the differences between subjects include not only their chronological age but also their life experiences such as education, nutrition and social climate. These other factors are known as cohort effects, and the results reported may be due to obsolescence in the context of a rapidly changing environment rather than true ageing effects. Figure 2.1 illustrates how cohort effects can appear to show decline when successive generations score better and cross-sectional methods are used.

Unfortunately, simply using a longitudinal method, in which groups are followed as they age, does not correct mistakes completely. Each group is subject to particular environmental influences and these may interact with ageing effects to produce spurious results. It is only when successive groups are studied over time that a true picture of the ageing process can begin to emerge.

Factors within the test situation itself are also influential. Younger people have generally had more exposure to the scientific setting and are more familiar with modern test methods than their elders. This general experience may well benefit them not only in doing

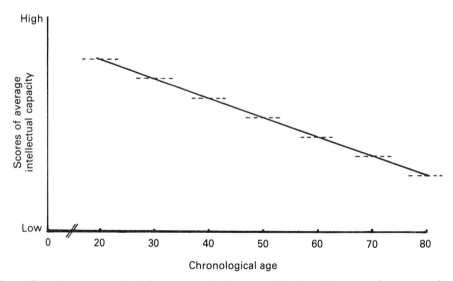

Fig. 2.1 Cohort effects in cross-sectional data: —— typical cross-sectional results; ----- cohort scores for each 10-year period.

the tasks presented but also in alleviating some of their test anxiety. High anxiety tends to have an adverse effect on performance. Test situations involve taking risks, particularly when time pressure is included. When the experimental conditions specifically require risky behaviour it seems that old people are as efficient as the young, but given a choice the older subject often performs more cautiously, often at the expense of lost marks. Commonly on tests our speed increases at the expense of mistakes. It seems that old people often prefer doing tasks thoroughly and carefully rather than rushing and risking more errors. A third matter for consideration in the test situation involves the attitudes of both the subjects and the experimenters. Since we know from general psychology that expectation of failure can depress performance and that experimenter characteristics affect results, it seems reasonable to suspect that young experimenters, often steeped in the decline literature, may bias results.

The materials used in experiments are of concern since they were often originally designed for a young age group. If it is possible that they include cohort effects than their application across age ranges is suspect. Many tests used appear petty and irrelevant. Gardner and Monge (1977) investigated the use of 'adult relevant' tests and found that whilst school-related tests were more poorly done by subjects in their sixties and seventies the adult relevant tests showed no such age decline.

A final group of influences on results involve factors inherent in the subject group. We have already noted that basic characteristics such as intelligence or educational experience can contaminate results. However, more subtle effects may also be involved. People generally show a drop in mental ability in the year before they die (Reimanis and Green 1971). Given that a substantial proportion of subjects in elderly groups may be near to death when tested, results can be biased towards a decline effect. Furthermore, undiscovered physical problems which are more common for elderly subjects, such as high blood pressure, may lead to an underestimate of average ability levels among the healthy (Wilkie and Eisdorfer 1971).

Problems of generalisability. One of the more striking facts about psychological experiments using older subjects is the range of ability levels they show. Typically the variance in an older group is much greater than in a young adult group. Figure 2.2 shows a typical pattern of results.

Given that average scores are often quoted and attempts are made to draw conclusions about individuals from them, the variability is often lost. Schaie (1973) presented data from a 14-year study which showed increasing,

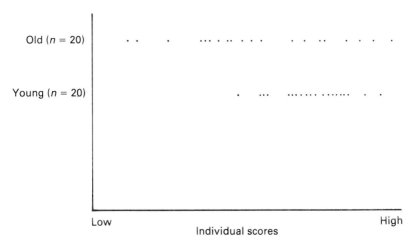

Fig. 2.2 Age and range of scores—typical data.

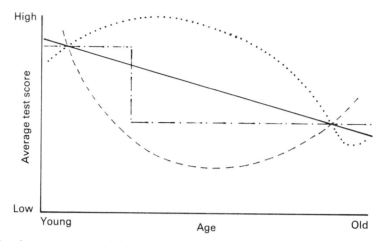

Fig. 2.3 Interpretation from two groups of data: —— commonly deduced 'trend'; —.— . . . . . ----- other possibilities.

decreasing and stable trends in performance in individual subjects. He suggests that the large range of scores often obtained from the elderly is due to varied patterns of ageing together with diverse life experiences. In sum, 'the elderly' are not a homogenous group, and yet we frequently discuss them and plan for them as if they were.

A second common mistake regarding generalisability involves the tendency to deduce a lifelong process from the measurement of two separate groups of subjects. Generally it is assumed that subjects who are midway in age between the groups studied will be midway in function, and that a trend based on the two measured groups can be expected to continue beyond the age range covered in the experiment. Figure 2.3 illustrates that mistakes may well arise from this. Along with this mistake is the problem of thinking of 'young' and 'old' as entities. Since both these terms are relative, in different experiments they may mean very different things. A 60-year-old is young in comparison with a person of 75 but old in relation to a teenager. Often it is not stated what 'young' or 'old' means.

It is common to draw general conclusions about aspects of psychological functioning which strictly speaking are far removed from the actual experimental basis. This is particularly true in problem solving and intelligence studies. This lack of accuracy should be studiously avoided, particularly in the field of intelligence where the work of such as Guilford (1956) suggests that intelligence is a very diverse set of abilities. Moreover we have no evidence that maturation has an equal effect on all aspects of ability.

A final consideration when generalising from research involves the characteristics of the subjects themselves. The sample groups used must be comparable both to each other and to those to whom we wish to apply the results. If a very aged group is involved can it be seen as representative or is it rather a peculiar group of 'survivors'? In longitudinal studies we need also to consider what conclusions may be drawn when some subjects die before completing the study.

Summary of changes

Support for the cultural stereotype of psychological decline in old age is at most equivocal. Many of the changes commonly thought of as part of the ageing process are by-products of role changes. These changes are imposed upon the elderly either by external events such as retirement or bereavement, or by the cultural mores which they are expected to conform to. It seems that people's individual reactions to these changes are extremely varied. Much of the experimental literature is suggestive of a cognitive decline in ageing (see

Table 2.1) but some studies do not agree with this conclusion. Much of the research which supports the decline hypothesis is cross-sectional whereas the longitudinal studies often report no decline. A variety of methodological issues are relevant to the consideration of the experimental data. Some personality studies suggest that negative personality traits are more common in old age, but again much of the literature supports the idea that personality is largely independent of age.

ADJUSTMENT

The issue of how people adjust to the changes involved in ageing will be examined in three parts. The first section will contrast two popular models of ageing. In the second section, adjustment will be considered in terms of the individual's lifespan, and finally personal adjustment to change will be examined.

Two models of adjustment

There are two well-known models proposed to explain the general processes of psychological adjustment which are associated with ageing. The two are particularly concerned with successful adjustment in retirement. The most striking aspect of the two models is that they have quite different implications for practical work with elderly people.

Disengagement

The most widely known model of adjustment in ageing was prepared by Cumming and Henry (1961) and is known as disengagement theory. The theory states that a process of mutual disengagement occurs during ageing in which both the individual person and the society in which that person lives withdraw from each other. To remain psychologically healthy and satisfied the elderly person retreats from the responsibilities and involvements which characterised middle life. Society

in turn withdraws from the individual by decreasing the demands made upon the person and by policies linked to chronological age such as enforced retirement. An example of this might be a factory worker who after retirement from work also curtails the social activities which are linked with ex-workmates. These ideas were based on a study carried out in Kansas Sity in 1955 which involved 172 people aged 50–70 years and 107 aged 70–90 years. The subjects were interviewed regarding their activities, general health, welfare and interactions. People who do not disengage, the theory implies, are likely to become frustrated and possibly depressed. It is acknowledged that not all people disengage at the same time. One experimental prediction from disengagement theory might be that feelings of control over life would wane with advancing age, but this has not been borne out by personality studies. The practical implications of this model, if adopted, would be enormous. To encourage disengagement would be to discourage active involvement, and in particular to discourage the initiation of new involvements.

Activity

The main alternative model to disengagement theory, activity theory, suggests that on the contrary successful ageing occurs when new or modified channels for a person's energies are found to replace pre-existing activities. This model is associated with Havighurst (1963). The pre-existing activities may be curtailed when society withdraws through retirement, or when the individual disengages because of factors such as ill health. An example of this might be the avid squash player who turns to golf when squash becomes too physically taxing. The activity model predicts that the frustrated depressed old people will be those who have been unable to find alternative outlets or interests. Some support for these ideas comes from Britton and Britton (1972), who reported that women who survived through the nine years of the study tended to be those who scored highly on measures of activity involvement and satisfaction.

These two contrasting theories have interesting parallels in the Health Service. Geriatric units usually pay lip service at least to activity theory, but often the day-to-day workings of a geriatric unit are more akin to those associated with disengagement theory.

Adjustment as a lifelong process

An alternative way of viewing the psychological adjustments made in later life, and the success or otherwise of these, is to look at the life-course overall. Erikson (1950) described eight stages of the life span each of which was concerned with a particular issue of psychological development. Thus the earlier stages include identity versus role confusion, an adolescent concern, and the issue of intimacy versus isolation which is central to development in young adulthood. The stages were seen as successive, each building on the structure constructed in earlier stages. The final stage which Erikson described was that linked to old age. Erikson labelled this stage 'ego integrity versus despair'. A state of ego integrity is achieved if the person in reflecting on her past life feels that life has been right and meaningful. Despair is the outcome if this is not the conclusion which results from looking back on life, and a fear of death is linked to this despair.

Lily Pincus (1981) says that the crucial aspect is the question of whether the world is different because the person has been in it. An integral part of the process is an attempt to survey and summarise one's life, looking back to past events and trying to make sense of the whole. The idea that an important part of the psychological 'work' of old age occurs via a life review was taken up by Butler (1963). He noted the strong tendency for old people to reminisce. He also noted that old people often enjoy this whilst their juniors often discourage it as 'living in the past'. Butler proposed that it was through activities like reminiscence that people worked on their life review, and so

came to terms with the meaning of their life and with their own mortality.

The theme of lifelong development is echoed both by Buhler (1961) and by Neugarten (1964) in her 'continuity theory'. Lily Pincus (1981) takes this same view in reviewing her own 83 years of life and when discussing case material from others. She sets out to examine what it is in an individual's life-history that determines his or her experience of old age. She pinpoints factors such as experience of loss, the family context, dependency, and relationships as being crucial.

A contrasting conceptualisation of successful ageing can be gleaned from Maslow's (1968) work on 'self-actualisation'. This state of 'full humanness' was achievable, he thought, when lesser human needs, for food, dominance, love etc. had been met and superseded. Self-actualising people were devoting their lives to what Maslow calls 'being' values, that is ultimate intrinsic values such as truth, beauty and simplicity. It is thought impossible to satisfy lower needs completely for many people, and only the middle aged or old can reach this state. Perhaps, then, the satisfied and successful old people are those who have transcended lesser matters and are self-actualising. This idea certainly gains support from a survey by Mary Spain which is quoted by Lily Pincus (1981). Two thirds of people aged 80 to 100 replied to her letter asking about their beliefs. Of these 200 people, only one mentioned their age in the reply. The rest were absorbed in issues outside of themselves and which gave meaning to their lives.

Adjustment to change

The broader issues of adjustment to change are probably best considered in relation to the major life changes of later life such as retirement, bereavement and death. The coping processes used determine to what extent changes are seen as gains or losses. Life events seem to be interpreted in relation to individual personality and life experience (Britton and Britton 1972). If adjustment is seen as a lifelong process, then successful adjustment to retirement rests on past experience of work and on the meaning of work to the individual. By contrast, bereavement reactions will be largely determined by the person's past experience of loss and by their relationship with the dead person.

Retirement

In recent years there has been a growing concern with preparation for retirement (Stott 1981). Such preparation involves both the practical aspects of sorting out financial matters and making decisions about where to live, and the psychological preparation for vast increases in leisure time and the loss of external time structure. Elwell and Maltbie-Crannell (1981) suggest that the role loss involved in retirement be considered as a stressor affecting both coping resources and life satisfaction. The study by Reichard et al (1962) found that a critical period of adjustment preceded the retirement date. Mary Stott points out that our retirement date is one of the few major decisions about life over which most of us have absolutely no influence. Kerckhoff (1964) looked at expectations and reactions to retirement among 108 husband and wife pairs in the United States. Most looked forward to the event, especially subjects from the middle and working classes, but few made definite plans. Once retired, the men experienced greater improvements than their wives. Those who had been retired more than five years tended to respond to Kerckhoff's questions more negatively. The husbands especially wished they had retired later. In terms of income group there was a positive association between income level and tendency to plan for retirement, and between income level and the likelihood of a positive experience of retirement.

Bereavement

Bereavement is not, as is so often assumed, an experience peculiar to the old, but it is, of course, a more common experience as one outlives friends and relatives. There seem to be definite stages through which the bereaved adult of any age passes (Murray Parkes 1975). The first stage of numbness leads on to a period of pining. This is followed by a stage of depression before recovery ensues. The modern western tendency to reduce the ritual of death and to discourage active mourning can interfere with the process. Mourning is often treated as if it were a weakness or a self-indulgence. Mary Stott describes the feelings which result on the death of a beloved spouse as not only 'loneliness of the most devastating kind, but a wilderness of pain and desolation impossible to imagine beforehand or to protect oneself against' (Stott 1981, p 68).

Death

Elisabeth Kubler-Ross (1975) describes the process of coming to terms with death as the final stage of growth. This thesis is similar to that of Erikson outlined earlier. Kubler-Ross identifies five stages of psychological adjustment which can be observed in the dying: denial, anger and guilt, bargaining, depression, and acceptance. A parallel is drawn with other life changes. Abandoning old habits and finding new ways of living is seen as a form of dying and regrowth. From this one might expect to observe similar stages as people adjust to the changes of ageing, but as yet we have only anecdotal evidence to support this.

Summary of adjustment

There is no universally accepted model of adjustment in old age. The two best-known models are contradictory. Perhaps this lack of agreement is a reflection of the enormous variability referred to earlier in this chapter. The most appealing conceptualisations of adjustment see it as a lifelong process but there is no hard evidence to support this. Objectively the life events of old age are characterised by loss but the subjective experience appears to depend on personal style. Some common stages of adjustment to bereavement and death can be outlined but beyond this the individual's personality and experience is the key to understanding the adjustment process.

THE HEALTH SERVICE CONTEXT

In coming into contact with the health services the elderly person becomes in some sense abnormal—either physically, socially or psychologically. Our primary concern as health care workers must be first to determine what has brought the person into contact with us. What has changed so as to bring them to our attention? Sometimes the main factor is a physical or social change which can be pinpointed. The focus of intervention is often determined by this. For example, the elderly person has broken a leg this morning, or the forgetful elderly person functioned well with the help of her spouse but the crisis has been precipitated by the spouse's death, or the usual home help is on leave and the eccentric person refuses to eat food provided by others. Sometimes the crucial change involved is in the patient's psychological functioning or in the interaction between this and other aspects of her condition.

The initial assessment of what has changed often shows us where we should aim our therapeutic efforts, particularly when the client appears to have multiple problems some of which are chronic and incurable. Sometimes we can effect useful changes in other areas too, but the focus for intervention needs to be carefully considered in the light of the client's personal needs, preferences and aims.

In this section we will examine first the informal and formal assessment of psychological functioning, and the application of this to decision making within the multidisciplinary context, before moving on to review the implications for the care of elderly people and of the individuality they show.

Informal assessment of psychological functioning

Whatever the patient's general condition, her mental functioning must always be noted. The physical and mental functioning will always interact and sometimes the indirect effects are considerable. This is amply illustrated by studies on the use of analgesics and recovery from surgery (Melzack 1973). Roughly speaking, the informal psychological assessment can be summarised in three simple questions:
1. To what extent does the client understand what is happening around her?
2. How does the client relate to other people?
3. Does the person learn new information (i.e. faces, names, the way around the ward) when regular events happen?

These factors need to be considered in a context which is personal for each client and which again can be summarised into two areas.
(a) Are physical factors affecting mental functioning? This can be crucial for patients in confusional states, depression and anxiety. We need to consider how good the patient's senses are. With regard to learning new information, we need to consider how readily available the information is.
(b) What was he/she like in earlier life?

These factors should be continually monitored by all those in contact with the patient, and need to be considered in the planning of interventions and, if appropriate, of future placement. The Health Service often considers these points intermittently and disjointedly, and we are usually woefully unaware of the person's past life and character. The positive as well as the negative factors must be recorded. At times the fact that a person is particularly easy-going and sociable, for example, is the single most important fact about them. This may be crucial in obtaining and maintaining a place in an old people's Home or in ensuring that neighbours continue to support the person at home. The introduction of the nursing process in this country should provide a more structured and consistent assessment of this sort. Julia Brooking uses such an approach in discussing the nursing assessment of confused and demented patient's (Chapter 18) and depression (Chapter 19).

In the course of this informal assessment

we need to be sensitive to the effects we ourselves are having. The change of role into patient or long-term patient may elicit particular responses. Institutionalisation is usually produced when people are admitted to hospital for more than a few days. Thus our own actions may have caused some of the withdrawal or dependency displayed by patients. We need to be aware of the extent that our actions and our health service regime disrupts this or interferes with normal routines. These observations must be taken into account when considering a person's abilities and difficulties. Particular areas of importance, especially any problems, will need a more detailed assessment, and usually a formal gathering of data is necessary.

Formal assessment

The most common formal assessment of psychological functioning required of a nurse is that of keeping precise records of some aspect of behaviour. The object of this may be to establish the pattern of existing behaviour before an intervention is applied. Such a record is known as a baseline. The formal recording of baseline data allows the precise effects of the intervention to be determined. Formal assessment may alternatively aim to determine the exact nature of the behaviour, to determine the quantity of that behaviour, to investigate the possibility that there may be a subtle pattern to the behaviour, or to determine the context of behaviour, that is what precedes it, whether it is environmentally linked, and what follows it. Nurses are also often required to fill out checklists or questionnaires about patient behaviour, or perhaps to complete a standardised assessment such as the Clifton assessment procedures for the elderly (CAPE, Pattie and Gilleard, 1979). The CAPE consists of a cognitive assessment scale and a behavioural rating scale, each of which indicate the dependency grade of the patient. The areas assessed include information and orientation, mental ability, psychomotor ability, physical disability, communication difficulties, apathy and social disturbance. There is also a shortened survey form. The object of these assessments is to obtain a precise measure of a specified aspect of psychological functioning. Sometimes when more than one person is taking measures it is necessary to run a check on how the people involved vary in the way they take measurements, and perhaps to standardise further the way in which it is done. These procedures make the conclusions drawn more reliable. Some tests have rigid instructions to follow and contain information on how other comparable clients' score. These co-called standardised tests allow the individual to be compared with an appropriate reference group.

A detailed nursing assessment of old people with dementia, confusion and depression is described by Julia Brooking in Chapters 19 and 20.

The multidisciplinary team

The data thus gathered will contributed to the planning and implementation of nursing care. Commonly though, it is in a multidisciplinary context that overall decisions are made. The contribution of each member is part of the group decision-making process. Clear presentation of the information gathered advances not only the management of a particular patient but also the understanding of the team as a whole regarding elderly people and their problems.

The team decision will usually be implemented by the team so that the nurse may be cast as therapist, researcher, or counsellor in turn in the management of patients with psychological difficulties.

Individuality

A recurrent theme of this chapter has been the great variability shown by elderly people in all aspects of psychological functioning. Their expectation, needs and coping skills are impossible to summarise meaningfully. Institutions work through standardisation and routine, and the Health Service is no exception to this. Even with the growing trend toward community work, encouraged by the 'rising tide' of people over 65 years of age, we often carry institutional practices and standardisation into people's homes.

The influence of this chapter should be to encourage the struggle towards reconciling the needs and rights of the individual old person with the system in which we work. The exploration of how far one can encourage individuality and personal expression in hospital wards without major interference with health care needs far more attention. The introduction of more personal possessions in hospitals, choice of meals, an flexible visiting times is part of this movement but we will have to go a great deal further to match the variability of our client group. Remember it is only really in the last decade that practices in children's wards have become more flexible and more in keeping with the psychological make-up of the clients. Let us hope the next ten years will see a similar revolution in geriatric wards.

In addition to these changes, another area for development concerns how to foster healthy adaptive processes in individual clients. More encouragement of active mourning, and of reminiscence, and the growth of the hospice movement for terminal care indicate that this development is beginning. We need further to consider how best to help people keep in touch with events in their own lives and in the outside world. Greater involvement of the family and of the informal network of carers, such as friends and neighbours, is an invaluable part of this (Pottle 1984). The use of reality orientation (RO) techniques to help people keep in touch with life is another essential element (Holden and Woods 1982).

CONCLUSIONS

This chapter has examined (a) the experimental evidence on the changes which accompany ageing, both of role and of individual psychology, and (b) the adjustments which occur during later life. We have seen in this review how limited a contribution these make to the working context. However, geriatric services would be radically changed if the meagre applications which do spring from the psychological studies were put into practice. A synthesis of how our knowledge of the psychology of ageing relates to the health service context has been attempted.

Our health care reflects the cultural stereotype of an inevitable and uniform psychological decline in ageing just the same as the rest of our society. Our institutions are geared to uniformity and standardisation. It is time to discard the ridiculous stereotype, to embrace the individuality of ageing, and to change our practices accordingly.

REFERENCES

Bayley N, Oden M H 1955 The maintenance of intellectual ability in gifted adults. Journal of Gorontology 10: 91–107
Birren J E 1963 Psychophysiological relations. In: Birren J E (ed) Human aging (USPHS Publ. 986). US Public Health Service, Washington DC
Birren J E, Botwinick J 1955 Age differences in finger, jaw and foot reaction time to auditory stimuli. Journal of Gorontology 10: 429–432
Blum J E, Fosshage J L, Jarvick L F 1972 Intellectual changes and sex differences in octogenarians: A twenty year longitudinal study of aging. Developmental Psychology 7: 178–187
Blythe R 1979 The view in winter—Reflections on Old Age. Penguin, Harmondsworth
Botwinick J 1973 Aging and Behavior. Springer, New York
Botwinick J, Storandt M 1974 Memory, related functions and age. Charles C Thomas, Springfield, Illinois
Britton J H, Britton J O 1972 Personality changes in aging: a longitudinal study of community residents. Springer, New York
Bromley D B 1957 Some effects of age on the quality of intellectual output. Journal of Gerontology 12: 318–323
Buhler C 1961 Meaningful living in mature years. In: Kleemeier R W (ed) Aging and leisure. Oxford, New York
Butler R N 1963 The life review: an interpretation of reminiscence in the aged. Psychiatry 26: 65–76
Canestrari R E 1966 The effects of commonality on paired associate learning in two age groups. Journal of Genetic Psychology 108:3–7
Cattell R B 1963 Theory of fluid and crystalized intelligence: a critical experiment. Journal of Education Psychology 54: 1–22
Chown S M 1962 Rigidity and age. In: Tibbitts C, Donahue W (eds) Social and psychological aspects of aging. Columbia University Press, New York

Craik F I M 1968 Short-term memory and the aging process. In: Talland G A (ed) Human aging and behavior. Academic Press, New York

Cumming E, Henry W E 1961 Growing Old: the process of disengagement. Basic Books, New York

Cunningham W R, Clayton V, Overton W 1975 Fluid and crystallized intelligence in young adulthood and old age. Journal of Gerontology 30: 53–55

Edwards A E, Vine D B 1963 Personality changes with age: their dependency on concomitant intellectual decline. Journal of Gerontology 18: 182–184

Eisdorfer C, Axelrod S, Wilkie F 1963 Stimulus exposure time as a factor in serial learning in an aged sample. Journal of Abnormal and Social Psychology 67: 594–600

Eisdorfer C, Wilkie F 1973 Intellectual changes with advancing age In: Jarvick L F, Eisdorfer C, Blum J E (eds) Intellectual functioning in adults. Springer, New York, p 21–29

Elwell F, Maltbie-Crannell A D 1981 The impact of role loss upon coping resources and life satisfaction of the elderly. Journal of Gerontology 36: 223–232

Erikson E H 1950 Childhood and society. Hogarth Press, London

Gardner E F, Monge R H 1977 Adult age differences in cognitive abilities and education background. Experimental Ageing Research 3: 337–383

Gilbert J G 1941 Memory loss in senescence. Journal of Abnormal and Social Psychology 36: 73–86

Gilbert J G 1973 Thirty Five year old follow up study of intellectual functioning. Journal of Gerontology 28: 68–72

Goldfarb W 1941 An investigation of reaction time in older adults and its relationship to certain observed mental test patterns. Contributions to Education no 831. Teachers College, Columbia University, New York

Green R F 1969 Age—intelligence relationship between ages sixteen and sixty-four: a rising trend. Developmental Psychology 1: 618–627

Guilford J P 1956 The structure of intellect. Psychological Bulletin 53: 267–293

Gunderson E K E, Rahe R H (eds) 1974 Life stress and illness, Charles C Thomas, Springfield, Illinois

Havighurst R J 1963 Successful aging. In: Williams R H, Tibbitts C, Donahue W (eds) Processes of aging, vol 1. Atherton Press, New York

Heglin H J 1956 Problem solving set in different age groups. Gerontology 11: 310–317

Holden U P Woods R T 1982 Reality orientation: psychological approaches to the 'confused' elderly. Churchill Livingstone, London

Huppert F A 1982 Does mental function decline with age? Geriatric Medicine 12:32–35

Kastenbaum R, Derbin V, Sabatini P, Artt S 1972 The ages of me: toward personal and interpersonal definitions of aging. Aging and Human development 3: 197–211

Kerckhoff A C 1964 Husband–wife expectations and reactions to retirement. Journal of Gerontology 19: 510–516

Kubler-Ross E 1975 Death. The final stage of growth Prentice Hall, London

Lehman H C 1953 Age and achievement. Oxford University Press

Levinson D J 1978 The seasons of a man's life. Ballantine, New York

Maslow A H 1968 Towards a psychology of being. 2nd edn. Van Nostrand, New York

Melzack R 1973 The puzzle of pain. Penguin, Harmondsworth

Monge R H, Hultsch D 1971 Paired-associate learning as a function of adult age and the length of the anticipation and inspection intervals. Journal of Gerontology 26: 157–162

Murray Parkes C 1975 Bereavement: studies of grief in adult life. Pelican Books, Harmondsworth

Neugarten B L 1964 Personality in middle and late life. Atherton Press, New York

Owens W A 1966 Age and mental abilities: a second adult follow up. Journal of Education Psychology 57: 311–325

Pattie A H, Gilleard C J 1979 Manual of the Clifton assessment procedures for the elderly (CAPE). Hodder and Stoughton, Sevenoaks, Kent

Pincus L 1981 The challenge of a long life. Faber, London

Pottle S M 1984 Developing a network oriented service for the elderly and their carers. In: Treacher A, Carpenter J (eds) Using family therapy. Blackwell, Oxford

Rabbitt P M A 1985 An age decrement in the ability to ignore irrelevant information. Journal of Gerontology 20: 233–238

Rabbitt P M A 1981 Talking to the old. New Society 140–141

Reichard S, Livson F, Peterson P G 1962 Aging and personality: a study of eighty-seven older man. Wiley, New York

Reimanis G, Green R F 1971 Imminence of death and intellectual decrement in the ageing. Developmental Psychology 5: 270–272

Savage R D, Britton P G, Bolton N, Hall E H 1973 Intellectual functioning in the aged. Methuen, London

Savage R D, Gaber L B, Britton P G, Bolton N, Cooper A 1977 Personality and adjustment in the aged. Academic Press, London

Schaie K W 1973 Methodological problems in descriptive developmental research on adulthood and ageing. In: Nesselroade J R Reese H W (eds) Lifespan developmental psychology: methodology. Academic Press, New York

Schaie K W, Marquette B 1972 Personality in maturity and old age. In: Dreger R M (ed) Multivariate personality research: contributions to the understanding of personality in honour of Raymond B Cattell. Clautors, Louisiana

Schaie K W, Strother C R 1968 A cross-sequential study of age changes in cognitive behaviour. Psychological Bulletin 70: 671–680

Schonfeld D 1974 Translations in gerontology—from lab to life: utilising information. American Psychologist 796–800

Schonfield D, Robertson B 1966 Memory storage and aging. Canadian Journal of Psychology 20: 228–236

Smith D K 1967 The Einstellung effect in relation to the variables of age and training. Dissertation Abstracts 27B:4115

Stott M 1981 Ageing for beginners. Blackwell, Oxford

Talland G A 1965 Three estimates of the word span and

their stability over the adult years. Quarterly Journal of Experimental Psychology 17: 301–307

Terman L W, Oden M H 1959 The gifted group at mid-life: thirty five years follow up of the superior child. Genetic studies of genius, vol. 5 Stanford University Press, Stanford, California

Wechsler D 1944 The measurement of adult intelligence, 3rd edn. Williams and Wilkins, Baltimore

Wetherick N E 1964 A comparison of the problem solving ability of young, middle-aged and old subjects. Gerontologia 9: 164–178

Wilkie F, Eisdorfer C 1971 Intelligence and blood pressure in the aged. Science 172: 959–962

Young M L 1966 Problem-solving performance in two age groups Journal of Gerontology 21: 505–509

Young M L 1971 Age and sex differences in problem solving Journal of Gerontology 26: 330–336

G. C. J. Bennett

3

The physiology of ageing

INTRODUCTION

In the sixteenth century a Spanish conquistador, Ponce de Leon, went searching for the Fountain of Youth. He was probably not the first and was certainly not the last, and the search has been going on ever since. Brown Séquard (1899) theorised that we aged secondarily to our gonads and he claimed rejuvenation after administration of testicular extracts. In the early 1900s, Metchnikoff (1907) advocated yoghurt diets to decrease intestinal toxins. However, eunuchs do not live longer and one's maximum lifespan is not altered by eating yoghurt. Comparatively recently, Aslan et al (1965) in Romania have claimed to rejuvenate humans (decreasing symptoms of ageing, not increasing the lifespan) by the use of a substance called gerovital H3. This solution is a weak inhibitor of monoamine oxidase and as monoamines have chemical actions in the brain, especially the hypothalamus, more research is being carried out into these claims (Macfarlane 1975). Much has been written about parts of the world where populations are said to be extremely long lived—the Caucasus mountains, Vilacabana in the Equadorian Andes and the Karakorum mountains in the Kashmir Himalayas. These areas are all high altitude and involve the elderly in hard physical work on a low protein and fat diet. Also these areas are remote with poor demographic records and there is very

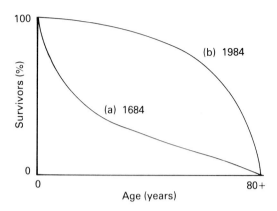

Fig. 3.1 Age survival curves.

little evidence that extreme old age is common.

Figure 3.1 shows that advances in public health (housing, sanitation, diet, etc) have caused the phenomenon of more people surviving to be elderly (curve b). This is the rectangular curve described in Chapter 1. Populations living under severe life conditions have a different survival curve (curve a)—a constant force of mortality.

The younger age groups are no longer dying but the maximum life span thereafter remains constant (Fig. 3.2, curve a). Moving the curve to the right (curve b) involves research into the physiology of the ageing process itself to see if this process can be slowed down or postponed.

Man being the longest lived species makes

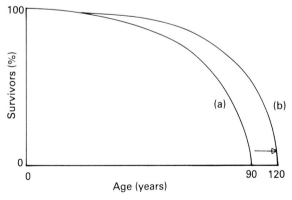

Fig. 3.2 Maximum lifespan.

longitudinal studies (over a lifetime or a period of time) of ageing research unrealistic. Animal or cross-sectional studies (looking at groups of different ages) are more commonly used. Changes caused by ageing, however, must be separated from those which are due to other factors. Strehler (1962), an American gerontologist (gerontology—the study of ageing) proposed that any physiological ageing phenomenon met four criteria—universality, intrinsicality, progressiveness and deleteriousness. This means that an ageing process must occur in everyone, must not be due to outside factors (such as ultra violet rays from the sun), must be progressive and must do the person some harm. Although hypertension, for example, is common in the elderly in our society, high blood pressure is not universal amongst all elderly people. It may be due to external factors (e.g. high salt intake) and is not always progressive. Hence it is an age difference and not an age change.

The search for the knowledge base of ageing is exhaustive. There is no single generally accepted theory, but all the theories fall into two broad groups. One, variously termed the random, extrinsic or epiphenomenalist theory, argues that ageing is due to the effects of living, basically wear and tear. There may be an accumulation of waste products or increasing chemical changes affecting DNA, etc. The other main group of theories, pacemaker, death-clock and fundamentalist, all state that ageing is basically genetically programmed.

BIOLOGICAL AND PHYSIOLOGICAL THEORIES OF AGEING

Random theories

Leo Sziland (1959) claimed that ageing is due to the background radiation (from the sun, rocks, etc.) randomly hitting chromosomes and causing harmful mutations. Leslie Orgel (1963, 1970) and Medvedev (1966) extended this idea so that errors (however caused) in the DNA protein synthesis chain could produce faulty templates. Thus faulty proteins such as enzymes could compound the error resulting in an 'error catastrophe' and cell death. However, if ageing is due to this error accumulation the abnormal protein should be detectable in the elderly. Collagen is different in old tissue, i.e. aged collagen, but newly formed collagen in the elderly is normal. In normal cell physiology chemical reactions take place producing compounds called free radicals. These may damage cell constituents and hence cause errors in protein synthesis. Substances called antioxidants limit this damage. As collagen ages, it increases the number of cross-linkages (also seen in other proteins). This changes its properties but the accumulation of these damaging links has been shown to be delayed or even prevented by antioxidants. It has been proposed that ageing may be due to these cross-link effects and that this may be slowed down by taking the antioxidant vitamin E.

Evidence that cells accumulate waste products, altering the cell function, is said to be shown by the fact that old cells (in man and other species) commonly have a pigmented material called lipofuscin within them. Lipofuscin has been termed the 'ageing pigment'. McCay et al (1939) showed 40 years ago that one can prolong the life of rats by 25% if their diet is restricted in early life and puberty delayed. Children, however, can develop mental retardation with dietary restriction. The lifespan of the fruit fly (Drosophila) can be doubled or halved by either lowering or raising the temperature and it has been shown that mice with lowered body temperatures can live twice as long.

Programmed ageing

The first specific genetic programme determining life span was proposed by August Weismann in Salzburg in 1881. He theorised a limitation in the number of cell generations for somatic (body) cells. Leonard Hayflick (1965) has shown that normal human diploid cells cultured in vitro (outside the body) possess a limited clonal (group of cells all descended from a single individual asexually) life span. Within a species senescence has a fairly predictable onset and as separate species have different but also predictable lifespans some genetic programming seems likely. Programmed ageing has been variously called the ageing clock (Everitt 1973), or the ageing pacemaker (Finch and Hayflick 1977), whereas Denckla (1974) hypothesised an ageing hormone. The favoured site for ageing control is the hypothalamus within the brain with its nervous system and endocrine links.

Studies have shown that the age at death is closer in monozygotic rather than dizygotic twins hence implicating the importance of heredity. Pearl (1934) has a dictum—'the best way to achieve a long life is to choose long-lived grandparents'.

PHYSIOLOGICAL CHANGES WITH AGE

The ageing brain

Viewed from above, the brain is an egg-shaped mass, broader behind and widest in the parietal region. The two halves of the brain are incompletely separated by a deep median cleft, the longitudinal cerebral fissure. Each half contains a central cavity—the lateral ventricle—in which the cerebrospinal fluid which bathes the brain is formed by the choroid plexus. The two halves of the brain are joined in the mid-line by the corpus callosum which in the adult is about the size of the little finger. Up to the age of four months the embryonic brain is smooth but from them on it develops an irregular surface with prominent folds (gyri) separated by grooves (sulci). This means that the total area of grey matter is 30 times greater than the skull size. To the naked eye nerve cells form the grey matter and nerve fibres the white matter. A typical nerve cell in the cerebral cortex has a number of processes, one of which (the axon) transmits impulses away from the nerve cell. The others are receptors (the dendrites) which branch into intricate patterns. Millions of brain cells form the grey matter. With age, the brain volume gets smaller (as measured at post-mortem) but this age atrophy could be a cross-sectional difference. Old brains usually have more prominent gyri and deeper sulci and larger ventricular systems. Brain weight falls by about 10% between the ages of 25–75 years, though it is debatable whether or not brain cells are lost with age.

Comparatively little is known of the function of the brain of the normal adult and even less of the changes with age. Most methods of testing, e.g. the Weschler Adult Intelligence Scale, (WAIS) are speed related. It is known that the speed of response declines with age and this probably explains the perceived decline in intelligence quotient (IQ). There is a loss of ability to recall sequences of nonsense symbols or unrelated words with age. Retrieval capacity (especially for recent memories) and speed of recall declines, although the ability to remember complex concepts and relationships and to categorise items is not impaired. Basically, elderly people need shorter lists and more time to recall. The effect, or lack of effect, of age on intellectual functioning is discussed in more detail in Chapter 2, The Psychology of Ageing.

The changes that occur with age are both physiological and pathological. The brain of a 75-year-old will usually show meningeal thickening and some degree of cerebral atrophy and ventricular enlargement. Microscopic changes include lipofuscin deposition in all cells. In neurones there will be loss of ribonucleic acid (RNA) and mitochondrial enzymes in the cytoplasm. There are also tissue degenerative changes in the neurones characterised by senile plaques, neurofibrillary tangles and granulovacuolar degeneration. These changes are not distributed uniformly in the brain in normal ageing. They are seen in excess in pathological conditions such as senile dementia of the Alzheimer type. Other age-related neuronal inclusions include hyaline and eosinophilic elements and Lewy bodies (inclusion bodies first noted in idiopathic cases of Parkinson's disease). Atheromatous changes occur in both cerebral vessels and the major extra-cranial vessels (carotid and vertebral arteries).

Ageing and the skin

The epidermis (the most superficial layer of the skin) is composed of stratified squamous epithelium which varies little with age. The dermis is thicker and contains mucopolysaccharide ground substance, collagen, elastin fibres, fibroblasts, macrophages and mast cells. The amount of skin collagen decreases with age (a decreased rate of production by fibroblasts) and there is a loss of elasticity. Each collagen molecule is made up of a triple helix with two different types of chain, alpha and beta. Each chain has more than 1000 amino acids, of which proline and hydroxyproline constitute one third. This helix is held together by cross-linkages which increase with age. Loss of skin elasticity means that minor skin trauma can produce an extravasation of blood due to capillary rupture. The lack of dermal support allows spreading of the blood and the 'senile purpura' retains its colour because it is deoxygenated blood. Lack of skin fibroblasts means that it is not degraded quickly.

The ability for light to pass through skin (transparency) increases with age in both sexes. Wrinkles are closely associated with age changes in the dermis and both aged skin and sun-damaged skin lose tone and elasticity giving rise to sagging and wrinkling (Fig. 3.3). Nude sunbathing may be popular when young but regretted later when wrinkles develop early. Wrinkles are evident where the skin folds frequently and resorption of the maxilla and mandible lead to furrowed pockets at the corners of the mouth (especially noticeable in the edentulous).

Normal aged skin is thus relatively dehydrated with loss of elasticity and strength. The loss of subcutaneous fat has caused wrinkles and lines and there is also a loss of vascularity. Decreasing seborrhoeic glands make the surface dry and hence friable and more susceptible to trauma and especially pressure. There is some evidence for a gradual deterio-

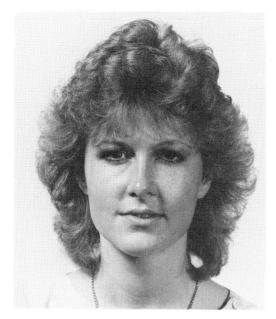

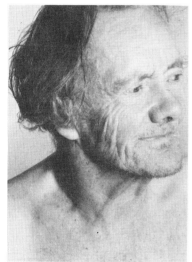

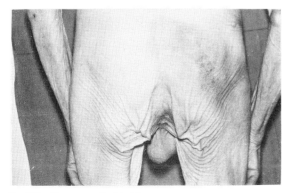

Fig. 3.3 Young and old skins.

ration in peripheral nerve function causing some reduced sensation and reflexes, again increasing the tendency to skin injury.

Even this aged skin represents an effective barrier to infection. However, once breached minor trauma can cause large wounds owing to the lack of elasticity, decreased vascularity and infection. These factors account for the fact that wound healing can be delayed especially when the initial trauma was due to pressure. The decreased vascularity may have important implications in body heat regulation (see Chapter 13, Maintaining Body Temperature).

Greying of hair (canities)—owing to lack of pigment in the cortex—is normally distributed in the population and usually begins at the temple. It is determined by an autosomal dominant gene. Temple recession occurs in 100% of men and 80% of women. Females have the same tendency to baldness as males but to a lesser degree.

Nails become increasingly brittle and hard with age, often ridged longitudually. They usually have a matt finish rather than the lustre of young nails but can become pathologically hard and curved—a condition called onychogryphosis (see Chapter 9, Care of the Foot).

The ageing musculoskeletal system

Bone

Bone is composed of living cells and a bone matrix (mainly collagen) upon which bone salts are deposited. Throughout life, even after longitudinal growth ceases, cancellous and cortical bone is constantly being replaced. In both sexes the amount of bone in the body increases until the fourth decade, then declines—more rapidly in women. Some individuals, however, have more bone at the age of 80 than others have at age 30.

There are many factors influencing the amount of bone formed but it is probably true to say that the amount of bone in old age is determined by how much was present at maturity. The quantity of bone present at maturity depends upon sex, race, height, body build, posture, exercise, endocrine factors, supply of calcium and general nutrition. There is a poorer skeletal development in girls (they have a relatively lower bone mass). This may be a factor in the higher incidence of osteoporosis (thin bones) in older women.

Endosteal envelope phenomenon. Bone material lies outside the bone cells and remodelling takes place from the surfaces, upon which the cells active in remodelling reside. Three surfaces or envelopes have been defined. The periosteal surface lines the outside of all bones, the endosteal surface lines the marrow cavities and covers the trabeculae of cancellous bone while the intracortical, or Haversian, surface lines the Haversian canals. The periosteal surface is predominantly a bone-forming surface so the external diameter of bones increase with age. The endosteal surface is mainly a resorbing surface so the marrow cavity also enlarges with age.

Bone collagen and salts. The function of collagen is mainly mechanical and throughout the body collagen fibres are stabilised by a system of covalent interchain cross-links. Both intra- and intermolecular cross-links increase with age. It is not known whether the increasing cross-linkages which strengthen the bone are eventually deleterious. Approximately 90% of bone is fibrous collagen protein, the remainder being mainly calcium and phosphorus.

Accurate measurement of bone in the skeleton is very difficult. Radiographs provide only an approximate indication of bone density. Modern methods include photoelectric densitometry and photon absorption. The loss of bone from the skeleton with the atrophy of this tissue (as seen in all other ageing tissues/organs) has some specific features in the elderly. Kyphosis (forward bending) increases in frequency with age subsequent upon the above processes occurring in the spine. This has relevance when dealing with both posture and locomotion of old people. Bone resorption occurs noticeably around the jaw—the so-called shrinking jaw—causing dental problems especially when false teeth

are worn and hence become loose and uncomfortable, with subsequent effects on diet and nutrition.

Muscle

For 50 years it has been accepted that there is decrease in physical strength due to physiological ageing. Recently this view has been questioned because low serum potassium levels found in many elderly people predispose to impaired muscle strength. Lack of vitamin C, being found increasingly in the elderly, can also lead to muscle weakness.

The ageing cardiovascular system

Ageing of the cardiovascular system has long been thought to be the basis for the general physiological decline that is part of ageing.

Anatomy

There are progressive changes in the aorta with decreasing elasticity and an increase in calibre. Heart valves characteristically accumulate lipid, undergo collagen degeneration and an increase in calcification. The classic age changes in the myocardium (heart muscle) are 'brown atrophy', the accumulation of lipofuscin (age pigment) and a decrease in heart weight. Accumulation of amyloid is also said to occur with age—so called 'senile amyloidosis'. In the conducting system there is a decrease in the number of pacemaker cells in the sino-atrial node with a decrease in muscle fibres and an increase in fibrous tissue and fat.

Function

The effect of age on the resting heart rate is equivocal and there is probably little alteration. The heart rate increase in response to exercise and stress, however, is less effective with increasing age. As a consequence of the atrophy of the aortic elastic tissue there is an increase in pulse and systolic pressures with age but not the diastolic pressure. There are vascular changes that in themselves could lead to raised blood pressure with age but some individuals and populations can compensate by bringing other factors into play. In the short and long term, lifestyle changes such as diet and physical exercise can reduce blood pressure. In healthy individuals cardiac output drops off in linear fashion, approximately 1% per year, when measured with the individual at rest. This is due to a reduction in stroke volume with heart rate being unaltered.

Organ perfusion can be said to decrease with age using data on peripheral resistance, blood flow and clearance of substances. Compensatory mechanisms such as vaso-dilation and increased vascularisation may occur in some sites with increasing age. Changes in organ perfusion could be secondary to less blood being supplied to the capillaries because of changes in cardiac output or due to atherosclerosis of large vessels. Peripheral resistance increases with age and this probably plays an important role in decreasing blood flow. A change in one part of the cardio-vascular system influences every other and it is difficult to distinguish primary from secondary age changes. However, most of the changes with age are probably due to a small number of factors which are intrinsic.

The ageing respiratory system

Determining true ageing processes in the lungs is extremely difficult because they bear the brunt of modern living (the inhalation of smoke and fumes, etc) and yet have a great ability for self-repair. There is increasing calci-fication of the costal cartilages with age, increased anterior-posterior diameter of the chest and kyphosis (forward bending). Alveolar duct volume increases with age, producing wider ducts, a condition known as ductectasia. A diffuse loss of elastic fibres in the supporting tissue of the lungs occurs with some thick-ening of the pulmonary artery walls. However, after inhalation it is not elastic recoil that is the main retractive factor. The principal compo-nent is the surface-active forces developed at the air-tissue interface—the force maintained by surfactant. Age changes on this aspect of the recoil process are not known. Bronchial mucous glands increase with age but the lining cilia are fewer and hence the 'ciliary escalator' for debris evacuation is less efficient.

Lung volumes of the elderly have been thoroughly studied. Total lung capacity is unchanged though the various subdivisions are markedly different with age. There is a progressive fall in vital capacity (20–30 ml per year) and as the total lung capacity remains constant the residual volume must increase. The ratio of residual volume to total lung capacity (RV/TLC) increases with age (25% aged 20, 40% aged 70) resulting in gradual hyperexpansion. The forced expiratory volume in one second (FEV_1) also declines with age. Lung compliance (the change in volume per unit change in pressure) increases with age so that lungs of the elderly have increased expan-sibility (are less 'stiff').

Prior to old age the lower lobes of the lung are preferentially ventilated. In old age, blood perfusion (Q) at the bases remains good but ventilation (V) is poorer, resulting in a ventilation/perfusion V/Q mismatch, or physiological shunt. This contributes to the arterial oxygen level being lower for the normal elderly. Cardiopulmonary reserve decreases in old age and hence the elderly are less able to tolerate situations requiring increased oxygen requirements (e.g. exercise, shock).

The ageing kidney and bladder

The functional unit of the kidney—the nephron—comprises the glomerulus, the proximal tubule, the loop of Henle, and the distal tubule. The glomerulus is a filter and in a healthy young adult 180 litres are filtered daily, most of which is reabsorbed to leave about 1.5 litres of urine per day. This volume depends on the hydrostatic pressure, the rate of blood flow through the glomerular tuft and the integrity of the filtering membranes. The proximal tubule carries out most of the active reabsorption and excretion processes. The loop of Henle with the distal tubule is the main site of urine concentration.

Change in structure and function

Aged kidneys are generally smaller than young. Non-hypertensive vascular changes occur with reduplication of elastic tissue and thickening of the intima. The nephron and tubular basement membranes also thicken. There is, however, a poor correlation between glomerular numbers and age. Increasing numbers of diverticula occur in the distal tubules probably from herniation through the basement membrane. The most important change in renal function occurring with age is the loss of urine concentrating power (hence fluid cannot be conserved efficiently). Tubular excretory function begins to fall off in the third decade and precedes any demonstrable fall in glomerular filtration rate. Both subsequently decrease at the same rate with the glomerular filtration rate tending to fall off increasingly after the age of 70 years. There is some evidence that the ageing nephron fails as a unit.

Bladder

Muscle tone declines in the ureters, bladder and urethra lending to some impairment of complete emptying of the bladder, residual urine often causing urinary tract infections. Bladder capacity declines from an average 500 ml in young people to approximately 250 ml in the elderly, hence the bladder will need to be emptied more frequently. Furthermore, as there is evidence that the stretch receptors become less sensitive, then the urge to urinate will occur later, when the bladder is full, causing urgency and nocturia.

The spinal reflexes that cause bladder contractions are usually inhibited by the cerebral hemispheres. If there is diminished cerebral function or degeneration of the inhibiting nerves, then the bladder may empty involuntarily under the influence of the uninhibited reflex contractions. These uninhibited contractions occur more frequently with increasing age.

Ageing of the alimentary system

Age changes occur in the gastrointestinal tract but function is usually adequate. In the elderly peridontal disease is the main cause of loss of teeth (dental caries is the main reason in the young). Peridontal disease is accelerated by lack of saliva (ageing salivary glands), age atrophy of the alveolar bone and epithlial atrophy of mucus membranes. By 60 years of age 60% of people are edentulous and this percentage increases with increasing age. Reduced saliva production also predisposes to oral infections. Varicosities on the undersurface of the tongue are seen in 40% of people over 70, their significance is unknown but maybe related in a few cases to vitamin C deficiency.

There are changes in the senses of taste and smell as we age. The number of taste buds decline with a subsequent increase in the threshold levels needed to achieve 'taste', especially for sweet taste. Hence elderly people will often apply far more flavouring to food (sauces, spices, etc.) to achieve the desired effect. The sense of smell also declines and the two senses are intricately combined in the appreciation and enjoyment of foods. Lack of smell also means lack of taste. The vanilla test proves this: hold your nose and then place vanilla extract on your tongue—it has no taste until you release your nose. Hence the provision of enjoyable food for the elderly requires a knowledge of these sensory changes and compensation in certain cases.

The oesophagus conveys foods from the mouth to the stomach aided by peristalic waves or contractions. Primary waves occur after swallowing and secondary waves arise when the upper oesophagus is distended by food. Tertiary contractions are ring-like non-peristaltic waves occuring increasingly in old age and occasionally producing symptoms of dysphagia (difficulty in swallowing). In presbyoesophagus (a specific swallowing problem in old age) the normal swallow is not followed by a primary wave but by non-propulsive contractions and uncoordination of the lower oesophageal sphincter relaxation. Atrophic gastritis occurs increasingly in old age and is associated with pernicious anaemia (vitamin B12 deficiency) and stomach cancer. In the small bowel the proximal jejunal villi tend to be broader and shorter with decreased cell production in the jejunal crypts. Diverticulae (pouches through muscular walls) occur increasingly with age. Changes in absorption in the small bowel are complex but basically fat absorption is delayed and reduced. Vitamin B12 absorption is normal and protein, calcium and iron have been insufficiently investigated.

The large bowel is probably the part of the gut most affected by age changes. The colon receives ileal contents, absorbes water and sodium chloride and secretes potassium, bicarbonate and mucus and then stores the faeces until evacuation. Histological age changes include mucosal cell and muscle layer atrophy, and an increase in connective tissue. Ingestion of food stimulates gut motility via the gastrocolic hormonal reflex. The response is enhanced by physical activity and there is little propulsive activity in an immobile person. This relationship between reduced colonic motility and physical inactivity is one of the main factors in constipation occurring in old age. Using radio-opaque markers or dyes, elderly people have been shown to have a slower transit time of faeces.

Ageing of the reproductive and endocrine systems

Female

The menopause at about 50 years of age marks the end of child bearing with the menstrual periods becoming irregular and then stopping. After the menopause there appears to be a physiological acceleration of the ageing process.

Hormonal changes. In the reproductive years oestradiol is the main ovarian oestrogen produced. After the menopause, however, the amount of oestradiol declines. The main postmenopausal oestrogen is oestrone, derived from conversion of an adrenal cortical hormone androstenedione. The conversion takes place in fat and increases with age. The low levels of oestradiol means there is no negative feedback on the hypothalamus (and possibly pituitary) and hence the levels of circulating and urinary gonadotrophins (follicle stimulating hormone—FSH, and luteinising hormone—LH), are raised.

Ovary. The number and quality of the oocytes in the ovary declines with age as shown by an increase in damaged chromosomes in women approaching the menopause—the most notable result being trisomy of chromosome 21 resulting in babies with Down's syndrome. Possibly, oocytes that spend a long time in the ovary prior to conception are more prone to radiation/infection/autoantibody damage (see Theories of Ageing). The human post-menopausal ovary has little response to gonadotrophic hormones and eventually it becomes fibrotic.

Vulva and vagina. There is a shrinkage and wrinkling of vulval skin. Tissue atrophy in the vagina causes shortening and decreases the size of the lumen. A loss of elastic tissue plus the fact that vaginal muscle is replaced with fat predisposes to uterovaginal prolapse. The epithelium becomes thin, pale and dry.

Uterus. For a few years before the menopause the uterus increasingly fails to support a pregnancy, probably owing to changes in the uterus itself and altered hormonal balance. Post-menopausally the uterus slowly atrophies—with a sparse endometrium (inner layer) and fibrous myometrium (muscle layer)—to as little as 1 cm in diameter in extreme old age.

Breasts. From about the age of 35 years there is replacement of glandular breast tissue with fat. There is an increasing risk of malignancy in the ageing breast with evidence that some types of carcinoma may depend on hormone stimulation (oestrogens and prolactin).

Male

The ageing of the male reproductive system is a gradual process. It probably has a variable period of onset and although there is some evidence for a 'male menopause' it usually passes without major physical or psychological side-effects.

Testes. There is no decline in the size or weight of the testes. Spermatozoa continue to be produced into old age. The secretion of testosterone decreases in elderly men.

Prostate. From puberty to the fifth decade the prostate shows secretory activity but then degenerative changes begin which increasingly lessen secretions. Nodular hyperplasia is common after the age of 50 years, while the cause of the hypertrophy is unknown.

Function. The ageing male reproductive system can keep enough functional capability so that reproduction remains possible (a 94-year-old man has been a 'successful' father.) Sex drive is said to lessen with age and time to ejaculation lengthens. The first changes occur in the penis at about the age of 40 years, with fibroelastosis of the trabeculae in the corpus spongiosum, followed by progressive sclerosis of arteries and veins.

The endocrine system

The adrenal response to stress declines with age. Underactivity of the adrenal gland (Addison's disease) occurs in the elderly whereas overactivity (Cushing's disease) is extremely rare over the age of 70. Insulin deficiency is strongly age related and glucose tolerance tests indicate that many elderly people have problems coping with a glucose load rendering them at least transiently 'diabetic'.

From a functional point of view the thyroid gland of even very elderly people maintains adequate function. The secretion of T4 (thyroxine) decreases with age whilst plasma T4 levels do not. The TSH (thyroid stimulating

hormone) response is unchanged. There are markedly lower levels of plasma T3 (tri-iodothyronine) and if this is the circulatory 'active' hormone, then there may be a decrease in the effective hormone with ageing. But since TSH levels do not rise, there may also be deficiency in the negative feedback.

Ageing in the immune system

Lymphoid tissue

Thymus. This reaches its maximum weight at puberty and decreases with age (following sexual maturation). Histology of the ageing thymus shows cortical atrophy and replacement by connective tissue.

Spleen. There is a decrease in the amount of white pulp and a relative increase in red pulp with a reduction in follicular tissue. Germinal centres are absent in the elderly.

Lymph nodes. There is a reduction in the weight of lymph nodes with thinning of the cortex, absent or reduced germinal centres, an increase in the macrophages in the medulla and dilatation of the medullary sinuses. Organised lymphoid tissues undergo regression with age but the amount of diffuse lymphoid tissue throughout the body increases (lymphoid follicles in bone marrow, salivary glands, portal triads and lung parenchyma).

Cells

Stem cells. There are adequate numbers of stem cells (cells which will later differentiate into either T or B cells) but ageing may produce defects in differentiation.

T cells. T lymphocytes are responsible for delayed hypersensitivity reactions and for providing immunity against virus, fungal and mycobacterial infections. There is a reduction of peripheral T lympocytes and a reduction in the delayed hypersensitivity response to skin tests. This means that Mantoux tests often produce negative results in the elderly. Helper cells occur in normal numbers. Cytotoxic T cells are reduced in number, therefore the ability to kill target cells such as cells infected with virus is reduced. Suppressor T cells limit the immune response and occur in reduced numbers, while the frequency of autoantibodies increases.

B cells. The numbers of circulating B cells (which mature into plasma cells and produce antibody) are probably unchanged.

There is some evidence to suggest that the decreased immune surveillance by T cells may be responsible for the increased incidence of neoplasia (cancers) seen with age and if suppressor T cells are reduced more auto-immune diseases are likely to be expressed.

Humoral immunity

Serum immunoglobulins. The total amount of immunoglobulin in the serum does not change with age, but the amounts of specific immunoglobulins does alter with an increase in levels of IgG and IgA in the fit elderly and 'normal' IgG levels in the elderly near to death.

Mucosal immunity. IgA is the principal immunoglobulin in human exocrine secretions and may occur in reduced concentrations in the nasal secretions of aged people. The meaning in terms of function of the changes in serum immunoglobulins and mucosal immunity is not known.

The ageing auditory system

Hearing is impaired with advancing age both from physiological effects and by pathological changes. Presbyacusis is the term used for the changes in the auditory system occurring with age. Functional abnormalities include impaired sound localisation, decline in discrimination (especially of speech), a decrease in time-related processing abilities and also tinnitus (an abnormal buzzing/distracting sound in the ear).

From the third decade onwards the threshold of normal hearing begins to deteriorate and, as high frequency hearing is the most susceptible to damage, high frequency loss occurs first in both ears. This high frequency loss contributes significantly to the difficulty in understanding speech. Slight impairment can be corrected for with a slightly louder voice but moderate to severe impairment can seriously hamper communication. Hearing-loss graphs for the elderly indicate a probable maximum (physiological) hearing loss at each decade. There are also age changes in the middle ear conducting system with thickening of the tympanic membrane and loss of elasticity. See Chapter 5 for a more detailed discussion on the prevalence of hearing loss in the elderly.

The ageing eye

Eyes of the elderly are somewhat sunken (due to loss of orbital fat) predisposing to droopy eyelids (ptosis). The pupil is small and the cornea surrounded by a dense white ring, the arcus senilis (gerontoxon). Visual acuity and visual fields decrease with age, the acuity problems being termed presbyopia (old age visual loss). Light impinging on the eye is first focused by the cornea (to a much greater extent than was once realised) and then the lens. Fine focusing is achieved by relaxation of the suspensory ligament—allowing the lens to change shape and focus rays. The lens, however, is unique in that new lens fibres are constantly being formed while old fibres are not lost. These old fibres lie deeper and the lens increases in size which results in increased rigidity. Clarity for near objects is only achieved by increasing the focal length (moving the object away—such as holding a book at arm's length). Eventually one's arms are no longer long enough to hold the object far enough away and an artificial lens has to be used (in the form of reading glasses) to correct the presbyopia.

Cataract

The increase in the layers of the lens with age is progressive (and hence considered by some to be a physiological ageing process, or at least a process where physiology and pathology overlap), and successive layers compress the central area of the lens. The centre becomes hard and has a high refractive index, i.e. it becomes opaque (a process termed nuclear sclerosis). The posterior pole of the lens is a common site for this compression process, and with the added problem of a small pupil allowing in a narrow beam of light the cataract forms a visual plug resulting in an incapacitating loss of vision (even when small). Peripheral (cartwheel) cataracts may be less disabling initially but the cataract disperses light and in bright light causes a marked flashing and glare effect (hence the use of peaked caps or card-dealer's shades to minimise this phenomenon).

There is a reduction in the metabolic activity of the lens with increasing age and a tripeptide, glutathione, which is present in high concentrations in the normal lens, is reduced as the cataract forms. Soluble proteins are reduced in concentration and are thought either to be changed to insoluble complexes or leaked out via the capsule. A diabetic is six times more likely to develop a cataract and the concentration of the sugar, sorbitol, in the lens of diabetics is markedly abnormal.

The mean pressure inside the eye increases with age and hence elderly people will be in the 'high pressure group' at risk from open-angle glaucoma. The elderly with high pressure will often have a strong family history. The increasing lens thickness mentioned previously also leads to a shallowing of the anterior chamber and here the main danger is the provocation of acute-angle closure glaucoma. The resting pupil size decreases with age. There is also increased fibrosis of the iris with a reduced response to accommodation with reduced light access.

The loss of orbital fat can cause the lower lid to curl in and the eyelashes irritate the cornea (entropion). This is easily remedied by taping down the lower lid so that it curls outwards until a minor surgical procedure can be performed. The laxity of the eyelids aids the mechanism of ectropion where the eyelids fall away resulting in poor tear syphoning and excessive tear production to compensate (epiphora).

CONCLUSION

The knowledge concerning the physiology of ageing is still in its infancy. True ageing processes are difficult to distinguish from pathological processes yet it is this difficult area which we must aim to clarify. Growing old must be seen to be a success if ageism is to be combated. It can only be a success if doctors and the elderly themselves are clear about what is normal ageing and what is an illness process. For too long the elderly have been existing with ill health and frailty under the umbrella of 'old age'. The pioneering work into the physiology of ageing, gerontology and geriatric medicine will enable much of this frailty to be seen for what it really is—hopefully a reversible disease process.

REFERENCES

Aslan A, Vrabiescu A, Domilescu C, Campeanu L, Costiniu M, Stanescu S 1965 Longterm treatment with procaine (gerovital H_3) in albino rats. Journal Gerontology 20: 1–8
Brown Séquard C E 1899 Des effets produits chez l'homme par des injections sous cutanees d'un liquide retire des testicules frais de cobayes et de chiens. Comptes rendus de la Societe de Biologie 4(1): 415–422
Denckla W D 1974 Role of the pituitary and thyroid glands in the decline of minimal O_2 consumption with age. Journal Clinical Investigation 53: 572–581
Everitt A V 1973 The hypothalmic-pituitary control of ageing and age-related pathology. Experimental Gerontology 8: 265–277
Finch C E, Hayflick L (eds) 1977 Handbook of the biology of ageing. Van Nostrand Reinhold, New York
Hayflick L 1965 The limited in vitro lifetime of human diploid cell strains. Experimental Cell Research 37: 614–636
Macfarlane M D 1975 Procaine HCl (gerovital H_3): a weak reversible, fully competitive inhibitor of monoamine oxidase. Federation Proceedings 34: 108–110
McCay C M 1939 Retarded growth, lifespan, ultimate body size and age changes in the albino rat after feeding diets restricted in calories. Journal of Nutrition 18: 1–13
Medvedev Z A 1966 Protein biosynthesis. Oliver and Boyd, Edinburgh
Metchnikoff E 1907 The Prolongation of life. Optimistic studies, Heinemann, London
Orgel L E 1963 The maintenance of the accuracy of protein synthesis and its relevance to ageing. Proceeds National Academy of Science (Washington) 49: 517–521

Orgel L E 1970 The maintenance of the accuracy of protein synthesis and its relevance to ageing: a correction. Procedes National Academy of Science (Washington) 67:1476

Pearl R, Pearl R de W 1934 The Ancestry of the long-lived. Milford, London

Strehler B L 1962 Time, cells and ageing. Academic Press, New York

Sziland L 1959 On the nature of the ageing process. Proceedings of the National Academy of Sciences of the USA 45: 30–45

FURTHER READING

Comfort A 1979 The biology of senescence, 3rd edn. Churchill-Livingstone, Edinburgh

Behnke J A, Finch C E, Moment G B (eds) 1978 The biology of ageing. Plenum Press, New York

Brocklehurst J C (ed) 1978 Textbook of geriatric medicine and gerontology, 2nd edn. Churchill Livingstone, Edinburgh

Finch C E, Hayflick L 1977 Handbook of biology of ageing. Van Nostrand Reinhold, New York

PART TWO

Nursing elderly people: their needs and problems of living

4

J. Macleod Clark

Communicating with elderly people

It is ironic that in old age, when people have more time to communicate for pleasure, they often develop problems which make communication more difficult. The desire to communicate is a central human drive and the need for communication increases in situations of stress and uncertainty.

For many elderly people, the experience of becoming a patient is an extremely stressful, often frightening event. However, several research reports have highlighted the fact that nurses spend only a small proportion of their time actually communicating with their elderly patients (Stockwell 1972, Norton et al 1975, Wells 1980) and it is essential for nurses to develop the skills necessary to communicate as well as possible with such patients. This chapter begins with an overview of the elements of verbal and non-verbal communication which mesh together to produce successful interaction skills. This is followed by a description of some of the most common communication difficulties that the elderly may have to cope with. These difficulties are discussed in the context of the most appropriate ways to assess them, and where possible, overcome them.

ELEMENTS OF COMMUNICATION

Communication between human beings involves a meshing of verbal and non-verbal behaviours. The principal components of communication include:

— Verbal communication—the words that are spoken or written.
— Intonational communication—the stress, pitch and intensity which give words extra meaning.
— Paralinguistic communication—laughter, crying, coughs and spluttering.
— Non-verbal (kinesic) communication—body and facial movements.

Non-verbal communication is particularly important when caring for the elderly (Burnside 1973, Hardiman et al 1979). There are many elements of non-verbal behaviour including facial expression derived from movements of the eyes, eyebrows and mouth; eye contact and gaze, head movements such as nods; gestures of hands, head, shoulders; posture which can indicate attitudes and emotional states; proximity and body contact and touch. It is the flexibility of non-verbal communication which makes it so valuable in communication with old people. If speech, hearing or sight is limited then skilful use of non-verbal communication, particularly touch, can ensure that patients are aware that they are being cared for. Observation of the patient's use of non-verbal behaviours can also be vital to the accurate assessment of physical and psychological needs.

THE COMMUNICATION NEEDS OF THE ELDERLY

The communication needs of the elderly will not necessarily differ from those of any individual in hospital (Fig. 4.1). It is often felt that old people are lonely and therefore have special needs for social contact. However, they may also be used to their own company

---

1. The need for social contact and interaction
2. The need for explanation, confirmation
3. The need for advice, education, support
4. The need for comfort and reassurance

Fig. 4.1 Patients' communication needs.

and can find the public life of a hospital, nursing or residential Home confusing and disturbing.

The nurse's primary role is to become skilled at recognising and assessing the extent of each patient's needs for different types of communication and in planning care appropriately. For some old people, the need for social contact can be met simply through the knowledge that others are around them. They do not necessarily require conversation. For others, their main need is for someone to talk to (or often for someone to listen to them).

In order to assess a patient's needs and to communicate effectively it is essential that nurses have the appropriate skills.

Communication skills needed to assess and meet the needs of elderly patients

The listed communication skills given in Figure 4.2 are essential prerequisites for effective assessment and communication with the elderly. By observing, listening and attending to what the patient says and does (the patient's verbal and non-verbal communication) the nurse will be able to build up a picture of the patient as an individual. Active listening will also help the nurse to recognise and respond to the patient's direct questions and, more importantly, their indirect questions, statements or cues. Macleod Clark (1981) found that 80% of surgical patients' requests for information are indirect or subtle, and this may be even higher for the elderly who can be diffident and unsure of themselves. The skill of asking questions appropriately is essential if a patient's needs are to be assessed accurately. If the intention is to explore how someone is really feeling, then open questions will be most useful. However, if the patient has difficulty in speaking or hearing then simple closed questions requiring a Yes or No answer may be the most appropriate. Old people tire easily and have a limited memory span, so it is vital to choose the right moment to give important instructions or information. It is also a good idea to repeat the information and, possibly, to write it down, using short

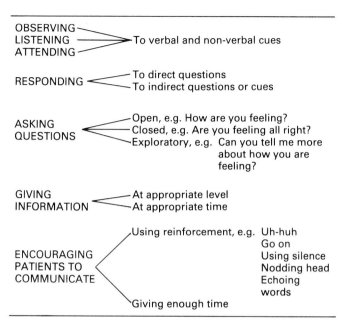

Fig. 4.2 Some communication skills necessary for assessing patients' needs.

sentences, and avoiding jargon.

One of the most valuable communication skills is that of being able to encourage other people to talk. Many old people become withdrawn and may need a great deal of encouragement to talk freely. Using reinforcement strategies such as saying 'When?', 'Go on', 'I see', will always help the patient to carry on talking. Nodding your head and repeating important words back to the patient are also very effective. The skill of staying silent and giving time for an elderly person to think and answer will also facilitate communication.

However, for many old people communication does become a problem for a variety of physical and psychological reasons. Trying to overcome these problems requires even more skill on the nurse's part and this is discussed in the following section.

REASONS FOR COMMUNICATION PROBLEMS OF ELDERLY PEOPLE

The process of ageing is accompanied by degeneration of neuronal tissue in the central nervous system, although whether these changes occur as a result of ageing itself or of pathology is not altogether clear (see Chapter 3, The Physiology of Ageing). In consequence, the reactions of elderly people become slower. Sensory inputs are reduced and this is particularly noticeable in relation to the special senses of vision and hearing. When sight and hearing are impaired, then communication becomes more difficult.

Other factors also create problems and these include the increase in sensory and social deprivation that often occurs in old age. The elderly can be confused and disoriented and many develop speech difficulties. Such difficulties are often related to diseases such as Parkinsonism, or pathology such as cerebral vascular accidents and atheroma.

Problems caused by visual impairment

With the passage of time, the power of visual accommodation diminishes and there can be particular difficulty with accommodating to darkness. Presbyopia, or farsightedness, is an almost universal phenomenon so that nearly all elderly people require glasses for seeing things that are near. Ageing also brings an increased incidence of intraocular pressure and thickening of the lens causing glaucoma and cataracts, and, in extreme cases, blindness (see Chapter 3). Problems of sight are also discussed by Bob Greenhalgh in Chapter 6.

Assessing patients' visual acuity and overcoming problems

Since the majority of elderly patients will have some limitations of vision it is necessary for the nurse to establish the extent of disability and to try to compensate for this where possible.

All patients (or their relatives) should be asked about their sight and the use of spectacles. Many old people do not have their eyes tested regularly and as a consequence their prescription lenses may not be effective. If you suspect that the patient's glasses are ineffective and if the patient is in hospital for any length of time an attempt should be made to get her sight retested and new lenses prescribed. If the patient does wear glasses she should be encouraged to wear them at the times when she would normally wear them at home. They should also be checked to make sure they are clean.

— When communicating with patients with poor vision it is essential to introduce yourself before you speak as the patient may not be aware of your presence.
— Sit or stand in a position which suits the patient best.
— Do not sit or stand too close. This can be uncomfortable for old people whose eyes cannot focus or accommodate to very near objects.
— Non-verbal communication is vital, especially touch and the use of clear intonation.
— Try to keep the patient's environment as consistent and familiar as possible.

Problems caused by hearing impairment

The incidence of deafness increases with age and, as discussed in detail in Chapter 5, 60%

of people over 70 years are deaf (Gilhome Herbst and Humphrey 1981). Hearing is a vital means of orientation, giving information on proximity and distance. However, degeneration of this sense (presbyacusis) is also an inevitable concomitant of ageing. Cochlear problems include diminished hearing and tinnitus while vestibular problems result in disturbance of balance. Irreversible physiological changes to the hearing mechanism typically begin sometime after the age of 30 years, with a gradual loss of acuity for high frequency sound. This loss steadily increases and gradually encroaches upon lower sound frequencies and both ears are usually affected at much the same rate.

The elderly often complain that they are unable to 'understand' rather than not being able to hear, and this difficulty in discrimination is usually experienced initially when the environment is noisy or when speech is rapid. As the ageing ear becomes incapable of reacting to higher sound frequencies, the perceived quality of sound also changes. As increase in loudness cannot compensate for missing sounds, hearing aids may be of limited use. With progressive inability to hear various speech sounds, the total speech flow becomes less intelligible. Lip-reading (or speech reading) may be the only practical form of help available but if hearing loss is accompanied by impaired vision then lip-reading will have limited value.

It is easy to understand why acquired hearing loss is often strongly associated with feelings of depression and isolation. It is hard to feel 'part of things' when you cannot hear well or understand.

Coping with hearing problems

Many people feel that the answer to deafness is to provide a hearing aid. However, it is clear that a hearing aid is not the ultimate answer for every elderly person who is hard of hearing. When there is high frequency hearing loss the aid will do very little to help discrimination of sounds—it merely amplifies sound. It is important for nurses to remember that hearing aids amplify all sounds in the vicinity, not just speech. Many patients cannot and should not tolerate their aids being switched on permanently.

Elderly patients often seem to have difficulties with their aids. Practical difficulties can arise as a result of the patient's poor vision, when they are unable to set the aid appropriately or insert it correctly. Poor memory can result in the patient forgetting which ear takes the aid, forgetting to turn it off or on as appropriate, forgetting to change the battery, forgetting the right settings and getting the old and new batteries mixed up. Deficiencies in manual dexterity, caused, for example, by arthritis, can result in difficulty in manipulating and inserting the aid and in changing the batteries. As a consequence the elderly deaf may require a good deal of sensitive and practical assistance from the nurses who care for them. These issues are discussed in greater detail by Katia Gilhome Herbst in Chapter 5.

As hearing loss does affect the majority of elderly patients, all nurses looking after old people should routinely assess their patients' hearing and plan care to facilitate communication. There are many practical steps that can be taken to recognise the extent of deafness and these include:

— Observation of the patient's behaviour with nurses, with other patients and with visitors
— Observation of the patient's response to noises, particularly loud noises, in the environment.
— Observation of the patient when in conversation with you:
  Does the patient appear withdrawn?
  Does the patient seem inattentive?
  Does the patient appear to respond with inappropriate irritation or anger when spoken to?
  How does the patient respond to your touching her?
  Does the patient move in response to your change of position?
  Does she have difficulty in following instructions?
  Does she ask for things to be repeated

or say 'What?' 'Pardon?', etc. frequently? Does she tend to turn one ear towards you?
  Is her voice monotonous, unusually loud or soft?
— If the answer to any of the above questions is Yes, then it is likely that your patient has some degree of hearing impairment. Having established this, it is necessary to make sure that any hearing aid is working, worn and switched on. In the absence of a suitable aid, arrangements should be made for a hearing assessment to be done.

If the patient is deaf, the extent of the deafness should be documented clearly in the Kardex and in the care plan. If a hearing aid is available, this should also be documented. It is essential that everyone involved with the patient knows that he or she is hard of hearing.

Whatever the extent of deafness, all communication with the patient must be carefully planned. Various strategies to improve communication are suggested in Chapter 5, such as always sitting or standing where the patient can see you and your lips, and making sure the patient has his or her glasses on before you speak. Other important points to remember are:

— Try to avoid distracting extra noises by going to a quiet room or corner.
— Turn off the television or radio before speaking.
— Ensure the hearing aid, if it exists, is switched on and working.
— Write important messages clearly on a piece of paper.
— Repeat your message if you do not think you have been understood.
— Give your patient time to think about what you say and respond to it.
— Ask simple, clear questions.
— Use short sentences.

Problems caused by sensory deprivation

Many elderly people lead isolated and lonely lives, with 45% of women and 17% of men living alone (Office of Population Censuses and Surveys 1982). Some elderly people live in circumstances which could be described as seriously deprived, in the sense that their environment is restricted to a level of dull monotony. The combination of environmental monotony and reduced sensory acuity can result in the elderly being assessed inappropriately as confused or demented.

It has been demonstrated that sensory deprivation tends to exaggerate existing personality traits and can distort perceptions of shape, size, colour and time (Vernon et al 1961). Emotional changes can also occur such as increased boredom, restlessness, irritability, anxiety and panic (Soloman 1961). In extreme circumstances marked behaviour changes can take place, such as hallucinations, delusions, and confusion of sleeping and waking states. Hebb (1949) demonstrated that monotony produces a disruption of the capacity to learn and the ability to think and in the absence of adequate stimulation the brain functions less efficiently.

Once the problem of sensory deprivation has been recognised it is often possible to produce a good response by increasing stimulation in the environment. However, stimulation should be introduced gradually as rapid increases can result in emotional outbursts (Lambert and Lambert 1979) and an apparently negative reaction to attempts to make life more interesting. It is important for nurses to be aware of this reaction and assess each patient's needs for stimulation individually and to pace the introduction of stimulation accordingly. It has been found that sensorily deprived patients respond best initially to gentle and consistent stimulation such as touching, stroking and being talked to quietly (Wolanin and Phillips 1981).

For the institutionalised, privacy and space can become inaccessible luxuries. Roberts (1973) suggests that old people work hard to maintain a sense of personal space using strategies such as accumulating clutter, props or significant personal items and possessiveness. Nurses can respect and facilitate this need in

a number of ways. These include moving slowly into private space or private thought, encouraging the collection of personal items, avoiding transferring the patient to another bed or room, unless requested and not moving any personal items without permission.

Problems of disorientation and confusion

> If a man does not keep pace with his companions perhaps it is because he hears a different drummer. Let him step to the music which he hears, however measured or far away (Thoreau 1845, p 285).

Confusion occurs when present reality is distorted but the term is easily misplaced when applied to patients. It can often be the nurse who is confused. When patients are confused it is important to identify the source of confusion.

Distortion of time perception

Keeping track of time requires an individual's attention and interest and these are easily diverted by physiological factors or psychological stress. This disordered time perception is often the first aspect of disorientation to be manifest with patients being unclear about 'real' time. Being unclear about time puts the individual out of step with the rest of the world. Reality orientation in this case can be attempted by developing a regular daily routine and providing cues in the form of clocks, cards, calendars and name boards (Conroy 1977).

Distortion of place perception

This type of perceptual disorientation usually occurs following a physical change of environment such as moving from one house to another, or from a house to a nursing home or even from one room to another room. Patients who are disoriented in this way will often try to fit events or characteristics of the new location to their old way of life.

Often there is confusion about time and

place and when this happens elderly people can slip into the familiarity and security of the distant past: 'My mother is cooking dinner.' It can be very frustrating and distressing when patients persistently claim they are in a different place or call for someone who is not there (as often as not, someone who is dead). Arguing with the patient does not work and it is important to try to increase orientation. This can be attempted in the following way:

1. Assess the patient's needs for stimulation, remembering that too much may cause stress and too little facilitates the delusion.
2. Make frequent visits to the patient, introducing yourself each time and explain what you want to do.
3. Try to find objects that provide comfort and security such as pictures, photographs.
4. Use cards or labels to identify important items such as clothes, spectacles, etc.

Old age brings an inevitable decrease in physical mobility and the resulting immobility can also have an effect on mental alertness. Petrov and Vlahlijska (1972) found that groups of elderly residents in nursing Homes were able to think and verbalise more clearly and coherently after taking part in exercise groups. This may be a strategy which could be used effectively in other settings to increase the effectiveness of reality orientation programmes.

Problems caused by speech impairment

Speech can be impaired in elderly people for a variety of reasons. Sometimes the impairment is a result of serious pathology, but there are a number of simple and practical interventions that can improve speech.

Unclear speech can be related to severe hearing loss, and if this deafness has been previously unrecognised then improving hearing will also improve speech. Another common cause of speech difficulty in the elderly is that of ill-fitting or absent dentures. Speech is inevitably more difficult in the absence of teeth, and dentures which do not fit adequately can cause a variety of speech peculiarities. One old lady was quite imposs-ible to understand until it discovered that she had to keep her tongue on the roof of her mouth all the time she was speaking in order to keep her top denture in place.

Another common cause of speech problems in the elderly is confusion, or disorientation. This can be exacerbated by distraction and noise in the environment, especially from televisions and radios. Such distractions make it impossible for the confused elderly to concentrate and their speech may become disjointed and inappropriate. Those for whom English is not their first language have added difficulties. There is a tendency for the elderly to revert to their native language, certainly in terms of their thoughts (Cumming and Henry 1961) and this can make verbal communication more problematic.

One of the most difficult problems is that related to the inherent isolation and social withdrawal of many old people. They quite simply get out of the habit of talking and communicating and it can take some time for them to become used to a more public existence. It has been suggested that those who have spent many years alone may also have forgotten the 'rules' of social interaction, especially in terms of when to speak and what to speak about (Panicucci et al 1968).

Speech problems can also occur as a result of pathology or disease such as cerebral atrophy, atheroma, Parkinsonism or stroke. Patients who have suffered from a stroke can present a special challenge in terms of coping with overcoming the communication problems that occur.

Communication difficulties caused by stroke

The incidence of stroke, or cerebrovascular accident, rises steadily with age affecting approximately three persons in every 1000 of those aged under 65 years, eight persons in every 1000 of those aged between 65 and 74 years, and 25 persons in every 1000 of those aged over 75 years. The sexes appear to be equally affected (Harris et al 1971).

For most of the many thousands of elderly

patients who suffer a stroke, communication becomes a major problem. It has been estimated that over two thirds of those suffering from a right-sided hemiplegia will have a significant degree of speech impairment. A similar proportion of those suffering from a left-sided hemiplegia will suffer from more obscure but equally distressing communication difficulties. As Smith (1967) says: 'Loss of control over one side of the body is a disaster, loss of the ability to communicate is a catastrophe.'

Difficulty with communication can be aggravated by a variety of factors such as sensory or perceptual decrements, intellectual changes, impaired memory span, reduced ability to concentrate, fatigue, emotional lability and apathy. For the stroke patient and his or her family, an overwhelming concern is whether the stroke victim will be able to communicate again (Jenning 1981).

Stroke patients depend upon nurses in the immediate post-stroke period for all aspects of care and support (Christo 1978). The potential role that nurses have for helping and encouraging these patients to cope with their communication difficulties cannot be overestimated. The pathology underlying speech and communication difficulties after strokes is complex. The terminology used is confusing and the explanations for different types of disability is still a matter of some debate (Licht 1975). However, the communication problems that a stroke patient has to cope with are determined by the size and site of the cerebrovascular accident, and the side on which weakness is manifested.

Right-sided hemiplegia

A lesion occurring in the left hemisphere of the brain may result in a right-sided hemiplegia and, very commonly, a degree of speech loss or impairment. The terms most frequently used to describe this impairment are as follows:

1. Dysarthria. This term is used to describe disorders of articulation where the mechanisms which produce sounds and speech are faulty. Dysarthria is thus a speech impairment resulting from a disruption of the neuromuscular control of speech. The degree of dysarthria can range from slight slurring of the speech to total inability to articulate any sounds.

2. Aphasia. Strictly interpreted this term means complete absence of speech but it is frequently used instead of the term dysphasia.

3. Dysphasia. This term encompasses any degree of impaired or partial loss of speech ability. As most people have left hemisphere dominance, strokes in the left side of the brain are most likely to produce dysphasia. It is believed that lesions in different parts of the cortex disturb speech in certain ways. The most common classification is that of:

(a) Broca's aphasia (motor or expressive dysphasia). Broca's area lies close to the motor cortex and a lesion in this area is said to result in an inability to translate speech concepts into meaningful articulated sounds. Speech is often limited initially to one or two words and the patient may say the opposite to what is meant. Emotional expressions or expletives may be unaffected. If the lesion is restricted completely to Broca's area then comprehension is said to be unimpaired.

(b) Wernicke's aphasia (sensory or receptive dysphasia). Wernicke's area lies in the auditory cortex (the left superior temporal gyrus) and lesions in this region are said to impair the comprehension of speech, so that the meaning of words received in the auditory cortex is not understood. If such lesions are localised then the production of speech is unimpaired and that patient will produce speech which is fluent and rhythmic but the content is abnormal. This is because the patient is unaware of the words being used and in severe cases may only produce a stream of meaningless words.

(c) Global aphasia or global dysphasia. This label is given to speech disorders where there appear to be deficits in terms of expression and reception of words. This situation is thought to occur when there is an extensive lesion in the patient's dominant cerebral hemisphere involving both frontal and temporal lobes.

It has been suggested that most patients suffering from dysphasia have expressive and receptive deficits (Karis and Harenstein 1976) and there is a continuing controversy about the theory of localised lesions (Gonzalez 1977). This controversy highlights the importance of assessing each individual patient's speech impairment or difficulty. In summary, the patient who has suffered a left hemisphere stroke and whose speech has been affected is likely to have some or all of the following problems: poor speech, impaired word recognition, impaired word retention and recall, difficulties in articulation, impaired comprehension. Although speech is poor and may initially be absent, it is probable that overall intellectual activity and mentation are generally quite good.

Left-sided hemiplegia

A lesion occurring in the right hemisphere of the brain may result in a left-sided hemiplegia with no obvious speech loss or impairment. However, this does not mean that the stroke patient with a left-sided paralysis will not have any problems with communication. Paradoxically, these patients are often able to express themselves well and no intellectual damage is apparent. In reality the disruption to their sensori-motor, conceptual and spatial abilities can be very severe and cause more difficulties in communication and rehabilitation than the lack of speech.

Patients with a left-sided paralysis can suffer from a disturbance in body image, spatial judgment, time judgment, impaired drawing and writing and mathematical ability, and an inability to understand the written word. All these problems inhibit communication and such patients are often labelled as 'difficult', particularly as they seem to be unaware of the mistakes that they have made.

It is clear that in order to help their patients who have suffered a stroke, wherever the lesion is sited, nurses must develop the skills and strategies which will encourage and facilitate communication.

Physical rehabilitation is a crucial part of eventual recovery in terms of communication. Efforts to encourage the patient to chew and swallow food efficiently will result in an increased ability to articulate sounds and words.

Patients must be encouraged to utilise all auditory, visual, tactile and emotional inputs. Some language problems are common to most dysphasic patients and these problems include a very limited vocabulary (maybe restricted to emotional speech only), reduced verbal memory span, grammatical and semantic confusions, varying degrees of ability to understand written as well as spoken words and, of course, varying degrees of difficulty in writing.

Guidelines for communicating with stroke patients

— Ensure that you have obtained the patient's attention before speaking.
— Ensure that the patient can see and hear you.
— Tell the patient you are trying to help her to speak.
— Speak directly to the patient, talking clearly and slowly but with normal intonation and phrasing.
— Use simple sentence structure, incorporating one idea at a time.
— Commands can be given in single words, e.g. watch, listen, wait, swallow.
— Repeat key words, rephrase if necessary.
— Do not shout.
— Label important items, e.g. cup, glass, spectacles.
— Ask simple closed questions so that the patient can answer with one word, e.g. 'Would you like tea or coffee?'
— If the patient cannot answer Yes or No, try to devise a gesture or sign language for these words, e.g. thumbs up for Yes and thumbs down for No.

— Do not push your patient too hard; learn to pick up signs of distress such as perseveration (meaningless repetition of a word or act), loss of concentration, eye blinking, irritability and sweating.

— Do not underestimate the patient's comprehension or potential capacity to communicate.

— Avoid distractions, especially noise.

— Give enough time for the patient to respond.

— Find out what interests the patient (from relatives or visitors if necessary) and talk about these things.

— Promote 'ritual' communication. Familiar phrases reduce stress and improve performance.

— Involve relatives and friends in all stages of care and teach them to help the patient communicate.

— Use alternative methods of communication such as communication boards, written instructions, picture cards, etc. Encourage patients to use the unaffected hand for writing or drawing.

People who have recovered from a stroke are very consistent in their descriptions of the problems and frustrations they suffered. Nearly all these problems focus upon aspects of communication. Skelly (1975) found that the most common complaints from 50 stroke patients were as follows:

— Their ability to comprehend what was said was reached sooner than those caring for them realised.

— Input was too fast and too dense with nurses and doctors speaking too quickly and with too much complexity.

— Not enough time was given for patients to try to reply to questions, etc.

— Noise level was generally too high and made the patients feel irritable.

— They felt there were too many people to interact with.

— They were not told what was happening and speech difficulties were not discussed with them by nurses or doctors, only by speech therapists if and when they saw one.

This list of complaints emphasises the importance of communication with all patients who have speech problems or indeed any difficulty in communicating with others. The responsibility for initiating appropriate care and encouraging and maximising communication with such patients lies squarely with the nurse. It is nurses who spend most time with patients and who are in a position to give the most consistent help and support.

It has been demonstrated that early encouragement with communication results in better levels of speech recovery after stroke (Leutenegger 1975), and it is essential that encouragement with communication is seen as an active part of the nursing care plan in the immediate post-stroke period. Once a clear plan or strategy has been designed then all those involved with care can provide consistent and regular support and teaching. Where patients have concerned relatives or friends they should be included in all activities which encourage the redevelopment of communication ability.

Aronson (1983) has demonstrated that speech and language therapy in the immediate post-stroke period produces significant improvements in speech rehabilitation. The speech therapist obviously has an important role to play in the rehabilitation of speech-impaired stroke patients. However, the service provided in most National Health Service hospitals is limited and often does not continue after discharge from hospital (Bailey 1983). It is therefore the nurse who must act as the co-ordinator of this aspect of care for stroke patients.

CONCLUSION

This chapter has covered a range of issues which can result in problems of communication for the elderly. Impairment in the ability to communicate can be viewed as possibly the greatest burden of all for old people. Diminution of visual and auditory acuity will limit the reception of both spoken and written information. Changes in the tongue, jaw and lip movements combined with cerebral degeneration or disease will impair expressive function. Such changes will reduce elderly people's ability to express needs and emotions and to understand the world about them. This will inevitably lead to problems of social adjustment, which in turn can lead to withdrawal and isolation. The nurse's role is paramount in assessing the extent of any impairment and in planning care so as to minimise isolation and withdrawal and maximise the patient's ability to communicate.

REFERENCES

Aronson A 1983 Aphasia therapy on trial. Proceedings of First European Conference on Research in Rehabilitation. Edinburgh
Bailey S 1983 The response of general practitioners to the problems and rehabilitation of stroke patients with communication handicaps. Proceedings of First European Conference on Research in Rehabilitation. Edinburgh
Burnside I (ed) 1973 Psychosocial nursing care of the aged. McGraw-Hill, New York
Christo S 1978 Nursing approach to adult aphasia. Canadian Nurse 74(7): 34–39
Conroy C 1977 Reality orientation: a basic technique for patients suffering from memory loss and confusion. British Journal of Occupational Therapy 40(10): 250–251
Cumming E, Henry W 1961 Growing old. Basic Books, New York
Gilhome Herbst K R, Humphrey C H 1981 Prevalence of hearing impairment in the elderly living at home. Journal of Royal College of General Practitioners 31: 155–160
Gonzalez D E 1977 Receptive-expressive aphasia. Does it really exist? Journal of Neurosurgical Nursing 9(3): 122–3
Hardiman C, Holbrook A, Hedrick D 1979 Non-verbal communication systems for the severely handicapped geriatric patient. Gerontologist 19(1): 96–101
Harris A, Cox E, Smith C 1971 The handicapped and impaired in Great Britain. Part 1. Office of Population Censuses and Surveys. HMSO, London

Hebb P O 1949 The organisation of behaviour. Wiley, New York
Jenning S 1981 Back to basics. Communicating with your aphasic patients. Journal of Practical Nursing 31: 22–23
Karis B, Harenstein K 1976 Localisation of speech parameters by brain scan. Neurology 26: 226–230
Lambert V, Lambert C 1979 The impact of physical illness and related mental health concepts. Prentice Hall, Englewood Cliffs, N.J.
Leutenegger R 1975 Patient care and rehabilitation of communication impaired adults. Charles C Thomas, Springfield, Illinois
Licht S 1975 Stroke and its rehabilitation. E, Licht Waverly Press, Baltimore
Macleod Clark J 1981 Nurse patient communication. Nursing Times 77(1): 12–18
Norton D, McLaren R, Exton-Smith A N 1975 An investigation of geriatric nursing problems. (Reprint.) Churchill-Livingstone, Edinburgh.
Office of Population Censuses and Surveys 1982 General household survey for 1980. HMSO, London
Paniccuci C, Paul B, Symonds J, Tambellini J 1968 Expanded speech and self-pacing in communication with the aged. ANA clinical sessions. Century Croft, New York
Petrov I, Vlahlijska L 1972 Cultural therapy in old people's homes. Gerontologist 12:429
Roberts S 1972 Territoriality: space and the aged patient in intensive care units. In: Burnside I (Ed.) Psychosocial nursing care of the aged. McGraw-Hill, New York
Skelly M 1975 Aphasic patients talk back. American Journal of Nursing 77(7): 1140–1144
Smith G W 1967 Care of the patient with a stroke. A handbook for the patient's family and nurse. Springer, New York
Solomon P et al 1961 (ed) Sensory deprivation. Harvard University Press, Cambridge, Mass
Stockwell F 1972 The unpopular patient. Royal College of Nursing, London
Thoreau H 1845 From Walden XVIII. Conclusion. (Reprinted 1946.) Dodmead, New York
Travis L E (ed) 1971 Handbook of speech pathology and audiology. Appleton, New York
Vernon J et al 1961 The effect of human isolation on some perceptual and motor skills. In: Soloman P et al (eds) Sensory deprivation. Harvard University Press, Cambridge, Mass
Wells T 1980 Problems in geriatric nursing care. Churchill-Livingstone, Edinburgh
Wolanin M, Phillips L 1981 Confusion: prevention and care. Mosby, St Louis

K. Gilhome Herbst

5

Hearing

THE STIGMA OF DEAFNESS

One of the great tragedies of deafness is that it is traditionally accepted as a suitable subject for music-hall jokes and is therefore not taken seriously. Indeed, when in 1953 Barker and his colleagues published their now famous study on jokes about handicap, deafness was reported as being the third most joked about physical defect. It came third after 'having an unattractive face' and 'fatness' (Barker et al 1953). Note, for example, that much of the humour of 'Steptoe and Son' on television was derived from Steptoe's deafness.

In addition, deafness is generally accepted as a hoax disorder. It is often understood to be aggressive behaviour, with overtones of deliberate withholding of communication ('Old Mrs So-and-So seems to hear only when, and what, she wants to'). Hence that well-known saying, 'None so deaf as those who will not hear.' The implication is that the deaf could manage if only they pulled up their socks. No parallel proverb exists which accuses the blind of peeping when they particularly want to see. Furthermore, it would be considered very poor taste to laugh at a blind woman because she bumped into things. But not so with deafness.

What is it that is so special about deafness? Why are attitudes to deafness so negative?

It is important to consider this quite seriously since nurses, doctors and their elderly patients are all members of our society and, to that extent, will tend to hold prevailing attitudes to the disorder. Recent research by the author and colleagues has indicated that negative attitudes to deafness, coupled with a very hazy idea of the true psychosocial implications of the disorder, inhibit demand for deafness-specific services by the elderly deaf themselves and inhibit referral to other services by the general practitioner or nurse (Humphrey et al 1981, Gilhome Herbst 1982a).

There are many factors which contribute to prevailing negative attitudes to deafness. These are too varied and wide ranging to be discussed thoroughly here, but have recently been the subject of a review paper by the author (Gilhome Herbst 1982b).

The fundamental problem with deafness, which puzzled the ancient Greeks (Aristotle, *History of Animals* BK IV, No. 9) and still puzzles the general public today (Bunting 1981), is that it is very difficult to distinguish between the symptoms of deafness and those of some types of mental disorders (particularly defects of reason). These symptoms—indistinct speech, not answering when spoken to, answering inappropriately or out of context, pitching the voice incorrectly—often encourage people to talk to and treat the hearing impaired as if their cognitive abilities were also impaired. Regrettably, deafness has in consequence, become a disorder to be ashamed of: 'I felt as if I were living in a twilight world. Deafness seemed a badge of shame.' (Jack Ashley, MP, 1973).

The second problem is that one cannot see deafness. It has to be volunteered by the handicapped person if it is to be known. It can be, and more frequently than not is, hidden. Hiding one's deafness is undoubtedly detrimental for both the hearing impaired person and those with whom she wishes to communicate. The normally hearing person may not realise what the cause of the communication problem is and jump to his or her own conclusions. At the same time (s)he will, in all probability, feel ill at ease, frustrated, finally resigned and even embarrassed. Unfortunately, we tend to laugh at things that embarrass us.

Our work has shown that such responses are well perceived by the deaf of all ages, but particularly by the elderly who are most sensitive to being considered 'senile' (Gilhome Herbst 1983). It is the embarrassment and the sense of shame and stigma that prevent people from announcing what the problem is. Such feelings apparently affect people from all walks of life. Beethoven suffered terribly: 'Yet I could not bring myself to say to people, "Speak up; shout, for I am deaf". . . . Oh, I cannot do it' (Beethoven 1802).

The third crucial reason for the general dislike of deafness is undoubtedly its popularly accepted, and well-founded, association with ageing. Intuitively we all 'know' that many elderly people are deaf. This knowledge has been used by playwrights and novelists throughout the centuries when depicting old age. It is much more strongly associated with ageing than is poor sight. Regrettably, it is often used in an allegorical sense to represent a breakdown in meaningful communication with the world.

Thus people will often resist any acceptance that they might be deaf for as long as possible—in part because they do not wish to be seen to be suffering from an age-related disorder and in part because they do not wish to be mistaken as being of unsound mind.

Thus we have a disability which is stigmatised in its own right and associated very closely with two other 'conditions' which are equally stigmatised, mental disorder and old age. Indeed, in our ageist society, it could be argued that much of the dislike of deafness is derived from its very synonymity with old age and its attendant frailties. To admit to deafness is tantamount to admitting to being old and of unsound mind, although the common belief that deafness is associated with confusion and dementia is not supported if the effect of age is eliminated (Gilhome Herbst and Humphrey 1980). It is this stereotypical fusion between deafness and old age that is probably the root cause of the neglect in reporting and treating the disorder.

Being deaf does make elderly people feel differently about themselves. They say that deafness makes them 'feel closed in', 'feel inferior', 'get frustrated or depressed', 'tend to evade other people'. These sentiments express the feeling of personal degradation associated with being deaf (Gilhome Herbst 1983).

Yet another problem is the patchy auditory performance so typical of acquired deafness (particularly in the elderly) whereby, apparently for no reason, conversations, words, names in particular, are clearly understood. This, of course, fuels the none-so-deaf-as-those-who-will-not-hear school of thought. Interestingly enough, the very (apparently freak) conditions in which improved hearing occurs in this way are those which those who live and work with the elderly should foster.

PREVALENCE OF DEAFNESS

Denial of deafness by young and old alike has been noted since early times by psychologists and researchers (Menninger 1924, Wilkins 1948, Gregory 1961, Townsend and Wedderburn 1965). It has generally been assumed that the stigma of being deaf was the prime factor behind this denial. It is a major force to contend with and one that has been ill-understood. For doctors and nurses who are responsible for setting in motion rehabilitation and care of deafness of the elderly, probably the central problem will be to detect the deafness in the first place. Some discussion now of the probable prevalence of deafness in old age, and how estimates of the prevalence have been arrived at, will expose the scale, and importance, of the problem of denial.

Estimates of hearing loss of the elderly have traditionally been undertaken in order to establish the probable numbers of elderly people likely to require hearing aids under the National Health Service. Thus we are talking about a level of bilateral impairment that would, by convention, be deemed to require amplification from a hearing aid.

Community studies of the elderly which have included questions concerning hearing loss are numerous. A review of 15 such studies by the author confirmed the conventionally held belief that between 30% and 40% of all persons of retirement age are hearing impaired to the extent that they would benefit from amplification (Gilhome Herbst and Humphrey 1981, Gilhome Herbst 1983). All these studies assess the presence of hearing loss either by asking the elderly person some question associated with their hearing (Sheldon 1948, Harris 1962, Kay et al 1964, Brockington and Lempert 1966, Abrams 1978) or by the assessment of the clinician or interviewer (Stockport County Council, 1958, Williamson et al 1964; Sheard 1971, Cumbria County Council 1973).

These estimates, whilst accepted as being of questionable validity (Rawson 1973, Haggard et al 1981), are nonetheless still used by the Department of Health and Social Security when considering rehabilitation services for the hearing impaired (DHSS 1977).

A wide-ranging and thorough review of the literature reveals no estimates of prevalence of deafness of the elderly based upon thorough audiometric assessments of the elderly until the work of the present author (Gilhome Herbst and Humphrey 1981). In her study (inter alia), the prevalence of hearing impairment in a community sample of the elderly aged 70 years and over was assessed using pure-tone audiometry. 'Deafness' was defined as an average loss over the speech frequencies at 1 kHz, 2 kHz and 4 kHz of 35 dB* or more in the better ear. The proportion found to be 'deaf' was 60%. A statistically significant association between increasing age and the incidence and severity of deafness was also found (Gilhome Herbst and Humphrey 1981):

Such that of all those aged		
70 yrs+	60%	were deaf
75 yrs+	69%	were deaf

* Sound frequency, or pitch, is expressed in numbers of vibrations (cycles) per second. By convention these vibrations (cycles) are called Hertz. kHz means thousands of cycles of sound per second. Output of sound is measured in decibels (dB). By convention, hearing loss is measured in terms of the output (dB) necessary for sounds at certain pitches (kHz) to be heard.

80 yrs+   82% were deaf
85 yrs+   84% were deaf

In addition, a further 14% of the sample were found to have a unilateral loss of 35 dB or more. Under auroscopic examination, wax in both ears was observed in 25% of the sample. The presence of wax was not significantly related to deafness.

The findings of that study challenge conventionally held assumptions about the prevalence of hearing impairment in old age, which until very recently have resulted in the scale of the disorder being considerably underestimated, in both professional and official thinking. Preliminary results from the National Study on Hearing confirm these findings (Haggard et al 1981). It is of particular interest to the present discussion on the problems of detecting deafness to note that, in that same study, the conventional kind of question 'Do you think you are at all deaf?' (as used in all other studies which attempted to estimate the prevalence of deafness by questionnaire techniques) yielded similar results (Gilhome Herbst and Humphrey 1981). This is displayed on Table 5.1 The discrepancy in the results is important. It shows the discrepancy between 'true' impairment and the number of elderly persons who either do not notice that they have any problems or who wished to hide it. Whilst to some extent this discrepancy may be due to genuine ignorance of the fact, it is likely that deliberate denial of the problem was present. Those studies which provide results of the prevalence of deafness based upon the clinician's or researchers' assessments provide results which are equally at odds with those based upon audiometric findings as are those based on self-estimate.

Table 5.1 Estimates of prevalence of deafness in an elderly person (N = 253)

	Age in years			
	70+	75+	80+	85+
Based on self-estimate	38%	39%	54%	69%
Based on pure-tone audiometry	60%	69%	82%	84%

It is very difficult for the general practitioner, nurse and caring others to recognise the disorder when it is not volunteered by the patient. This is firstly because the very high prevalence of deafness amongst the elderly renders it almost synonymous with old age, and secondly because its major effects—namely impoverished communication and a subsequent tendency to withdraw from social intercourse—may too readily be mistaken for so-called 'normal ageing'.

In our study, of those elderly people found to be significantly bilaterally hearing impaired, 26% refused to accept any suggestion that they might be hearing impaired despite the evidence of their audiograms. The mean dB loss of this group was 43.9 dB in the better ear. A further 25% admitted to the interviewer that they knew that they had a hearing loss but had never mentioned this to their doctor. The mean dB loss of this group was 51.9 dB in the better ear. Thus over half the deaf elderly population under investigation had never mentioned their deafness to their general practitioner (Humphrey et al 1981). Yet, as a group, they were substantially impaired. This gives some indication of the size of the problem facing doctors and nurses.

DEAFNESS AND SOCIAL THEORIES OF AGEING

An awareness of the synonymity of deafness and ageing can provide some useful insight into social theories of ageing, particularly Cumming and Henry's disengagement theory (Cumming and Henry 1961). This theory strives to explain the observed phenomenon of social withdrawal which may often accompany advancing years. It suggests that ageing people naturally and voluntarily withdraw from too great involvement with others, thus also diminishing their emotional investment in personal relationships. It also suggests that the elderly are generally satisfied with comparatively casual, surface social contacts and proposes that this diminution in social involvement is convenient for the young—society being content to release its elderly from the normal demands of responsibility and accountability. The emphasis is on this being a 'natural' and 'mutual' process and one to be condoned and promulgated. Such a theory seems to draw directly, if unwittingly, on the effects of deafness as a communication interrupter. Deafness supports, or at least explains, the observed phenomenon of mutual release, or should one say breakdown, in communication between young and old. Consequently, from a disengagement perspective, deafness can be seen as a normal and natural part of ageing which may not therefore demand attention.

The opposing view, sometimes known as the activity or continuity approach to explaining the observed social changes that accompany old age, is that the diminishing world of the older person is largely societally constructed and reinforced. It suggests that in fact people continue throughout their lifespan with very much the same social and emotional requirements (e.g. Abrams 1979) and that it is therefore fallacy that older people are content with less because they are old and physically less robust.

Thus the very recent interest in the social implications of deafness in ageing goes hand in hand with the widespread rejection of disengagement. Indeed there is a general antagonism to the acceptance of any of the disorders of ageing as unalterable and inexorable. Deafness must now be seen as another physical disorder requiring treatment and care for which our understanding of the social and psychological implications of the disorder is a necessary prerequisite.

ASSESSMENT OF HEARING LOSS

One certainty results from our research—when a person complains of hearing loss they are very likely to be correct in their assessment and should be encouraged, before time is lost, to make use of appropriate services. In our study, such people were substantially bilaterally impaired with average loss of between 56.3

and 69.5 dB in the better ear (Humphrey et al 1981).

Certain very simple strategies may help to disclose poor hearing amongst those who do not volunteer it (though severity of loss is difficult to judge). The two best are speaking in a normal voice to the patient with the back turned and simultaneously, or in addition, asking unexpected questions or questions that may be slightly out of context. These are rough and ready techniques and no more to be firmly relied upon than are the simple techniques used by health visitors when testing infants. Our own work has shown that with care and regular calibration of the audiometer, simple pure-tone audiometry can successfully and accurately be carried out in a non-clinical setting by suitably trained staff.

REHABILITATION

Improving communication

The following conditions and strategies will improve communication with an elderly person who is hearing impaired:
— Ensure that light is on the face (of the speaker) so that the whole face, and in particular the lips, are clearly seen.
— Improve visual acuity, by encouraging the elderly person to wear her spectacles—it will help her to lip-read and in consequence to understand speech better.
— Ensure that the face of the speaker is not obscured (by hands) or distorted (by eating or smoking).
— Ensure that the elderly person is concentrating on what is to be said and is not doing something else which may distract her.
— Talk clearly, and enunciate clearly. If the voice is raised, be sure not to shout as this both distorts the mouth and face (which can be interpreted as aggressive behaviour).
— Shouting can cause pain. It is characteristic of sensorineural deafness (which is the kind of deafness most frequently associated with ageing) that the transition from hearing little or nothing, to hearing sounds

very loudly (called recruitment) is abnormally abrupt. Pain is caused by over-boosting those frequencies which are not impaired.
— Use familiar words and phrases. This reduced guess-work.
— Use words in context—single words repeated again and again with no clues offered will be more difficult to 'hear'.
— Talk slowly.
— Talk with kindness and sympathy. The tone of the voice will be understood even if the word is not (remember that children understand tone well before they understand language. Even animals understand tone).
— All people perform best in an atmosphere of sympathy. It is crucial to reduce stress on both the part of the hearing impaired and the normally hearing. When difficulties arise, try and laugh.

Wearing a hearing aid

Researchers have found that the earlier a person is referred for a hearing aid the more likely they are to learn to benefit from and continue using their aid (Pedersen et al 1974) well into advanced age (Gilhome Herbst 1983). Those elderly who do have aids (who represent a minority of the elderly deaf) have been found to use their aids about as frequently as do people of employment age (Humphrey et al 1981). Poor hearing aid usage is not specific to the elderly, though their reasons for poor usage may be different from younger people. It is, rather, a sad reflection on the state of hearing aid services in this country and the complex nature of sensori-neural deafness.

It is unfortunate that sensorineural deafness, which characterises hearing impairment in old age, is progressive, associated with recruitment and tinnitus and lends itself but grudgingly to amelioration with the use of a hearing aid. Nonetheless, for a substantial number of persons, even the elderly, some benefit is to be derived from wearing an aid and it should be tried. Furthermore, access to

other services—from volunteers, the hearing therapist and even the social worker for the deaf—is often to be found through referral from the hearing aid clinic. Domiciliary visits from the hearing aid clinic are available and crucial for the very old and frail amongst whom deafness is most prevalent.

It seems probable that nurses and general practitioners take a rather similar view to that of the elderly, and indeed society at large, about the inevitability of deafness in old age and the futility of attempting much in the way of rehabilitation. Ironically, to some extent they are being realistic in doubting the value of the rehabilitative service for the elderly in the present circumstances. The problem is circular so long as, for the reasons discussed above, the elderly tend either to defer demand for aids indefinitely or at least postpone it for as long as possible, the majority who do come forward are liable to be very old, very frail and almost 'stone deaf' (Brooks 1979, Ward et al 1979). It has been suggested (Alberti 1977) that attempting to initiate aural rehabilitation with such subjects is largely a waste of time. Rumour of the failure of rehabilitative measures when undertaken with the very deaf and very old may well contribute one further reason for the elderly deaf not to bother to come forward in time to benefit from rehabilitation. It certainly lowers morale within the hearing aid service. A strong case is therefore made for the encouragement of early intervention and an improvement in the service available.

Indeed, the NHS hearing aid service has improved dramatically since the behind-the-ear (BE) programme (BE10 series) was introduced in 1974 with the BE11 model (Fig. 5.1). By 1981, there were four more aids in the BE10 series: the BE12, BE13, BE14 and BE15. The Be13 has a forward-facing microphone. Otherwise there is little difference in performance between the aids. The main reason for such a choice of aids in this series is the purchasing policy of the DHSS, who tries to ensure that it does not depend on a single manufacturer to supply all NHS aids (Johnson 1981).

The BE30 series of high power, high gain

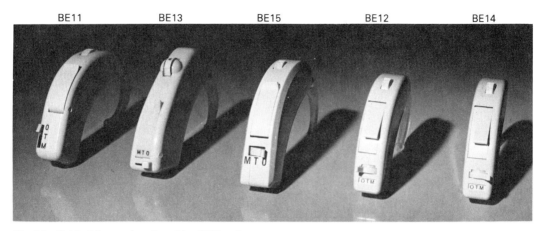

Fig. 5.1 Behind-the-ear hearing aids: BE10 series.

aids is intended for patients who are unable to use the BE10 series because of insufficient output (Fig. 5.2). It is also intended for those persons who can only use the BE10 series when set at maximum output. There are two models in this range—the BE31 and BE32. The BE32 is slightly more powerful and has a forward-facing microphone. Aids in this series have been available since December 1980.

A further series, the BE50 series of aids, was launched in the spring of 1982. These aids are more powerful than the BE30 series (Fig. 5.3).

With the introduction of the BE50 series, the programme of development is seen to be at an end, although thought is being given to still further types of aids with more facilities. This does not exclude the planned updating of obsolescent models, but it does mean that the

Department of Health and Social Security is sufficiently confident that NHS aids will be of a wide enough range to fit all types and degrees of hearing loss now that all restrictions on the supply of commercial aids through the NHS have been lifted. As from 1 July 1980, health authorities have been empowered, at their own discretion, to make arrangements for the supply of commercial models to patients of any age who have exceptional medical need and for whom a standard NHS aid is not satisfactory. As a temporary measure the DHSS made arrangements for private sector hearing aids to be available under the NHS for persons who would

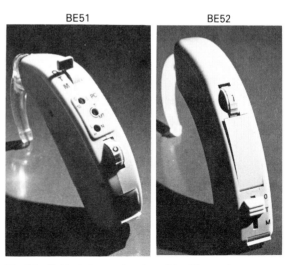

Fig. 5.2 Behind-the-ear hearing aids: BE30 series.

Fig. 5.3 Behind-the-ear hearing aids: BE50 series.

normally be deemed to benefit from the new BE50 series.

The old body-worn Medrescos (OL56, OL58, OL66), which were the only hearing aids available under the NHS until November 1974, are being replaced by new body-worn aids under the BW60 and BW80 series (Fig. 5.4). The range of body-worn aids available under the NHS will be kept up-to-date by introducing new aids when necessary. Both series are intended for patients with very severe hearing losses who need high power and high gain particularly in the lower frequencies. Bone conduction fittings are available with the BW80 series

Ear moulds, batteries, leads and all servicing and repairs to hearing aids have always been and still are offered free of charge under the NHS. Hospital nurses often do not realise that these items can be obtained from the audiometric department and hearing therapist. Acoustic aids (non-electric), the descendants of the old-fashioned ear-trumpet, are particularly useful where patients find it difficult or impossible to handle sophisticated hearing aids. They are available to the hearing impaired on the recommendation of an ear, nose and throat consultant in exactly the same way as are electric hearing aids and are

particularly useful for very fail elderly or disabled persons. They are also particularly valuable for all professionals working with the elderly, and it is wise to keep one on the ward.

There are four types of non-electric aids available: the OL340 telescopic plastic ear-trumpet; the OL370 plastic ear-trumpet (otherwise known as the London horn); the OL301 standard auricle in plastic with an adjustable head-band; the OL38001 conversation tube with a swivel joint ear-piece (Johnson 1981). The ear-trumpet is simply held to the ear by the hearing impaired person. The standard auricle is much like an ear-trumpet, but instead of being hand-held to the ear is mounted on a head-band. It is binaural. The conversation tube fits directly into the ear of the hearing-impaired person—the other end is held to the lips of the speaker, thus enabling high levels of sound to be delivered. A recent review of the acoustic gain which can be obtained from these aids suggests that there is considerable potential for development of these so-called old-fashioned aids (Grover 1977).

Other services available

There may be many circumstances where environmental aids and adaptations to the home are far more, or as, relevant to the elderly. People often will buy them, but if funds are a problem, statutory provisions for the deaf and hard-of-hearing can be made. These are to be found in Section 2 of the Chronically Sick and Disabled Persons (CSDP) Act. Local authorities can provide: alarm bells or light systems to enable hard-of-hearing persons to know when a caller is at the door; special attachments for radio and television so that volume can be raised to an adequate level for the hard-of-hearing without disturbing others;* assistance to travel to club meetings and lip-reading classes and assistance with fees for such classes; assistance in obtaining

BW61   BW81

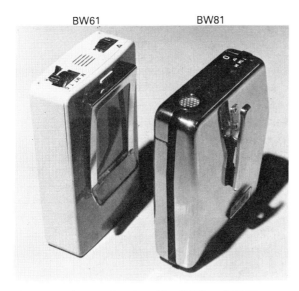

Fig. 5.4 Body-worn hearing aids: BW60 and BW80 series.

* The Royal National Institute for the Deaf (RNID) publishes two special booklets offering advice on the purchase and installation of these aids.

special attachments for the telephone including an amplifier or extra head set where necessary.[†]

Sections 4, 7 and 8 of the CSDP Act require local authorities to wire all public and recreational halls with a loop system for the convenience of hearing aid wearers and to put up signs to show that this service is available.

Nowhere is it specified who should be the responsible officer for ascertaining need for environmental aids. By convention this task has always been performed either by social workers, occupational therapists, or other local authority personnel. Where a hearing therapist is in post at the hearing aid clinic, this task may be carried out by her or him. The actual level of provision of aids for the deaf under Section 2 of the CSDP Act is extremely difficult to ascertain from national returns.

Although hearing aids have been available free under the NHS since its inception, a substantial number of elderly hearing impaired people do not know of this service (for example, as many as a third of a sample of elderly deaf people under study by the author and colleagues were ignorant of the free service (Humphrey et al 1981). Ignorance of the service must inevitably dampen reportage of deafness to the general practitioner. Steps can be taken by doctors to advertise the existence of the service.

Patients (and relatives) should be encouraged to try NHS hearing aids before embarking on the very expensive and often hazardous purchase of hearing aids from the private sector. However, if such action is preferred, the RNID offers a free service to the general public on how to set about buying a hearing aid.

The situation is far worse as regards environmental aids and adaptations. A truly tiny proportion of elderly deaf people know that they exist. General practitioners and district nurses have a central responsibility in this regard to ensure that the social worker for the deaf has been notified of elderly deaf patients—in particular, the most vulnerable deaf, who are those living alone. As has been said, for the very old and those living alone, environmental aids may be far more relevant than the personal hearing aid which must be worn all the time to be of any value for hearing the telephone or the doorbell. Because of the fragmentation of services for the deaf, referral to the hearing aid clinic does not ensure that the social worker for the deaf or responsible officer within the local authority has been notified.

Awareness of the problems deafness causes is slowly gaining public attention. Many shops, offices and banks now display a Sympathetic Hearing Scheme symbol which shows that deaf people can obtain discreet help in these premises. The scheme was set up by four charities for the deaf and they are keen that more shops, offices and places of amusement carry the symbol.[*]

THE CONSEQUENCES OF DEAFNESS

Why does all this matter? After all, deafness is not a matter of life or death. How seriously should it be taken? The evidence from our own research showed a significant association between deafness in old age and depression. This association remained when the effects of age and socioeconomic status were eliminated (Gilhome Herbst and Humphrey 1980). In addition, a significant overall association was found between deafness and low socioeconomic status, advanced age, poor health, reduced out-of-doors activity owing to fears of managing with poor hearing, loss of friends and loss of enjoyment of life. Indeed there was sufficient evidence to support the notion that deafness in old age is strongly associated

[†] British Telecom now publish a well-illustrated booklet entitled: *Help for Handicapped People* (British Telecom 1981, Code DLE550), in which telephone aids produced by the GPO and for purchase by local authorities under the CSDP Act, 1970 are laid out. However, availability of devices is patchy throughout the country.

[*] More information on the scheme can be obtained from the Sympathetic Hearing Scheme, 7/11 Armstrong Road, London W3.

with isolation, but not necessarily loneliness, and an artificially imposed loss of personal autonomy and physical independence. These associations were not necessarily perceived by the elderly themselves.

Deafness of the elderly poses many challenging problems for nurses and doctors. There is no single foolproof course of treatment to adopt that will solve the problem. It is largely a social malady caused by a physical impairment. In addition, the sheer prevalence of deafness amongst the elderly (hitherto known only intuitively) which renders it almost synonymous with ageing in both the popular and professional mind, is undoubtedly daunting. Nonetheless, the scope for early intervention with an aid is evidently wide and the scope for intervention with environmental aids even wider. Regrettably, disinterest by physicians is reflected in the disinterest of nurses and other paramedical staff and ignorance of the extent of the problem suppresses interest at policy level. Of all health care staff, the primary health care team holds the crucial role in the rehabilitation of the elderly deaf.

REFERENCES

Abrams M 1978 Beyond three score and ten. Age Concern Research Publications, Mitcham

Abrams M 1979 Transitions in middle and later life. Paper presented to the British Society of Social and Behavioural Gerontology, Keble College, University of Oxford

Alberti P W 1977 Hearing aids and aural rehabilitation. Journal of Otolaryngology 6: suppl no. 4

Ashley J 1973 Journey into silence. Bodley Head, London

Barker R G, Wright B A, Myerson L, Gonick M R 1953 Adjustment to physical handicap and illness: a survey of the social phychology of physique and disability, 2nd edn. Social Science Research Council, Bulletin 55, New York

Beethoven L 1802 Heiligenstadt document. Stadtbibliothek, Hamburg

Berry G 1933 The psychology of progressive deafness. Journal of the American Medical Association 101: 1599–1603

Brockington F, Lempert S M 1966 The social needs of the over-80s. Manchester University Press

Brooks D N 1979 Hearing aid candidates—some relevant features. British Journal of Audiology 13: 81–84

Bunting C 1981 Public attitudes to deafness. Social Survey of the Office of population Censuses and Surveys. HMSO, London

Cumbria County Council 1973 Survey of the handicapped and impaired and elderly over seventy-five in Cumberland. Cumbria County Council

Cumming E, Henry H E 1961 Growing old: the process of disengagement. Basic Books, New York

Department of Health and Social Security, ACSHIP 1977 Report of a sub-committee appointed to consider the role of social services in the care of the deaf of all ages. Advisory Committee on Services for Hearing Impaired People, London

Gilhome Herbst K R 1982a Some social implications of acquired deafness in ageing. In: Taylor R, Gilmore A J J (eds), Current Trends in British Gerontology Gower Press, London

Gilhome Herbst K R 1982b Social attitudes to hearing loss in the elderly. In: Creber A (ed) Barriers to communication: a national seminar on acquired hearing loss in elderly people. Beth Johnson Foundation, Keele University

Gilhome Herbst K R 1983 Psycho-social consequences of disorders of hearing in the elderly. In: Hinchcliffe R (ed) Medicine in old age—hearing and balance. Churchill Livingstone, Edinburgh

Gilhome Herbst K R, Humphrey C M 1980 Hearing impairment and mental state in the elderly living at home. British Medical Journal 280: 903–905

Gilhome Herbst K R, Humphrey C M 1981 Prevalence of hearing impairment in the elderly living at home. Journal of the Royal College of General Practitioners 31: 155–160

Gregory P 1961 Deafness and public responsibility. Occasional Papers on Social Administration, no. 7, Codicote Press, Welwyn

Grover B C 1977 A note on acoustic aids. British Journal of Audiology 11: 75–76

Haggard M, Gatehouse S, Davis A 1981 The high prevalence of hearing disorders and its implications for services in the UK. British Journal of Audiology 15: 241–251

Harris A 1962 The social survey. Health and welfare of older people in Lewisham. Central Office of Information, London

Humphrey C M, Gilhome Herbst K R, Faruqi S 1981 Some characteristics of the hearing impaired elderly who do not present themselves for rehabilitation. British Journal of Audiology 15: 25–30

Johnson J A 1981 National Health Service hearing aids. Hearing 36(1): 8–13

Kay D W K, Beamish P, Roth M 1964 Old age mental disorders in Newcastle upon Tyne. I: A study of prevalence. British Journal of Psychiatry 110: 146–158

Menninger K A 1924 The mental effects of deafness. Psychoanalytic Review 11: 144–155

Pedersen B, Frankner B, Terkildsen K 1974 A prospective study of adult Danish hearing aid users. Scandinavian Audiology 3: 107–111

Rawson A 1973 Deafness: report of a departmental enquiry into the promotion of research. DHSS, HMSO, London

Sheard A V 1971 Survey of the elderly in Scunthorpe. Public Health London 85: 208–218

Sheldon J H 1948 The social medicine of old age. Report of an enquiry in Wolverhampton. Oxford University Press, London

Stockport County Council 1958 Report on the survey of the aged in Stockport. Stockport County Council

Thomas A J, Gilhome Herbst K R 1980 Social and psychological implications of acquired deafness for adults of employment age. British Journal of Audiology 14: 76–85

Townsend P, Wedderburn D 1965 The aged in the welfare state. Occasional Papers on Social Administration no. 14, G Bell, London

Ward P R, Gowers J I, Morgan D C 1979 Problems with handling the BE10 series hearing aids among elderly people. British Journal of Audiology 13(1): 31–36

Wilkins L T 1948 The social survey. Survey of the prevalence of deafness in the population of England, Scotland and Wales. Central Office of Information, London

Williamson J, Stokoe I H, Gray S, et al 1964 Old people at home: their unreported needs. Lancet 1: 1117–1120

6

R. Greenhalgh

Sight

Sight is the most important of our five senses. We rely on our eyes to provide us with visual information about our physical and social environments. Our eyes give us access to numerous 'pieces' of information simultaneously, whereas our other senses will only give us access to the information in a sequence. For example, if we look at an object we can identify a number of characteristics and our task is to select the one that interests us. The characteristics from which we select might include

Size
Shape
Colour
Speed of movement
Direction of movement
Location in space

If we are unable to look at the object, then we have to use our senses of hearing, touch, smell and taste to identify the information we require, but simultaneous reception will not be possible.

We are bombarded with visual information all the time we have our eyes open, but much of that information is redundant—its existence is a luxury rather than a necessity. We frequently prove this for ourselves when we drive a car at night or in fog. On these occasions we have access to a greatly reduced bank of information, but still manage to function effectively using our sense of sight. If sight is significantly impaired it can lead to disability. In other words there will be one or more of the normal tasks of daily life which we cannot perform effectively. It is that group of elderly people with significantly impaired sight which concerns us here.

THE PREVALENCE OF VISUAL IMPAIRMENT

There are two registers held by local authorities concerned with people who have significantly impaired vision: the blind register and the partially sighted register. Certification for both registers must be undertaken by an ophthalmologist of consultant status. Once certification has taken place, the information is passed on the local authority where registration takes place. Registration is completely voluntary. For the purposes of registration, a blind person is someone who is 'so blind as to be unable to perform any work for which eyesight is essential'. A partially sighted person is someone who is 'substantially and permanently handicapped by defective vision caused by congenital defect, or illness, or injury'.

There are numerous advantages both in terms of service provision and financial aid for people who are registered as blind, but there are few real benefits for those who are registered as partially sighted. It is suggested by the Department of Health and Social Security (1979) that for this reason the blind register is likely to be more complete than the partially sighted register. The same report says that 'studies such as Graham et al (1968), Brennan and Knox (1973) and Cullinan (1978) suggest that the true prevalence of blindness in adults might be 10% to 40% higher than is shown by the registers and that the true prevalence of partial sight might be twice as high as that shown in the registers'.

The number of people registered as blind in England remains fairly constant at about 100 000 (DHSS 1979). About 12 000 people are registered blind each year and about the same number are taken from the register when they die. In 1976, 73% of people on the blind register were aged 65+ years

and 54% were over the age of 75 years.

The number of people who are registered as partially sighted is rising slowly and at the present stands at about 50 000 in England (DHSS 1979). The partially sighted register consists largely of people who are elderly, 65% of people being over the age of 65 years in 1976. Visual impairment is clearly a problem associated with ageing (see Chapter 3, 'The Physiology of Ageing'), and as the elderly population increases, so will the number of people who are registered either as blind or partially sighted.

The criteria for registration are based largely on visual acuity (the ability to see detail in visual material) and field of vision (the ability to see the whole picture). Registration is based on the ability to perform specific clinical tests and is not concerned with functional ability. There may be many elderly people who do not meet the criteria required for registration who might still be considered to be severely visually impaired.

ASSESSING VISUAL ABILITY

Performance does not necessarily improve as visual acuity rises. There are many factors related to the ability to perform tasks efficently and these include motor function, intelligence, motivation and social experience. To individuals with similar visual status will not be consistent in the way each can perform specific tasks. For instance, one may be able to perform reading tasks easily, but be in great difficulty when it comes to tasks involving movement. Unfortunately, it is quite impossible to be prescriptive when predicting performance based on an individual's visual ability. Each individual must be assessed independently, although there are indicators which might help us to eliminate inappropriate steps in the assessment process. Registration is therefore not a good indicator of whether an individual will be able to function effectively using vision. Our assessment must consider the functional ability of the individual to perform tasks using vision and the ability to receive visual stimulation.

Failing sight is frequently perceived as being a consequence of increasing age, and indeed this is so with some eye diseases such as macular degeneration. We become more reliant upon visual information as we get older and it is therefore important to ensure that the sense of sight is maximised wherever possible. A functional examination of visual ability should include questions such as:

Can you read the print in the newspaper?
Can you read the headlines in the newspaper?
Can you see the cup on the table?
Can you see the chair over in the corner?
Can you see the picture on the television screen?
Can you tell me the colour of the curtains?
Can you pour water accurately from the jug to the cup?
Can you walk to the door at the other end of the room?

These are not merely questions involving answers, they involve tasks which need to be demonstrated. The demonstration will often indicate the severity of a visual impairment.

TYPES OF VISUAL IMPAIRMENT

People with a significant visual impairment can be divided into two groups, each having quite different kinds of needs.

Firstly, there is a group of people without functional vision. This group requires help at the level of vision substitution, particularly through sound and touch. We have deliberately avoided using the word 'blind' to describe this group as it can be a confusing term and is usually used very loosely as part of our labelling system. There are relatively few people who are completely without functional vision, probably less than 15 000 in England. Most elderly people with failing sight will retain some useful functional vision throughout life.

The second broad grouping consists of those people who have a significant visual impairment, but who retain useful functional vision. These people require strategies based on vision enhancement rather than vision substitution. There are some people who will be able to undertake some tasks using vision, who for other tasks will require vision substitution techniques. People who lose a significant amount of vision, tend to experience either a loss of visual acuity or a loss in the field of vision. The most common type of loss for elderly people, which is in some ways less disabling, is a loss of visual acuity.

Our ability to see detail in visual material is determined by the efficiency of the macular area of the retina. A deterioration in the functioning of the macula, a degeneration of the cone receptors, results in a loss of ability to read effectively and to undertake fine discrimination tasks such as threading a needle. However, mobility should be relatively unimpaired. Consequently, a loss of visual acuity—that area in the centre of the field of vision—is a nuisance, but should not prevent an old person from carrying out most of the tasks of daily life, other than those demanding the resolution of fine detail. Unfortunately, elderly people are more likely than others to require good visual acuity as they are more inclined to spend considerable lengths of time reading, sewing and undertaking other solo tasks.

A loss of the field of vision can be extremely disabling as it almost inevitably has the effect of reducing one's ability to negotiate the environment effectively. In its most severe form, a loss of the visual field is commonly called 'tunnel vision' and is rather like spending one's life looking down a long tube. Visual acuity available at the macular area is used to identify the characteristics of objects in the environment. Peripheral vision is used for detecting movement, for seeing in dull lighting conditions and in alerting the person to hazards within her path. A loss of peripheral vision is likely to be particularly disabling for someone who is elderly because the reduction of motor function which can occur with increasing age, demands good early warning of hazards.

FACTORS INFLUENCING SIGHT

There are three important factors which influence the ability to see: light, contrast and size.

Eyes function on light and it is therefore a very important factor in determining whether we are able to see properly. Generally, we appear to need more light as we get older in order to see well, and people with a visual impairment often function more effectively if lighting is increased. General lighting used to illuminate a whole room should be sufficient to allow people in the room to distinguish its major features and be able to move around it in comfort. Local lighting, or task lighting, allows us to bring an intensive source of light near to the material we want to view. Desk lamps and table lamps provide excellent sources of local lighting, but they should not be used in a room where there is no general lighting present, because our eyes take time to adapt from one lighting condition to another. Using a desk lamp in an otherwise darkened room could prove hazardous to elderly people when they need to move around. Illumination throughout a building should be as constant as possible so that movement from one area to another one will not prove too hazardous. Lighting can increase visual acuity considerably and may be the complete solution to the sight problems of many elderly people.

Contrast is the second factor which can help people to see more effectively. It is a way of making things visible by making them stand out from their background. We usually think of contrast in terms of colour, and used intelligently it can make a great deal of difference to the visibility of some objects. For example, white crockery on a white table may cause elderly people with significantly impaired vision a lot of difficulty because they cannot distinguish the edge of the plate from the white table and may therefore spill food. If the

surface under the plate is dark then it will greatly enhance the visual characteristics of the task. The addition of contrast is not expensive, as in the example above, it can be done by using a table-cloth, a table-mat, or even a piece of coloured paper. The use of contrast involves imagination rather than expense. The principle can be adapted to many situations and can help to improve the quality of life for many elderly poeple. It can be applied equally well in an individual's own home or in an institutional setting.

The third factor which can help to improve our ways of seeing things is size. There are a number of ways of manipulating the apparent size of objects, though in many ways this is the most difficult of the three factors to deal with. The easiest way to increase the apparent size of an object is to move closer to it. If you move from a distance of 10 feet from a television screen to a distance of 2 feet, then the apparent size of the screen will have increased in size five times as far as the retinal image is concerned. The same principle applies to any visual task. Elderly people find it difficult to accept the idea of reading with the material held very close to the eye. This reluctance probably stems from some of the long-held myths about vision which unfortunately still persist. It is not uncommon to find people who believe they will harm their sight if they read in a dim light or if they peer closely at written material. We cannot damage our eyes by using them. Generally, what we describe as eye strain is no more than fatigue in the muscles that move the eyes in their orbit. A short rest will soon allow the muscles to regenerate their strength so that work can be resumed. We do not hear people talking about brain strain when they have been thinking about problems for any length of time. Certainly, we rarely think it possible to wear out organs of the body in the way that we consider the possibility of eye sight wearing out. Even people with significantly impaired sight will not damage their eyes further by using them.

The second way of changing the apparent size of visual material is through optical magnification. Unfortunately, elderly people tend to have unrealistic expectations of magnifying aids. It is fairly common to be asked for a lens which will be high powered and which will cover a complete page of a book or a newspaper. The reality is that the larger the aperture of the magnifier the smaller is the amount of magnification. Inevitably, people who require high levels of magnification will have to cope with a small field of view through the aperture of the magnifying aid. Elderly people need to learn how to use magnifiers effectively. Reading speed will be reduced and there will be more likelihood of muscular discomfort through taking up an unusual viewing position. Elderly people need continuing help once an aid has been provided. Like many other technological aids, provision of an aid does not mean it will be used.

The most difficult method of providing magnification is by enlarging the actual size of the objects. This principle can be seen in large-print books, large-print playing cards, and so on. It is not possible to enlarge the size of everything one wants to see. The greatest disadvantage is probably the size of the enlarged material. Large-print books tend to be heavy and cumbersome to handle. Many elderly people may find that they require a reading stand as they are unable to hold a heavy book for any length of time.

Environmental techniques of assistance should be used in preference to special aids whenever possible. Special aids often require special training and are much more likely to be rejected by an elderly person than the adaptation of the normal environment.

IMPAIRMENT, DISABILITY AND HANDICAP

The objective when intervening in the visual difficulties of elderly people is to reduce the consequences of disease to a minimum. The consequences form a continuum through impairment, disability and handicap. The individual can move along the continuum in either direction. The effects of a disease can lead to the presence of a handicap without the intermediate steps of impairment and disability. A visual impairment is a function of the organ of sight. A visual disability is a function of the individual and some tasks cannot be undertaken in a manner which is perceived as 'normal'. A visual handicap is a function of society as there will be a perceived 'normal' role which the individual is not able to undertake because of the problems within the visual system.

Appropriate intervention can reduce a handicap to the level of disability. This might be done by encouraging an elderly person to explore her surroundings rather than to stay in bed. It is still possible to visit institutions where patients are allowed to vegetate by being the recipients of well-intentioned over-protective care. A disability might be reduced to the level of impairment by teaching the patient to carry out tasks independently or by manipulating the environment to facilitate its use by people with a significant visual problem.

REHABILITATION

Work with people who have a visual disablement is both interdisciplinary and multidisciplinary. No single worker can resolve all the associated problems when an elderly person is admitted to institutional care. Rehabilitation demands the mobilisation of a variety of skills if it is to be successful. The kinds of worker likely to be instrumental in the rehabilitation of someone with a visual disablement are:

    Ophthalmologist
    Optician
    Nurse
    Occupational therapist
    Social worker
    Technical officer
    Mobility officer

Rehabilitation can be divided into three distinct phases, although there is constant overlap as the patient progresses and regresses and new problems are identified.

The first phase may be seen as medical, and during this phase there is medical and surgical intervention to maximise the patient's physical capability. This may be done by surgically removing a cataract or by prescribing an appropriate optical aid in the form of spectacles or a low vision aid. A range of medical and surgical strategies might be used to develop latent physical abilities.

The second phase is educative, when the patient, either within a hospital or within her own community, is taught new skills and strategies for coping with the tasks of everyday life. The technical officer, usually employed by the local authority social services department, might teach cooking skills, reading techniques or leisure activities. The mobility officer from the same department might teach the patient how to travel independently either by using a white cane or by making the most effective use of any remaining vision. This educative phase is one of growth, when skills are re-established and an effective coping repertoire is developed.

The third phase, which overlies the other two, is psychological support. Both medical and educative interventions can be rendered irrelevant if the psychological care is inappropriate. If an elderly person is at the point of acquiring a permanent visual disablement because medical intervention can be of no further help, the patient will be in great need of psychological support. She should be given ample opportunity to discuss what is happening and what is likely to happen. If she is to be registered as a blind person she may wish to know the prognosis—is she going to lose her sight completely? She needs to know that there are many strategies which can be employed to help her. If appropriate psychological support is not available at this stage, then later rehabilitation will be much more difficult. Other people who have come to terms with their own loss of sight can be a great help in the recovery of psychological well-being of the patient.

Nurses play an important part in the rehabilitation process. They provide continuity by forming a link between all members of the therapeutic team, and between hospital and the community. They should be active in the rehabilitation process by continuing the care prescribed by specialists, by patient teaching, and by evaluating the effects of therapy and the patient's progress.

Aids and services

There are literally hundreds of aids and services for people with a visual disablement. Some are intended to maximise a small amount of sight, and some to act as a substitute for sight. Aids range from simple templates to enable someone with poor sight to complete a cheque or sign a pension book, to sophisticated communication devices for enlarging print or producing Braille type. The suitability of a particular aid or service will depend upon a range of factors such as age, ability to learn, mobility, manual dexterity, and so on. The most helpful strategy is to identify the problem—be it communication, mobility or a daily living task—and then seek out a solution through the appropriate agency or by reference to one of the resource books. There are two agencies in England primarily concerned with people who have a visual impairment. The Partially Sighted Society, Queen's Road, Doncaster, South Yorkshire DNI 2NX, is prepared to accept any general or specific queries relating to the problems of people who have some sight, however small that amount may be; requests for help which cannot be resolved by the society are referred to more appropriate sources. The Royal National Institute for the Blind, 224 Great Portland Street, London W1A 6AA, has particular expertise in vision substitution and is prepared to accept both general and specific requests for help; again, when requests cannot be responded to directly, referral will be made to a more appropriate source.

Resources, which give general information about the problems of people with visual impairment are British Broadcasting Corporation (1982), Partially Sighted Society (1979), Electricity Council (1981) and the Royal National Institute for the Blind (1983).

REFERENCES

British Broadcasting Corporation 1982 In touch. BBC Publications, London
Cullinan T R 1978 The epidemiology of visual disability: studies of visually disabled people in the community. HSRU Report No. 28. Health Services Research Unit, University of Kent, Canterbury

Department of Health and Social Security 1979 Blindness and partial sight in England 1969–76. Reports on public health and medical subjects, No. 129. HMSO, London
Electricity Council 1981 Lighting and low vision. Electricity Council
Partially Sighted Society 1979 Light for low vision. Partially Sighted Society, Doncaster
Royal National Institute for the Blind 1983 How to guide a blind person. RNIB, London

7

A. Stokes-Roberts

Maintaining activities and interests

THE NEED TO MAINTAIN ACTIVITIES AND INTERESTS

People are living longer and are being forced to retire before they are ready to give up paid work. It is so important for society to develop an awareness of the difficulties associated with enforced leisure, and how it can best give constructive help. Life does not end at retirement but certain adjustments have to be made. All elderly people have certain needs which must be fulfilled in order to maintain a satisfactory quality of life. These might include physical and emotional health, adequate income and accommodation, congenial friends and neighbours with whom to enjoy absorbing interests, and an adequate personal philosophy of life. Those who have something to live for, a positive outlook on life and who maintain some level of continuity with their past, despite all the other changes associated with old age, seem to be the most successful at managing their old age.

To withdraw from life because one cannot adjust is a loss for the individual and for society. Boredom, depression and isolation may be symptoms of withdrawal, as is an apparent apathy when activity is reinstated. It is a great mistake, however, to think that because an elderly person is not obviously doing something (s)he is doing nothing. Silent reminiscence is important, as will be discussed later in this chapter, and so is the need for peace, quiet and solitude. Bromley (1974) observed that, with advancing age, activities selected by individuals show a trend towards spectatorship (such as watching television) rather than participation and that they are self-paced (for example, gardening, reading).

Many old people, like younger people in our society, see ageing in terms of failure. The maintenance of activities and interests provides opportunities for achievement which can improve an old person's confidence and self-esteem, and can preserve her identity and individuality.

FACTORS INFLUENCING THE ELDERLY PERSON'S ABILITY TO KEEP OCCUPIED

Time factors

For some, retirement can be a new beginning, a chance to indulge in activities and hobbies for which there has previously been too little time. For others it is like a life sentence. The value of planning and preparing for retirement is well documented and the increase in pre-retirement courses reflects a recognition of their role in assisting people to adjust to this period of their lives. As well as retirement from work there may be a change in family obligations. For example, many couples today have over 15 years to enjoy together after the marriage of their last child.

For those who have never had 'spare time', learning how to develop a new routine and the constructive use of the time they now have is especially important. Some old people use activities as a method to pass time and avoid loneliness. They need help, for it is an indication of a lack of adjustment to the circumstances in which they find themselves. Time in retirement is rarely all leisure since daily chores still have to be done, and these may be much the same as those done before the issue of the old age pension. Education and recreational activities may now become priorities, and there are opportunities for elderly folk to put their abilities to good use and to explore new areas of involvement, such as participating in community work.

Physical factors

Old age is not synonymous with illness, but there will be a certain slowing of function and increase in frailty for elderly people over the age of 75 years. Problems with mobility are particularly likely to affect the ability of the elderly to participate in leisure activities (Glyn-Jones 1975). Disability resulting from acute and chronic conditions will affect an individual's ability to perform any task. It is often a struggle just to cope with the activities of daily living, let alone indulge in other interests. For those with chronic conditions the knowledge that they will never get better may be very hard to come to terms with. Their self-confidence is low, an element reinforced by repeated failure, and they may, for good reason, be extremely difficult to motivate.

The blind and the deaf have special problems, primarily of communication. They may lack appropriate aids and not have had any expert advice. Those around them may be unaware of how to make the most of their other abilities. For the blind (see Chapter 6), mobility especially in unfamiliar surroundings, is difficult and disorientating; it may be less frightening to stay at home. For the deaf (see Chapter 5), verbal communication may be almost impossible, and misinterpretation and ignorance by others may contribute to their isolation. Similarly, with the incontinent (see Chapter 12), a person might prefer to withdraw from human relationships than face possible rejection, avoidance, pity or ridicule (Kastenbaum 1979). These reactions are evoked by many other physical problems as well.

Psychological factors

The capacity of the elderly to learn is underestimated, by the elderly themselves as well as those around them. Many left school early, to go to work or to war, and apparently lack the background to attempt new tasks in retirement. Even so, provided activities are presented in the right way and the elderly are motivated to undertake them, there are few obstacles to success.

Any visual, auditory or sensory impairment will affect a person's ability to write, speak and gesticulate in some way or another. Communication skills are often taken for granted and problems in this area are rarely easily solved. Anyone who has tried to talk to a person with dysphasia, dysarthria or articulatory dyspraxia knows the frustration involved not only for the listener but also for the person who is struggling to communicate. Many give up and withdraw. People vary in their degree of articulateness and this will influence their ability to participate with confidence in activities. Non-verbal clues, such as an uneasy posture, may provide important information in these instances. Jill Macleod Clark in Chapter 4 discusses communication in more detail.

The outgoing affable person who joins in and enjoys activities is welcomed in any circle, the introverted, socially unskilled one less so. In a study of ageing and personality, Reichard et al (1962) identified five personality types: the 'rocking chair' passive person, the 'armoured', vigorous, physically and socially active person, and the 'mature', well-adjusted person who had all adapted to their role in society; the other two types, the 'angry' and the 'self-haters', demonstrated a maladaptive pattern to ageing and were lonely and depressed as a result. Although this study was limited to men, on an intuitive basis, it seems equally applicable to women.

A person who has a flexible and adaptable temperament and who is willing to seek out new areas that will give her satisfaction, will probably get more out of life than the passive individual who waits for events to happen. Some of those who have successfully adjusted to old age seem to be able to accept help when necessary, but others do not. Being brought up in an era of self-help when the state did not provide either financially or practically, they find turning to bureaucratic establishments for help unpalatable and depressing.

The majority of the elderly feel that people are concerned about them and see themselves as exceptions to a generally dreary picture. An important part of their activity is getting out and about, the most frequent reasons being to shop and visit friends. Many, given the chance, would have stayed on at work. These attitudes of the elderly are important considerations for those involved in their care (Age Concern 1974a).

Old habits die hard, which is why preparation for retirement is so vital. Loss and bereavement increase with age; friends, family, health and belongings are all affected. The changes wrought by their loss can be devastating and disruptive. Kastenbaum (1979) describes a sense of panic and disintegration that an old person sometimes feels, and one of the outward manifestations may be a lack of motivation towards joining in activities and interests.

Cultural and religious factors

Certain expectations and beliefs concerning the elderly are prevalent. The stereotype is to consider them as physically frail, mentally inept, inflexible, dependent and unproductive.

Old age is viewed as a negative period preceding death, an approach described by Butler (1974) as 'ageism'. However, some of the men who dominate world politics and some very well-known musicians are good examples of another side to the elderly which contrasts vividly with the picture of the 80-year-old demented person in a long-stay ward. It is not surprising that the ambivalent attitude of society to the elderly makes them so reluctant to ask for any form of assistance.

In certain cultures the elderly are regarded as the head of the family whose role is to pass on historical information and customs to the younger folk. In Britain this no longer occurs, and for the elderly belonging to ethnic minorities the insecurity of a new environment and the remoteness of the family left behind in the country of origin are additional problems. For them the problems of growing old are compounded by special difficulties, such as unfamiliar language and a very different way of life. They also suffer from discrimination and prejudice at the hands of the host community (Age Concern 1974b), factors which all contribute to their problems of survival, let alone the difficulties involved in maintaining their activities and interests. Getting help is equally difficult, as not only have they little or no knowledge of the services available but they frequently are unknown to health and social workers.

The lifestyle of old people belonging to ethnic minorities is, to a large extent, dictated by their religion, just as it is for many of the elderly in western cultures. The spiritual and social support to be gained through contact with the church should not be underestimated. An Age Concern survey (1974a) found that over 40% of those they questioned had some interest in, or contact with, the church. Religion may or may not have provided continuity throughout life, but in old age it may give special security and comfort. Beliefs, especially with regard to taboo subjects, can have an inhibitory effect on elderly people's ability to conduct their affairs as they would wish. Old folk on the whole are not afraid of death, whereas those around them often are. The process of coming to terms with life and accepting the prospect of death is often discouraged by younger relatives, friends and health workers, when what the old person really needs is support, understanding, and discussion of an inevitable and fairly imminent part of life.

Another subject considered to be taboo is sex. Comfort (1974) put the problem in a nutshell: 'Old folks stop having sex for the same reasons they stop riding a bicycle—general infirmity, thinking it looks ridiculous, no bicycle—and of these reasons the greatest is the social image of the dirty old man and the asexual, undesirable older woman.' The attitudes of society inhibit expression of sexual desires even though such desires may remain as strong as ever. The intimacy of those who have shared a long life of joys and sorrows is both precious and life affirming and should be respected as much as they are for the young. Expressing sexuality is discussed in more detail by Christine Webb in Chapter 16 of this volume.

There exist many stereotypes concerning the activities and interests which old people can enjoy. Men apparently have no interest in self-expressive activities such as dancing, painting and cooking, and women only enjoy those concerned with homemaking. Members of the upper classes, having been managers and executives, belong to clubs and bridge circles, whilst those from the working classes, the skilled, semi-skilled and manual workers, play bingo and go to the pub. These are exaggerated examples, but give an idea of the generalisations that tend to be made.

Studies have shown that home-centred activities tend to revolve around cooking, housework, gardening, radio and television (Tunstall 1966). Those most commonly undertaken outside the home include shopping, visiting friends or going out for the day (Age Concern 1974a). The social and economic background of an individual does have a tremendous influence on the activities and interests pursued. Each person's interests should be considered individually in order that maximum fulfilment and satisfaction can be achieved.

Climatic and environmental factors

Winter heralds a period of decreased activity, the cold and damp slow both function and motivation. The risk of falling is higher and the potential danger of venturing out after dark is a greater problem than in the summer. Most of the elderly who visit relatives or who travel for social and recreational purposes use public transport. Those in rural areas are particularly vulnerable as services are unreliable and infrequent. Some 40% of journeys made by the elderly are for shopping (Age Concern 1978) but the reduction of public transport in many areas has put access to public facilities out of reach for many people. Local shops are often expensive, which leaves less money for recreational pursuits.

Public facilities are rarely designed to suit elderly users. Steps instead of ramps, few handrails, poor lighting, lack of seating and toilet facilities, and little chance of assistance make any trip a daunting prospect. Fortunately, society is gradually becoming aware of the needs of the elderly and the disabled, and many local authorities now issue information guides which pinpoint suitable facilities.

The problems that can be created by an institutional environment are probably even greater. In physical terms, facilities may be less than ideal: high beds, toilets with difficult access, unsuitable chairs, no lift, etc. The psychological effects of living in an institution may be even more traumatic. The stripping of individuality and status which occurs when an elderly person enters an institution is well documented (e.g. Goffman 1961). The loss of role, personal belongings, support of family and friends and a sense of personal control over one's life, all contribute to a feeling of insecurity and isolation. A strange environment and a new routine can be extremely disorientating, their constraints leaving little time or inclination for the pursuit of activities and interests. Such a person may subside rapidly into a state of 'learned helplessness', when the motivation to carry out any activity, even though capable of it, has gone (Schulz 1980).

Economic factors

Although pensions today may be supplemented by income from odd jobs, private investment or savings, they are frequently the sole source of income. Wedderburn (1973) found that half Britain's pensioners were living at or below the government-defined poverty level. An old person's main outgoings are usually rent, food and fuel, the latter being a particularly difficult expense to bear. No old person wishes to add to the financial burdens of her family but she may feel she has nowhere else to turn. There is considerable lack of knowledge about benefits and aids available, and when offered, these are too often accepted reluctantly, or refused as charity. The state pension provides a minimum fixed income and is not linked to inflation and the cost of living. Pension increases are dependent on the priorities of the government in power, and old people are frequently confused and worried about their future financial status. When it comes to pri-

orities, food and warmth take precedence over recreational activities. Hendricks and Hendricks (1977) provide a comprehensive discussion of the myths and realities of ageing in modern mass societies.

WHAT CAN BE DONE

To keep old people in the environment of their choice

Assessment of function

The ability of an elderly person to perform activities of daily living often means the difference between being independent or dependent. Information should, where possible, be substantiated by careful observation and practical assessment, because sometimes the elderly are unrealistic about their capabilities. The purpose of assessing functional abilities is to establish which activities of personal care a person is able to perform: to assess how that ability, if necessary, can be improved, and to decide the best methods to use in order to achieve their maximum potential (Turner 1981). As well as the physical ability of an individual, psychological and social functioning should also be assessed.

Mobility is the area of physical function that is likely to have the most effect on an old person's ability to cope, and is covered in detail in Chapter 8. Transfers, sitting, standing and walking safely are the primary considerations. Together with physiotherapists, decisions are made as to what, if any, aids (walking-stick, walking-frame, etc.) are most likely to achieve maximum mobility. An integral part of treatment and advice on mobility is the assessment of the environment, with particular reference to such details as the height of chair, bed and toilet, floor coverings, stairs and steps. Adaptations to existing equipment, such as chair, bed and toilet 'raises' and rails can be invaluable for old people who have difficulties, as well as the employment of new methods.

Wheelchairs can give a chairbound old person considerable mobility. They can be self-propelled (manual or electric) or attendant-propelled. Careful assessment is necessary to ensure that the wheelchair suits both the mental and physical capacity of the individual and the environment in which (s)he lives. Many models are available either on prescription or by private purchase. A full description of all hand-propelled chairs available on prescription is given in Department of Health and Social Security (1982).

Eating and drinking are often the first activities in which a disabled person can achieve independence. When assessing, it is necessary to consider the effects of muscle weakness, tremor, spasm, lack of co-ordination and any chewing or swallowing difficulties. An awareness of factors such as positioning and table heights is essential. For some, specially designed or adapted cutlery or crockery may be necessary. More detailed information on this subject can be found in Wilshere (1976).

Dressing and grooming should be assessed as soon as possible. Abilities here can boost patients' morale and enable them to look and feel normal. Undressing is easier than dressing and attention should be given to individual sequence, the way a person has dressed for the last few decades. There are often severe problems and much patience and practice may be required before a patient achieves independence. Clothing adaptations should only be attempted when all other techniques and methods have been tried. On the whole, it is better to buy loose fitting, front fastening, easily laundered clothes. Maximum independence may be possible but unrealistic, especially when there is a wife or husband who always helps. In order for confidence and self-esteem to develop, it is essential that an old person is encouraged to take pride in his or her appearance, by paying special attention to the care of hair, teeth and nails, and by encouraging the old person to shave regularly, or use make-up, if done so in the past.

Toilet management. For many elderly people in hospital being able to use the toilet is crucial for attaining personal independence and for fulfilling the requirements for resettlement. The hospital environment may be responsible for an old person's incontinence (see Chapter 12). Sometimes easy practical solutions can be found, for example toilet raises, rails at the side of the toilet, or simply advice on easily managed clothing. Night-time management should also be assessed; a commode at the side of the bed, or a urinal may be of help. For those alone at home with a toilet outside or one that is otherwise inaccessible, a chemical commode may be of use. Further details are to be found in Wilshere (1978).

Personal hygiene. Some old people live in properties that do not have bathrooms, and which also lack hot water. This may mean they have to boil kettles in order to wash which presents additional problems. Those who do have the facilities may find bathing a difficult and strenuous process even with aids or the assistance of a bath attendant. Nevertheless, cleanliness and thorough washing should always be encouraged, and a shower might be easier than a bath.

Domestic tasks may include house-cleaning, meal preparation, cooking and serving, laundry, budgeting and shopping. Assessment of the old person's ability must be realistic and undertaken with knowledge of a patient's home situation, such as the help available (family, home help or meals-on-wheels). The kitchen is usually the area that causes most concern to relatives because of the risks involved, such as lighting gas or carrying boiling water. It is also an area where the assessment of certain patients, such as those who are blind or partially sighted, can effectively be undertaken only in their home. Much practice may be needed to reinforce retraining, or to encourage the learning of new methods. A publication from the Disabled Living Foundation which provides comprehensive information and advice is *Kitchen Sense for Disabled or Elderly People* (Foott et al 1975).

A proportion of the patients being assessed will have communication difficulties of one sort or another. In conjunction with the speech therapist, the occupational therapist should be able to provide assistance with speech, hearing, reading and writing, and give advice on appropriate aids. Additional information may be found in Wilshere (1980).

Assessment of home conditions

Once the assessment of a patient's function is complete, it is essential to have first-hand experience of that person in their own home, where several areas can be assessed. Home visits are usually done by an occupational therapist who may take a student nurse with her. Sometimes the physiotherapist or social worker will come too and a representative from the community services might attend.

The primary area to be assessed is the patient's physical capacity to cope with the accommodation and furniture, and its suitability in relation to the short and long-term consequences of the patient's disability. General mobility and transfers, and a person's ability to cope with the environment, for example plugs and heating, are assessed. Potential hazards such as loose carpets and poor lighting are also examined. Observations of what, if any, aids/adaptations have been or could be provided to enable a patient to manage are also made. The most commonly supplied aids are to raise chair, bed and toilet and there is frequently a need for rails. Help from outside agencies such as the gas or electricity boards may be required.

What does the patient think about her home environment? Is she well oriented? Does she feel able to cope? All these demonstrate a person's attitude and the level of adjustment to her condition.

It is important to assess the level of physical and psychological support that exists as well as that which would be required to get the patient home from hospital. Social services, such as meals-on-wheels, friends, neighbours, day centres, church and voluntary bodies all come into this category. It is important also to identify the attitudes of the family and neighbours to having the old person at home and services that may be involved. Those people directly concerned may require counselling and reassurance, and to know that help is available. Those less directly concerned, for example families who live some distance away, may feel guilty, and should be given the opportunity to discuss their feelings with someone who knows the patient well.

Once the home visit has been done, considerable liaison is necessary in order to plan and co-ordinate future care and resettlement. The importance of thorough and detailed communication between all those involved cannot be overstated. Many discharges have failed as a result of poor organisation, and it is always the elderly person who suffers.

Services and equipment available

The services provided vary tremendously from area to area, and there is considerable confusion as to which organisation is responsible for a particular service. The local social services department of the local authority should know whom to contact. This department is usually responsible for the major support services, for example meals-on-wheels, home help, laundry services and chiropody. They also run social clubs, day centres and luncheon clubs and help with transport facilities, as well as providing aids and adaptations to the home. Other services, such as the district nurses, are provided by the health authority. They may also be involved with medical loans and the supply of some aids and gadgets.

Many elderly people rely on help from voluntary sources such as Good Neighbour schemes, Women's Royal Voluntary Service, and local schools and church organisations. These services give tremendous back-up support to those provided by the state. There are several national organisations which can be called upon for advice or assistance, such as Age Concern, Help the Aged, Royal National Institute for the Blind and the British Red Cross Society.

Booklets focusing on the needs of the elderly are now being produced by several areas giving a guide to local facilities; these should help increase awareness of the assistance that is available. There are many aids to daily living which can be borrowed, bought or made. The demand is such that many large chemists and stores stock a range of specialist aids and equipment, and items that were once provided for the disabled are now available as convenience items; for example one-handed whisks and non-slip bowls. It is worth remembering, however, that the elderly often abandon their aids once they return to their own homes as they tend to revert to their old habits. It is therefore essential that the use of anything new is carefully taught and its value reinforced by all those involved with the care of that person.

Occupational therapists can advise on the use of aids as well as on adaptations to the home, such as stair rails and larger items of equipment like hoists and stair lifts. These may require liaison with housing and other social services departments. In his book *Designing for the Disabled* Selwyn Goldsmith (1976) gives detailed descriptions of those aspects that require attention.

The primary objective for the elderly person is to get home as soon as possible with minimum disruption to her environment. Counselling and reassurance of friends and relatives, and demonstration by the old person of her capabilities is vital if she is to manage at home. Many old people discharged from hospital fail to cope because of the anxiety of the carers, which affects the confidence of the patient. A level of risk has to be accepted, and absolute guarantees cannot be given.

Recent evidence (Cloke 1983) highlights the stress involved in caring for elderly relatives, and the fact that the elderly themselves may be at risk of ill-treatment (see Chapter 27 by Alison While for further discussion of elderly abuse). The support, in both physical and psychological terms, and advice given to the carers by all members of the multidisciplinary team is becoming increasingly important, as is the need for thorough co-ordination of effective support services on discharge from hospital.

What can be done to encourage and enhance well-being in institutions

The majority of people working in institutions underestimate the abilities of the frail elderly. The attitudes of staff to their patients are probably one of the most important factors to consider in regard to the patient's well-being and quality of life. Millard and Smith (1981) found that lack of personal belongings increased the likelihood of an elderly person's being perceived in a negative way. If a person is approached as being less able than others, it is likely that the more decrepit aspects of their behaviour will be reinforced. As mentioned earlier, the elderly need to take a positive attitude to their lives and so do the staff who tend them. Showing an interest in an old person as an individual and reinforcing the positive aspects of her abilities can do much for her self-esteem and confidence. Pride in personal appearance and the opportunity for choice about which clothes to wear, facilities to use, activities to pursue, etc. are most important.

Activities

Isolation and disorientation are common problems for people in institutions, and the use of individual and group activities can be of great benefit as well as enhancing a sense of well-being and satisfaction. The renewal of old and exploration of new interests and hobbies should be an intergral part of institutional life. McCormack and Whitehead (1981), in their study of engagement levels of long-stay patients, found that engagement levels were consistently higher when activities were provided, with group activities on the whole being more successful than individual activities. They concluded that patients' engagement levels are usually low, not because they lack ability, but because they are not given the opportunity or encouragement to practicipate in any activity.

When doing any activity, it is important to remember certain points which will affect the level of engagement and participation of those involved. Activities should be purposeful and enjoyable. No one will do something they see as pointless or join in for the sake of doing something. Wherever possible, use should be made of any previous experience and the activity tailored to the ability of the participant. There should be opportunities for choice, and patients should never be forced to join in an activity as it is likely to elicit an angry response or further depress someone who is already withdrawn. Encourage them to watch, however, and curiosity will often win the day. Old people frequently find groups threatening; it takes time for them to relax in such a setting, and initially their concentration will be low.

The thorough planning and preparation of an activity is essential; if disorganised, the participants will neither co-operate nor concentrate. Consideration must be given to environmental factors, staffing, types of patients and activity itself. The venue for the group, such as dayroom, ward, occupational therapy department, and the amount of space available will affect the choice of activity. The suitability of furniture also requires assessment, and factors that may act as distractors, like television, should be avoided. The number of staff available will affect the activity that is done, as some require much higher staff/patient ratios than others. A great deal of enthusiasm and resilience is necessary, and it is important that the quality of the teaching is as high as possible. The patients themselves need both encouragement and support, and not all activities will suit all patients. In order to avoid increasing their sense of failure an activity should be offered to those who will get the most enjoyment out of it and who will cope fairly well with the task. Some patients need a lot of help in order to achieve success, but it is important to give them the opportunity. There is a tremendous range of activities which can be used in original or adapted form. There are those provided by specialists, such as art and music therapists and local authority teachers, and many others which may be provided by occupational therapists, physiotherapists, nurses and voluntary helpers. The value of many of the craft activities used by occupational therapists is clearly demonstrated by Hamill and Oliver (1980). Traditional activities are included such as knitting, embroidery and woodwork, and a wide variety of new ideas for creativity are explored (Fig. 7.1).

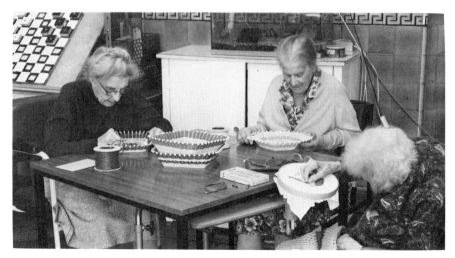

Fig. 7.1 Basketwork and embroidery.

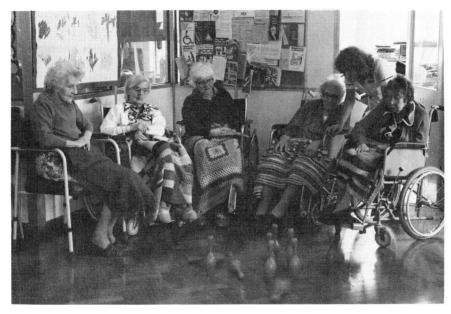

Fig. 7.2 Skittles.

Occupational therapists together with other specialists provide many other types of activities which aim to be physically, socially and educationally stimulating as well as assisting orientation. Many good examples are cited by Comins et al (1983) and Cornish (1983). Exercises and games are popular, the enjoyment of the participants is evident, and the opportunity to 'let off steam' especially during team games appears to be most welcome (Fig. 7.2). Powell (1974) showed exercise to be beneficial for the cognitive and behavioural capacities of the aged. For this reason, Salter and Salter (1975) emphasised recreational activities involving exercise in their study of the effects of an individualised activity programme on elderly patients. The use of music and movement has proved invaluable in many institutions, not only for the physical benefits achieved but also for the sheer pleasure that is created. Copple (1983) gives striking evidence to support the work of Mary Bagot Stock who instigated a scientifically graded and recreational exercise system involving a rhythmic musical accompaniment. Although this particular project was community based, it could apply equally well in institutions.

The elderly people in hospital are frequently withdrawn and isolated. The stimulation of social interaction is therefore most important. Table games, sing-alongs, cookery, bingo, quizzes and discussions are a few examples (Fig. 7.3). Many activities used to this end also have features which are instructive. In the book *Care of the Long-Stay Elderly Patient* (Denham 1983) the potential of occupations such as poetry, art and music are explored (Fig. 7.4). They provide 'the opportunity to be, to act, to express, to manipulate, to rehearse, to listen, to participate, to practise, to perform. In such circumstances the patient is not the object of attention, the dependent one, but is to an increasing extent, the chooser, the mover, the doer' (Jones 1983, p 126).

The value of music and art as 'therapy' has in the past been underestimated since both have been regarded as mere entertainment. But many of the problems of old age such as adjustment, physical handicap, lethargy, apathy, loneliness and depression, can in part, at least, be alleviated by the use of these activities.

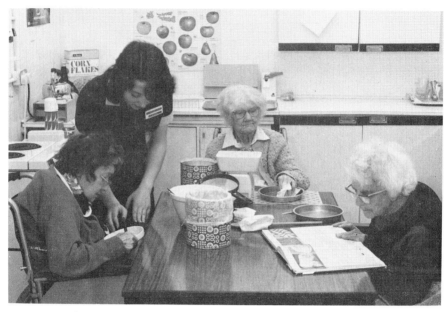

Fig. 7.3 Cookery.

Reality orientation

The majority of the activities already mentioned can, in one way or another, be employed as aids to orientation, but in recent years, the use of Reality Orientation (RO) has become an increasingly popular technique. An account of this method of treating confusion, disorientation and memory loss of the elderly, is provided in Chapter 18, by Julia Brooking.

Reminiscence and life-review

RO may involve a comparison of life present

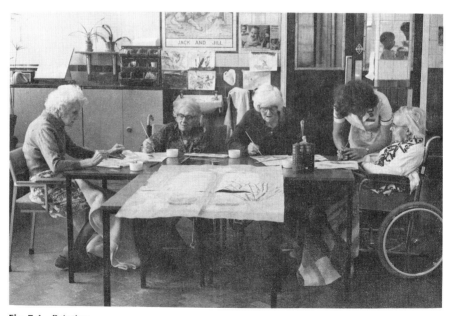

Fig. 7.4 Painting.

with life past. The role of reminiscence as part of the life-review process is well recognised but not always viewed positively, the elderly being accused of preoocupation with the past. Butler (1974) felt the life-review process to be preventative and therapeutic for the mental, social and physical well-being of the elderly. It is a method of coming to a conclusion about the value of life and the balance of achievement within it. Reminiscence is a normal and valuable part of that process (Kastenbaum 1979). Sharing reflections of the past can give a great deal of pleasure to both the listener and the teller (Fig. 7.5). It is an opportunity to look at the past objectively and thereby perhaps encourage a more positive assessment of one's past life. Preoccupation with the past is only detrimental if the past is denied, when it contributes to isolation.

Old people can be helped to reminisce simply by using tangible reminders of their past such as personal possessions; for example family albums, scrap-books and old letters (Holzapfel 1982). Help the Aged (1981) have produced a tape/slide programme called 'Recall' which covers topics from childhood (pre-First World War) to the Space Age. Other organisations are developing ideas along similar lines which focus on their local area and community. The familiar pictures and sounds draw lively and informative discussions which are much enjoyed by all those involved. Sessions can be supplemented by items of everyday use or records of old-time music, which can be especially evocative. Family and friends, too, have an important role to play and this is frequently forgotten in the routine of institutional life. They hold many keys to the past and may be able to help reinforce the identity and individuality of the person in care. Their involvement may also help them to view their relationship more positively. Many carers feel very guilty when an old person is taken into an institution. They need support and reassurance in order to adjust to their new role and to be reconciled with their relative. Their participation in reminiscence and RO can be invaluable.

Much of what we do every day with our patients contains constituents of both RO and reminiscence, and arises from a philosophy of care that involves a belief in the potential worth and value of old people. The elderly in institutions are, on the whole, dependent

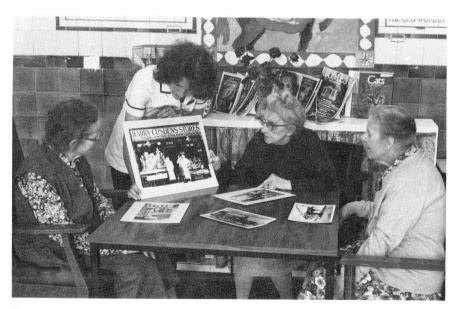

Fig. 7.5 Reminiscence.

on other people in order to achieve life satisfaction. Unfortunately, interprofessional conflicts and inadequate organisation of institutional routines often seems to work against the initiation of activity programmes (Davies 1982) even though their value is well recognised (Salter and Salter 1975). Change and overlap of roles are regrettably regarded as threatening instead of being viewed positively. Quality of life is a difficult concept to describe in concrete terms (Denham 1983) but its constituents are as applicable to us as to the old people we work with. We are the elderly of the future. If we recognise our own needs, likes and dislikes, we will see and understand many of theirs.

REFERENCES

Age Concern 1974a The attitudes of the retired and the elderly. Age Concern, London

Age Concern 1974b Elderly ethnic minorities. Age Concern, London

Age Concern 1978 Profiles of the elderly, their mobility and use of transport. Age Concern, London

Bromley D B 1974 Personality and adjustment in middle age and old age. In: Bromley D B (ed) The psychology of human ageing, 2nd edn. Penguin, London, p 235–240

Butler R 1974 Successful ageing and the role of life review. Journal of the American Geriatrics Society 12: 529–535

Cloke C 1983 Old age abuse in the domestic setting—a review. Age Concern, London

Comfort A 1974 Sexuality in old age. Journal of the American Geriatrics Society 12: 440–42

Comins J, Hurford F, Simms J 1983 Activities and ideas. Winslow Press, Buckingham

Cornish P 1983 Activities for the frail aged. Winslow Press, Buckingham

Copple P 1983 The concept of exercise. Nursing Times 79(32): 66–69

Davies A 1982 Research with elderly people in long term care: some social and organisational factors affecting psychological interventions. Ageing and Society 2: 285–298

Department of Health and Social Security 1982 Handbook of wheelchairs and bicycles and tricycles. DHSS, Blackpool

Denham M J (ed) 1983 Care of the long-stay elderly patient. Croom Helm, London

Foott S, Lane M, Mara J 1975 Kitchen sense for disabled or elderly people. The Disabled Living Foundation. Heinemann, London

Glyn-Jones A 1975 Growing older in a south Devon town. University of Exeter

Goffman E 1961 Asylums: essays on the social situation of mental patients and other inmates. Doubleday, New York

Goldsmith S 1976 Designing for the disabled, 3rd edn. RIBA, London

Hamill C, Oliver R 1980 Therapeutic activities for the handicapped elderly. Aspen, London

Help the Aged 1981 Recall. Help the Aged Education Department, London

Hendricks J, Hendricks C D 1977 Ageing in mass society, myths and realities. Winthrop, Cambridge, Mass

Holzapfel S 1982 The importance of personal possessions in the lives of the institutionalised elderly. Journal of Gerontological Nursing 8(3): 156–158

Jones S 1983 Education and life in the continuing care ward. In: Denham M J (ed) Care of the long stay elderly patient. Croom Helm, London, p 122–148

Kastenbaum R 1979 Growing old—years of fulfilment. Harper and Row, London

McCormack D, Whitehead A 1981 The effects of providing recreational activities on the engagement level of long-stay geriatric patients. Age and Ageing 10: 287–291

Millard P, Smith C 1981 Personal belongings—a positive effect? Gerontologist 21: 85–90

Powell R R 1974 Psychological effects of exercise therapy upon institutionalised geriatric mental patients. Journal of Gerontology 29: 157–161

Reichard S, Livson F, Peterson P G 1972 Ageing and personality. Wiley, New York

Salter C de L, Salter C 1975 Effects of an individualised activity programme on elderly patients. Gerontologist 15: 404–6

Schulz R 1980 Ageing and control. In: Garber J, Seligman M E P (eds) Human helplessness: theory and applications. Academic Press, New York

Tunstall J 1966 Old and alone. Routledge and Kegan Paul, London

Turner A (ed) 1981 The principles of the activities of daily living in the practice of occupational therapy. Churchill Livingstone, Edinburgh, p 31

Wedderburn C 1973 The aged and society. In: Brocklehurst J C (ed) Textbook of geriatric medicine and gerontology. Churchill Livingstone, Edinburgh, p 692–717

Wilshere E R 1976 Home management In: Equipment for the disabled, 3rd edn. Oxfordshire Area Health Authority, Oxford

Wilshere E R 1978 Personal care. In: Equipment for the disabled, 4th edn. Oxfordshire Area Health Authority, Oxford

Wilshere E R 1980 Communication. In: Equipment for the disabled, 5th edn. Oxfordshire Area Health Authority, Oxford

8

L. Batehup, A. Squires

Mobility

THE CONCEPT OF MOBILITY AND PREVALENCE OF IMMOBILITY

To be mobile implies the ability to move around. It is a wide and diverse term which encompasses mobility required to care for one's self and the home environment, to move around outside the home in order to obtain the necessities for living, to take part in the social life of a community and recreation, and to be able to visit friends and relatives. The wide aspect of mobility is reflected in the way it is defined. According to Ebersole and Hess (1981) 'mobility is the pattern of how and where one moves about in personal and life space'. Barker and Bury (1978) stress the social aspect of mobility when they state that mobility is the key to active access to community, neighbourhood or friendship involvement, and that to be housebound tends to be a state of non-participant dependence, while mobility means self-sufficiency and engagement. Norman (1981) emphasises the relative qualities of mobility, what may be relative immobility to one can be regarded as high level mobility to another. In this era of 'constant movement' and ease of travel over long distances, those who cannot move so easily are increasingly at a disadvantage.

Loss of mobility is a common problem for ageing persons. A survey by Abrams (1978), which amongst other things enquired about the domestic mobility of two groups of elderly people, found that for the age group 65–74 years, 11% of the sample had a problem getting around the house, with this proportion rising to 25% for the 75+ years age group. For the 65–74 years age group 8% had difficulty getting out of bed, and this rose to 15% for the 75+ age group. Limitations of mobility affect all aspects of daily life including washing, dressing, eating and going to the toilet. An earlier survey by Harris (1971) found that of the total population over 65 years of age, 27% suffered some impairment which limited their daily activities of living, and this proportion rose to 37% for those aged 75 years and over.

Prevalence of immobility

The level of mobility an individual is able to achieve is usually classified into: (i) the ability to move alone without difficulty; (ii) the need to have help going out; (iii) those who are housebound; (iv) those who are bedfast or chairfast. Within these groups there are wide variations. Those who are independent are usually able to negotiate pavements and roads and use public transport, while those who have difficulty are usually restricted to walking unless taken in a car. Those who are housebound or bedfast may be so temporarily because of ill health, but there still remains a group who are permanently either housebound or bedfast. The study by Hunt (1978) found that 1.9% of the over 85 years age group were permanently bedfast, and 18.7% were permanently housebound. In addition, 25% of the housebound lived alone and were therefore dependent on others to bring them the necessities for living. Furthermore, 42.5% of the bedfast and housebound had not been out of their houses for over a year, and 18.9% had not been out for three years. The conditions that are responsible for most mobility problems are of a chronic nature. These are arthritis and rheumatism, heart and lung conditions such as congestive cardiac failure and bronchitis, circulatory diseases, stroke illness, Parkinson's disease and problems with vision (Abrams 1978, Hunt 1978). There are, however, many people with mobility problems who report no illness or disability. Hunt (1978) reports that 44% of all men over 65 years, and 43.5% of all women 65 years and over with no illness or disability.

The role of physical fitness in maintaining mobility

Before discussing reasons for loss of mobility, the concepts of prolonging and maintaining functional capacity, especially of locomotor activity, into old age are briefly explored.

There is some agreement that in the absence of overt pathology there is often a slow decline in function with age, although individuals age at different rates. Also, different tissues and systems within a person demonstrate differences in rates of ageing (Weg 1975). One of the most critical age-related differences is the ability to respond to stress, both physical and emotional, and the rate of return to pre-stress levels of homeostasis (Selye 1970). This decrease in homeostatic capacity is most marked in neuroendocrine interaction. For the elderly person, stress reveals a declining capacity to achieve responses in, for example, heart rate, and blood pressure, and whether it be physical stress, as in exercise, or emotional stress, as in fear and anxiety, the rate of recovery by the individual is slower with increasing age. Gerontologists agree that there is a decline of approximately 1% per year in functional capacity in most organ systems *Shock 1962*, but it has been demonstrated that not all functional changes in older people are due to ageing. Some may be due to misuse or disease (de Vries 1970, 1974, and see Chapter 3).

Age-related changes in bone, muscle, and nervous tissue result in a decreased work capacity for the body. There is an overall decrease in bone mass which drops steadily from about the age of 45 years, and occurs more rapidly in women than in men (Exton-Smith 1978). This leads to a greater predisposition to fracture. There may be some thinning or even collapse of intervertebral discs. Muscle strength and size apparently diminish with age. There is prolongation of contraction time, latency period, and relaxation period by about 13%, and a decrease in the maximum rate of tension development (Goldman 1979). There are many changes with ageing in the nervous system, and also notable is the decrease in the overall co-ordinator–integrator role for the body's muscular, neuronal, glandular and circulatory systems (Shock 1962). Reduced efficiency of the heart muscle and contractile strength are reflected in a smaller cardiac output which is adequate for the average older person to function until additional and unaccustomed physical activity puts the individual under stress. When this happens, lower contractile strength, smaller cardiac output, and reduced enzymatic performance, cause the heart to respond to the work demand with less efficient performance and a greater energy expenditure than would be required by the same person years earlier (Ebersole and Hess 1981).

It is true in most western societies that habitual activity of a person declines as she becomes older, and at retirement she is expected to slow down and take things easily. The decline in physical activity with age is more evident in leisure occupations. A general finding is that the types of leisure activity change little with age, but as people grow older they spend less time in physical recreation and engage in them less energetically. A man in his twenties spends about five hours weekly in physical activities during his leisure time, but this is reduced to about three hours weekly when he is in his sixties (Lange et al 1978). A study by Wessel and Van Huss (1969) showed that age-related loss in physiological variables important to human performance were more highly related to the decreased habitual activity level than they were to age itself. The term 'hypokinetic disease' was first used by Kraus and Raab (1961) to describe the various bodily and mental derangements induced by inactivity, and may be one important factor involved in bringing about an age-related decrement in functional capacities (de Vries 1975). There is some support for this in a study by Saltin et al (1968), which describes changes similar to the age-related

changes mentioned above in well-conditioned young men after three weeks of enforced bed-rest. It was found that maximal cardiac output decreased by 26%, maximal ventilatory capacity by 30%, oxygen consumption by 30% and the amount of active tissue decreased by 1.5%. Thus it seems that inactivity can produce losses in function entirely similar to those brought about more slowly in the average individual when he grows more sedentary as he grows older. This brings into question the losses of function attributed to ageing, and raises the question of how much of the functional loss is due to long term deconditioning, and the sedentary life of the older individual.

There is now some interest in the possibility of improving the physical capacity of older individuals by exercise training. A study by de Vries (1970) looked at 112 men aged 52–87 years. These men took part in a vigorous exercise programme and were tested at regular intervals on the following parameters: blood pressure, percentage of body fat, resting neuromuscular activation, arm muscle strength and girth, maximal oxygen consumption and oxygen pulse at heart rate of 145, pulmonary function, and physical work capacity on the bicycle ergonometer. A subgroup were also tested for cardiac output, stroke volume, total peripheral resistance, and the work of the heart at a workload of 75 watts on the bicycle. The most significant findings were related to oxygen transport capacity. Oxygen pulse and minute volume at a heart rate of 145 improved by 29.4% and 35.2% respectively, and vital capacity improved by 19.6%. A subsequent study looked at older women aged 52–79 years who participated in a vigorous three month programme, and again physical fitness was improved (Adams and de Vries 1973). It seems that physical conditioning of the healthy older person can bring about significant improvements in the cardiovascular system, the respiratory system, the musculature and body composition. In general the result is a more vigorous individual who can also relax successfully. Other health benefits are likely to include a lower blood pressure and lower percentage of body fat, with concommitant lessening of the risk factors attributed to the development of coronary artery disease (de Vries 1975).

FACTORS AFFECTING MOBILITY

Psychological and socioenvironmental factors

For those individuals who are able to get out and about quite a high level of mobility is required. According to the Department of Transport (1975) 52% of journeys made by people over 65 years are made on foot, and it is the more frail elderly who rely on walking as opposed to using public transport. Use of buses requires the mastery of considerable obstacles particularly associated with getting on and off and moving about within a travelling bus (Robson 1978). The elderly pedestrian is more likely to be involved in a road traffic accident than the younger adult pedestrian, with a casualty rate for those aged 70 years and over being five times that of the 25–39 age group (Goodwin and Hutchinson 1976). The difficulties encountered are those of coping with fast traffic when crossing roads even at pedestrian crossings and traffic lights, in negotiating hills, narrow uneven pavements, and steps and kerbs.

The internal environment of the home can harbour hazards to safe mobility, including poor lighting, narrow dark stairs, and slippery rugs. The danger of this type of hazard will be mentioned later in relation to falls. It is possible to prolong independent mobility for the elderly by simple adaptations such as handrails and correct seat heights. In a survey of mainly elderly and arthritic people living at home, it was found that ease in rising was rated as the most important factor in their choice of an easy chair (Munton et al 1981). Compared with young adults, older people are observed to take longer to rise from a chair and to rely on handgrip for balance, and to use thrust from arms and leg muscles (Shipley 1980). Loss of muscle strength, and the effects of illness on joint flexibility and muscle co-ordination may be part of the reason for difficulties in rising from a chair, but the problem may lie with the

chair itself. Greater joint flexion and thrust will be needed if the seat platform and armrest are low, or the upholstery does not give firm support. A backward tilt in the angle of the seat or back support will require greater leaverage (Finlay et al 1983). Though not in itself sufficient, ease in rising is clearly necessary for mobility.

The effects of an institutional environment such as a hospital ward or nursing Home can be detrimental to the elderly person. Lieberman et al (1971) found that patients placed in a cold dehumanised dependency-fostering environment show decline. Marlowe (1973) compared two groups of patients in two different institutions, and found that those who became more active were in environments which encouraged autonomy and a personal approach, did not foster dependency by doing things for individuals that they could do for themselves, encouraged community integration and social interaction, and did not expect passivity and docility.

A home routine which includes walking to local shops, visiting friends or regularly walking a dog, may keep an elderly person fairly mobile. Admission to hospital for whatever reason will cut off these normal everyday reasons for getting out and about. Levels of mobility may rapidly deteriorate. It is probably true that many institutions, be they hospital wards or community Homes, foster dependency, unless it is a progressive atmosphere that encourages self-sufficiency. This may be related to the environment itself, or to the attitudes of the care staff. There is a tendency to overprotect elderly persons in institutions, to prevent them from moving around at will. This is a reflection of the fear for the person falling and sustaining an injury which will be blamed on inadequate supervision by nursing staff or relatives at home. If the mobile elderly person is not to deteriorate, and the rehabilitation of the person with impaired mobility is not to be impeded, then it is surely necessary to allow the individual more freedom of movement. Ensure that the environment is as safe and supportive as possible; by having beds chairs, toilets, at heights which make it easy to get in and out, on and off; by having non-slip floor surfaces, handrails good lighting, identification of doorways; and by making sure that the person has her glasses, hearing aid, and walking stick available if these are used. The choice to live dangerously is the prerogative of us all, and this should not be less so for elderly people.

Whether an individual retains a good functional level of mobility into old age is not totally reliant on physical ability or fitness, although it appears that medical problems are the major source of difficulties (Hunt 1978). Many people are mobile even though they suffer chronic conditions which cause much pain and discomfort, whilst others who are physically better may withdraw and become housebound. An individual's past experiences and others' perceptions and expectations of her and her abilities can together result in a reduction in mobility and activity. Loss of friends and relatives can reduce motivation required to make the effort to get out and about. Old people who on retirement move to a different geographical area can become isolated from their family and friends and become lonely, and this may be a cause of reduced mobility. Restriction or loss of mobility affects the ability of the individual to care for themselves adequately, and this may result in social isolation.

Physical factors

An individual's mobility and independence are reliant to a great extent upon the normal functioning of the nervous, musculoskeletal, circulatory, and respiratory systems in a co-ordinated and integrated manner to produce a normal gait and posture. Injury or disease of one or more of these systems may lead to impairment of gait with subsequent reduction or difficulty with mobility (Imms and Edholm 1981). Disorders of gait, balance, and posture are common in the elderly, and they account for a large number of admissions to medical, geriatric, and orthopaedic wards (Nayak et al 1982). The term gait is defined by Galley and Forster (1982) as 'the manner of walking', and

it includes locomotion or the act of moving from place to place. A 'gait cycle' consists of a step each by the right and left legs through the 'stance' and 'swing' phases. In normal walking, when approximately 50 to 60 steps/minute are taken, the stance phase comprises about 60% of the cycle and the swing phase 40%, with the two periods overlapping when the two feet are on the ground together for about 25% of the time (Galley and Forster 1982).

The gait of elderly people has been studied and compared with young normal subjects. Healthy old people showed on average a slower walking speed, shorter step length and lower frequency of stepping, with little difference in stride width (Guimaraes and Isaacs 1980). The slowing of the gait happened as a result of lengthening of the stance and double support phase, the period when both feet are on the ground simultaneously, with little change in the length of the swing phase. According to Azar and Lawton (1964) this alteration in gait seems to be a physiological concomitant of ageing and it differs between the sexes. Women typically adopt a narrow walking and standing base and walk with a waddle, whilst men use a wide walking and standing base and a small stepped gait. On the other hand, results of a study of gait and mobility of the elderly (Imms and Edholm 1981) suggest that chronological age has only a minor effect on gait and mobility with pathological changes being more important. Findings by Visser (1983) show that patients with senile dementia of Alzheimer's type walked more slowly, took shorter steps, had a lower frequency of stepping, and a higher double support ratio when compared with matched normal controls. These gait characteristics closely match those described for normal healthy old people, and so it is probably the degree to which these changes have taken place in various groups that are the important factors. Support for this comes from Guimaraes and Isaacs (1980), who found that a group of patients who were hospitalised following falls had shorter steps, narrower stride lengths, slower speed, wider range of frequency of stepping, and a wider degree of variability of step length when compared with patients who either had not fallen or had fallen and were not admitted. All the groups showed some features of abnormal gait, with the highest level of abnormalities occurring in the oldest most disabled group. The commonest gait abnormalities have been listed by Caird and Judge (1976):

1. Abnormal elevation of the hip of the moving limb owing to a stiff hip.
2. Elevation of the moving limb due to a stiff knee.
3. The waddling gait of patients with bilateral hip disease or proximal muscle weakness.
4. The circumduction of a spastic hemiplegic leg in which the foot moves in an arc of a circle during forward movement.
5. The scissors gait, with crossing of the feet due to adductor spasm from bilateral pyramidal lesions, or more rarely, osteoarthrosis of the hips.
6. The apparent unequal length of steps in a person with some degree of pyramidal tract disorder. The movements of the unafffected leg seem to carry the foot further than those of the affected leg.
7. The abnormal elevation of the limb, sometimes also with a little circumduction occuring in the presence of foot drop.
8. The shuffling gait with small hesitant steps particularly when beginning to walk and turning, of the patient with Parkinsonism. She also tends not to swing the arms normally.
9. The wide-based staggering gait of the person with cerebellar disease.
10. The shuffling and tottery gait with small steps of the patient with severe brain disease whether vascular or non-vascular, and severe intellectual impairment. In general, those with vascular brain disease tend to have increased muscle tone and reflexes, and those with non-vascular disease mild rigidity and slowing of movement, with reduced reflexes. Both gaits may be difficult to distinguish from the gait of Parkinson's disease, although the patient with severe brain disease does not tend to have any greater difficulty in turning.

It is well to remember that old people are likely to have more than one abnormality, and previous traumas and congenital deformities should be noted.

Gait should be assessed with the patient wearing her normal footwear, and the shoes or slippers themselves should be examined for particular areas of wear. All parts of walking, including starting, turning, and stopping need assessment on different types of flooring, but essentially in as similar condition to the patient's home as possible if assessment in the home is not possible.

GAIT AND MOBILITY PROBLEMS RELATED TO PATHOLOGICAL CAUSES

Parkinson's disease

Parkinsonism is a clinical syndrome characterised by a combination of rigidity and bradykinesia, and frequently including the following: resting tremor, a disorder of posture and balance, automonic dysfunction and dementia (Broe 1982). This syndrome produces a series of highly characteristic features which affect mobility. The standing posture is one of flexion of the knees, hips, trunk, neck, and elbows, with adducted shoulders. This posture has the tendency to push the centre of gravity too far forward resulting in a continuous acceleration of forward movement (festination) in order to prevent a forward fall. Or else the gait tends to be slow with small shuffling steps (Sabin 1982). Reduced ankle movements causes 'scuffing' of the toes, loss of heel strike, and the whole trunk and arms are moved as one unit with resultant loss of arm swing and shoulder rotation (Murray et al 1978).

This type of gait is highly unstable and falls are common. Individuals with this type of gait abnormality find it difficult or impossible to rise from a chair or bed. The sitting person fails to flex her legs close to her centre of gravity when trying to stand up, and so falls backwards. During walking, defective balance and righting mechanisms may cause the individual to lose balance when jostled, hurried, or when turning. The failure to lift the feet high enough off the ground means that tripping on such familiar and everyday things such as the edge of a carpet or a small irregularity on the floor, is likely. Difficulty in locomotion, i.e. inability to initiate or continue the forward shift of the body, can cause the person to remain rooted to the spot until given a small push which allows her to move her legs forward (Rosin 1982). Individuals may also have a tendency to run with small teetering steps—the 'festinating gait'.

It is obvious, therefore, that the range and speed of movements in Parkinsonian patients alter their ability to control locomotion, and it is thought that this gait pattern may be the result of adaptation to gain control of forward movement and balance with the actual power of motor control (Knutsson 1972). The effects of Parkinsonism vary in the degree to which they are seen in different individuals with only the severist sufferers displaying all these features. Patients with mobility problems related to Parkinson's disease require careful assessment in order to identify the abnormal patterns, and this should be followed by a programme of techniques and training to help alleviate the problem.

Hemiplegia

The effects of a stroke on mobility are usually catastrophic, ranging from complete immobility, bedfast or chairfast, to a highly unstable staggering type of gait. From various studies it is understood that the inability of the hemiplegic patient to walk in a normal fashion appears to be related to:

1. Abnormal muscular activity resulting in loss of selective movement patterns.
2. A disorder of the normal postural mechanism—the righting and equilibrium reflexes.
3. A sensory deficit (Wall and Ashburn 1979).

The abnormal muscular patterns are usually characterised by increased flexion of the muscles of the upper limbs, trunk and neck, and increased extension of the muscles of the lower limbs. If the patient is able to walk, the hip is retracted with the leg hitched forward at the pelvis and with the toe or sole of the foot hitting the floor first rather than the heel. There may also be toe drag and inversion of the ankle. The affected leg is 'favoured' with the patient spending more time supported on the unaffected side. Disordered balance mechanisms result in an inability to sit without falling to the affected side, or to walk without leaning and perhaps falling to the affected side. These patients seem to be incapable of the integrated action necessary to align the body segments and bring their centre of gravity into balance with their feet below it (Adams 1974). The problems are further compounded by deficits in sensation and proprioception, so that signals from peripheral muscles and joints and from the environment are misinterpreted or not attended to at all. The combination of all these effects results in varying degrees of mobility restriction with loss of ability to attend to a wide range of activities of living. These patients require an intensive programme of retraining. Methods of therapeutic exercise described by Bobath (1978) aim to facilitate normal patterns of movement in response to tactile and proprioceptive stimuli, whilst inhibiting abnormal patterns of muscular activity. In addition, many activities of living have to be relearnt and a safe and stimulating environment provided. There are several sources that describe rehabilitation methods for stroke patients (Johnstone 1977, Bobath 1978, Batehup 1983, Myco 1983) and further discussion can be found later in this chapter.

Arthritic conditions

The commonest type of arthritic conditions which affect the elderly are osteoarthrosis and rheumatoid arthritis (Wright 1983), and it is generally acknowledged that these conditions are an important cause of mobility problems for the elderly.

Osteoarthrosis can be radiologically detected in almost all ederly people though it may be symptomless (Lawerence et al 1966). Generalised osteoarthrosis describes a widespread pattern of synovial joint involvement including as well as hips and knees, terminal interphalangeal joints and thumb bases, with ankles and shoulders usually spared (Bird 1983).

Rheumatoid arthritis is a chronic systemic disorder affecting primarily the peripheral joints through inflammation and proliferation of the synovial membrane (Stevens 1983). The pattern of joint involvement is additive and symmetrical especially affecting proximal interphalangeal and metacarpophalangeal joints, wrists, knees, and small joints of the feet, but may also affect elbows, ankles, shoulders and hips (Stevens 1983). With some exceptions, the elderly person with inflammatory rheumatoid disease will have reached a 'burnt out' stage (Agate 1983), and, in common with osteoarthrosis, the most serious effects for an individual's mobility arises from problems in the main weight-bearing joints of the hips and knees. Pain and flexion contractures of hips with instability in the knee joints contributes particularly to immobility. To rise out of a chair or climb stairs, for example, requires a 90° range from almost full extension, and for ease in performing these activities a range of 110° flexion is necessary (Chamberlain 1983) in at least one leg.

Restoration of lost mobility can be especially difficult when the cause is arthritis of the rheumatoid type. Too often a permanent contracture in flexion of the knee for example has become established, and taking weight through such an abnormal joint is often very painful. It appears that attempts to correct flexion deformities with exercise or surgery for elderly patients is not wholly successful for a variety of reasons (Agate 1983), and prevention of this type of contracture in youth or middle age determines what capabilities exist when the patient reaches old age. This relies on enlightened care from doctors, nurses and physiotherapists. Much of what has been said also applies to osteoarthrosis, but it may be easier with the elderly osteoarthritic patient to reverse the immobility resulting from disuse.

This can only be done by controlling pain, persuading the patient to stand and extend bent knees and hips, and straighten back and neck, and if necessary to walk with the help of some sort of aid. If in bed, patients should be encouraged to extend their knees and hips and to avoid pillows under the knees. It is usually the case that the aim is not to return the person to work or some other form of outside activity, but rather to enable her to walk slowly and safely on one floor of a house, dress, and manage the toilet. Attention should also be paid to techniques of rising from and sitting down in chair, bed or toilet. This limited range of mobility may be the difference between dependence and independence.

Amputation

Seventy-five per cent of new lower limb amputees are over the age of 60 years, and most have lost their limbs because of peripheral vascular disease or diabetic gangrene (Van de Ven 1984). These patients often have the associated problems of cardiac involvement, low exercise tolerance, arteriosclerosis with possible hemiplegia and diminished mental ability.

In the early stages after surgery it is important that attention is given to the position of the stump which should be extended at hip and knee and not raised on a pillow. A board under the mattress will help. According to Nichols (1976) the three main factors contributing to the development of contractures after amputation are: pain, spasm, and immobility and bad posture either in bed or chair. Effective pain relief should help the muscle spasm. It is important that the stump should be positioned as stated, and lying prone with a pillow under the trunk for short periods throughout the day also helps to prevent contractures. Control of oedema in the stump by effective bandaging is essential to promote healing (Van de Ven 1984).

The team will decide on the most appropriate mobility regime and the condition of the remaining leg is an important factor. If an artificial limb is to be provided for mobility or aesthetic purposes, it should be worn as much as possible in order to maintain the shape of the stump. Protective footwear is advisable for the other leg. Wheelchair mobility may be more realistic for some elderly patients. A stump board on which the chair cushion is placed so that the stump can be extended, will prevent oedema and contractures. Boards can be provided for bilateral stumps, and can be folded down when the patient transfers or stands. The psychological benefits of being able to move around again should not be underestimated. Even though wheelchair mobility has to be accepted for some frail elderly persons, rehabilitation should never lack urgency, because in its own terms it can be highly successful in returning the person to an appropriate, largely domestic routine (Crowther 1982). Once mobility begins, it should continue as part of the day's routine. The patient should be encouraged to maintain an upright posture with weight bearing through the stump, so reducing the possibility of a circumduction gait. Some patients find the loss of one leg gives balance problems because of the altered weight distribution, and double amputees may find a similar problem in sitting because they feel unbalanced.

Falls

Falls are a major problem for elderly people. It is not unusual to find that a person suffering from recurrent falls becomes housebound, even chair- or bedbound, immobile, demoralised and dependent upon the support of the social services (Exton-Smith and Overstall 1979). The majority of falls in old age result from a combination of factors. The ageing process, disease, drugs, and external hazards may all contribute (Campbell et al 1981). The rates of falls occurring in various settings have been reported in many studies. Exton-Smith (1977) found, in a survey of elderly people at home, that 31% of men and 47% of women over the age of 80 years reported falling. Brocklehurst et al (1978) found that in a group over the age of 85 years 46% had fallen during the previous year, and Overstall et al (1977)

reported that 50% of his subjects aged 60 years and over had fallen for various reasons. This is obviously a problem of some magnitude. The outcome of falls is not always of a serious physical nature, but undoubtedly always causes some loss of confidence. The most common serious consequence of a fall for an older person is a fracture of the proximal femur (Fernie et al 1982).

Activity at the time of fall

Falling at home occurs most often in the bedroom or sitting-room, or when going to the toilet (Brocklehurst et al 1976, Wild et al 1981b). The study by Wild et al (1981b) shows that high numbers of falls occur on change of position such as getting up from bed, chair or toilet, going up stairs or walking on an irregular surface. There are also a large number of falls which happen unexpectedly with no accompanying symptoms or external hazards. In institutions most falls are associated with getting in or out of bed, on or off a chair, and when using the toilet or commode (Rodstein 1964, Ashley et al 1977).

Causes of falls

There is agreement that falls of the elderly can be attributed to extrinsic or intrinsic factors or a combination of both. Extrinsic factors include a wide range of environmental hazards such as loose carpets, trailing wires, dark stairs, uneven floors. Intrinsic factors include postural hypotension, cardiac dysrhythmias, muscle weakness, cervical spondylosis, and balance and righting problems. According to Wild et al (1981a) the concept that a fall in old age has 'a cause' is inadequate, and they contend that the attribution of falls to perceived pathogenic mechanisms is often conjectural. Doctors rarely witness the fall, and so the 'cause' is often diagnosed from a combination of the patient's statement and the doctor's physical findings. Their evidence suggests that the patient's statements even when most carefully collected are not by themselves a very good guide to the possible cause. The elderly people in this study used the terms dizziness, giddiness, blackout, and light-headedness when describing what happened, but all these terms lack a precise and unambiguous meaning. Falls result from uncorrected displacement of the body from its support base, which implies a difficulty with control of balance and posture.

Balance and falls

The term 'loss of balance' is frequently used in two different ways. It describes the single fall of a healthy person which is not otherwise explained by an accidental trip, and it describes those recurrent falls of a person who cannot maintain the upright posture unsupported. (Isaacs 1982). It is also a term frequently heard in relation to elderly people, and implies usually that balance has been lost.

Balance is the set of functions which keeps the body upright during stance and loco-motion by detecting and correcting displacements of the line of gravity beyond the support base (Isaacs 1982). The centre of gravity is the equivalent point within the body at which the whole body-weight may be considered to act, and in the upright position it lies within the pelvis at approximately the upper sacral region anterior to the second sacral vertebra (Galley and Forster 1982). It is beyond the scope of this chapter to describe the components of the balance mechanism in any great detail, but briefly these include:

1. *Afferrent mechanisms*, which detect displacements; these include vision, vestibular, and proprioceptive organs.
2. *Central mechanisms*, which receive and integrate information from the periphery and issue corrective instructions; these include stretch reflexes, righting reflexes, long loop reflexes which help to control gait and posture, unexpected disturbances and voluntary movement, and tend to restore conditions to their previous state before displacement occurred (Grimm and Nashner 1978).
3. *Efferrent mechanisms*, which transmit instructions to the muscles, including cells in the motor cortex and their connections with the spinal motor neurones, motor units, muscle fibres.

The rate of falls of the elderly has already been mentioned and it corresponds closely with failure of the balance mechanism in old age. The mechanisms involved in balance are particularly susceptible to age-related changes. According to Hasselkus (1974), although feedback is impaired by changes in joints, muscle spindles, and peripheral nerves, it is the slowing of central processes in the brain which perceive and integrate proprioceptive signals that is mainly responsible for increased reaction time. Therefore, the elderly person who stumbles finds that the speed of her postural reflexes is too slow to prevent a fall, and she has failed to correct the displacement of the body from its support base. Wild et al (1981a) have devised a classification of falls which is based on this idea. A fall or displacement can be of two types—initiated and imposed—and of two degrees—ordinary and extraordinary.

Initiated displacements are falls which the person herself induces in the course of her activities such as rising from a chair or bed, or during walking when the line of gravity is momentarily displaced beyond the support base. An 'ordinary initiated displacement' might result from an error on standing up, whilst an 'extraordinary initiated displacement' could be a fall from a chair or ladder or a sudden change of direction.

Imposed displacements are falls which occur from factors in the outside world such as irregular surfaces, and unexpected obstacles like pets and small grandchildren. There is normally sufficient capacity in the recovery mechanism for the detection and correction of the displacement, but as the balance mechanism becomes less efficient in later life the range and speed of recovery is reduced. An 'ordinary imposed displacement' might result from a trip on a loose carpet. An 'extraordinary imposed displacement' could occur when slipping on a patch of ice or a wet floor, or if a dog runs unexpectedly into one's path. Various medical factors such as reduced visual and vestibular function, reduction in proprioceptive mechanisms, pathology in the brain or spinal cord, and diseases of the peripheral nerves and muscles, may impair the balance mechanism. The advantage of this classification is that it becomes possible to categorise a fall on the basis of the information obtained from the patient or other onlookers, and may therefore be of some help in the prevention of falls (see Table 8.1).

Advanced old age is accompanied by an increased probability of falling even in quiet domestic surroundings. The elderly adjust their gait to diminish the danger of falling by shortening and slowing the pace, broadening the base and lowering the height of their step (Murray et al 1978). Those at risk of falling are people aged 75 years and over who are housebound, who walk with shuffling irregular steps, and have a fear of falling whilst on their feet. Little evidence was found to support the statements frequently made that falls in old

age are often caused by cervical spondylosis, vertebrobasilar ischaemia, etc. (Wild et al 1981b).

ASSESSING AND MANAGING IMMOBILITY

The multiple pathologies associated with ageing bring with them multiple problems, and for rehabilitation to be effective, a thorough functional assessment of the patient is essential to identify the real barriers to independence and facilitate discharge. It is important to be realistic about the potential for rehabilitation, and predicting the potential has been examined in Scotland, where it was found that bowel and bladder control, and the ability to walk, together with minimal loss of mental clarity, was significant in the discharge potential of elderly patients (Stewart 1980).

The physiotherapist's assessment is aimed mainly at the components required for

Table 8.1 Prevention of falls

Displacement	Example	Causes	Prevention
Extraordinary imposed	Patch of ice Dog running into path	Environmental hazards	Avoid hazard Improve environment. Accidental falls due to an unsafe environment such as loose carpets, wet floors, dark stairs, account for a third to a half of all falls (Exton-Smith and Overstall 1979). Slippers and bare feet contribute to falls (Wild et al 1981)
Ordinary imposed	Trips on rug or carpet	Trivial hazard Impaired perception of displacement	Correct hazard Patients with a history of falls place their feet unpredictably and may induce a displacement of which they are unaware (Guimaraes and Isaacs 1981). Perception of unsafe gait and retraining may be possible
Extraordinary iniated	Sudden movement of head	Hurried action	Teaching to help match activities to balance mechanisms, so that range and speed of activities is diminished to remain within the person's reduced competence
Ordinary iniated	Error on standing up	Disease Drugs	Identify cause The importance of psychotropic drugs in causing impaired balance of old people is increasingly recognized (Macdonald & Macdonald 1977). Wild et al (1981) found that fallers were taking significantly more hypnotics, tranquilizers, and sedatives than were a matched control group

mobility, whilst the occupational therapist will focus attention on the daily living needs for that person. Assessment is a continuing process and needs constant review. The initial assessment provides a baseline for the evaluation of subsequent treatments (Parry 1980). All professional staff have a legal and moral responsibility to do what is right for the patient, and failure to assess thoroughly may be viewed as negligence (Association of District and Superintendent Physiotherapists 1984). It is important to remember the atypical disease presentation, and biological factors which may affect rehabilitation, such as reduced exercise tolerance (Payton and Poland 1983). Also, an elderly person with a limited life expectancy may have different priorities to those of a younger person.

Occupation

The term old age pensioner gives no insight into the life of the person being assessed. Time spent enquiring into the occupations held by the patient will give a fascinating view of a disappearing era, and may also indicate the physical tolerance likely to be available from either the work or recreational pursuits described. The last or current job held by an old person has been described as an 'end occupation' such as caretaker or commissionaire, and previous occupations or hobbies should be investigated. There may have been contact with lead in metalwork or paint, leaving the patient with signs of neurological dysfunction; or with dust, resulting in chest diseases. Industrial accidents and occupational hazards may have left the person with joint damage or limb deformity, and the neurological signs indicating the tertiary stages of syphilis, such as tremor and spastic paresis together with dementia, should not be overlooked.

Diagnosis

Pathology increases with age which means that a single symptom such as a stiff joint may have more than one cause. In addition, co-existing disorders may require treatments which are acceptable for one problem, but contraindicated for another. An example here is rheumatoid arthritis and spastic hemiplegia. Passive movements may be contraindicated in the former because of soft tissue involvement, but necessary in the latter to try to prevent contractures forming. The therapists must decide which problem poses the greater risk and select the appropriate treatment for each individual patient.

Brief history

This can reveal the main problem if time is taken to investigate. In many cases breakdown in the person's ability to cope at home leads to hospital admission, and setting up domiciliary services may be more beneficial than rehabilitating someone who was managing quite well at home. On the other hand, the breakdown may reveal a situation that has been deteriorating for some time, and illness of the home help prevents the elderly person carrying on. The practice of domiciliary visiting by geriatricians to elderly patients at home, following a general practitioner's request, has reduced hospital admissions by up to 59% when alternative help was offered (Arcand and Williamson 1981).

Social circumstances

As the majority of elderly patients are referred from home, knowledge of the accommodation and available support is essential. Realistic rehabilitation cannot occur without information of door widths for walking aids, number of stairs and the siting of the toilet, etc. Relatives, friends, community nurses and social services staff can often provide valuable information, and a visit to the home by a member of the team, preferably with the patient, early during her hospital stay is an advantage. The treatment of the patient within her own home has obvious advantages, but has yet to be fully developed in terms of community physiotherapy, and the social advantages of attending for outpatient treatment should not be overlooked.

Motivation

This is really the key to whether treatment is going to be effective or not, and motivation is just as necessary for the staff as for the patient. When one considers the incentives of the company, warmth, and interest provided in a hospital, it is not surprising that discharge home may sometimes be resisted. A similar situation may occur when a community nurse visits a lonely person at home and is her only visitor.

Communication

It is essential to check that the assessor and the patient can communicate with each other. This not only means checking speech, sight and hearing, but also language and dialect. The increasing number of people from ethnic minorities now reaching old age in this country is posing a challenge for health professionals. The old person may not have learnt English, or if a second language it may have been lost, which happens to people suffering with dementia or a stroke. An assessment of the patient's mental status should have been completed at the time of admission and this will be a useful indication of the level of mental ability that can be expected. Reassessment at intervals is essential and can reveal improvements in mental ability as the patient settles down to her new environment and becomes less confused. Denham and Jeffreys (1972) showed that a more realistic rehabilitation programme could be planned when the intellectual ability was known.

Physical assessment and management

Neck

This can be a potent source of problems for old people. Intervertebral discs begin to degenerate from the second decade of life. The mechanics of the cervical spine are therefore altered and abnormal movement produces an increase in osteophyte activity and may subsequently cause cervical spondylosis. The increased bone formed can cause pressure on nerve roots, vertebral artery or even the spinal cord, with the resultant problems of altered sensation, muscle weakness and reduced blood supply to the brain. The lower vertebrae tend to be more affected, and the first signs reported by the patient are usually weakness in the legs (Jeffreys 1980).

Unfortunately, little can be done except to advise less movement of the neck. Surgical collars have little to offer as they seldom fit and cannot be easily applied and removed. A cheaper and aesthetically more acceptable, and probably more benefical, solution is to wear a thick scarf which will act as a warmer and will remind the patient not to turn her head too quickly. If the elderly person spends lengthy periods sitting in an armchair, this may increase the tendency to a flexion deformity of the neck, and a chair which allows relaxation in an upright posture may be more suitable.

Trunk

Thoracic deformities rarely start in old age and are usually congenital problems which were untreated owing to lack of facilities or finance. The main exceptions are deformities resulting from osteoporosis (Caird and Judge 1976). The consequences of thoracic deformity are that chest expansion will be reduced owing to calcification of the cartilages, and exercise tolerance and a powerful cough may also be reduced. Again the condition cannot be reversed, but giving advice to the patient on posture in front of a mirror may prevent further deterioration, and diaphragmatic breathing can be taught so that as much of the lung capacity as possible is used. A wary eye should be kept on the deformity in case a pressure sore should develop on the apex of the curve, and attention to seating may be needed. Pain may be present from spinal deformity or joint degeneration, or wedge fracture of the vertebrae which occurs spontaneously in osteoporotic spines. One in 20 people over the age of 70 years experiences crush fractures of the spine (Nordin 1983). Surgical corsets may give some relief but are expensive, cumbersome and seldom worn correctly, and are often welcomed mainly for the warmth they offer, or worn out of habit. The elasticated abdominal support corsets can provide some support also to the lumbar and lower thoracic spine, and are easier to put on, washable, cheaper and warm, and can be supplied 'off the shelf'. Should a treasured corset be worn, it should be checked and renewed if necessary. Abdominal weakness is common in old age owing to poor posture and lack of exercise. Anyone undertaking a frantic keep fit campaign after Christmas excesses will know the exceptional amount of effort required to strengthen these muscles, and although some strength can be regained by 'bridging exercises' on the bed and 'sit forwards' on the chair, it may be that aids such as a bed ladder to get out of bed, and a wheeled frame to walk with will be needed as well.

Upper limbs

Assessment of the upper limbs will depend on the patient's requirements. A person living alone will need to be able to dress, cook and eat independently, whilst a patient living in sheltered accommodation may have help with some of these activities.

In old age the hands in particular can often provide a vivid picture of the life that has been led, showing callus formation, deformities and scars. In terms of function we must know what the patient needs to do and what is preventing her from doing it. An assessment of joint range and muscle power and sensation will show deficiencies, especially if compared with the opposite limb; and treatments to relieve pain, improve strength and range can be devised for the individual patient. Elevation of the arm will provide an indication of shoulder range and strength. Gripping the assessor's hand and trying to pull her or push her, will assess grip strength and elbow mobility. The patient's hand should also be assessed for fine movements such as picking up a small object such as a pencil, or doing up a button. The ability to bring the hand to the mouth for eating will also assess range, strength, and co-ordination.

Muscle power is best assessed by comparing it with the opposite limb. The Medical Research Council gradings can be a useful baseline from which to work:

Grade 0 No contraction felt or seen
Grade 1 Flicker of activity felt or seen
Grade 2 Production of movement with gravity eliminated
Grade 3 Production of movement against gravity
Grade 4 Production of movements against gravity and an additional force
Grade 5 Normal power.

The hemiplegic patient who has had a severe stroke is likely to have a painful dislocated shoulder owing to the loss of muscle tone (Lind 1982), and so great care should be taken when handling and moving these patients. The patient may be unaware of the affected side and may even disown it, and she should be taught to attend to it by being encouraged to look for it, and handle and exercise it. Oedema is also a problem, and elevation throughout the day and night on a pillow will usually reduce it by means of gravity, but a lapse in surveillance allowing the patient's hand to become dependent for even a short time will undo all the work the elevation achieved.

Massage may improve fluid absorption and venous return, and excellent results have been reported with pressure therapy units. The limb is elevated and placed within an air pressure sleeve, and air pumped into the sleeve provides gentle pressure on the limb so that similar effects to massage are achieved. The pressure can be individually selected for each patient, and can be constant, pulsed, or sequential in mode (Pflug 1975). Slings have gone out of favour in recent years as they

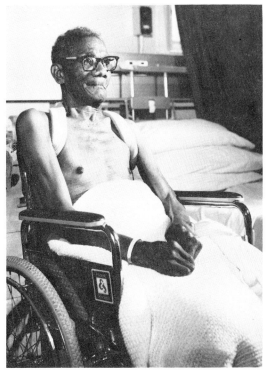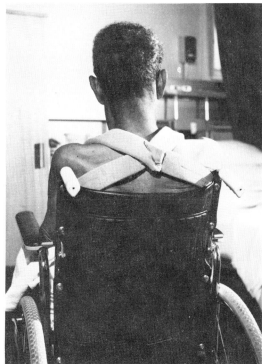

Fig. 8.1 Shoulder support for left hemiplegic patient: (a) front view; (b) rear view.

reinforce the flexor spasticity of the hemiplegic arm, which may be in flexion, adduction, pronation, and internal rotation, and it is this spasticity which may contribute to subluxation (Bobath 1982). The arm is also prevented from functioning whilst encased in the sling. A more useful support is the 'figure of eight' bandage traditionally used for a fractured clavicle (Fig. 8.1), with the addition of a roll of foam placed in the axilla of the affected side. This supports the shoulder and leaves the arm free for exercise (Bobath 1982).

Lower limbs

The lower limbs also require a functional assessment of joint range, strength and sensation. If the patient has to use the stairs, then hip, knee, and ankle mobility is necessary. The ability to rise from a chair and walk on the level must be assessed. There may be reduced range of movement of the ankles, and compensation for this may have to be taught, such as lifting the feet slightly higher to prevent tripping. Some deformities may be found, particularly of the knee, but perseverance by the patient and therapist, and application of innovative splints by the orthotist can overcome tremendous odds. In addition, the patient's feet must be examined, as painful feet will not welcome walking practice at any age, and may have been the cause of immobility in the first place.

Oedema of the lower limbs is a frequent problem for the elderly, and this may be gravitational owing to inability to get into bed and elevate the legs at night. This should be investigated, especially if the patient is attending hospital as an outpatient and practices at home are not known. Pressure therapy has been found to be effective in oedema of the lower limbs (Pflug 1975), and the patient should be encouraged to elevate the legs during the day between treatments and to go to bed at night.

The advice of the chiropodist should be

sought. Shoes must be suitable and often attempts at rehabilitation are wasted when insufficient attention is paid to footwear. Suitable shoes that can be put on and taken off by the patient unaided are available. Slippers with adequate support and non-slip soles are also available for those with limited mobility, or for protection, and patients and relatives need advice before buying footwear. Shoes which will require any adaptation such as a raise or caliper must be well constructed, and advice should be sought. Unequal leg length should be checked and a decision made as to whether a raise should be applied or not. The patient may have adapted to long standing shortening, but recent shortening, particularly from hip surgery needs correction.

A caliper, if worn, should be examined and the repairs organised early. Fewer calipers are supplied these days as different treatment approaches have emerged, but some patients require supports, and the possibility should not be overlooked. The ability of the patient to get the caliper on and off and actually function with it must be assessed, and practice should be encouraged as with all daily living activities.

Skin condition

Although the nurse will be aware of any skin condition that the patient has, the other members of the team may not, and sharing this information is essential. For instance one method of teaching transfers from a wheelchair to bed is to slide from one position adjacent to another. If a gluteal sore is present or likely, such friction will make it worse. Another method of transfer could be used, such as standing up from the chair, turning and sitting down on the adjacent bed, and this would prevent the friction risk. Any suspect areas should be discussed to ensure no further risk is entailed. For example, although bandaged leg ulcers of female patients wearing skirts are visible, those concealed under trousers are hidden and should be brought to the therapist's attention.

Assessment scales

Assessment of physical activities and abilities after a stroke has presented many problems which are due mainly to the complexity of recovery patterns and difficulties in achieving objective and valid measurement tools. The assessment of other disabling conditions such as arthritis, Parkinson's disease, and amputation, in common with stroke illness, includes such aspects as activities of living, mobility, independence, motor deficit and neuromuscular performance. A discussion of assessment scales for stroke recovery therefore has relevance for the assessment of other chronic conditions.

Many scoring devices have been described to grade functional capacity and improvement during the rehabilitation process. Generally, these have been divided into organ system assessments, such as skeletal neuromuscular assessments (DeSouza et al 1980, Sheikh et al 1980, Ashburn 1982), and assessment of purposeful activities, such as eating, dressing, standing, walking, usually referred to as activities of living (ADL) (Katz et al 1963, Mahoney and Barthel 1965, Schoening and Iversen 1968, Sheikh et al 1979). For the purposes of research, it has been the practice for each study to develop its own assessment tools, and this tendency is criticised in a report by a group reviewing rehabilitation research and methods (Lancet 1982). This group identified 27 ADL scales, all of them representing minor variations on a common theme. Yet, if different therapeutic interventions in different settings are to be compared, a core of agreed measures has to be developed. In addition, many hospitals and rehabilitation centres have their own assessment tools which are used in physiotherapy and occupational therapy departments, and which are in the main untested.

Two assessment tools which may prove useful for widespread use are the motor assessment form for measuring physical disabilities following stroke (Ashburn 1982), and the ADL index devised for the Northwick

Park stroke rehabilitation trial (Sheikh et al 1979), which has since been used for assessing disability across a wide range of conditions in a rehabilitation centre (Parish and James 1982). A combination of these measures would provide a comprehensive picture of a patient's progress towards recovery, and in addition could be used for comparing different therapeutic techniques. Accurate measurement of disability is an essential component of rehabilitation, it provides a clear record of the patient's functional abilities, and should lead to the patient being discharged into a setting which is appropriate to her needs.

Problems associated with loss of balance, co-ordination and gait

The factors affecting balance have been described earlier. For treatment to be effective, a thorough clinical examination is necessary and it should be remembered that similar symptoms can be produced by several pathologies occurring together.

The problems related to loss of balance and co-ordination which can be treated by physiotherapy include the following conditions.

Pain. Pain can be reduced by heat or ice, both of which produce vasodilation which relieves vascular congestion and causes a reduction in the activity of the pain receptors (Lee and Warren 1978). Pain often causes muscle spasm and can therefore affect balance. Pain relief can also be achieved by transcutaneous nerve stimulation and by massage, which stimulate large diameter nerve fibres to close the 'gate' and reduce pain transmission (Melzack and Wall 1965).

Spasticity. Spasticity arises from hyperexcitability of the strech reflex following an upper motor neurone lesion such as a cerebrovascular accident (Young and Delwaide 1981). The increase in skeletal muscle tone can produce patterns of abnormal flexion or extension. The posture and anxiety level of the patient at the time of assessment will affect the degree of spasticity. Spasticity is never confined to a single muscle but affects various muscle groups. Treatment by ice depresses the nerve conduction in the afferent nerves and reduces muscle tone (Lee and Warren 1978). Exercise of the muscle group antagonistic to those in spasm will reduce the spasticity (Knott and Voss 1968). Rhythmical passive movements through a normal pattern may also help (Cash 1977). The most important component in promoting mobility of patients with spasticity is to start from a stable base, and patients should not be encouraged to mobilise until they have achieved a stable sitting and standing balance.

Reduced sensory input. A reduction in the activity of any of the senses which affect posture can occur in old age. Because of visual changes, older people may have trouble in assessing adequately environmental hazards. For example, there is a decline in visual acuity, with the pupil decreasing in size and becoming less responsive to changes in light (Riffle 1982). The older person requires more illumination in order to see well. With ageing, depth perception may become impaired (Riffle 1982), so the elderly person needs to be made aware of this change in relation to stepping off kerbs or stairs, and place her foot more consciously than before. Physical methods should be used to compensate wherever possible, for instance wearing spectacles and hearing aids. It is difficult, however, to compensate for lack of skin sensation and proprioception but knowledge that they exist is important.

Imbalance of muscle power. The treatment of muscle weakness is by repetitive exercise, preferably in the normal pattern for that part of the body, such as in proprioceptive neuromuscular facilitation techniques. Sensory stimulation over the working muscles increases input to the motor neurone pools, and techniques incorporating a stretch stimulation will also increase the input. Joint traction force assists flexion patterns, and joint compression facilitates extension patterns, as can be seen in normal weight bearing where the extensor patterns of the leg are brought into action. Stimulation can also be gained by using the body's natural righting reflexes (Atkinson 1977).

The Bobath method, which is suitable for a mixture of flaccid and spastic muscles as seen in hemiplegia, gives emphasis to re-educating movement in a bilateral way. The aim is to normalise tone and facilitate normal movement. The patient should be discouraged from using the unaffected arm and leg to compensate for the affected limb. Elderly patients with multiple pathology, which may include poor intellectual functioning, must be carefully assessed for a treatment regime which will be realistic for their needs. The whole team must be advised of the plan and must apply it continuously, from positioning of the unconscious patient through to mobilisation.

Positioning the hemiplegic patient

Following a stroke the patient is left with a variety of sensory and motor deficits including loss of sensation, visuospatial disturbances, disorders of body image, muscle paralysis, posture and balance disturbances, and abnormalities of muscle tone. By adequate positioning and handling of the patient, it is possible to prevent an undue increase in spasticity, contractures and shoulder pain (Parry and Eales 1976, Bobath 1982). The approach to positioning the stroke patient should be a co-operative effort with an informed patient and carer working with the nurses and physiotherapists to provide a consistent positioning routine.

It is helpful if the bed is firm and of variable height with locking wheels. This provides support for the whole body and aids the patient when transferring from bed to chair. If possible the bed should be placed to allow for an adequate amount of stimulation to the affected side.

Lying on the back (Fig. 8.2). This position should be used as little as possible because it encourages extensor spasm (Johnstone 1977). The patient's head should be supported on one pillow and follow the straight line of the spine. The affected arm should be extended alongside the patient's body with the shoulder elevated. This can be achieved by placing a pillow lengthways under the shoulder and arm. The affected hip is supported on a pillow to prevent retraction and external rotation of the leg. Nothing should be placed in the patient's hand or against the sole of the foot as this encourages flexor spasticity. This applies to all positions.

Lying on the affected side (Fig. 8.3). The patient's head should be supported on one pillow and follow the straight line of the spine. The affected arm should be eased forward with the palm of the hand uppermost. The affected leg is extended at the hip with the knee slightly flexed. The other leg is

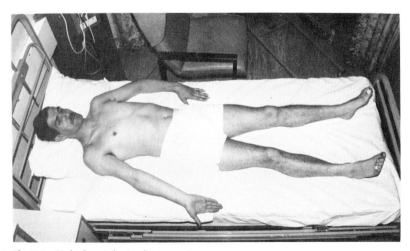

Fig. 8.2 Right hemiplegia: lying supine.

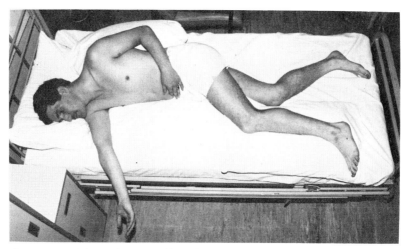

Fig. 8.3 Hemiplegia: lying on affected side.

supported on a pillow. A pillow may be used to keep the trunk aligned.

Lying on the unaffected side (Fig. 8.4). The patient's head should be supported on one pillow and follow the straight line of the spine. The affected arm is brought forward with the palm facing down. The affected leg is brought forward, slightly flexed at the knee, and supported on a pillow. A pillow may be used to keep the trunk aligned and prevent the patient rolling backwards.

Sitting up in bed (Fig. 8.5). The patient's head and trunk should follow a straight line well supported by sufficient pillows to prevent

sagging. The posture should be as erect as possible. The affected shoulder should be brought forward, and this can be achieved by interlacing the fingers and extending the arms. The arms should be supported on one or two pillows. Both legs are extended.

Sitting in a chair (Fig. 8.6). The chair should be of a height to allow the patient's feet to be placed flat on the floor with the knees at an angle of 90°. The back of the chair should be upright, and the armrests wide. The patient should sit upright in the chair, and, if the chair is suitable, supporting pillows should not be necessary. The shoulders should be placed

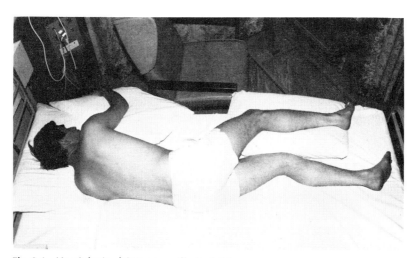

Fig. 8.4 Hemiplegia: lying on unaffected side.

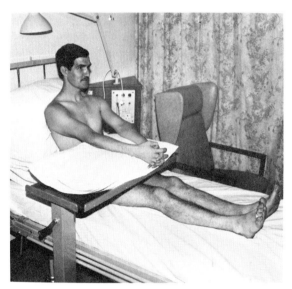

Fig. 8.5 Hemiplegia: sitting up in bed.

forward, hands clasped and resting on a table.

Problems with shoes, feet and walking aids. All these need assessment and attention. Calluses and bunions can alter the body's

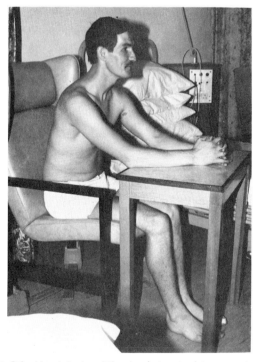

Fig. 8.6 Hemiplegia: sitting in chair raised to correct height for patient.

balance, and the patient should be seen by the chiropodist. In a survey of walking-sticks used by the elderly, it was found that only 22% had been measured and of these only two thirds were the correct length, most of the others being too long (Sainsbury and Mulley 1982). Of the patients assessed in the survey who were fallers, 75% had sticks of an incorrect height. A survey by Kinsman (1983) showed that 75% of fallers wore slippers compared with 4% who wore lace-up shoes. Kinsman (1983) also found that 95% of the fallers were unsteady on their feet, but 48% improved after physiotherapy treatment.

Managing poor balance

When this is practised safely it ensures that someone can get up from a chair, or toilet, and can sit down on it safely. The prerequisites are a suitable chair (height, arms, slant of back and seat), a non-slip floor, adequate strength and joint range and a reason to move. The chair most likely to be used at home can be adapted if necessary.

The usual method of chair drill is for the patient to position her feet parallel, slightly apart and slightly under the chair with her hands on the arms of the chair. She then wriggles towards the front of the chair, leans forward and pushes up from the chair and when upright places her hand on the aid if used. The reverse is performed when sitting down, in that the patient approaches the chair and turns around until the backs of the legs are touching the chair. She then feels for the arms of the chair with her hands, and gently lowers herself into the chair by bending in the middle. The same procedure should be followed when sitting or getting up from the toilet (Fig. 8.7).

Walking. The patient may walk incorrectly because an aid is used, particularly a frame. The patient should lift the frame (or push a wheeled frame), a pace in front of her and move first the weaker leg, and then the other leg up the frame but not inside it. She is then able to lift the frame again. Walking sticks are usually held in the hand opposite to the leg

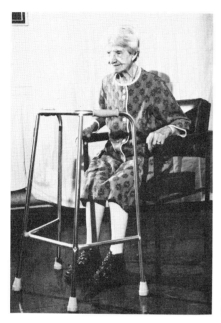
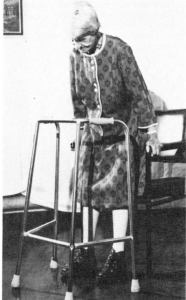
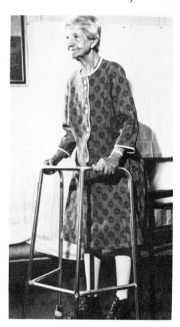

Fig. 8.7 Chair drill: (a) suitable chair, feet under and apart, hands on chair arms, lean forward; (b) push up from chair and lean forward; (c) hands on walking aid when upright.

which is weaker or giving pain, but habits die hard and if an elderly person has always used a stick in the right hand she will probably continue to do so.

The re-education of gait should relate to the patient's needs. Muscle strength, joint range, balance, correct walking aid, and footwear have all been discussed. The steps should be even in length, with even pace and even weight distribution, adequate abduction to prevent the legs crossing over and encouragement of a heel toe pattern (Lee 1978). The patient should practise going up and down steps and stairs if they are to be used at home. Provision of rails, or altering the house so that a one-level existence can be achieved may be wise since two thirds of the falls in the elderly occur on stairs (Caird and Judge 1976), and the majority of these occur when descending (Overstall 1978).

Patients should be encouraged to look ahead when walking and not at their feet, as this neck flexion results in a total body flexion pattern with bent knees and hips. A mirror or video system can be used so that the patient can see how she walks and can learn to control and improve it.

Mobility aids. These must be selected to ensure that the patient can move about safely and there is a variety of aids on the market. Gait will be abnormal with any support in the hands as this is not the natural gait for the human, but if an aid is necessary it must be suitable for the home as well as in hospital. Some wheeled varieties are not suitable on carpets. The aids must be carefully selected to meet individual needs, and those already in use should be checked for suitability and safety.

It has been suggested that the correct aid height is achieved when the handle is level with the distal crease of the wrist when the arm is down by the side of the body (Sainsbury and Mulley 1982). The patient's balance can be improved by raising or lowering the aid, and it is essential that only the aid that has been prescribed for the patient is used. The aid should be easily available to the patient on the ward if unaided mobility is to be encouraged. Further information can be obtained from the physiotherapy and occupational therapy departments.

Methods of getting up after falling. Isaacs (1979) estimated that three millon old people fall each year and yet little has been written about methods of getting up after falling. Priorities are warmth and calm, and a pre-arranged method of summoning help should be used. The elderly person living alone is the most vulnerable and should benefit from being taught different methods of getting up.

Roll and crawl. The faller must be able to roll onto her front, get on to all fours, and crawl to a chair which she then uses as a support to get up. The most frequent obstacle to this method is knee pain and weakness. The faller if hemiplegic should roll onto her front and push herself up into a side sitting position using the unaffected side. She then shuffles on the floor in this position using the unaffected leg and arm until reaching a chair. Then using the unaffected arm and leg she can push herself up onto the chair (Robinson 1980).

Backwards shuffle. The faller gets into a sitting position on the floor and then, using her arms and legs, shuffles backwards to a low stool, ramp, or bottom stair and pushes herself up onto it until in a position to get up. This is particularly effective on the stairs as gradual progression up the stairs will bring the person to a good height to attempt to stand up.

Rescue chair. A mechanical device has been developed on the 'fork-lift truck' principle (Fig. 8.8). The seat of the chair can be lowered to the ground by the faller, who then shuffles back onto it and raises it electrically to a suitable height from which to stand up. It can also be used to lower a patient onto the floor from the sitting position so that conventional methods can be practised (Squires 1983). The faller should be encouraged to sit still for a while and recover before attempting to walk again. Remembering to pull the mobility aid along with her when moving across the floor after falling is wise so that it is ready by the chair when needed.

The long-stay patient

There will always be some patients who will

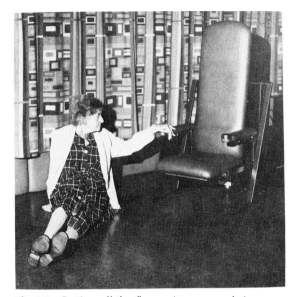

Fig. 8.8 Getting off the floor using rescue chair.

have reached the limit of their physical capacity and for whom maintenance treatment is appropriate (Denham 1983). Passive movements to assist in nursing care may be undertaken by the therapist or taught to nursing staff where suitable. Hip abduction for hygiene, knee extension to prevent heel pressure, ankle movements to maintain circulation and upper limb movements to assist washing and dressing are fundamental. Full range passive movements to the joints of the limbs should be undertaken twice daily, taking care to support the limb throughout, to hold it and not pinch, and especially to be receptive to messages from the muscles or from the patient in terms of spasm or pain. A working knowledge of normal joint range is necessary and advice should be sought from the physiotherapist before undertaking passive movements if there is any doubt as to suitability or the range and pressure necessary (Martin-Jones 1962).

Where possible, standing will help by giving stimulation through the feet and initiating an extensor thrust movement which will prevent flexion patterns developing. Standing also aids bowel and bladder function and is particularly useful in preventing the accumulation of bladder calculi. Passive movements, handling and standing can be taught to interested relatives.

Patients being rehabilitated for discharge from hospital

These patients need constant advice, encouragement and supervision, which should be withdrawn gradually as the discharge date approaches. Communication between all the carers involved is necessary to ensure continuity of treatment and to prevent the problem of being too helpful. Activities achieved with the therapist should be continued by the nurses and other helpers every day. In a survey by Livesley and Graham (1983) it was found that of patients readmitted to hospital after discharge, the earliest admissions were due to insufficient notice being taken of the therapist's assessment and advice, whereas the later readmissions were generally for unavoidable clinical deterioration.

Lifting disabled old people

Research relating to nurses shows that low back pain is a major problem, accounting for between 35% and 47% of job-related injuries. The commonest alleged precipitating cause is lifting patients—this is implicated in 49–79% of all low back injuries (Stubbs and Osborne 1979). Although a variety of lifting methods is used, basic principles should be observed, as follows (Lloyd et al 1981):

— Assess the situation and see if the patient does need to be lifted, and if so how much can she do to help.
— Be aware of the medical condition present. Explain to the patient and any helper what you are going to do.
— Use mechanical aids if available and desirable.
— Ask for help if in any doubt of your physical limitations.
— Clear the area of hazards, wear safe shoes, prepare the destination.
— Position the feet correctly.
— Keep the patient as close to you as possible.

— Keep your back straight.
— Use your body as a counterbalance.
— Keep good time with your partner.

The shoulder lift (Fig. 8.9)

This has been shown to halve the back stress as compared with other methods (Stubbs and Osborne 1979), and can be used to move the patient up and down the bed, from chair to bed, and from floor to bed. Two lifters are needed. They face the patient, one on each side, place their shoulders nearest the patient under his axillae and their arms under his thighs, and clasp hands. The patient rests his arms along the backs of the lifters, or if this is not possible because of shoulder pathology the lifter on the affected side supports the patient's back with her other hand. The lifters point their leading feet in the direction they are moving and use their spare arms to press down on the bed, or hold the bed-head if going that way, which lessens the stress (Scholey 1982). The lifters lift and move the patient together, keeping their backs straight and bracing their free arms. It is essential to lift the patient and not drag him along the bed, so causing shearing forces on the skin. Lowering the bed will make this lift easier as the lifter's back legs can kneel on the bed and give additional support.

The Bobath stand (Fig. 8.10)

This is an excellent method for standing and turning a patient, for example from bed to chair, when only one person is needed. It was developed for hemiplegic patients but can be successfully used for elderly people with other conditions. With the patient sitting on the edge of the bed either with bare feet or in non-slip footwear and feet slightly apart, the lifter places her feet outside those of the patient and her knees against hers, slightly to the lateral side. The patient can either place her hands around the lifter's waist, or around her neck with the weaker hand being grasped by the stronger. When everything is ready, the patient is encouraged to lean forward whilst

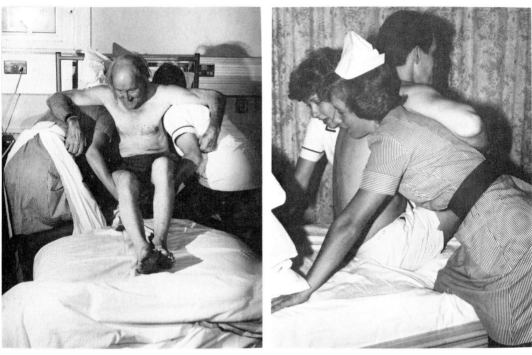

Fig. 8.9 Shoulder lift: (a) showing position of patient's arms and operators' arms; (b) method with leading hand on bed.

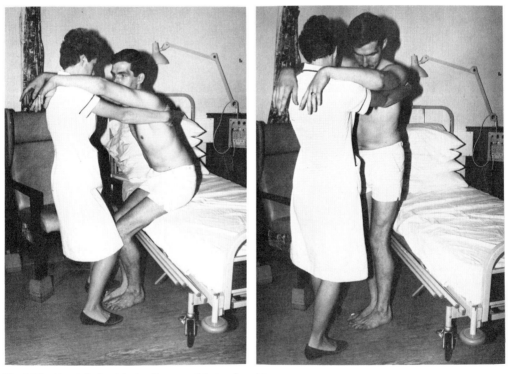

Fig. 8.10 Hemiplegia: (a) standing up; (b) stand and turn.

the lifter uses her body weight to counter-balance and help the patient to a standing position. When balance is gained, the turn is controlled by the lifter and the patient is lowered by reversing the movements into the adjacent chair (Bobath 1982).

This method can be used to sit a patient back into a chair when she is slipping out, by helping her to stand and applying pressure to the knees which will push the hips back in the chair. When transferring patients from chair to bed and vice versa, both pieces of furniture must be stable and unable to move with the brakes on if available.

STROKE UNITS

Stroke patients account for 6% of all hospital running costs, 13% of all general medical bed-days, and 25% of geriatric bed-days (Carstairs 1976). The care of stroke patients in the United Kingdom with some exceptions is poor, and has failed to keep pace with developments in North America.

The question of stroke units is controversial, but there does seem to be agreement that changing the organisation of stroke care to provide intensive care equipment, facilities and staffing, has no impact on overall mortality during the immediate period following the event (Akhtar and Garraway 1982). Therefore, interest has centred on the period following the acute phase, and the most effective means of organising rehabilitation for the patients that have survived it. There is evidence that care in a specialised stroke unit is more effective for some patients than the care provided in a general medical unit. McCann and Culbertson (1976) found that those patients at 'level three' (those with severe impairment), attained significantly better results than similar patients on medical wards, although patients with moderate and profound impairment were no different.

Stroke severity ratings (McCann and Culbertson 1976)
1. Mild   Patient has minor disabilities which slightly restrict ability to function at home and in community, can live independently.
2. Moderate Patient has moderate disabilities, needs assistance of another person to help with some activities.
3. Severe   Patient has severe disabilities, needs supervision to function at home and in community.
4. Profound Patient is completely dependent upon assistance of at least one person to carry out daily needs, not functionally competent in the home or community.

A study by Feigenson et al (1979) compared stroke unit patients with non-stroke unit patients, and found that more stroke unit patients were discharged home, walked better than non-stroke unit patients, but there was no difference between the two groups in ability to perform activities of daily living. There was also no difference between the two groups in length of stay in hospital. A British study supports these findings (Garraway et al 1980a). A higher proportion of patients discharged from the stroke unit compared with those from the medical unit, were assessed as independent, although these findings were not supported at one year follow-up (Garraway et al 1980b). On the other hand, studies by Peacock et al (1972) and Waylonis et al (1973) did not support improved function of stroke unit patients. There are also advocates for stroke care at home (Smith 1981, Wade and Langton Hewer 1983) and as an outpatient (Smith et al 1981). Clearly then, the question of where stroke rehabilitation takes place remains unanswered, but there are some tentative conclusions that can be reached.

1. The group of patients in the middle range of impairment would probably do better in a disability oriented stroke unit than in general medical or geriatric wards.

2. Those with minimal impairment will usually recover 'spontaneously' wherever they are, and those with very severe impairment will not recover more function if treated in a special unit.

3. Stroke units provide an environment in which communication between different members of the multidisciplinary team is extremely effective, so providing a more consistent approach to stroke care than might be found in medical and geriatric wards.

4. Stroke units should improve patient interaction when participating in group activities with others suffering from similar disabilities.

5. Stroke units should improve carer knowledge and participation in the recovery process.

6. Stroke units have an important role in studying the value of different diagnostic and therapeutic interventions (von Arbin et al 1979).

Stroke rehabilitation

There are conflicting views on the effectiveness of rehabilitation after stroke. Recent studies which attempt to evaluate rehabilitation methods for stroke patients are comparing mainly quantitative aspects of therapy such as the relative amounts of physical, occupational, and speech therapy received by patients in a controlled stroke unit/ward, with the amount received by patients in general medical wards (Garraway et al 1980, Smith et al 1981, Stevens et al 1984). An example of the amounts of physiotherapy, occupational therapy, and speech therapy received by patients in a stroke rehabilitation ward as compared with therapy received by a group of patients in general wards is given by Stevens et al (1984):

A variety of remedial techniques may have been used in these studies but they have not been described. Modern exercise therapy for stroke patients takes into account the principles of neuromuscular facilitation. Various methods of facilitation have been developed (Brunstromm 1970, Kabat 1977, Bobath 1982), with each emphasising a different aspect of the neurophysiological approach.

Neuromuscular facilitation

The neuromuscular mechanism which includes the muscles, nerves, neural pathways and brain centres, iniates and achieves movement in response to a demand for activity (Gardiner 1981). To facilitate is to 'make easier', and neuromuscular facilitation is the process by which the response of the patient's neuromuscular mechanism is made easier. This is done by the therapist using specific techniques. The techniques developed by Bobath and Bobath (1950) and described by Bobath (1982) for the treatment of spastic hemiplegia, have received attention and recognition in the United Kingdom. This method is based on the concept that there exists a hierarchy of functions in the human nervous system, with a range from stereotyped and obligatory responses at the spinal cord level, to more variable selective ones integrated at subcortical and cortical levels. The influence of sensory stimuli and subsequent feedback from the motor response produced, upon the integrative process is the basis of the treatment. Damage to the upper motor neurone, as in stroke, results in abnormal postural reflex activity with spasticity and disturbances in

| | (SRW) Patients | | General ward | |
	Patients Treated	Hours	Patients Treated	Hours
Physiotherapy	112	4463	104	1486
mean		40		14
Occup. therapy	47	654	24	212
mean		14		8
Speech therapy	37	633	27	188
mean		17		7

balance and righting mechanisms. The techniques are designed to increase, decrease or maintain muscle tone during a motor activity, and to facilitate active movements from a controlled posture (Flanagan 1967). Proprioceptive neuromuscular facilitation (PNF) (Kabat 1977) is another facilitation technique which relies mainly on stimulation of the proprioceptors for increasing the demand made on the neuromuscular mechanism to obtain and facilitate a response. Treatment by these techniques is very comprehensive and involves application of the principles of PNF to every aspect of the patient's handling.

There is doubt concerning the value of rehabilitative and physiotherapy procedures and the influence of therapy on recovery in the damaged central nervous system (Langton Hewer 1972). The major criticism is that the techniques of physical therapy for stroke patients, such as facilitation techniques, have not been evaluated in controlled trials. There are many factors which make research in the area of stroke recovery problematic, including cognitive and perceptual impairment, and spontaneous recovery (Lind 1982), but there still remains need for evaluation of specific methods of remedial therapy especially in the light of doubts expressed by physicians and others.

REFERENCES

Abrams M 1978 Beyond three score years and ten. Age Concern Publications, London
Adams G F 1974 Cerebrovascular disability and the ageing brain. Churchill Livingstone, Edinburgh
Adams G M, De Vries H A 1973 Physiological effects of an exercise programme upon women aged 52–79. Journal of Gerontology 28: 50–55
Association of District and Superintendent Physiotherapists 1984 Spring report. ADSP, London
Agate J N 1983 Physiotherapy problems and practice in the elderly: a critical evaluation. In: Wright V (ed) Bone and joint disease in the elderly. Churchill Livingstone, Edinburgh
Akhtar A J, Garraway W M 1982 Management of the elderly patient with stroke. In: Caird F I (ed) Neurological Disorders in the Elderly. Wright, Bristol
Arcand A, Williamson J 1981 An evaluation of home

visiting of patients by physicians in geriatric medicine. British Medical Journal 283: 718–720
Ashburn A 1982 A physical assessment for stroke patients. Physiotherapy 68(4): 133–149
Ashley M J, Gryfe C I, Amies A 1977 A longitudinal study of falls in an elderly population II: Some circumstances of falling. Age and Ageing 6: 211–220
Atkinson H 1977 Principles of treatment. In: Cash J (ed) Neurology for physiotherapists. Faber, London
Azar G J, Lawton A H 1964 Gait and stepping as factors in the frequent falls of elderly women. Gerontologist 4:83
Barker J, Bury M 1978 Mobility and the elderly: a community challenge. In: Carver V, Liddiard P L (eds) An ageing population. Hodder and Stoughton in Association with the Open University Press, Sevenoaks, Kent
Batehup L 1983 How teaching can help the stroke patient's recovery. In: Wilson Barnet J (ed) Patient teaching. Churchill Livingstone, Edinburgh
Bird H A 1983 Osteoarthrosis. In: Wright V (ed) Bone and joint disease in the elderly. Churchill Livingstone, Edinburgh
Bobath B 1978 Adult hemiplegia: evaluation and treatment, 2nd edn. Heinemann, London
Bobath B 1982 Adult hemiplegia: evaluation and treatment, 3rd edn. Heinemann, London
Bobath K, Bobath B 1950 Spastic paralysis: treatment of by the use of reflex inhibition. British Journal of Physical Medicine 13: 121–127
Brocklehurst J C, Exton-Smith A N, Lempert Barber S M, Hunt L, Palmer M 1976 Fracture of the femoral neck. Report No 1 to the Department of Health and Social Security, London
Brocklehurst J C, Exton-Smith A N, Lempert Barber S M, Hunt I, Palmer M K 1978 Fracture of the femur in old age: a two centre study of associated clinical factors and the cause of the fall. Age and Ageing 7: 7–15
Broe G A 1982 Parkinsonism and related disorders. In: Caird F I (ed) Neurological disorders in the elderly. Wright, Bristol
Brunstromm S 1970 Movement therapy in hemiplegia: a neurophysiological approach, Harper and Row, New York
Caird F, Judge T 1976 Assessment of the elderly patient. Pitman, London
Campbell A J, Reinken J, Allan B C, Martinez G S 1981 Falls in old age: a study of frequency and related clinical factors. Age and Ageing 10: 264–270
Carstairs V 1976 Stroke: resource consumption and cost to the community. In: Gillingham F J, Maudsley C, William A E (eds) Stroke. Churchill Livingstone, Edinburgh
Chamberlain M A 1983 Mobility of the elderly. In: Wright V (ed) Bone and joint disease in the elderly. Churchill Livingstone, Edinburgh
Crowther H 1982 New perspectives on nursing lower limb amputees. Journal of Advanced Nursing 7: 453–460
Denham M 1983 Care of the long stay elderly patient. Croom Helm, London
Denham M, Jefferys P 1972 Routine mental testing in the elderly. Modern Geriatrics 2:275
Department of Transport, National Travel Survey 1975/6.

Department of Transport, Marsham Street London SW1P 3EB

De Souza L, Langton Hewer R 1980 Assessment of recovery of arm control in hemiplegic stroke patients. International Rehabilitation Medicine 2: 3–16

De Vries H A 1970 Physiological effects of an exercise training regime upon men aged 52–88. Journal of Gerontology 24: 325–336

De Vries H A 1974 Vigour regained. Prentice Hall, Englewood Cliffs, NJ

De Vries H A 1975 Physiology of exercise and ageing. In: Woodruff D S, Birren J E (eds) Ageing: scientific perspectives and social issues. Van Nostrand, New York

Ebersole P, Hess P 1981 Toward healthy ageing. Mosby, St Louis

Exton-Smith A N 1977 Functional consequences of ageing: clinical manifestations. In: Exton-Smith A N, Grimley Evans J (eds) Care of the elderly: meeting the challenge of dependency. Academic Press, London

Exton-Smith A N 1978 Bone ageing and metabolic bone disease. In: Brocklehurst J C (ed) Textbook of geriatric medicine and gerontology. Churchill Livingstone, Edinburgh

Exton-Smith A N, Overstall P W 1979 Geriatrics. MTP Press, Lancaster

Feigenson J S, Howard S, Gitlow S, Greenberg S D 1979 The disability oriented rehabilitation unit—a major factor influencing stroke outcome. Stroke 10: 5–8

Fernie G R, Gryfe C I, Holliday P J, Llewellyn A 1982 The relationship of postural sway in standing to the incidence of falls in geriatric subjects. Age and Ageing 11: 11–16

Finlay O E, Bayles T B, Rosen C, Millig J 1983 Effects of chair design, age and cognitive status on mobility. Age and Ageing 12: 329–335

Flanagan E M 1967 Methods for facilitation and inhibition of motor activity. American Journal of Physical Medicine 46: 1006–1011

Galley P M, Forster A L 1982 Human movement. Churchill Livingstone, Edinburgh

Gardiner M D 1981 The principles of exercise therapy. Bell and Hyman, London

Garraway W M, Akhtar A J, Prescott R J, Hockey L 1980a Management of acute stroke in the elderly: preliminary results of a controlled trial. British Medical Journal 281: 1040–1043

Garraway W M, Akhtar A J, Hockey L, Prescott R J 1980b Management of acute stroke in the elderly: follow-up of a controlled trial. British Medical Journal 281: 827–828

Goldman R 1979 Decline in organic function with age. In: Rossman I (ed) Clinical geriatrics, 2nd edn. Lippincott, Philadelphia

Goodwin P B, Hutchinson T P 1976 The risk of walking. In: Elkington P, McGlynn R, Roberts W (eds) The pedestrian: planning, and research. Transport and Environment Studies, Unpublished report by University College (London) Traffic Studies Group

Grimm R J, Nashner L M 1978 Progress in clinical neurophysiology 4:70

Guimaraes R M, Isaacs B 1980 Characteristics of the gait in old people who fall. International Rehabilitation Medicine 2: 177–180

Harris A 1971 Handicapped and impaired in Great Britain, Part 1. Social Survey Division, Office of Population Censuses and Surveys, London

Hasselkus R 1974 Ageing and the human nervous system. American Journal of Occupational Therapy 28:16

Hunt A 1978 The elderly at home—a study of people aged 65 and over living in the community in England in 1976. Social Survey Division, Office of Population Censuses and Surveys, HMSO, London

Imms F J, Edholm O G 1981 Studies of gait and mobility in the elderly. Age and Ageing 10: 147–156

Isaacs B 1979 Thoughts from a bathchair. Physiotherapy 65: 338–340

Isaacs B 1982 Disorders of balance. In: Caird F I (ed) Neurological disorders in the Elderly. Wright, Bristol

Jeffreys E 1980 Disorders of the cervical spine. Butterworth, London

Johnstone M 1977 The stroke patient: principles of rehabilitation. Churchill Livingstone, Edinburgh

Kabat H 1977 Studies in neuromuscular dysfunction. In: Payton O D, Hirt S, New R A (eds) Neurophysiologic approaches to therapeutic exercise. Davies, Philadelphia

Katz S, Ford A B, Jackson B A, Jaffe M W 1963 Studies of illness in the aged: the Index of ADL, a standardized measure of biological and psychological function. Journal of the American Medical Association 184: 914–919

Kinsman R 1983 Falls in the elderly. Unpublished audit, Barnet Health Authority

Knott M, Voss D 1968 Proprioceptive neuromuscular facilitation. Harper and Row, New York

Knutsson E 1972 An analysis of Parkinsonian gait. Brain 95: 475–486

Kraus H, Rabb W 1961 Hypokinetic disease. Thomas, Springfield, Illinois

Lancet 1982 Research aspects of rehabilitation after acute brain damage in adults. Lancet 2: 1034–1035

Lange K, Anderson R, Masironi R, Rutenfranz J, Seliger V 1978 Habitual physical activity and health. World Health Organization, Copenhagen

Langton Hewer R 1972 Stroke units. Lancet 1:52

Lawrence J S, Bremner J M, Bier F 1966 Osteoarthrosis. Annals of the Rheumatic Diseases 25: 1–24

Lee J 1978 Aids to physiotherapy. Churchill Livingstone, Edinburgh

Lee J, Warren M 1978 Cold therapy. Bell and Hyman, London

Lieberman M A, Tobin S S, Slover D 1971 The effects of relocation on long term geriatric patients. Final report of Department of Mental Health, State of Illinois Project 17 328 (mimeo)

Lind K 1982 A synthesis of studies of stroke rehabilitation. Journal of Chronic Diseases 35: 133–149

Livesley B, Graham H 1983 Can readmissions to a geriatric medical unit be prevented? Lancet 1: 404–406

Lloyd P, Osborne C, Tarling C 1981 The handling of patients. Back Pain Association and Royal College of Nursing, Shears, Hants

Macdonald J B, Macdonald E T 1977 Nocturnal femoral fracture and continuing widespread use of barbiturate hypnotics. British Medical Journal 2: 483

McCann B C, Culbertson R A 1976 Comparison of two systems for stroke rehabilitation in a general hospital. Journal of the American Geriatrics Society 25: 211–216

Mahoney F I, Barthel D W 1965 Functional evaluation: the Barthel Index. Maryland State Medical Journal 14: 61–65

Marlowe R A 1973 Effects of the environment on elderly state hospital relocatees. In: 44th Annual Meeting of the Pacific Sociological Association, Scotsfale, Arizona (Mimeo)

Martin-Jones 1962 Passive movements: physiotherapy helps nursing. Nursing Times Publication, London

Melzack R, Wall P D 1965 Pain mechanisms: a new theory. Science 150: 971–978

Munton J S, Ellis M, Chamberlain A, Wright V 1981 An investigation into the problems of easy chairs used by the arthritic and the elderly. Rheumatology and Rehabilitation 20: 164–173

Murray M P, Sepic S B, Gardner G M, Downs W J 1978 Walking patterns of men with Parkinsonism. American Journal of Physical Medicine 57: 278–295

Myco F 1983 Nursing care of the hemiplegic stroke patient. Harper and Row, London

Nayak U S L, Gabell A, Simons M A, Isaacs B 1982 Measurement of gait and balance in the elderly. Journal of the American Geriatrics Society 30: 516–520

Nichols P J R 1976 Rehabilitation medicine: the management of physical disabilities. Butterworth, London

Nordin B 1983 Preventing osteoporosis. Geriatric Medicine 13: 873–876

Norman A 1981 Barriers to mobility. In: Hobman D (ed) The impact of ageing. Croom Helm, London

Overstall P W 1978 Falls in the elderly: epidemiology, aetiology and management. In: Isaacs B (ed) Recent advances in geriatric medicine. Churchill Livingstone, Edinburgh

Overstall P W, Exton-Smith A N, Imms F J, Johnston A L 1977 Falls in the elderly related to postural imbalance. British Medical Journal 1: 261–264

Parish G, James D N 1982 A method for evaluating the level of independence during the rehabilitation of the disabled. Rheumatology and Rehabilitation 21: 107–114

Parry A 1980 Physiotherapy Assessment. Croom Helm, London

Parry A, Eales C 1976 Handling the early stroke patient at home and in the ward. Nursing Times 72: 1680–1688

Payton O, Poland J 1983 Ageing process—implications for clinical practice. Physical Therapy 63(1): 41–47

Peacock P B, Lampteon T D 1972 In: Stewart G J (ed) Trends in epidemiology. Thomas, Springfield, Illinois

Pflug J 1975 Intermittent compression in the management of swollen legs in general practice. Practitioner 215: 69–76

Riffle K L 1982 Promoting activity: an approach to facilitating adaptation to ageing changes. Journal of Gerontological Nursing 8: 455–459

Robinson G 1980 Multiple sclerosis—simple exercises. Multiple Sclerosis Society, London

Robson P 1978 Profiles of the elderly: their mobility and use of transport, vol 4, no 6, Age Concern Publications, London

Rodstein M 1964 Accidents among the aged—incidence, causes and prevention. Journal of Chronic Diseases 17: 515–526

Rosin A J 1982 Parkinsonism. In: Isaacs B (ed) Recent advances in geriatric medicine. Churchill Livingstone, Edinburgh

Sabin T D 1982 Biologic aspects of falls and mobility limitations in the elderly. Journal of the American Geriatrics Society 30: 51–58

Sainsbury R, Mulley G P 1982 Walking sticks used by the elderly. British Medical Journal 284:1751

Saltin B, Blomquist G, Mitchell J H, Johnston R L, Wildenthal K, Chapman C B 1968 Response to exercise after bedrest and after training. American Heart Association Monograph H23. The American Heart Association, New York

Schoening H A, Iversen I A 1968 Numerical scoring of self-care status: a study of the Kenny self-care evaluation. Archives of Physical Medicine and Rehabilitation 49: 221–229

Scholey M 1982 The shoulder lift. Nursing Times 78:12, 506–507

Selye H S 1970 Stress and ageing. Journal of the American Geriatrics Society 18: 669–690

Sheikh K, Smith D, Meade T, Goldenberg E et al 1979 Repeatability and validity of a modified ADL Index in studies of chronic disability. International Rehabilitation Medicine 1: 51–58

Sheikh K, Smith D, Meade T, Brennan P et al 1980 Assessment of motor function in studies of chronic disability. Rheumatology and Rehabilitation 2: 83–90

Shipley P 1980 Chair comfort for the elderly and infirm. Nursing 20: 858–860

Shock N W 1962 The physiology of ageing. Scientific American 206:100

Smith A 1981 When home management of stroke was a success. Geriatric Medicine May: 65–70

Smith D S, Goldenberg E, Ashburn A, Kinsella G, Sheikh K, Brennan P J et al 1981 Remedial therapy after stroke: a randomized controlled trial. British Medical Journal 282: 517–520

Squires A 1983 Rescue chair. Multiple Sclerosis Society Bulletin 104: 1456

Stevens M B 1983 Rheumatoid arthritis. In: Wright V (ed) Bone and joint disease in the elderly. Churchill Livingstone, Edinburgh

Stevens R S, Ambler N R, Warren M D 1984 A randomized controlled trial of a stroke rehabilitation ward. Age and Ageing 13: 65–75

Stewart C 1980 A prediction score for geriatric rehabilitation prospects. Rheumatology and Rehabilitation 19: 239–245

Stubbs D A, Osborne C M 1979 How to save your back. Nursing 3: 116–124

Van De Ven C M 1984 Amputations: Cash's textbook of general medical and surgical conditions for physiotherapists. Faber, London

Visser H 1983 Gait and balance in senile dementia of Alzheimer's type. Age and Ageing 12: 296–301

Von Arbin M, Britton M, de Faire U, Helmers C, Miah K, Murray V, Wester P. O 1979 A stroke unit in a medical department. Acta Medica Scandinavica 205: 231–235

Wade D T, Langton Hewer R 1983 Why admit stroke patients to hospital? Lancet 1: April 9 807–809

Wall J C, Ashburn A 1979 Assessment of gait disability in hemiplegics. Scandinavian Journal of Rehabilitation Medicine 11: 95–103

Waylonis G M, Keith M W, Aseff J W 1973 Stroke rehabilitation in a mid-western county. Archives of Physical Medicine and Rehabilitation 54: 151–174

Weg R B 1975 Changing physiology of ageing: normal

and pathological. In: Woodruff D S, Birren J E (eds) Ageing: scientific perspectives and social issues. Van Nostrand, New York

Wessel J A, Van Huss W D 1969 The influence of physical activity and age on exercise adaptation of women 20–69 years. Journal of Sport Medicine 9: 175–180

Wild D, Nayak U S L, Isaacs B 1981a Description, classification and prevention of falls in old people at home. Rheumatology and Rehabilitation 20: 153–159

Wild D, Nayak U S L, Isaacs B 1981b How dangerous are falls in old people at home? British Medical Journal 282: 266–268

Wright V 1983 Bone and joint disease in the elderly. Churchill Livingstone, Edinburgh

Young R R, Delwaide P J 1981 Spasticity. New England Journal of Medicine 304:1 28–33

9

M. C. Hobday

Care of the foot

THE PREVALENCE OF FOOT PROBLEMS

Painful and deformed feet are very common problems for the elderly. Ebrahim et al (1981) surveyed 100 patients in an acute geriatic assessment and rehabilitation ward and found just one patient who presented no problem with her feet. Most of their sample had three or four specific foot problems which, apart from pitting oedema, excluded complications of systemic disease. Earlier, Hobson and Pemberton (1955) concluded that four out of five elderly people had foot disability on examination though not all complained of pain. Vetter et al in an as yet unpublished study of a much larger sample of people over 70 years of age found that over half of their interviewees had difficulties with their feet and that as would be expected the incidence of problems increased with age. Clark (1969) found that three quarters of people over 65 years reported trouble with their feet and the proportion recorded as having foot problems increased when they were professionally inspected. The attitudes of the elderly explain the difference between their perceived need for chiropody treatment compared with the actual need for treatment and is well documented (Townsend and Wedderburn 1965). Foot disability is frequently unreported by the elderly. It is seen as an inevitable accompaniment of ageing and many old people fail to seek help because of this (Williamson et al 1964, Kemp and Winkler

1983). The attitudes and expectations of patients have proved a difficult factor in many studies which seek to establish the incidence of foot problems in the population. The elderly, particularly, seem to expect to have to endure painful feet with increasing years.

It is quite clear from surveys that a large majority of the elderly population do have problems associated with foot disorders. Kemp and Winkler (1983) found that some 88.7% of the elderly population was in need of foot care, if prophylactic advice and education were to be included in the concept of need.

Agate (1963) states that if a normal gait is to be preserved in the elderly then it is vital that the feet should not be painful or deformed. Vetter et al's study shows a clear relationship between foot problems and immobility of the elderly. Collyer (1981) concludes that an old person with painful feet may very easily become house-bound and lose mobility, and this view is supported by Suvarna (1981). Mobility can be severely restricted by relatively simple foot problems. Most of these problems fall within the scope of practice of the state registered chiropodist, who can do much to alleviate these problems with palliative treatment and patient education. Loss of mobility will frequently exacerbate other problems from which a patient may be suffering, and general debility may be increased. Many common foot conditions which impair foot function can lead to, or contribute towards, falls (Helfand 1966).

There are many problems which can impair an elderly person's ability to cope with routine hygiene and care of the foot. Neglected feet are frequently an early sign of physical or mental deterioration. These problems include poor eyesight, rheumatic disease affecting the ability of patients to reach their feet or affecting the dexterity of the hands, obesity, neurological conditions and muscular weakness, hypertension, cardiac and pulmonary disorders which prevent old people from bending down to reach their feet.

Women over 65 years have a higher incidence of foot disorders than men over 65

(Clark 1969). The most prevalent problems which affect the elderly are corns and callouses, trouble with toenails, foot deformities resulting from badly fitting shoes in youth, and arthritis. Clark (1969) found that 34% of the elderly in her sample had difficulty in cutting toenails. Ebrahim et al (1981) found that of the 100 patients examined, 66 complained of difficulty in cutting toenails, 38 complained of onychogryphosis (thickening and deformity of the nail plate) and nine had ingrowing toenails. These are all high incidences when compared to the younger population. Clark (1969) found that 26% of elderly men and 49% of elderly women complained of corns, and that 25% of elderly men and 34% of elderly women complained of troublesome hard skin. Ebrahim et al found that 30 of the 100 patients exhibited corns and callous and 15 complained of pain from corns and callosities. Heloma (corn) and hyperkeratotic lesions are caused by excessive pressure and are frequently secondary to badly fitting shoes, forefoot dysfunction and deformity of the toes. Hallux valgus has been found in 24% of people over 65 years old (6% in men, 35% in women), and lesser toe deformities in 70% of those over 65 years (Clark 1969). This figure for deformity of the lesser toes may well be low, as a hallux valgus angle of greater than 16° will in many cases impair the function of the adjacent toes. A compromised function of these toes, together with the deformity of the first metatarsal segment, will in most cases lead to pressure lesions under the central metatarsal area and give rise to metatarsalgia.

The expertise and scope of practice of the state registered chiropodist is today far wider than generally understood. This presents real difficulties for other members of the health team concerned with foot care, who are uncertain whether or not to refer a problem to a chiropodist. As Kemp and Winkler (1983) state, 'The relationship of chiropody to the other foot care services remains ill-defined and hence the allocation of patients between them haphazard.' They tabulate a foot care spectrum (Fig. 9.1) which gives some indication of the scope of practice of chiropody.

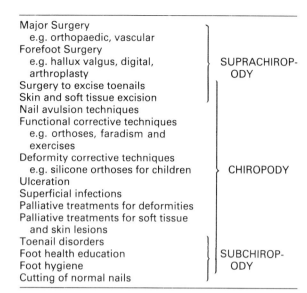

Major Surgery
  e.g. orthopaedic, vascular
Forefoot Surgery
  e.g. hallux valgus, digital,
  arthroplasty   } SUPRACHIROP-ODY
Surgery to excise toenails
Skin and soft tissue excision
Nail avulsion techniques
Functional corrective techniques
  e.g. orthoses, faradism and
  exercises
Deformity corrective techniques
  e.g. silicone orthoses for children   } CHIROPODY
Ulceration
Superficial infections
Palliative treatments for deformities
Palliative treatments for soft tissue
  and skin lesions
Toenail disorders
Foot health education   } SUBCHIROP-ODY
Foot hygiene
Cutting of normal nails

Fig. 9.1 The foot care spectrum. (*Kemp and Winkler 1983.*)

The variable degree of debility of the elderly makes some surgical chiropodial procedures inappropriate. Chiropodists are trained to a high level of proficiency to recognise and evaluate the state of a patient's general health and the factors which make the administration of local analgesics and various topical drugs contraindicated. Most elderly patients want to be made free of discomfort and pain and are intolerant of radical therapies. As a result, much of the chiropodial treatment of the foot problems of elderly patients is of a palliative nature and is concerned with the lower half of the spectrum of treatments shown in Figure 9.1.

Ulceration, corn and callus

The aetiology of foot ulceration in the elderly is usually multi-factorial. Infection of skin abrasions frequently leads to intractable ulcerative lesions which require systemic antibiotic therapy because of compromised vasculature in the lower limb. A major factor, the importance of which is often underestimated, is trauma. Wall (1978) applies the work of Barton (1977) to the pathogenesis of foot ulceration which stresses the effects of pressure on

the micro-circulation. The pressure from ill-fitting shoes and from mattresses is an easily recognised problem. Less recognition has been given to skeletal deformity of the foot which can result in localised concentrations of pressure from footwear or from normal weight-bearing when standing or walking (Chodera and Cterceteko 1979, Snowden 1979), and ulceration associated with hyperkeratotic lesions results. Many of these ulcerations become secondarily infected (Hobday and Swallow 1973).

If an evaluation of the prognosis requires referral, then good teamwork is essential. A patient may well require systemic antibiotics, pathology and radiography examination or consultation with orthopaedic, diabetic or rheumatology specialists. Having made this assessment, the chiropodist will treat the ulceration by debridement of hyperkeratosis and necrotic tissue and with application of polyurethane sponge padding to dissipate high gradients of pressure which fall onto the lesion. Materials of higher density, or a combination of materials, may also be used.

Pressure ulcers on the foot differ from other pressure sores in several ways, the most important being their association with hyperkeratotic growth and their predilection to macerate because of the enclosed environment of hosiery and footwear. Because of these factors, together with the problems of reducing trauma to the ulcer, many of the topical drugs and applications used for gravitational ulcers and pressure sores prove disappointing. Most chiropodists will remove the overlying and surrounding hyperkeratotic tissue because it is a contaminant and so that evaluation of the state of the ulcer can be more accurately made. The calloused mass frequently becomes macerated with exudate and necrotic. The sedentary oedematous limb presents particular problems with maceration of such lesions.

Of particular importance in the treatment of plantar ulceration is the redistribution of pressure away from the ulcer site. Chodera and Cterceteko (1979), studying diabetic patients with and without peripheral nerve

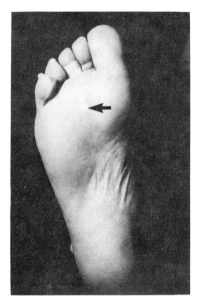

Fig. 9.2 Moderately severe heloma (arrowed) beneath the second metatarsal head.

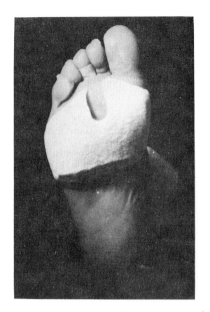

Fig. 9.4 The same foot with a felt protective pad.

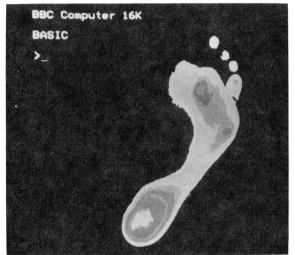

Fig. 9.3 Pedobarograph picture of the foot in Fig. 9.2

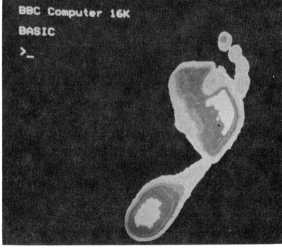

Fig. 9.5 Pedobarograph picture showing a reduction of pressure on the second metatarsal head area.

pathology, showed that an ulcer is always found at the site of localised maximum pressure with a steep pressure gradient. There is always a structural deformity and usually some loss of muscle function to the toes.

Padding such lesions, whether by application directly to the foot or in the form of an insole, is a major aspect of chiropodial treatment and is also used in the treatment of corn and callus. Figure 9.2 shows a foot with a moderately severe pressure lesion beneath the second metatarsophalangeal joint area. Figure 9.3 is a pedobarograph picture of the same foot in a static position showing that the calloused area has a high level of pressure and that there is a steep gradient of pressure. Figure 9.4 shows the foot after the hyperkeratotic mass has been removed and a felt pad has been applied to the forefoot to protect the area when weight bearing. Figure 9.5 is a pedobarograph picture which demonstrates the effectiveness of such a pad in deviating pressure away from the lesion.

Superficial infections

Plantar or digital warts are often asymptomatic on the foot of the elderly and it might be unnecessary to treat. They can be painful if periungual, and respond well over a period to applications of a mild caustic.

Pyogenic infections are usually associated with trauma which breaks the integument allowing opportunistic infection (Hobday and Swallow 1973). Serious infections with coagulase-positive staphylococci and haemolytic streptococci frequently develop cellulitis and lymphatic involvement and osteomyelitis of phalanges and metatarsals. The chiropodist visiting the elderly housebound patient is often the first to see such cases and will initiate medical supervision. Minor infections and septic paronychia are routinely treated topically and rarely give cause for concern, except for the severely debilitated and immunity compromised patient. The chiropodist frequently identifies maturity-onset diabetes or established diabetics who are not stabilised through treating such infections. Chiropody treatment is frequently incriminated in causing foot infections and subsequent gangrene (Gaunt et al 1984). State registered chiropodists who receive a three-year full-time course of training are very aware of these problems. Care must be taken to refer patients to practitioners who are state registered.

Foot deformity

Pronation of the foot at the subtaloid joint complex resulting in a variable degree of valgus foot is most commonly the result of compensation for abnormality of the lower limbs or the result of rheumatic desease. In the young, biomechanical examination and treatment is of great benefit for this condition

but, for the elderly, palliative relief of symptoms is often the most appropriate. There is a positive correlation between valgus foot and the incidence of hallux valgus with all the secondary forefoot problems associated with this. Soft protective insoles with adequate footwear, toes protected from trauma and debridement of corns and calluses give relief from pain and prevent ulceration of traumatised areas. Wright and Haslock (1977) found that 49% of their sample of rheumatic sufferers required chiropody. Many rheumatic diseases affect the feet in the early stages. The elderly rheumatic patient is therefore likely to present with severe foot deformity and the above treatment regime is essential for the management of these cases. This treatment is particularly appropriate for people with rheumatoid arthritis but is also helpful for diabetics and other groups with microangiopathy and peripheral neuropathy.

Pes cavus, talipes conditions and other deformities of neurological origin will produce areas on the foot with very concentrated pressure lesions. Orthoses or pads designed to deviate weight bearing or shoe pressure away from these lesions may be fitted for pain-free walking to take place.

Hallux valgus, hallux rigidus, dorsally dislocated lesser toes, hammer toes and clawed toes all present problems of disturbed forefoot function and adequate accommodation in footwear. Chiropodial orthoses for individual toes or multiple deformities prove useful for long-term management provided the patient can reach her feet. Otherwise protective dressings can be applied to the toes but these are of limited use. Digital or forefoot amputees may be fitted with either a prosthesis which fits to the foot or is incorporated into an insole to sit inside the shoe.

Soft tissue conditions

The most prevalent soft tissue conditions encountered by the elderly are bursitis, chilblains and the degenerative effects of atrophic changes with vascular impairment.

An inflamed bursa may occur in the foot

over any prominent bony deformity but is most frequently associated with the medial aspect of hallux valgus. Treatment is aimed at the alleviation of initiating mechanical stresses and the prevention of ulceration, sinus formation and sepsis. The danger is for penetration to occur into the joint space where the prognosis, with sepsis, almost always requires referral for orthopaedic procedures. Most uncomplicated cases of bursitis respond well to conservative measures.

The treatment of chilblains and the effects of cold and draughts on the feet of elderly rely largely on prophylaxis. Thermo-insulating insoles issued in the autumn, together with advice on suitable hosiery and footwear are relatively simple preventive measures. However, patients who annually develop extensive or ulcerative chilblains should receive advice on diet and help with their living accommodation. Topical applications of rubefacients and other proprietory creams may give ephemeral relief of symptoms but are of unproven prophylactic use.

Most elderly chiropody patients exhibit degenerative changes of the soft tissues of the foot and lower limb. The ageing process and atrophic changes lead to fragility and loss of elastic properties of the skin and diminished adiposity of the superficial fascia. This loss and modification of the soft tissue under the principal weight-bearing areas of the foot, the heel and metatarsal heads, may lead to inflammatory conditions or pressure lesions. It is often important to compensate for this thinness of the feet by recommending microcellular rubber-soled footwear and/or soft cushioning insoles.

Plantar fasciitis, tenosynovitis, strains and sprains are less frequent local conditions seen by chiropodists working with the elderly. Interdigital maceration of the toe webs is more common, especially in neglected cases, and also poor hygiene and leg oedema.

Toe nails

The management of normal nails of old people should present no problem for friends, rela-

tives or health care personnel provided the general state of the patient's feet is considered and simple guidelines are followed. Normal nails will not be painful to touch, will not be excessively brittle, thickened, friable, discoloured or dystrophic (structurally affected by changes to digital blood supply). The lateral margins of the nail plate will be free of each sulcus and the transverse and longitudinal curvature will not be exaggerated.

After cleansing, three or four separate cuts using toenail nippers should be used rather than attempting to cut in one. A cut from each corner towards the middle should be made first and then the residue trimmed straight across the free edge of the nail plate. Nails should not be cut too short. A common fault in nail cutting is to cut towards the sulci, leaving a rough spike within the sulcus. This penetrates the skin causing onychocryptosis, that is, an ingrown toenail where the nail has penetrated the soft tissue of the nail sulcus. In the debilitated person this can lead to a serious infection. After cutting, any roughness at the free edge should be filed smooth using a nail-file or emery board to prevent inadvertent excoriation of the skin of the leg or adjacent foot whilst the patient is in bed.

Pathological nails require the attention of a chiropodist. Onychogryphosis and onychomycosis (fungal infection of the nail plate) are probably the most frequent local conditions which cause difficulty with cutting nails. A chiropodist will reduce the thickness of these nails by using a nail drill, which is a skilled exercise (Figs. 9.6 and 9.7). In cases of neglect, gryphotic nails may attain such length as to curve under or over the toes preventing walking and frequently leading to ulceration. If traumatised, subungual ulceration or paronychia may result if onychogryphosis is not treated.

Partial or total nail avulsion techniques (sterilisation of the nail matrix) for onychocryptosis have a high success rate with the younger patient but are not often appropriate for the elderly, and conservative management is most often employed. The excision of the penetrating nail spike must be achieved

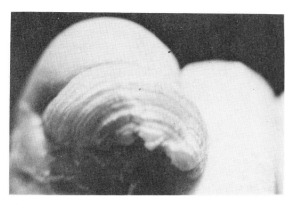

Fig. 9.6 Onychogryphosis before chiropody treatment.

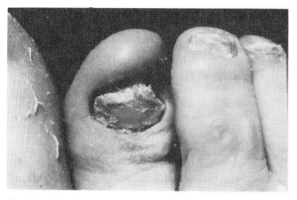

Fig. 9.7 Onychogryphosis after treatment.

before resolution occurs.

Arterial impairment and vasospastic disorders cause dystrophic thinning and sometimes absence of the nail plate. Residual slow nail growth and periungual roughness should be reduced with an emery board rather than nippers or scissors and an emollient cream applied.

FOOT CARE ADVICE

Much of the foot care advice needed by elderly people is fundamental and common sense but enquiry by patients is rarely made until signs and symptoms are present. This can be well into adult life, if not old age. Swallow (1976), writing about the problems that diabetics have with their feet, gives extremely good advice, much of which is relevant to old

people in general. They should be encouraged to wash their feet daily, or on alternate days, in warm water (40–45°C), but not to soak them, which causes excessive dryness. The feet should be dried using a soft towel with particular attention given to the interdigital spaces but without forcing the toes apart. If feet are moist or hyperhidrotic (affected by excessive sweating) then a spirit-based swab followed by a light dusting of talc should be recommended. If the feet are dry, the patient should use a hand cream or emulsifying ointment, but not between the toes if moist.

This routine hygiene can present a problem for many elderly housebound patients because of disability. The help of members of the household or friends and relatives should be sought to carry this out. Certainly, debilitated patients should inspect their feet or have them checked weekly for abrasions, blisters, colour changes, swelling or any suppurative lesion, especially if they have loss of sensation in the feet or lower limb.

Any open wound should be covered with a sterile dressing, and if healing is delayed or infection ensues then it must be brought to the attention of the health care team. Housebound patients should have a telephone number or address readily available and the reticent should be actively encouraged to seek medical help.

Burns on the feet of elderly people with sensation loss are common and often lead to intractible ulceration. Hot-water bottles should be discouraged unless used only to warm the bed before retiring and bath water should not be too hot. Accidental scalding of the feet is not uncommon. A relatively large number of old people have erythema ab igne of the legs and feet. This is a brown-red reticular patterned discoloration owning to exposure to heat. These patients should be advised to use a rug or blanket over their legs to prevent burning when sitting by a fire.

Socks and stockings should be loose-fitting to avoid restriction to the superficial circulation particularly over the toes and heels. Garters should never be used. Patients should not walk about the house barefooted in case of injury, and many styles of bedroom slippers are unsuitable to wear for long periods of time or for anything but short walks around the house. Slippers are usually a poor fit to the foot and constrict the toes if too short and narrow or traumatise the toes when walking if too large. If carpet slippers are the footwear of choice they should be of a style which extends high up the dorsum of the foot with some form of fastening.

Patients will often purchase or be given proprietory products to ease painful feet. It is important to advise patients not to use corn plasters containing caustic medicaments, some solutions advertised to cure ingrown toenails and devices for cutting corns and callosities. Some of these products may be harmless but others contain strong keratolytics which may cause ulceration and lead to infection. Corn planes and other sharp instruments should not be used because of the danger of injury.

The chiropody service

The aims of the community and hospital chiropody service are to promote pain-free healthy feet and maintain the mobility of the disabled and elderly population; to evaluate the effects of local and systemic disorders; to educate the patient in foot health, and to liaise with members of the health care team for overall patient management.

An efficient and successful foot care service for the elderly relies on a multidisciplinary approach involving surgeons, doctors, nurses, physiotherapists, chiropodists, other paramedicals, voluntary bodies, friends and relatives. Co-ordination of personnel to respond to the needs of elderly people usually operates through the patient's general medical practitioner. State registered chiropodists employed within the National Health Service are in extremely short supply and the chiropody service is inadequate to meet the demand for treatment of the priority groups (Department of Health and Social Security 1979). The *Survey of Manpower Resources in the NHS Chiropody Service* (Association of

Chief Chiropody Officers 1980) revealed that in order to give an adequate service, more than double the number of practitioners is needed. The ACCO calculation is an underestimate of manpower shortage as it did not take account of the true prevalence of foot problems of the elderly. The adequacy of the chiropody service for old people varies according to residence. Wade et al (1983) reported that 75% of residents in private nursing Homes found the service adequate, compared with 63% of old people living at home, 38% in hospital and 36% in local authority residential Homes.

It is impossible for the chiropody service to achieve its aims and potential and play a full part in the foot care team. Nurses are in a particularly good position to help old people with general foot care, whether they are in hospitals, residential Homes or at home. Whilst it is recognised that hospital and community based nurses have a heavy workload, it would be an easy, efficient and inexpensive exercise to organise training programmes for nurses. Nurses have good opportunities to gain insight into the elderly patient's circumstances and problems and could deal with hygiene and the cutting of normal nails, footwear advice and the recognition of serious lower limb conditions which require medical attention. This would free the chiropodist to utilise his or her time more effectively and ensure that more elderly people receive chiropodial foot care. It would also keep more old people mobile, independent and at home.

Adendum

The following organisations are a useful source of information and educational leaflets and materials.
— Association of Chief Chiropody Officers, 3 New Road, Aston Clinton, Aylesbury, Bucks HP22 5JD.
— Chiropodists Board, The Registrar, Council for Professions Supplementary to Medicine, 184 Kennington Park Road, London SE11.

— Disabled Living Foundation, 346, Kensington High Street, London W14 8NS.
— Health Education Council, 78 New Oxford Street, London WC1A 1AH.
— Shoe and Allied Trades Research Association, Rockingham Road, Kettering, Northants NN16 9JH.
— Society of Chiropodists, 53 Welbeck Street, London W1M 7HE.
— Society of Shoe Fitters, Carlisle House, 8 Southampton Row, London WC18 4AW.

REFERENCES

Agate J 1963 The practice of geriatrics. Heinemann, London

Association of Chief Chiropody Officers 1980 Survey of manpower resources in the NHS chiropody service. ACCO, Aylesbury, Bucks

Barton A A 1977 Prevention of pressure sores. Nursing Times 41: 1593–95

Chodera J D, Cterceteko G 1979 The application of the Pedobarogram in patients with diabetic neuropathic ulcers. A preliminary report, Biomedical Research and Development Unit, Bioengineering Centre, Roehampton, London

Clark M 1969 Trouble with feet. Occasional Paper on Social Administration, no. 29 G Bell, London

Collyer M I 1981 Maintaining the elderly patient's mobility. Geriatric Medicine 11(12): 27–30

Department of Health and Social Security 1979 staffing of the National Health Service (England): an analysis of the demand and supply position in the major staff groups. DHSS, London

Ebrahim S B J, Sainsbury R, Watson S 1981 Foot problems of the elderly: a hospital survey. British Medical Journal 283: 949–950

Gaunt N, Rogers K, Seal D, Denham M, Lewis J 1984 Necrotising fasciitis due to group C and G haemolytic streptococcus after chiropody. Lancet 1: 516

Helfand A E 1966 Foot impairment—an etiologic factor in falls in the aged. Journal of the American Podiatry Association 56: 326–330

Hobday M C, Swallow A W 1973 A pilot survey to investigate the incidence of bacterial types isolated from ulcerative lesions found on the feet of chiropody patients. Chiropodist 28: 260–266

Hobson W, Pemberton J 1955 The health of the elderly at home. Butterworth, London

Kemp J, Winkler J T 1983 Problems afoot: need and efficiency in footcare. Disabled Living Foundation, London

Snowdon C 1979 Pressure sores and patient support systems. Biomedical Research and Development Unit, Bioengineering Centre, Rochampton, London

Suvarna R R 1981 In: Neale D (ed) Common foot disorders: diagnosis and management. Churchill Livingstone, Edinburgh

Swallow A W 1976 Chiropody for the diabetic foot. British Journal of Hospital Medicine 23: 235–238

Townsend P, Wedderburn D 1965 The aged in the welfare state. G Bell, London

Vetter N J, Jones D A, Victor C R (Awaiting publication) Chiropody services for the over 70s: the problems and the response. Research Team for Care of the Elderly, Welsh National School of Medicine, St David's Hospital, Cardiff

Wade B, Sawyer L, Bell J 1984 Dependency with dignity: different care provision for the elderly. Occasional Papers on Social Administration no. 68. Bedford Square Press, London

Wall B 1978 The pathology of pressure sores and factors which influence their healing. Chiropodist 33: 442–445

Williamson J, Stokoe I H, Gray S et al 1964 Old people at home: their unreported needs. Lancet 1: 1170–20

Wright V, Haslock I 1977 Rheumatism for nurses and remedial therapists. Heinemann, London

10

A. Heslop

Breathing

A common problem for old people is difficulty with breathing. Breathlessness is a prominent symptom of both cardiovascular and respiratory diseases. It is accompanied by many feelings such as the fear of death, a sense of isolation, anger or humiliation. These feelings were expressed by patients in a research study offering respiratory patients with dyspnoea psychotherapeutic support with medical care (Rosser et al 1983). Unfortunately breathlessness is often poorly understood by health professionals which limits the support they are able to offer elderly patients.

This chapter aims to cover some of the facts about cardiovascular and respiratory fitness in both healthy and disabled elderly people. The hope is that this will enable those dealing with them to take a more positive attitude towards maintaining or regaining maximum independence and mobility in their lives.

CARDIOVASCULAR AND RESPIRATORY FITNESS IN OLD PEOPLE

Definition of fitness and exercise

Fitness may be defined in terms of maximal oxygen consumption per kilogram of body weight or more generally in terms of the capacity to enjoy moderate endurance without discomfort (Bannister 1969). The term implies optimal usage of oxygen transport systems which allow exercising man to use his own stored energy resources and those of his environment, to generate power output without undue strain. The superior performance of the athlete is achieved through such optimal usage. Performance is dependent partly on attributes that are distributed throughout the healthy population: such as variations due to sex and body dimensions which influence size of heart, lungs, and muscles to age, mainly influencing maximum heart rate and the haemoglobin content which affects the oxygen carrying capacity of the central circulation (Jones et al 1982).

Oxygen transport systems

  Steps in the chain
Getting air in and out of lungs
Gas exchange in lungs
Oxygen carriage in blood
Cardiac output
Local circulation to muscles
Utilisation of oxygen in muscles
  Faults that occur
Weak respiratory muscles, airways obstruction
Emphysema, pulmonary fibrosis
Anaemia
Ischaemic heart failure
Peripheral vascular disease
Unfitness
Insufficient exercise

Exercise is a stress to the system that increases the oxygen requirement of the exercising muscles. Exercise is limited for both normal people and those with cardiovascular factors. They stop exercising before approaching maximum ventilation because maximum heart rate is reached. For people with respiratory disease exercise is limited by respiratory capacity, and therefore they do not achieve maximum heart rate and reach, or nearly reach, maximum ventilation.

Aerobic exercise occurs when all the energy is provided by burning calories with oxygen, for example, when swimming, jogging or walking.

Anaerobic exercise occurs when the energy requirements are partly or totally supplied by metabolic activity not requiring oxygen, which leads to oxygen debt. This occurs with sports characterised by sudden high speeds, like squash, sprinting or football.

Limits due to the ageing process

Most old people will be less fit than the young because they take less exercise, and because of the effects of ageing and possible disease on their heart and lungs. In old age the heart becomes small and its cells are stained brown. With a gradual increase in fibrous tissue abnormal rhythms arise if conduction tissue is affected. In persons over sixty years of age the heart has experienced mechanical stress and normal wear and tear. This will lead ultimately to limited cardiac output and place restriction on exercise capacity. Thus an elderly person may walk slowly, though comfortably, up a hill, but is unable to run to catch a bus.

Assessing the effect of age on the lungs and respiratory tract is difficult as there is a high prevalence of chronic lung disease in the elderly. Pollution and smoking confuse the histological picture. Structurely, the lungs have less elastic recoil and there is alveolar dilatation. This leads to elderly people becoming more breathless on exertion even when lung disease is absent. Expectoration of secretions is more difficult (Hall et al 1978). Because of these changes the lungs (as measured by lung function tests) deteriorate with age. The predicted 'normal' values fall with age; this means less reserve of the lungs so that a degree of damage not causing symptoms in a young person could cause noticeable breathlessness in an old one. The ageing cardiovascular and respiratory systems are described in more detail in Chapter 3, The Physiology of Ageing.

Ageing, as well as its effect on the cardiovascular system and lungs, often leads to general 'fatigue' and reduced ability to perform physical activities because of decreased motivation. The contribution of this reduced motivation to overall loss of ability is difficult to gauge, but an attempt at this is an important facet of the overall assessment of an elderly person.

Forms of exercise commonly used by the elderly

Emphasis on the need to take exercise to improve health is a recent phenomenon, and it is now being given publicity and funds to create more sports facilities. Since 1950 there have been several social changes: a shorter working week, longer holidays and relatively higher incomes with women also earning. All these factors have helped to stimulate an interest in leisure. Increased mobility through car ownership enables more people to reach sports facilities.

Despite an increase in leisure time there are opposing factors which must be considered. Sport will continue to compete with other leisure activities which are more passive, for example bingo, betting shops or watching television. Also, Kelvin (1980) has argued that leisure cannot supply a structure to time or status to individuals that work can. Health professionals are not sufficiently committed, nor do they always recognise the value of exercise as a health benefit.

The elderly may not have had the opportunity to experience leisure and so may find constructive use of such time difficult to cope with. The usual forms of exercise they experience are domestic activities such as organising their day, which may encompass dressing, washing, housework, depending on their level of activity and ability. These tasks are often time-consuming and enervating for the disabled or chronically ill person. The more independent elderly shop or use social outings such as lunch clubs, day centres, visiting friends or walking the dog to take exercise. More importantly, an outing offers social contact and a reason to go out. Many of the elderly stress that they enjoy the company of young people as much as those of their own age.

An example of a recreational approach to exercise for the elderly is the organisation Extend. This offers exercise in a social setting which helps to promote the quality of life for the retired or elderly. Old people, whether active or not, are at risk of strain, and move-ment exercises require supervision from trained staff (Copple 1983).

The average person takes little exercise and work has become less physically active in recent years. This means that many old people begin their retirement unfit so that a gradual increase in their activities should be undertaken rather than a sudden energetic approach. Too sudden an approach can be hazardous and may discourage old people from attempting further exercise. Exercise is currently being advocated for all age groups (Sports Council 1982). It is important that opportunities for appropriate exercise for different ages be provided, and in this the elderly present a particular challenge.

Research on the effects of exercise on physical fitness of the elderly

There is very little available research in this area. Most literature describes exercise studies on young people. Exercise research with older people has paid attention to improved physical functioning ability in physical training programmes (Buccola and Stone 1975), and has shown a significant increase in muscle strength and decline in body fat (Sidney et al 1977). Improved cardiorespiratory fitness following exercise has been shown by Adams and de Vries (1973) and Sidney and Shepherd (1977). The research literature does not include studies with independent elderly people in non-institutionalized areas. Ray et al (1982) demonstrated that an exercise programme for older healthy adults significantly affected some areas of psychosocial functioning and physical abilities, but not their morale.

CARDIOVASCULAR AND RESPIRATORY MORTALITY AND MORBIDITY OF PEOPLE OVER THE AGE OF SIXTY

Ischaemic heart disease is a common cause of death for both sexes, but is relatively much lower for women under the age of 60 years (Fig. 10.1). The rates for elderly women

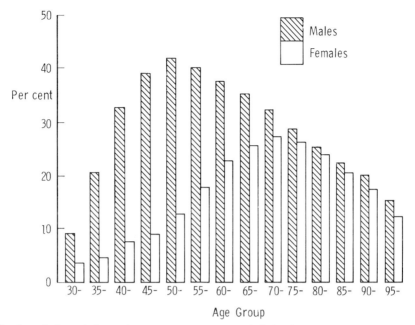

Fig. 10.1 Mortality from ischaemic heart disease as a percentage of all deaths in selected age groups, males and females, England and Wales, 1980.

Source: Office of Population Censuses and Surveys (Office of Health Economics 1982. Reproduced by permission of OHE).

increase, and after the age of 70 years they have almost caught up those of the men. In comparison, death from respiratory disease is less of a problem in that absolute rates are lower (Table 10.1). But, relative to younger age groups, respiratory deaths are high for elderly men, and they increase progressively with age up to 84 years.

These figures reflect morbidity from these diseases, but they do underestimate it. The description of disability associated with these chronic illnesses requires clear definition.

Table 10.1 Deaths for selected causes by age and sex plus per cent of total deaths, 1983—England and Wales. Source: Office of Population Censuses and Surveys, 1984 (reproduced by permission of OPCS)

Cause of death	Sex	Age group											
		Under 1 year		1–54		55–64		65–74		75–84		85 and over	
		No.	%	No.	%	No.	%	No.	%	No.	%	No.	%
All causes	M	3 654	100	29 008	100	47 315	100	88 622	100	91 531	100	29 289	100
	F	2 727	100	17 465	100	27 792	100	59 913	100	104 844	100	77 448	100
	P	6 381	100	46 473	100	75 107	100	148 535	100	196 375	100	106 737	100
Disease of the	M	19	0.5	25	0.1	7	0.0	6	0.0	5	0.0	—	—
respiratory tract	F	16	0.6	17	0.1	6	0.0	12	0.0	13	0.0	7	0.0
(ICD 460–465, 470–478)	P	35	0.5	42	0.1	13	0.0	18	0.0	18	0.0	7	0.0
Bronchitis (chronic	M	3	0.1	474	1.6	1 517	3.2	3 782	4.3	4 695	5.1	1 353	4.6
and unspecified emphysema) Asthma	F	9	0.3	352	2.0	690	2.5	1 335	2.2	1 696	1.6	1 149	1.5
(ICD 490–493)	P	12	0.2	826	1.8	2 207	2.9	5 117	3.4	6 391	3.3	2 502	2.3

ICD = International Classification of Diseases.

Health professionals and health policy makers need an integrated view and language for disability in order to establish optimal patterns of care and support (Office of Health Economics 1981).

Terminology to describe loss of functional capacity

The different aspects relating to incapacity have been defined with some precision (Office of Health Economics 1981).

Impairment describes specific physical damage whether to the nervous system or to any other part of the body.

Disability is the immediate consequence of impairment. It can be divided into functional limitations (for example, loss of ability to grip) and activity restrictions (for example, loss of ability to write, wash or feed oneself). The terms disability and disablement can also refer generally to the processes of impairment/disability/handicap described by the disability spectrum.

Handicap is used to refer to an individual's loss of a satisfactory social role, whether in work, leisure or domestic life. However, in certain instances, as in the widely used phrase 'mental handicap', it has a less precise meaning.

Factors which contribute to or aggravate cardiovascular and respiratory disease

Despite much known about coronary heart disease and the existence of considerable research, the cause of the disease is unknown. However, there are several factors which contribute to it, and there probably will be more than one of these present. The evidence (Department of Health and Social Security 1981) suggests that the main risk factors of coronary heart disease are smoking, raised blood pressure and a raised concentration of blood cholesterol. The secondary factors are:
— Family history of diabetes
— Obesity
— Stress/personality   evidence is equivocal

— Hard tap-water
— Lack of physical activity—good evidence to support this.

The main factors affecting chronic lung disease are:
— Cigarette smoking
— Air pollution and occupational dust—these may be primary causes of bronchitis and also responsible for exacerbating the condition when established.
— Respiratory disease in the first years of life may predispose to chronic bronchitis later in life (Royal College of Physicians 1981).

THE MANAGEMENT OF OLD PEOPLE WITH CARDIOVASCULAR AND RESPIRATORY DISORDERS

Assessment

> The idea of a man's interviewing himself is rather odd, to be sure. But then that is what all of us are doing. I talk half the time to find out my own thoughts, as a schoolboy turns his pockets inside out to see what is in them. He brings to light all sorts of personal property he had forgotten in his inventory. (Oliver Holmes.)

Nursing management begins with good assessment. Doctors and nurses differ in their assessment tools, but co-ordination is essential if a therapeutic plan with goals of care are to be tailored to the needs of the individual. Although we wish to give form or shape to our observations, it can be very constraining for an elderly person to be interviewed by a nurse checking a series of questions. Illness and disability sometimes cause people to feel a loss of identity, to lack confidence and to be afraid. Assessment by questioning during conversation will help a person reflect and will allow a picture of her life to emerge with biographical and health information. More objective information from the nurse's observations are also important.

When making an assessment a nurse will need experience and insight in observing a person's physical and psychological capacities in coping with illness and disability. Time and opportunity are necessary to form a relationship between nurse and patient.

Two examples will be used here to illustrate nursing assessment and management.

Example 1—in hospital

Mrs B is a 75-year-old widow who came into hospital with congestive cardiac failure and has the additional problem of painful knees from osteoarthritis. The last two weeks have proved difficult at home with decreased mobility and her general practitioner has asked for a medical review as her lifestyle has altered dramatically.

On assessment it was noted that Mrs B was dyspnoeic and only able to transfer from bed to chair with full support. Both feet were oedematous and she was troubled by constipation. She was pleased to rest, being clearly lethargic and somewhat depressed. Mrs B's daughter accompanied her, and, over several days, information was gathered from them both to assist her nursing care and to consider goals she would need to achieve prior to discharge. Normally she was independent with the aid of a stick and enjoyed going to a lunch club.

Mrs B's main problems	Aims/management 3–5 days
Unable to manage at home independently and learning to adjust to hospital	Responsibility for small decisions while recovering. Feel safe and comfortable in hospital
Lethargic and tired, mood despondent	Physical and mental rest
Dyspnoeic on slightest exertion	Less breathless through increased efficiency of myocardium and reduced cardiac workload
Appetite had diminished as food difficult to prepare at home	2–3 litres nutritious fluid in 24 hours, subject to weight and urine output. Reintroduction to no added-salt diet
Constipation	Bowel action on alternate days
Unable to perform personal hygiene (a) Pressure area discomfort	To feel cool, clean and comfortable with support Relief of pressure by repositioning
Unable to walk without aid, but able to transfer from bed to chair without help	Leg and breathing exercises to maintain physical activity. Periods in a chair. Confidence to use walking frame for transfer
(a) Oedematous feet	Reduced oedema in feet
(b) Painful knees	Less pain in knees

Summary of progress
Mrs B required time to recover mentally and physically.
1. Cardiac efficiency was established by the clinician's therapeutic plan of using digitalis and appropriate diuretics and nursing her by planning activities with appropriate rest and activity.

2. Rehabilitation and restoring functional abilities was achieved by gradually increasing exercises to maintain physical fitness. Nurses worked co-operatively with the physiotherapist and occupational therapist to simulate a therapeutic environment in the ward. Daily living activities such as washing, dressing and movement could be practised in order to achieve the long-term goal of independent mobility with a stick.

3. Controlling her future situation without unnecessary anxiety was an educative goal. She was taught to recognise physical deterioration in her cardiac state by recognising weight gain or increased dyspnoea. She learned to use scales and record her weight. She took her prescribed drugs with the knowledge about dose times and side-effects, using a calendar to tick off medications taken.

From admission emphasis was on discharge home, therefore the aim was to help her understand her condition and to participate in goal setting and planning her recovery. The services of the district nurse, home help, and reviewing aids for living were established during a home assessment visit prior to discharge.

Example 2—at home

Mr R was visited by the district nurse and general practitioner as he and his wife were very worried because he had lost movement in his legs overnight, and now felt he could not walk. Mr R had had chronic obstructive airways disease for three years and was supported by bronchodilators and oxygen therapy. He had given up smoking. He felt dyspnoeic, said his legs were heavy and that his nostrils were dry and sore. The general practitioner established that his legs were neurologically and physically in order and found no evidence of respiratory infection. It emerged that he had taken one of his wife's sleeping tablets because he had insomnia. Despite reassurance about resuming activities with his wife's support, Mr R remained in bed with very little exercise for two days. The district nurse invited a colleague with respiratory experience to visit and, after conversing with him and making an assessment, the following problems were defined and management planned.

Mr R's main problems	Aims/management—5 days
Total loss of confidence in ability to walk and unable to move around in his own environment	Regain confidence. Opportunity to talk with a nurse about restoring the ability to walk and the importance of exercise to maintain physical fitness and pulmonary ventilation. Short-term goal: walking frame, then walk with stick
Expressed fears that his legs had been paralysed and would not move properly again	Reduce fear by understanding the effects of sedation on sleep, his legs, and its dangers

Mr R's main problems	Aims/management—5 days
Dyspnoeic on exertion. Sore nostrils from oxygen therapy	Continue oxygen with comfort and portable oxygen for activity. Humidification introduced. Teach nasal cleansing
Unable to perform activities such as personal hygiene or movement, therefore totally dependent on his wife	Support from wife and nurse until confidence restored
Feels isolated, said his wife had too much to do	Acknowledge wife's role, but offer her additional support. Review use of wheelchair and recreational occupation

Summary of progress

1. Mr R was unable to achieve improved mobility until he regained his confidence and was given more understanding of the value of exercise. Emphasis was put on using oxygen (2 litres via nasal cannulae) for activity to improve exercise tolerance and comfort. Insight into the dangers of sleeping tablets was given.

2. His sleep improved with nasal cleansing done by himself, and his wife was taught how to set up his oxygen with humidification (which is not used much at home as it is usually unnecessary).

3. Targets were set for simple exercise to meet specific goals. He was able to move from his bedroom to the sitting room to watch television, and he was encouraged to do exercises, such as short walks to telephone or to the kitchen.

4. He chose to wear a track suit for easy dressing and some ideas for recreation were discussed—for example, clock repairing, which he used to enjoy.

Mr R did well at home with nursing and medical support. A recommendation has been made for the provision of a nurse or health visitor to support patients with chronic obstructive airways disease in the community (Royal College of Physicians 1981).

Clinical observation

The nurse's clinical observations will support a physician's plan and will provide a picture of the patient's health status to support the health data collected on first assessment. The following measurements should be recorded:

Oral temperature—frequency dependent on presence of pyrexia

Blood pressure

Radial pulse—if irregular, apex and radial pulse rate taken

Daily weight before breakfast if oedema present

Regular urinanalyses taken to detect abnormalities or check for glucose if steroids used in medical therapy

Height

Daily vitalography—represents

Forced expiratory volume (FEV) and Forced vital capacity of the lungs (FVC) } in one second

Peak flows—assess broncho-restriction and are used to evaluate the effect of medicines (e.g. a bronchodilator)

Maintaining physical fitness with a limiting disorder

Care and support should keep the disabled person in a state of optimum fitness. It is important for the disabled person to increase regular movement to whatever extent possible so that she can keep as fit as possible within her limitations. When planning an exercise programme for a patient at home the following points should be considered:

(a) Home environment—take advice from the occupational therapist. Rearrange furniture. Provide adequate warmth. Review bed height. Consider use of pillow support frame, comfortable chair, rails on staircase, suitable clothing—for example, a track suit.

(b) Promoting exercise—realistic goals: enquire what the patient wishes to achieve— perhaps reach front door, the next room, or garden gate, and then establish what is possible. Review aids to support activity: walking frame—rolator—walking stick. Teach simple, graded exercises with targets to reach. Encourage the patient to keep records of her achievement from her exercise programme.

(c) Planning activities—with periods of rest. Rest after meals or if dizzy.

(d) If oxygen is used, review how it is used. Education about oxygen prior and during activities improves exercise tolerance. Is portable oxygen available? or is the patient using long oxygen tubing to aid mobility? Is it safe?

Patients on long-term domiciliary oxygen may have oxygen concentrators which extract and filter oxygen from the atmosphere or oxygen cylinders. Concentrators are more convenient (Howard 1983).

(e) Social outlets—review opportunities to leave home by wheelchair or provide transport for journeys to reach club or friends (a two-hour oxygen cylinder is available for these purposes). Enjoyable activity to be considered a priority. Review recreational outlets.

(f) General advice—where necessary, give advice about weight reduction, giving up smoking and recognition of deterioration in health, and appropriate actions to take.

Planning activities within treatment regimes

This offers a patient choice and freedom which will lead to improved compliance and increase her sense of independence. It is important that a patient is educated to understand the purpose of treatment, how to use it, and to recognise the side effects of medication. The following lists how activity with rest can be planned:

Cardiovascular disease

If angina occurs, rest and take prescribed medication

Diuretic can be missed if outing planned

Encourage to take next day and recognise any deterioration, e.g. oedematous feet, dyspnoea

Respiratory disease

Prescribed oxygen or bronchodilator may be helpful prior to activity

Bronchodilator used in electric home nebuliser is useful to help expectoration and breathing during the morning prior to activity

Spacer * (for bronchodilator) useful for patient with poor hand dexterity or lack of co-ordination

---

* A spacer is a device which traps the medication briefly and obviates the need for accurate coordination of inspiration and aerosol activation.

The effect of exercise on cardiovascular and respiratory disorders

Cardiovascular disorders. Traditional medical care has advocated rest and caution when considering exercise for patients with cardio-vascular illness. However, in the past decade, a rehabilitative approach is considered to be more beneficial. Patients are mobilised earlier to prevent the deleterious effects of bed rest. Exercise is part of recovery; it improves the functional status and promotes a sense of well-being. Physical activity was reported to be valuable for patients with symptomatic coronary heart disease (Wenger 1983), and 90% of patients with peripheral vascular disease doubled their walking ability after training (Ekroth et al 1978). While exercise is essential to recovery, it is recommended that it is gradually increased in individually tailored programmes which are goal directed.

Respiratory disorders. There is no evidence that exercise improves lung function, but it does increase exercise tolerance, and increases functional ability in daily living activities (Cockroft et al 1981, Hedley Peach and Pathy 1981, Cockroft in press).

Defining the limits of exercise tolerance

Providing a patient remains well, she will need encouragement to maintain exercise in order to achieve safe and realistic goals. For example, if she cannot reach the lavatory because of distance, a commode should be located in a suitable place. She should be encouraged to take exercise until moderately breathless, to rest and start again. If she becomes ill, urge her to continue simple exercises—for example, leg exercises, and to try to spend periods sitting in a chair rather than in bed to prevent deterioration. Progress will be much slower if exercise is neglected for a few days.

Promoting independence and preventing deterioration is the essence of good nursing management of patients with breathing difficulties. Patients with dyspnoea associated with cardiovascular and respiratory disorders are likely to become progressively disabled, frail and have a shortened life. Nursing care requires the utmost skill in order that the old person achieves some independence, maximum comfort or can have a peaceful and dignified death.

Both the patient and her family will need much support in order to cope with the distressing aspects of dyspnoea. The family can contribute to the care of their relative and they often value the involvement. The nurse, patient and family must communicate effectively with each other in order to understand each other's roles. A telephone at home may be a life-line and a call bell at hand in hospital is essential. The presence of familiar faces and a feeling of confidence in those around promote emotional security and a physical sense of security for both the patient and her family.

A breathless patient has had long experience of trying to cope and illness increases anxiety. Anticipating these fears and helping the patient meet exhausting needs require sensitivity and skill. The patient's speech may be slow and laboured and time is necessary for listening. To breathe and to cope with small activities cost effort. Nursing management is directed at minimising oxygen requirements and promoting ventilation and comfort. Such management requires empathy, creative skill and continuous re-evaluation.

REFERENCES

Adams G M, de Vries H A 1973 Physiological effects of an exercise training regimen upon women aged 52 to 76. Journal of Gerontology 28: 50–55
Bannister R 1969 The meaning of physical fitness. Proceedings Research Society Medicine 62:1159
Buccola V A, Stone W J 1975 Effects of jogging and cycling programmes on physiological and personality variables in aged men. Research Quarterly 46: 134–138
Cockroft A in press Exercise for patients with respiratory disease. Update

Cockroft A, Saunders M J, Berry G 1981 Randomised control trial of rehabilitation in chronic respiratory disability. Thorax 36: 200–203
Copple P 1983 The concept of exercise. Nursing Times 70(32): 66–69
Department of health and social security 1981 Factors increasing the risk. In: Prevention and Health. Avoiding heart attack. HMSO, London, ch 4, p 27–30
Ekroth R, Dahllof A G, Gundewall B, Holm J, Schersten T 1978 Physical training of patients with intermittent clandication: indications, methods and results. Surgery 84:640
Hall M R P, MacLennan, Lye M D W 1978 The cardiovascular system: the ageing lung. In: Medical care of the elderly. H M & M Publishers, Aylesbury
Hedley Peach, Pathy M 1981 Follow up study of disability among elderly patients discharged from hospital with exacerbations of chronic bronchitis. Thorax 36: 585–589
Howard P, 1983 Oxygen in the home. Thorax 38: 161–164
Jones N L, Campbell E, Moran E J 1982 Clinical exercise testing, 2nd edn. W B Saunders, London
Kelvin P 1980 Work as source of identity. In: R Gilman (ed) The development of social psychology. Academic Press, London
Office of Health Economics 1981 Disability in Britain: the process of transition. OHE, London
Office of Health Economics 1982 Coronary heart disease: the scope for prevention. OHE, London
Office of Population censuses and surveys 1984 Personal communication
Panicucci C L 1983 Functional assessment of the older adult in the acute care setting. In: Shannon-Shine M (ed) The nursing clinics of North America, II: Gerontological nursing in acute care. W B Saunders, Philadelphia, vol 18 (2): 357–362
Ray R O, Gissal M L, Smith E L 1982 The effect of exercise on morale of older adults. In: Kiernat J N, Hasselkus B R (eds) Physical and occupational therapy in geriatics. Haworth Press, Boston Spa, vol 2
Rosser R, Denford J, Heslop A, Kinston W, Macklin D, Minty K et al 1983 Breathlessness and psychiatric morbidity in chronic bronchitis and emphysema: a study of psychotherapeutic management. Psychological Medicine 13: 93–110
Royal College of Physicians 1981 Disabling chest disease: prevention and care. Update Publishers, London, p 21
Sidney K H, Shephard R J 1977 Activity patterns of elderly men and women. Journal of Gerontology 32: 25–32
Sidney K H, Shephard R J, Harrison J E 1977 Endurance training and body composition in the elderly. American Journal of Clinical Nutrition 30: 326–333
Sports Council, 1982 The strategy. In: Sport in the Community, the next ten years. Sports Council, London, ch 8
Wenger N K, 1983 Uncomplicated acute myocardial infarction: Long term management. American Journal Cardiology 52: 658–660

11

S. Thomas

Eating and drinking

Until recent times knowledge of the dietary needs of the elderly was based largely on folklore and tradition. It was assumed that old people needed less to eat and that they enjoyed the mythical 'geriatric' diet. However, current thought suggests that old people may need less energy (kilocalories) than young, but their requirements for all nutrients is similar and, in some instances, actually increased (see Table 11.1). Yet, for a variety of medical and social reasons, many old people reduce not only their energy intake, but also their intake of many vital nutrients, resulting in malnutrition. What is the extent of malnutrition amongst the elderly in the United Kingdom? Prior to 1967, two major nutritional surveys had been carried out: Bransby and Osborne (1953) completed a survey of old people living alone or with their spouses in Sheffield, and Exton-Smith and Stanton (1965) carried out a smaller survey of elderly women living alone in two London boroughs. These surveys dispelled some of the rumours that old people exist mainly on a diet of bread, butter, jam, biscuits and cups of sweetened tea. However, more detailed research was needed in order to ascertain the actual extent of malnutrition which existed amongst the elderly.

In 1967 the Department of Health and Social Security undertook a nationwide nutrition survey of elderly people living in the community (DHSS 1972) in which they found that 3.2% of the subjects were suffering from

143

Table 11.1 Comparison between recommended daily amounts of food energy and nutrients for the elderly and younger age groups in the UK
Source: Department of Health and Social Security (1979a)

Age range years	Occupational Category	Energy		Protein	Thiamin	Riboflavin	Nicotinic acid equivalents	Total folate	Ascorbic acid	Vitamin A retinol equivalents	Vitamin D cholecalciferol	Calcium
		MJ	Kcal	g	mg	mg	mg	µg	mg	µg	µg	mg
Men												
18–34	Sedentary	10.5	2510	63	1.0	1.6	18	300	30	750	(i)	500
35–64	Sedentary	10.0	2400	60	1.0	1.6	18	300	30	750	(i)	500
65–74	Assuming a sedentary life	10.0	2400	60	1.0	1.6	18	300	30	750	(i)	500
75+		9.0	2150	54	0.9	1.6	18	300	30	750	(i)	500
Women												
18–54	Most occupations	9.0	2150	54	0.9	1.3	15	300	30	750	(i)	500
55–74	Assuming a sedentary life	8.0	1900	47	0.8	1.3	15	300	30	750	(i)	500
75+		7.0	1680	42	0.7	1.3	15	300	30	750	(i)	500

(i) No dietary sources may be necessary for children and adults who are sufficiently exposed to sunlight, but during the winter children and adolescents should receive 10 µg (400 i.u.) daily by supplementation. Adults with inadequate exposure to sunlight, for example those who are housebound, may also need a supplement of 10 µg daily clinical malnutrition. Five years later they repeated the study on those of the original sample still alive and willing to co-operate (DHSS 1979b). Seven per cent of the subjects had clinical malnutrition at the time of this survey. For the majority of these the malnutrition was found to be secondary to a medical or mental condition, which could lead one to conclude that a decline in physical or psychological well-being leads to a decline in nutritional status.

For every diagnosis of clinical malnutrition, there must be many more old people suffering from subclinical malnutrition. Overt clinical malnutrition only appears after a long latent period of inadequate food intake. During this time the body's nutrient stores are gradually depleted, but there are no outward signs of deficiency. However, when a crisis causing physiological stress occurs to such an individual, he or she has few nutritional reserves to draw on and thus slides into a state of malnutrition.

RISK FACTORS AFFECTING THE NUTRITIONAL STATUS OF THE ELDERLY

Based on a list drawn up by Exton-Smith (1978), the following risk factors may all predispose the elderly to malnutrition.

Loneliness

For some old people, dining alone heightens their feelings of solitude. Many women, used to a lifetime of cooking for their husbands and families, lose the incentive to cook for one.

Ignorance

The generation reaching old age today were brought up in times of great hardship, when financial limitations governed food choice. Housewives relied heavily on both sugar and fats in order to satisfy their family's appetites. This paved the way for a lifetime of poor eating habits. One of the groups of old people most at risk are widowers who, on the death of their wives, may be forced to fend for themselves with neither culinary skills nor nutrition knowledge.

Budget

Eating well on a pension demands that the individual be skilled at budgeting and motivated to shop wisely, taking advantage of special offers. Brockington and Lempert (1967) found that those old people with a supplementary income had a better diet than those who relied on their pension alone. Each person's priorities differ; to some, food may be less important than heating, bingo, alcohol or cigarettes.

Physical disability

Any disability, however great or small, can hinder the shopping, cooking or even eating of food. For example, one old lady who suffered from severe arthritis had her store cupboard well stocked with tinned food but ate none of it because she was unable to manipulate a can-opener.

Mental confusion and depression

Dementia affects 5% of the population aged 65 and over in this country. It brings with it a lack of awareness of the basic human needs—a confused old person may simply forget to eat, unless someone is there to remind them. Demented patients may demonstrate bizarre eating patterns, which, due to their poor nutritional balance, could lead to malnutrition. For example one patient was found drinking pickle and HP sauce, and another ate soap. Depression is also an important cause of anorexia in the elderly.

Iatrogenic factors

The continuation of special diets long after they are needed can cause malnutrition. For example, adherence to low fat diets 10 or 15 years after cholecystectomy can cause chronic weight loss and deficiency of the fat-soluble vitamins. The old 'gastric regime' for ulcers which excluded some fruit and vegetables could, in the long term, precipitate scurvy. The indiscriminate use of 'special' diets could also damage a patient with a precarious nutritional state. For example, overweight patients subjected to rigorous reducing regimes on admission to geriatric wards may well have an underlying subclinical malnutrition, which would be compounded by the diet. Many elderly people have a patchy knowledge of nutrition. This can lead to abstention from certain nourishing foods for no logical reason and a heavy reliance on other foods or vitamin pills, believing them to be the panacea of all ills. Both situations can lead to disaster.

Alcoholism

Alcohol may be drunk in excess quantity by an old person for pain relief, to dull loneliness, for warmth or, as one old man told me, for the maintenance of a last surviving vice. The elderly alcoholic may be difficult to detect because, like younger alcoholics, they tend to be secretive about their drinking habits. However, it is imperative that those with an excessive alcohol intake be identified in order to give appropriate nutritional supplements and advice, thus preventing the more harmful nutritional consequences of alcohol abuse. On investigating a patient suspected of drinking, a history from relatives, friends or the social services might be invaluable. One cachexic old man admitted to a geriatric unit in an acute confusional state was unable to give any sort of diet history. The doctors had rejected any thought that the patient was an alcoholic, but a routine call to the home help organiser, revealed that the only way the old man would eat his meals-on-wheels, was if the meal was delivered to the local public house, where he spent most of his day.

Deficiencies of the vitamin B complex, particularly thiamine and folic acid are commonly seen in the alcoholic.

Drugs

There are many harmful interactions between drugs and nutrition. Certain medications (e.g. digoxin, phenformin and chemotherapy agents) can cause nausea and loss of appetite. Others may induce depletion of the body's mineral stores, such as penicillamine with zinc, purgatives with phosphate, diuretics with potassium, zinc with magnesium (Roe 1977). Aspirins and salicylates may cause internal bleeding, leading to an iron deficiency anaemia. Certain other drugs can interfere with vitamin metabolism, but conversely the same vitamin, when given in therapeutic doses, can interrupt the drug metabolism, as with long-term use of anti-convulsants with folic acid and vitamin D (Dent et al 1970, Labadarios et al 1978).

Taste and smell perception

Whilst it is accepted that both sight and hearing might decline with ageing, the impairment in the senses of taste and smell is seldom considered. Other factors which contribute to a decline in taste and smell perception include disease state, drugs, poor oral hygiene and smoking. Food choice and appetite may be seriously affected by disorders of taste and smell, resulting in malnutrition.

Dentition

Lack of dentition or ill-fitting dentures may influence food choice, causing the elderly individual to select a diet high in soft starchy foods, at the expense of meat, fresh fruit and vegetables. Poor oral hygiene may mask taste perception.

Malabsorption

Malabsorption is a potent cause of malnutrition in the elderly. Conditions such as ischaemic bowel, post-gastrectomy syndromes and gluten sensitivity can all cause malabsorption, resulting in weight loss, with deficiency of folic acid, vitamin B12 and the fat-soluble vitamins.

Increased nutritional requirements

Elderly patients recovering from surgery, those on prolonged bed-rest and those with pressure sores may all have an increased nutritional requirement. However, it is just these patients who lose their appetite and eat less rather than more food.

Cultural and religious factors

Many of the Asian immigrants to Britain, particularly the elderly, have not adopted western eating habits, preferring to purchase their own familiar foods. Items such as imported leafy green vegetables are both costly and low in vitamin content owing to transportation problems. Many Hindu Asians are strict vegetarians, and a deficiency of iron and vitamin B12 may occur in those who take no animal products. Osteomalacia is also seen among the Asian community. Hindus fast on special festivals in their calendar and, in addition, many fast on one or two days each week. Muslims fast during Ramadan, and although they are exempt if ill many will insist on fasting, regardless of their condition. Such practices could compound an underlying malnutrition.

SPECIFIC NUTRITIONAL PROBLEMS

Anorexia

Loss of appetite, or anorexia, in elderly people is an important sign of loss of physical or emotional well-being, which needs thorough investigation. Whatever the cause, a sudden onset of anorexia, sometimes with total refusal of food, will result in a state of acute starvation within days of onset. A chronic loss of appetite can often go unnoticed, unless nursing staff are vigilant at mealtimes. Patients who survive on 500–600 kilocalories (kcal) daily or less can slowly slip into a state of semistarvation. In addition to the physical signs of starvation, with weight loss, poor wound healing and physical debility, the starved individual experiences mental changes. A starved patient may be withdrawn, depressed, emotionally labile and might express a death-wish. Treating this type of patient can be difficult and will be discussed further on.

Dehydration

A man can survive for some weeks without food, but without fluid he will die within a matter of days. Provided there is free access to water, the fluid balance is carefully regulated by the body and a balance between input and output maintained. The optimum fluid intake is 1.0–1.5 litres (6–9 cups) daily, yet many old people drink far less, some believing that they need less fluid as they grow older. Davies (1981) noted that certain old people limited the time of their last drink in the day, usually because they preferred not to get up in the night. Dehydration involves more than a change in water balance—there are also accompanying changes in electrolyte balance. When water supply is restricted, or losses excessive, owing to fever, vomiting, burns or haemorrhage, rate of water loss exceeds the rate of electrolyte loss. The extracellular fluid becomes concentrated and osmotic pressure draws water from the cells into the extracellular fluid in compensation.

In mild cases of dehydration, the encouragement of oral fluids may be all that is required. Offering tea, coffee, milk, fruit juice and carbonated drinks rather than water alone will encourage the patient to take fluids. In severe cases of dehydration, however, the patient may be unable to tolerate a sufficient quantity of oral fluids and intravenous infusion will be necessary.

Anaemias

Anaemia is the term used to describe any condition where the oxygen-carrying capacity of the blood falls below normal. Symptoms vary with the type and severity of the anaemia, but can include tiredness, breathlessness on exertion, dizziness, pallor of the mucous membranes, palpitations, ankle oedema and, occasionally, angina in the elderly.

Iron-deficiency anaemia

Iron deficiency causes a microcytic, hypo-chromic anaemia. In addition to the usual symptoms of anaemia described above, iron-deficient patients may have brittle, spoon-shaped nails (koilonychia) and a sore, red, smooth tongue. Iron-deficiency anaemia in elderly people is usually associated with chronic internal bleeding or acute haemor-rhage. Poor diet is rarely the sole cause of microcytic anaemia in this age group, but may be a contributory factor. Iron deficiency is usually treated with oral iron tablets, such as ferrous sulphate or ferrous gluconate. In severe cases blood transfusions are given. Advice on increasing the iron content of the diet is also important. Rich sources are liver and liver products such as liver paté and liver sausage, corned beef, kidney, red meats and eggs. Other good sources include whole-meal bread, fortified breakfast cereals, lentils and green vegetables.

Vitamin B12 deficiency anaemia

Vitamin B12 deficiency anaemia causes a megaloblastic anaemia. Other symptoms may include a red raw tongue, and, if advanced, there may be a subacute combined degener-ation of the cord, peripheral neuropathy and mental changes. The deficiency is caused by malabsorption owing to lack of intrinsic factor (pernicious anaemia) or chronic atrophic gastritis. It is also a long-term complication of partial or total gastrectomy. In rare cases, vitamin B12 deficiency has been diagnosed in people following Vegan diets, which exclude all animal products, including milk. Treatment is with monthly injections of vitamin B12 for life.

Anaemia due to folic acid deficiency

Folic acid deficiency also causes a megalo-blastic anaemia, and in addition to the symp-toms common to all anaemias, the patient may have a red, raw tongue. Unlike iron and B12 deficiency, this type of anaemia is often associ-ated with poor diet, particularly in the elderly. In the DHSS survey of the elderly in 1972 (DHSS 1979b), approximately one fifth of the men and one quarter of the women had evidence of long-term folate deficiency. There has been interest in the significance between dementia and poor folate status in the elderly (Sneath et al 1973). It is most probable that the dementia leads to inadequate dietary intake and, in turn, folate deficiency, although the likelihood that the folate deficiency itself leads to impaired mental function cannot be excluded. Rich sources of folic acid include liver and dark-green leafy vegetables. This vitamin is easily destroyed by prolonged cooking, and therefore those old people who rely upon institutional catering such as meals-on-wheels or hospital food, may have a low intake of folate. Treatment of this anaemia is with folic acid tablets and dietary advice.

Vitamin C deficiency

Scurvy, caused by severe vitamin C deficiency, is seldom seen today. However, occasional cases are still diagnosed amongst the elderly people, particularly old men living alone—hence the term 'widower's scurvy'. Symptoms include swelling and bleeding of gums (except in edentulous individuals), 'sheet' haemor-rhages in the skin of the arms and legs, anaemia and mental changes. One such case of scurvy was diagnosed in an old lady who was admitted to hospital from her own home. On admission she was emaciated, dehydrated and unable to respond to even the simplest command. 'Sheet' haemorrhages on both arms were noted and these spontaneously opened and bled within 24 hours of admission. Urinary saturation tests (Harris and Ray 1935) substantiated the provisional diag-nosis of scurvy, which was confirmed by the diet history obtained from relatives: three weeks' supply of meals-on-wheels were found, unopened, in the old lady's kitchen and the only other food in the house was half a packet of biscuits. There was also evidence that she had been drinking her own urine.

With rehydration, feeding and vitamin C this old lady made a remarkable improvement and soon became a pleasant, although slightly confused member of the ward. She chose not to return to her own home, but moved into a private nursing home.

Subclinical vitamin C deficiency is a more common finding in the elderly. Davies (1981) carried out research into the nutritional intake of elderly recipients of two meals-on-wheels per week in Portsmouth. It was reported that 40% of the subjects were taking less than the recommended daily amount (RDA) of vitamin C (DHSS 1979b), and that the vitamin C intake on the 'meals' days was less than on other days. The risks of rapid vitamin C destruction in institutional catering have long been recognised (Platt et al 1963) and yet vitamin C deficiency still occurs in institution-bound old people. Thomas et al (1982) reported that, of a group of elderly long-stay psychiatric patients, those who were not drinking a regular glass of orange juice had serum ascorbic acid levels suggestive of scurvy. Signs and symptoms of subclinical vitamin C deficiency are difficult to detect, but may in-include an increased tendency to bruising, poor wound healing and listlessness. Schorah et al (1979) reported that there was a slight but significant improvement in appetite, daily living activities and interest when a group of elderly long-stay patients, known to have low vitamin C levels, were given a one month course of this vitamin. A quick way to assess whether there is enough vitamin C in the diet is to find out whether the old person takes one of the following daily:
citrus fruit, e.g. orange or grapefruit; fresh orange juice; freshly cooked greens; raw tomato.
If none of these is included, a deficiency should be suspected. Useful suggestions of vitamin C foods for the housebound elderly and those not receiving regular supplies of fresh fruit and vegetables, include (fortified) blackcurrant juice, (fortified) dried instant fruit drinks and (fortified) instant mashed potato powder, all of which are fortified with extra vitamin C.

Vitamin D deficiency

From the age of 40 our bones begin to atrophy, although the speed with which this happens is subject to individual variation. This is an accepted process of ageing, known as osteoporosis, for which there is little remedy except to take regular exercise and to ensure an adequate calcium intake. However, a more treatable condition known as osteomalacia, or adult rickets, is also prevalent amongst elderly people, particularly those who are housebound. Anderson et al (1966) diagnosed oesteomalacia in 4% of female admissions to a geriatric unit. Aaron et al (1974) reported that 20–30% of women and 40% of men presenting with fractured proximal femur had osteomalacia. Thomas et al (1982) found that 43% of elderly psychiatric patients in long-stay care were at risk of osteomalacia.

Osteomalacia is caused by lack of vitamin D, which is needed to transport calcium from the diet to the bones. Symptoms of this deficiency disease include bone pain, muscle weakness and an increased susceptibility to falls and fractures. In Britain most of our vitamin D is derived from the action of sunlight on the skin, with a small contribution from diet. Osteomalacia can easily be prevented by adequate exposure to sunlight. Regular walks or rests in the sunshine should be encouraged. No stripping off is needed— open shirt collars and rolled-up sleeves are sufficient. Direct sunlight is not necessary—a seat in the shade will be adequate. For those who are completely housebound, a seat on a balcony or beside an open window would be beneficial. Serving afternoon tea in the grounds might encourage elderly residents of Homes and hospitals to take a little sunshine. Regular use of the foods containing vitamin D will help to boost the body's stores, particularly in the winter months when none can be derived from sunlight. Good sources of vitamin D include: oily fish; margarine; Ovaltine; liver; eggs; evaporated milk.

However, it should be remembered that diet alone will not prevent osteomalacia. If an old person is completely housebound, with no access to sunlight, then he or she should be referred to a doctor for vitamin D tablets. Finally, a word of warning, vitamin D can be extremely toxic and so self-medication should be discouraged.

Diet-related bowel disorders

Constipation

Causes of constipation in the elderly include lack of dietary fibre, lack of fluids, insufficient exercise, loss of muscle tone and the effects of drugs. Many patients during the first few days of hospital admission experience constipation. This is due to a change of environment, change of diet and emotional disturbance, but the constipation will usually settle within a few days.

The use of purgatives, although helpful in certain cases, should not become a ward routine. There are four different types of purgatives:
— Bulk-forming drugs, e.g. methylcellulose, Fybogel and Isogel.
— Stimulant laxatives which increase intestinal activity, e.g. bisacodyl, danthron (the active ingredient of Dorbanex), Senokot, castor oil.
— Faecal softeners which either soften the whole stool, e.g. Dioctyl sodium sulphosuccinate, or add lubrication, e.g. liquid paraffin.
— Osmotic laxatives maintain the volume of fluid in the bowel by osmosis, but do not act directly on the faeces e.g. magnesium sulphate, lactulose.

An adequate intake of fibre will help to prevent constipation. The diet should include wholemeal bread, high fibre breakfast cereals such as Weetabix, Shredded Wheat, Branflakes, Puffed Wheat and porridge, and plenty of fruit and vegetables. Whenever possible, encourage your patients to eat the skin of potatoes, tomatoes and apples as this will also supply valuable fibre. Bran should be included in the diet only if the high fibre foods alone have not regulated bowel habits. Old people should be encouraged to take plenty

of fluids (1.0–1.5 litre daily). Physical activity will help to stimulate the tone of the bowel muscle. Exercise classes for the elderly, whether in day centres, Homes or hospitals, can be very beneficial. Even the effect of laughter will stimulate the body. Constipation is discussed in more detail in Chapter 12, Eliminating.

Diverticular disease

Diverticular disease becomes more prevalent with increasing age and is common in old people. It is the presence of small pouches in the large intestine which are harmless in themselves, unless they become inflamed or, as occasionally happens, a diverticulum perforates. Evidence suggests that deficiency of fibre in the western diet is responsible for this disease. Treatment is based on increasing the fibre content of the diet, using both high fibre foods and added coarse bran (2–3 tablespoons daily).

Swallowing problems

Management of the patient with swallowing difficulties requires the joint skills of the nurse, speech therapist, occupational therapist and the dietitian. Patients most likely to have swallowing problems include those with head injuries, strokes, multiple sclerosis, motor neurone disease and Parkinson's disease. When nursing staff first notice that a patient has difficulties, a prompt referral to the therapists is necessary to prevent the patient suffering from starvation.

The physiotherapist will advise on the correct posture to facilitate easy feeding. Wherever possible the patient should sit in a chair, rather than in bed. Feet should be flat on the floor, ensuring good flexion of the hips. In the case of the stroke patient, the affected side of the body should be brought forward, by lifting the weaker arm onto the table. Non-stick mats will prevent the patient's plate from moving. Feeding cups should be used with caution, as certain conditions such as Parkinson's disease actually prevent the patient from being able to tip the head back sufficiently to drink from the feeding cup. A glass or cup and saucer with a straw may be more appropriate and less demoralising than a feeding cup. If a nasogastric tube is in place the patient may be unable to swallow normally (Waterhouse 1983). Nasogastric feeding is an essential nutritional support during the acute phase of illness, but should be discontinued as soon as the patient is taking sufficient oral nutrition. During the period of total dependence on tube feeding it is important regularly to moisten the tongue with drops of strong flavours, e.g. lemon juice, peppermint oil, in order to stimulate the taste buds. When patients are learning to bite (an essential pre-swallowing activity) allow them to practise on French toast or cream crackers wrapped in gauze. On the introduction of food, thought must be given to the correct texture required. A monotonous diet of sloppy foods such as mince will not help the patient's progress to normal eating. A variety of textures are preferable, but not mixed together as in stew, where solid lumps in a fluid sauce would create problems. Suitable main courses include boneless fish, chopped meat such as chicken, skinless sausages, corned beef and savoury egg custards. Root vegetables, cauliflower and tinned tomatoes are good accompaniments, but peas, cabbage and 'stringy' vegetables should be avoided. Desserts present less problems: tinned pears, icecream and yoghurts are all easily managed.

ASSESSMENT OF NUTRITIONAL STATUS

The primary cause of hospital admission is seldom identified as malnutrition, yet many old people are admitted with a subclinical malnutrition which may be overlooked. This can lead to poor wound healing, delayed recovery and inability to cope at home after discharge. A simple routine of screening all new admissions to the geriatric ward would identify those most likely to be malnourished and steps can then be taken to improve their nutrition and with it, their speed of recovery. Factors to be considered are listed below.

Diagnosis

The patient's diagnosed condition may hold a clue to malnutrition. For example, motor neurone disease or severe Parkinson's disease might cause physical difficulties in either eating or swallowing. A patient with bad pressure sores or leg ulcers may need extra nutrients for wound healing. A previous medical history of partial or total gastrectomy is worth noting, particularly if the patient is losing weight, as this might be due to the nutritional problems associated with gastric surgery.

Medication

In addition to recording the list of medications currently taken by the patient, ascertain whether purgatives are taken on a regular basis. An enquiry about any vitamin tablets or 'tonics' is also useful.

Weight

A record of each patient's weight on admission is essential and should be compared with the patient's normal 'healthy' weight, in order to assess whether there is any weight loss. Past medical notes may provide details of old weights. Each patient should be questioned about their normal healthy weight; many old people have little idea about recent weight, but may well remember their weight on entering the army/getting married or before having children. This is important information because, although the proportion of lean body mass to fat decreases with ageing, total weight should remain unaltered throughout adult life (Forbes and Reina 1970).

Social history

Routine questions about each patient's social status, home situation and social services are all relevant to the assessment of nutritional well-being.

Diet history

If the patient is a good historian, a simple diet history would be valuable. This should include the following points:

> Number of meals consumed daily.
> A brief account of the content of the meals.
> Does the patient take meals-on-wheels?
> — What time does (s)he receive them?
> — What time does (s)he actually eat them?
> Is fresh fruit or fresh fruit juice taken regularly?
> Does the patient drink alcohol? (specify type and amount)
> How much fluid is consumed daily (in cupfuls)?
> How many meals are eaten out each week?

If the patient is an unreliable historian, confirmation of the diet history could be obtained from relatives, neighbours or home help.

HELPING THE ELDERLY PATIENT TO EAT

Menu planning

Menus should be carefully planned, taking the special needs of elderly people into consideration. The nurse has a lot of expertise to contribute in this area, because she has a practical working knowledge of what her patients enjoy. The energy (Kcal) requirement is reduced for the elderly and this must be borne in mind when menu planning. Foods of a high nutritional quality should be encouraged and those of little nutritional value such as sugar and sugary foods should be discouraged. An excess of fried food, with its high energy value, should also be avoided. Small, frequent meals are ideal for those old people with little appetite. The menu should contain familiar foods, but bland dishes should be avoided. The frequently voiced complaint that 'food does not taste like it used to' is more likely to be a reflection of loss of taste and smell acuity than a complaint about hospital food. All patients should be offered a choice of menu

and this should include a soft dish for those who have difficulty in chewing. However, the use of puree food, sometimes known as 'geriatric' food, should be banned. If the menus and catering staff are flexible, advantage can be made of seasonal luxuries such as strawberries. Celebrations and festivities should be reflected in the style of meals served, in order to add variety to the ward routine and it should be remembered that meals are the focal point of the patient's day.

The dining environment

Communal dining can encourage sociability amongst the patients and help to increase the appetite. Round tables break down barriers between the diners. Tableclothes and flowers add style to even the plainest hospital fare.

If the hospital uses bulk food trolleys, why not acquire some serving dishes and allow the patients to serve themselves and each other with vegetables and gravy? The tactful segregation of the messy eater might save embarrassment. Serving the slowest eaters first will enable them to enjoy their meal, without feeling hurried. Feeding the dependent patients is a time-consuming task, but one which, if carried out with kindness and understanding, will strengthen the bond between patient and nurse.

The management of loss of appetite

Accurate nursing observation at mealtimes will provide essential information on the patient's progress. If a patient appears to be taking insufficient food and/or drink, it is useful to keep a food chart. This should record the amount of food/drink served to the patient and the quantity left on the plate, together with any special observations. This information, once collected by the dietitian, will form the basis of dietetic treatment.

The first step to take when loss of appetite has been observed, is to discuss it with the doctor, as this may be an important symptom of illness. Dietary supplements should be offered to the patient between meals. This could be a high protein milk drink such as Build-Up (Carnation Foods) or Complan (Farley Health Products), fruit juice and caloreen or a snack of daintily served sandwiches. A small amount of alcohol, such as a glass of sherry 20 minutes before a meal, may help to whet the appetite. In certain cases where the loss of appetite is due to acute illness or following surgery, a short course of appetite stimulants may be appropriate.

Tube feeding

Tube feeding should be considered as an interim means of nutritional support for the patient temporarily unable to sustain his or her own nutritional intake, for example, after major surgery or during the recovery period following a cerebral vascular accident. However, the decision to tube feed must be agreed by the whole care team and should not be considered when there is little chance of recovery. This method of feeding may also be beneficial to supplement oral intake for the semistarved patient. Bastow et al (1983) reported improvements in the clinical outcome of very thin patients with fractured neck of femur, when they were given supplementary overnight tube feeding.

The role of special diets

Special diets have a very limited role to play in the nutritional care of old people. Reducing diets should be limited to cases where obesity hinders the patient's mobility and rehabilitation. Initially the diet should exclude sugar and sugar-containing foods, such as sweets, chocolate, squashes, Lucozade and other carbonated drinks, because these supply 'empty' calories with little nutritive value. If a stricter diet is necessary, the dietitian should be asked to draw up a regime which will restrict Kcals whilst providing balanced nutrition. Elderly diabetics who are treated either by diet and tablets or by diet alone can usually be controlled by simple advice on eating regular meals and excluding sugar and sugar containing foods. However, those diabetics

taking insulin injections may need more extensive advice. Other special diets are seldom necessary the elderly, but if they are needed, diet sheets should be simple and concise.

NUTRITIONAL SERVICES IN THE COMMUNITY

The meals-on-wheels service which first began during the Second World War and was run by the Women's Voluntary Service (WVS, now Women's Royal Voluntary Service), is now organised jointly by local authorities and WRVS. It supplies a hot midday meal to 2.5–3.0% of the elderly population in Britain. The cost and quality of the meal varies between areas, as does its nutritional content. Hitherto the service also provided a valuable daily social contact with the housebound elderly, but as greater demands are put on the service that social contact has become minimal in some areas. Local authorities strive to provide between five and seven meals per week for many recipients but Davies (1981) suggests that it might be more beneficial to spread the net wider and offer two to three meals per week for a greater number of old people, and perhaps spur them on to cook for themselves on the other days. Davies also suggests that there should be more reassessment of the clients because some old people only need meals-on-wheels as a temporary measure, to help them over a period of illness or bereavement, but the meals may be continued longer than necessary. Home helps are invaluable in the maintenance of many old people's nutrition. In the limited time allocated to each client the home help might be asked to do both the shopping and cooking of food. Luncheon clubs and day centres can provide both company and a good meal for many mobile old people. A few centres provide wheels-to-meals, thus enabling the housebound elderly to enjoy the benefits of these facilities, rather than dining alone. Several adult education centres run 'cook and eat' classes, which have the dual purpose of teaching culinary skills whilst offering the students a well-balanced meal.

There is much to be done in the field of nutrition education for the elderly. Pre-retirement classes are excellent forum for nutrition teaching, because the individual is on the threshold of a major change in lifestyle and is often receptive to advice. Nutrition education is also disseminated via organisations such as Age Concern, by broadcasting and in the press. Education of the caring network available for dependent elderly people is essential if our aged population is to be well nourished.

DENTAL SERVICES FOR THE ELDERLY

Research into the dental requirements of the elderly suggests that they feel the need for dental care less and less with advancing age although evidence suggests that advanced periodontal disease in old people is a serious problem (British Dental Journal 1983). By the age of 65 years over 79% of the population are edentulous (Todd et al 1978). A large proportion of this age group wear dentures. These should be replaced every 5–10 years. However, in a survey carried out by Osbourne et al (1979) 16% of the respondents had been wearing their present dentures for 30 years or more. Neil (1972) concluded that masticatory performance was no better in subjects who wore dentures of indifferent quality than in edentulous individuals. The dental service makes no special financial concessions for old people who normally have to pay the full dental fees unless they are exempt from prescription charges. However, dentists do run a domiciliary service for the housebound elderly for no extra charge. Osbourne et al (1979) noted that many elderly people were reluctant to visit the dentist. Of the subjects who complained of dental problems, 32% never attended a dentist. Reasons cited included prohibitive cost of treatment, waste of time, difficulty in travelling and fear of the dentist. If the nurse could take time to ask about her patient's state of dentition and encourage them to seek expert help from the dentist, this may add to the pleasure of eating.

REFERENCES

Aaron J E, Gallagher J C, Anderson J, Stasiak L, Longton E B, Nordin B E C, Nicholson M 1974 Frequency of osteomalacia and osteoporosis in fractures of the proximal femur. Lancet 1: 229–233

Anderson I, Campbell A E R, Dunn A, Runciman J B M 1966 Osteomalacia in elderly women. Scottish Medical Journal 11: 429–435

Anonymous 1983 Do we fail our elderly? British Dental Journal 155: 6–179

Bastow M D, Rawlings J, Allison S P 1983 Benefits of supplementary tube-feeding after fractured neck of femur: a randomised controlled trial. British Medical Journal 287: 1589–1592

Bransby E R, Osborne B 1953 A social and food survey of the elderly living alone or as married couples. British Journal Nutrition 7: 160–180

Brockington F, Lempert S M 1967 The Stockport study: the social needs of the over 80's. University Press, Manchester

Davies L 1981 Three score years . . . and then? Heinemann, London

Dent E C, Richens A, Rowe D J F, Stamp T C B 1970 Osteomalacia with long-term anticonvulsant therapy in epilepsy. British Medical Journal 4:69

Department of Health and Social Security 1972 A nutrition survey of the elderly. Report by the Panel on Nutrition of the Elderly. HMSO, London

Department of Health and Social Security 1979a Recommended daily amounts of food energy and nutrients for groups of people in the United Kingdom. HMSO, London

Department of Health and Social Security 1979b Nutrition and Health in old age. HMSO, London

Exton-Smith A N 1978 Nutrition in the elderly. In: Dickerson J W T, Lee H A (eds) Nutrition in the clinical management of disease. Edward Arnold, London

Exton-Smith A N, Stanton B R 1965 Report of an investigation into the dietary of elderly women living alone. King Edward's Hospital Fund, London

Forbes G B, Reina J C 1970 Adult lean body mass declines with age some longitudinal observations. Metabolism 19: 653–663

Harris L J, Ray S N 1935 Diagnosis of vitamin C subnutrition by urine analysis. Lancet 1: 71–77

Labadarios D, Dickerson J W T, Parke D V, Lucas E G, Obuwa G H 1978 The effects of chronic drug administration on hepatic enzyme induction and folate metabolism. British Journal Clinical Pharmacology 5: 167–173

Neill D J 1972 Masticatory studies. In: A Nutritional survey of the elderly. DHSS. HMSO, London

Osbourne J, Maddick I, Gould A, Ward D 1979 Dental demands of old people in Hampshire. British Dental Journal 146: 351–355

Platt B S, Eddy T P, Pellett P L 1963 Food in hospitals. Nuffield Foundation, Oxford University Press

Roe D A 1977 Drug induced malnutrition in geriatric patients. Comprehensive Therapy 3(10): 24–28

Schorah C J, Scott D L, Newill A, Morgan D B 1979 Clinical effects of vitamin C in elderly patients with low blood vitamin C levels. Lancet 1: 403–405

Sneath P, Chanarin I, Hodkinson H M, McPherson C K, Reynolds E H 1973 Folate status in the geriatric population and its relationship to dementia. Age and Ageing 2: 177–182

Thomas S J, Millard P H, Storey P B 1982 Risk of scurvy and osteomalacia in elderly long-stay psychiatric patients. Journal of Plant Foods 4: 191–197

Todd J E, Walker A M, Dodd P 1978 Adult dental health survey UK. OPCS Volume 11. HMSO, London

Waterhouse C 1983 Feeding and swallowing problems after stroke. Geriatric Medicine 13: 433–435

C. Norton

12

Eliminating

INTRODUCTION

The passage of urine and faeces is, for most people in western society, a very personal and private function, which many are able to take for granted. Considerable control over micturition and defaecation is necessary for the commonly accepted criteria of continence to be met. This involves a complex neuro-muscular co-ordination, in conjunction with an awareness of societal norms. This control may become vulnerable for many older people, most especially at times of illness or disease, amongst the disabled elderly and those in residential or hospital care. The nurse has a key role, in both hospital and community settings, in identifying those elderly people at risk of elimination problems. By a thorough assessment of each individual's needs, appropriate care can be planned to maintain normal function and prevent problems, or to remedy those problems already apparent.

Traditionally, nurses have approached elimination care in a routinised manner—most nurses are familiar with bedpan rounds, bottle rounds, bowel books and four-hourly toileting regimes. Care of bowel and bladder tends to be seen as a low-status task which requires little knowledge or expertise, and is often left to the most junior or untrained staff. Working with the elderly is often identified as synonymous with an endless routine of changing incontinent patients and wet beds. Indeed, this may be partly responsible for the unfavourable image of geriatric nursing held by some nurses. Yet the majority of old people manage to maintain normal elimination function to the end of their days. Problems are not a necessary or inevitable concomitant of ageing and should never be passively accepted. Problems do not 'just happen'; there must always be a cause or reason. If this can be discovered it can often be remedied, or at least the effects upon the individual minimised.

Elimination is a difficult subject for most older people to talk about. Many were brought up with Victorian attitudes towards bodily functions—that these are somehow shameful and should never be mentioned in public. Commonly, failure to maintain normal function was thought to reflect adversely on the character of the sufferer. Elimination difficulties were a cause for shame, embarrassment and guilt and best kept hidden. Consequently, many people who have problems do not seek help. For example, only a tiny proportion of incontinent people reveal the fact to health or social service agencies (Thomas et al 1980). A nurse must approach the subject with the utmost sensitivity and tact if a good rapport and trust are to be established. She must also be alert to the possibility of problems with every patient, not just those with overt difficulties. Nurses may be reluctant to bring the subject into the open, either accepting problems as irremediable or pretending nothing is wrong in order to spare the patient's embarrassment. Schwartz (1977) has described this as an attitude of 'mutual pretence' between nurses and patients, leading to problems being coped with rather than constructively confronted. Nurses are notoriously good at 'coping' in unsatisfactory circumstances. This is not always in the patient's long-term interests. Elimination problems cause misery, discomfort, can be a burden to carers, and may even rob an individual of the ability to live independently. They merit a serious nursing effort to provide optimum care.

Elimination has repeatedly been identified as a major problem for geriatric nursing. From the time of Norton's study onwards (Norton et al 1962), it has been known that problems such as incontinence occupy a high proportion of nursing time and energy. Wells (1980) compared several studies which found between 4% and 8% of nursing activity related to elimination. Interestingly, she found that the amount of time spent 'promoting continence' was inversely related to the amount of incontinence on a ward. Trained nurses were found to have 'confused, inaccurate' knowledge about the causes of bladder or bowel problems.

Although bowel and bladder care is primarily seen as a nursing concern, the importance of other professions should not be forgotten. Ideally, the multidisciplinary team will work together to maximise function. This chapter will highlight the nursing component in the team's approach to care.

ELIMINATION NEEDS

Certain basic needs are common to both micturition and defaecation. Millard (1979) has argued that the individual must be able to identify an acceptable place for elimination; to be able to get to that place; and be able to hold excreta until that place is reached. The ability to empty the bowel or bladder easily, completely and in private once there, and to perform a number of toilet-related skills, could be added to this. This may sound obvious, but failure in these abilities is so common that each will be considered in turn, along with possible measures to solve problems.

Identifying an acceptable place

An older person's ability to identify correctly an acceptable place for elimination may be impaired in several ways. Most people expect to use a lavatory, behind a locked door. In unfamiliar surroundings, this presumes an ability to follow signposts and read and correctly interpret labels on doors. Impaired vision, dim lighting or unclear (or absent) signs will create difficulties. Sometimes male and female symbols can be difficult to distinguish. The problem is often compounded by a reluctance to ask for help. In some instances of cerebrovascular disease, the individual loses the ability to recognise the function of common objects (e.g. a lavatory). The confused or demented person may likewise experience difficulty correctly identifying right and wrong receptacles and may, for instance, use a sink or wash-basin in error. In hospital, expectations are different from those in general society, and people are asked to void into bedpans, bottles, commodes, behind curtains or doors without locks (or even without a door or any privacy). It is easy to see how a disoriented person may not be able to distinguish which is the 'acceptable' place. The very confused person may lose all 'socially acceptable' behaviour, and the concept of continence or incontinence becomes irrelevant to the individual.

Correct identification can be aided by clear explanations of what is expected, ensuring good lighting, signposting and labelling of facilities and, if necessary, improving vision by provision of spectacles. Gilleard et al (1981) have demonstrated how training can improve ward orientation with psycho-geriatric patients.

Ability to get there

It is no good knowing that there is a correct place for elimination unless that place can be reached. The problem may be an unsuitable environment or an individual's physical disabilities. At home, many elderly people have a lavatory which involves climbing stairs or is outside. It may be occupied if shared with others. Public lavatories are often difficult for anyone with even a slight disability to use and are usually in sparse supply. With council cutbacks they may be closed, or vandalised and not repaired. Many older women have a horror of public lavatories (believing that they risk catching diseases) and would rather avoid their use. It has been estimated (Scottish Home and Health Department 1970) that elderly people in hospital should be a

maximum of 12 metres from the lavatory. Yet many of our geriatric wards were built in the days when all patients were nursed in bed—lavatories have been built on as an afterthought, often at the opposite end of the ward to the dayroom and down a corridor or around a corner. The British Standards Institution (1979) has drawn up guidelines for recommended lavatory design for disabled people, but these seem seldom to be adhered to, even in new buildings or upgradings.

Mobility is essential in getting to the lavatory. This may be helped by ensuring that beds and chairs are of the correct height and design to aid rising; that routes are uncluttered with obstacles (e.g. loose mats in the house); and that the individual has the optimum mobility aid for her needs. Good footcare and well-fitting shoes can make a great difference. Opening the lavatory door and getting into the compartment may present problems if design is poor. The height of the lavatory and availability of grab-rails will often determine whether sitting and rising are possible. Manual dexterity is crucial in removal of clothing, positioning and cleansing. Appropriate clothing, a raised seat or a dressing aid can facilitate independent toileting.

Sometimes depression or apathy may result in lack of motivation to attempt to reach the lavatory. The individual with an impoverished social environment may simply cease to try. This is particularly a problem in long-stay care if incontinence has become the norm and no expectation is put upon the individual to attempt to be continent. Occasionally, incontinence seems to be a protest or sign of despair from an individual in an unacceptable personal situation. A positive atmosphere should be the aim.

Where physical disabilities are severe, an alternative such as a hand-held urinal (male or female) or a commode may be more appropriate, if privacy in their use can be ensured.

Ability to hold excreta

The individual needs to be able to control bladder and bowel contents reliably while getting to the lavatory. This requires competent urethral and anal sphincters and the ability to inhibit detrusor (bladder muscle) and rectal contractions. Any of these may be impaired by disease or ageing (see below). With increasing age, sensation tends to diminish and the individual gets less warning and often experiences increased urgency of micturition or defaecation. It is a cruel fact that this urgency may coincide with decreased ability to hurry.

Ability to empty

Constipation and bladder voiding difficulties are common in old age and have many possible causes (see below). Privacy is an important component in enabling complete evacuation.

Toilet-related skills

Sitting or standing in the correct position for long enough, using lavatory paper, flushing the lavatory, handwashing and many other incidental skills are all part of independence in toileting. The nurse's assessment will determine which, if any, of these prerequisites for successful elimination are lacking for each individual. Care should be planned which aims to maximise each individual's potential for independent continence. The physiotherapist, occupational therapist, chiropodist, optician and planner may each have a contribution. Wells (1980) has described how many nurses often accept an unsuitable environment without considering how it might be improved.

DEFAECATION

Many older people seem obsessed by their bowels. Having lived through an era when the medical profession extolled the virtue of at least one bowel motion per day and weekly purgation, many become distressed if they do not achieve this. In fact, the range of 'normality' is wide and lies between three

motions per day and one every three days (Connell et al 1965).

Assessing defaecation

Nurses often assess bowel function very superficially, simply determining whether the bowels have been opened or not. Wright (1974), in a study of bowel function of hospital inpatients, found that no ward routinely asked about a patient's usual pattern on admission, and that bowel problems caused considerable worry amongst the patients studied. Problems were most likely amongst bedpan or commode users and for old people, with one in three patients experiencing decreased bowel frequency in hospital.

Figure 12.1 gives a checklist which may be used to guide assessment of bowel function. Privacy is essential during this assessment. A common vocabulary must be established—most patients understand 'opening bowels', but this can never be presumed. By finding out the patient's usual bowel pattern the nurse will avoid imposing her own, possibly arbitrary, criteria for evaluating the success of bowel care. As far as possible care should conform to the individual's usual habit, providing this was problem-free. 'Constipation' may be used by the patient if an expected daily motion is missed, but more properly describes motions which are hard and difficult to pass as well as infrequent. Consistency of motions is difficult to assess accurately (Exton-Smith 1975), but generally distinction can be made between hard pellets (scyballae), soft motions and unformed diarrhoea.

If the patient has urgency, this must be considered in relation to mobility and the environment. Mobility itself is a major stimulant of colonic mass movements. Poor diet or low food intake may underlie problems. If dietary regulation is planned, the patient's preferences must be respected—spooning bran onto porridge uninvited may cause food to be left, rather than the intended benefit to bowel function. Many (possibly most) old people use laxatives (Brocklehurst 1978).

Name: Assessment
                               date:

Patient's usual term for
defaecation:
Usual frequency of bowel action: Range:
Usual time of day:
Any associated habits/events:

Does patient complain of
constipation?:
If so, what is understood by this?

Does patient get sensation of the
need to defaecate?
Average time taken for bowel
action:
Does patient have to strain?
Is defaecation associated with
pain?
Any bleeding: Fresh or altered
                   blood:
Mucus:
Problematic flatus: Continent
                       of flatus:
Scyballae: Ribbon
                       stools:
Usual consistency of faeces:
Usual amount of faeces:
Does patient experience urgency?   Time of warning:

Diet: Any food taken for bowels:
      Any food avoided for
      bowels:
      Average daily fluid intake:

Laxative use: Present:
              Past history of use:
Any constipating drugs taken:
History of perianal problems:

Faecal incontinence?:
If yes: Nature of soiling:
        Sensation of incontinence:
        Frequency of incontinence:

Result of rectal examination if
done:
Any recent change in bowel
habits?

Toilet facilities
      Problems with using
      lavatory:
      If bedpan/commode used,
      reaction to this:

Ability to cleanse after
defaecation:
Mobility impaired?

Are any bowel problems
anticipated with current
illness/condition?

Fig. 12.1 Assessment of defaecation.

Often this is for no good reason and can be stopped, especially if diet is improved (Bass 1977, Battle and Hanna 1980). A long history of laxative abuse may lead to colonic damage. Any alteration of an established regime will need to be carefully monitored.

Recording defaecation

Accurate records are vital in assessing the success of bowel care. If the patient cannot communicate, or is thought to be an unreliable witness, the nurse must inspect excreta. A simple Yes/No response is inadequate; note should also be made of amount, consistency, ease or difficulty of passage, whether laxatives were used, and if the patient feels the rectum has been cleared. If constipation or impaction is suspected, a digital rectal examination will confirm this. Immobile, confused patients with a tendency to impaction should be examined regularly to check that the rectum is not becoming loaded with faeces.

Planning care

Bowel care should involve active nursing policies, not an assumption that all is well until problems arise. A routine which is sensitive to each person's needs should be planned, and changed over time if those needs change. Table 12.1 gives a sample care plan which illustrates that comprehensive care often involves many different aspects.

Constipation

There is little evidence that constipation is an inevitable accompaniment to old age (Brocklehurst 1978). Many of the reasons older people experience infrequent, hard, difficult motions are reversible. A variety of physiological causes may underlie constipation; for example, a bowel lesion, neurological or metabolic disease, or psychological illness (e.g. depression). These will be aggravated by immobility, poor diet or fluid intake, inappropriate environment, drug side-effects, and ignoring the call to stool (Exton-Smith, 1972). Constipation should be investigated and

Table 12.1 Sample care plan—Mrs SW

Date	Problem	Goal	Planned action	Review date	Outcome
17.1	Admitted incontinent of fluid stool many times each day. Found to be faecally impacted	Faecal continence within one week	Administer one phosphate enema each morning until no further return	24.1	No further return from enemas. Faecal continence now restored
17.1	Embarrassment at communicating need to defaecate	Able to ask for lavatory facilities	Explain hospital terms. Frequent, discreet enquiries of needs. Ensure privacy	21.1	Seems less shy but still will not ask for lavatory. Continue to ensure she is asked if she needs to go
19.1	Worried other patients will be offended by smell when uses commode	Patient is less worried about other patients	Avoid use of bedpan or commode. Take to lavatory at quiet times. Reassure	22.1	Patient happier using lavatory, but feet do not reach the floor
19.1	Inability to reach lavatory independently	Independence in reaching lavatory within one week	Refer to physiotherapist for advice on mobilisation. Ensure correct height bed and chair	23.1	Can walk slowly with walking frame. Requires encouragement and sometimes becomes disoriented
19.1	Difficulty removing clothes and wiping bottom because of arthritic hands	Independence at toilet within 2 days	Refer to occupational therapist. Allow time and give encouragement for independence	21.1	Patient provided with more suitable pants and a wrap over skirt, which she finds easier to remove. Uses bottom-wiper
20.1	Need to prevent future constipation and recurrence of impaction	Frequent (every 1 or 2 days), soft, easy motions	Encourage fluid intake (at least 1500 ml/24 h). Add fibre supplement (bran—2 heaped tablespoons) each day	25.1	Motion achieved on alternate days but still hard and difficult to pass. Dislikes bran and fluid intake
22.1	Feet do not reach floor when on lavatory	Patient reaches optimal position for easy defaecation	Provide foot block	24.1	Foot block aids bowel evacuation—continue use
26.1	Dislikes bran and high fluid intake	Takes acceptable alternative to prevent constipation	Obtain prescription for laxative. Provide preferred drinks (Bovril or lemonade)	30.1	Motions now softer and more regular. Patient understands importance of this continuing after discharge from hospital

appropriate treatment instigated for any of these problems.

The virtues of a high-fibre diet have been extolled in the prevention and management of constipation. The evidence for the efficacy of this diet is far from unassailable (Pollman et al 1978). For the elderly, caution should be taken against intestinal obstruction, metabolic effects and lowered food intake due to satiety. Most studies have measured success of fibre by a decrease in laxative use, but often without evidence that laxatives were necessary in the first place.

Where constipation is known to be a problem, prophylactic laxatives may be of benefit. Godding (1972) reviewed the mode of action of the commonest laxative agents, which are essentially bulking, lubricant or stimulant in function (see Chapter 11 for further discussion). Evidence on the criteria for selection is sparse and seems to rest largely on the physician's preference. It is now well established that liquid paraffin should not be used because of the risk of inhalational pneumonia and paraffinomas.

Faecal incontinence

Faecal incontinence may be a symptom of a number of different disorders, e.g. severe diarrhoea, neurogenic bowel, muscular damage or, most commonly in the elderly, faecal impaction with overflow incontinence or spurious diarrhoea (Parks 1980). Impacted faeces, resulting from chronic constipation, can usually be presumed to be the cause of faecal incontinence in the elderly, especially those in long-term care. Action of mucus and bacteria cause diarrhoea-like discharge which seeps around the faecal mass. If the rectum is chronically distended the anus becomes patulous and allows free passage of this and small pieces of formed stool. Hard (or occasionally soft, putty-like) faeces can be felt digitally in the rectum in 98% of instances. Treatment involves relief of the impaction, usually with a course of enemas (e.g. 7–10 days of a daily phosphate enema) until the colon is cleared (this may be checked by plain abdominal radiography) and then care provided to prevent future constipation.

If the faecal incontinence is neurogenic in origin (i.e. a failure to inhibit rectal emptying), then management by induced constipation with planned evacuation (e.g. alternating a constipating agent with suppositories) may help keep incontinence under control. This, of course, requires meticulous monitoring if problems are to be avoided, and a regime must be evolved to suit each individual.

Case report

Mr FC was an 82-year-old resident in a Part III residential Home. A chronic schizophrenic, his usual behaviour pattern had been inactive, passive and co-operative according to the staff. When this changed and Mr FC became noisy, restless, aggressive and doubly incontinent, he was referred for geriatric care, as the Home felt they could no longer cope with him. On examination he was found to be faecally impacted. The district nurse visited the Home daily and eight consecutive enemas were given before the bowel was cleared. Thereafter Mr FC became his old self again. Future problems were avoided by increasing his fluid intake and mobility, adding more fruit, vegetables and high-fibre bread to his diet and administering a 10 ml dose of Dorbanex at night if no good bowel action had occurred in the previous 36 hours.

MICTURITION

Disorders of micturition become increasingly common with age. Nocturia (rising at night to pass urine) affects most old people. Many also experience diurnal frequency, urgency and, between 10–20%, some degree of urinary incontinence (Brocklehurst et al 1968, Yarnell and St Ledger 1979, Thomas et al 1980, Vetter et al 1981). Between 16% and 19% of people in residential care are regularly incontinent (Masterton et al 1980), and in geriatric wards 30–60% of patients, with an average of 44%, are reported to be incontinent (Gilleard 1981). In psychogeriatric wards, complete continence has been found to be rare (McLaren et al 1981). Urinary tract infection is present in 17% of older people (Brocklehurst et al 1968) and up to 50% of those in institutional care. One in 10 men are likely to experience symptoms attributable to prostatic hypertrophy.

As with bowel problems, causation is often complex and multifactorial. Each patient requires a detailed assessment of his individual needs and problems prior to planning of care. Figure 12.2 illustrates a checklist which covers the different aspects of this assessment. An accurate chart will supplement and clarify this assessment and reveal any pattern to problems.

Bladder dysfunction in old age

Most people with urinary symptoms have an underlying bladder dysfunction. Indeed, in old age two or even three separate problems may be present in combination. It is important to obtain an accurate diagnosis, as the treatments are different. Usually a careful history and examination will indicate the cause, but if in doubt urodynamic studies are necessary to distinguish the bladder dysfunctions.

Name:	Assessment date:
Patient's usual term for micturition:	
Daytime frequency:	Range:
Nocturia:	
Urgency:	Time of warning:
Urge incontinence:	
Stress incontinence:	
Passive incontinence (just wet):	
Nocturnal enuresis:	

If patient is incontinent:
    When did this start?
    How much is leaked?
    How often?
    What events cause
    incontinence?

Symptoms of voiding difficulty:
    Does patient experience bladder
    sensation?
    Hesitancy?
    Is stream good?
    Straining to void?
    Post-micturition dribbling?

Dysuria:
Haematuria:
Medical conditions which might
affect bladder:
Drugs:
Parity:

Any mobility/dexterity problems?
Observe toileting and comment on
problems:

Examinations:
    MSSU result:
    Skin condition:
    Rectal examination:
    Atrophic vagina or prolapse:
    Post-micturition residual urine
    volume:

Fig. 12.2 Assessment of micturition.

Detrusor instability

Detrusor instability, or the 'unstable bladder', is the commonest bladder dysfunction in old age, and may, indeed, be the norm for elderly people (Brocklehurst and Dillane 1966). The patient, usually because of neurological impairment (e.g. cerebrovascular disease), loses the ability to inhibit reliably detrusor (bladder muscle) contractions and so experiences urgency and frequency. If this is severe, or the sufferer is immobile, asleep or no lavatory is at hand, incontinence may result. This is treated most successfully by a combination of anticholinergic medication (e.g. imipramine 10–25 mg at night) and bladder training (see below).

Incompetent sphincter

This complaint is commonest for post-menopausal, parous women and may be associated with atrophic changes in the vagina and urethra or prolapse. It causes symptoms of stress incontinence (leakage upon physical exertion such as cough). If incontinence is slight, relief can be gained from pelvic floor exercises with hormone replacement therapy if indicated. The patient is taught to interrupt micturition midstream to identify the sensation of a pelvic floor contraction, and then to practise this contraction on a very regular basis (Harrison 1975). More severe stress incontinence usually requires surgical correction, for which advanced age is no contraindication (Stanton and Cardozo 1980). Sometimes a vaginal ring pessary will produce symptomatic relief.

Outflow obstruction

Prostatic enlargement in men is the commonest example of outflow obstruction. It may occur in both sexes because of faecal impaction or a pelvic mass. The patient usually experiences frequency and difficulty voiding. A residual may develop and overflow incontinence usually presents as a continuous non-specific dribbling. Treatment involves relief of the obstruction.

Atonic bladder

If the detrusor muscle fails to contract for micturition, or if the contraction is not sustained until the bladder is empty, a chronic residual may be present. This may become infected and lead to overflow incontinence. Common in both diabetics and demented people, this may be a feature of any neurological disease. The use of intermittent (in—out) catheterisation to drain off this residual is widespread for younger patients with this problem. Its use for the elderly has not yet been widely reported, but initial results are promising. Some patients can be taught to self-catheterise; for others, a relative or nurse must do the catheterisation. Some patients seem to regain detrusor tone with this management and resume normal voiding; for others, the intermittent catheterisation must be a long-term management, usually once or twice a day.

Urinary tract infection (UTI)

The presence of 'significant' bacteruria (commonly accepted as 100 000 organisms per ml of urine) is so high (Brocklehurst et al 1968, Milne et al 1972) that it must call into question the criteria of significance adopted for younger people. Milne et al could find no symptoms clearly associated with infection, and Brocklehurst et al found that infection correlated with frequency and difficulty in passing urine. Neither study demonstrated a relationship between incontinence and urinary tract infection (UTI).

Probably the most useful way to treat UTI is to distinguish between acute and chronic infection. The patient with a sudden onset of the symptoms of cystitis—dysuria, pain, frequency, pyrexia and possibly confusion—should receive the appropriate antibiotic therapy. The chornic infection is often asymptomatic, will not respond to antibiotics, or will soon return, and should seldom be treated (Brocklehurst 1977). Routine treatment of UTI, regardless of symptoms or needs, risks the emergence of resistant organisms and should be avoided.

It is wise to remember that for older women, symptoms of atrophic urethritis may mimic cystitis. Inspection of the vulva will reveal classic atrophic changes.

Incontinence in institutional care

Incontinence in patients in Homes or hospitals is often associated with multiple, undiagnosed and untreated problems (King 1979, 1980, Lepine et al 1979) which, if remedied, lead to restoration of continence for a proportion of patients. It cannot be overemphasised that an individual assessment is the crucial first step in any nursing intervention. If the patient is confused, a behavioural assessment is indicated (Turner 1980) and a psychologist can be invaluable in examining behavioural causes of incontinence. A behaviour modification programme, which rewards the desired behaviour (continence) and gradually extinguishes the unwanted behaviour (incontinence) may be devised and is often successful if implemented consistently (e.g. Grosiki 1968, Hartie and Black 1975, Barker 1979).

Promotion of continence

Where incontinence levels are high, there is much evidence that the situation can be improved considerably by the introduction of a more reality-oriented, therapeutic environment (Volpe and Kastenbaum 1967, Storrs 1982). Even without any specific elimination management, continence can be promoted, it seems, by motivating patients and stimulating an interest in life and activities. Much depends on the attitude and ethos of care and it should be remembered that elimination care will not be beneficial unless general care is individualised in intent and content.

Toileting and changing

Both Reid (1974) and Ramsbottom (1980) have studied toileting and changing routines in hospital, and describe the sacrifice of privacy and dignity to speed, with care delivered in a purely routine fashion. Ramsbottom concludes 'care is not focused on patients' needs but on routines which might or might not be appropriate for each patient'. Nursing auxiliaries were observed to give most care. It is still common for a ward or home to have toileting times (e.g. before or after meals) when everyone is toileted, regardless of needs. For some people whose elimination exhibits no pattern, this might be the best policy, but it is hardly likely to suit a whole group of people who are likely to have a variety of requirements.

Reid (1974) identified the ward environment as a major obstacle to better care once incontinence has occurred. The problem is particularly acute where an increasing number of patients are ambulant and spend a proportion of each day in a communal day area with no facilities for changing wet pads or clothes. This problem needs further attention and the development of nursing practices to cope with it.

Cleansing of the skin after incontinence is likewise a rather hit or miss affair. Only one study has compared skin cleansing agents (Willington et al 1981), and often anything which comes to hand is used, with as yet unmeasured effects upon the vulnerable skin of incontinent people.

Bladder training

Bladder training is a very misused term in nursing. Many nurses claim to be implementing 'bladder training' when really all that is happening is that the patient is toileted at pre-set intervals, usually at times which fit the ward routine. This might train staff not to forget toileting, but does little to 'train' a bladder. Routine toileting at rigid intervals has a place for patients who have not responded to bladder training, and may decrease incontinence. Bladder training refers to a more specific management (e.g. Clay, 1978). The individual's own pattern of micturition and incontinence is carefully charted on a baseline chart and then individualised toileting times devised to anticipate these needs. This may need to be frequent initially, and the interval may vary (e.g. more often in the morning after a dose of diuretic, less often in the evening). Gradually the intervals between toilet visits should be extended until a more normal and convenient pattern is restored. This training is most suitable for patients with detrusor instability and may be used in hospital and community settings.

MANAGEMENT OF INTRACTABLE INCONTINENCE

Even with the best available management and care, some patients remain incontinent. It is important that this is recognised as inevitable and that nurses do not feel guilty about it. The individual can usually be helped to maintain dignity and comfort is some way. The nurse should teach the patient, or her family, the most suitable management techniques, and she has an important supportive role in care.

Incontinence aids

A good incontinence aid will enable the incontinent person to be socially accepted and to lead a relatively normal life. Despite the huge range and variety of aids now available (Association of Continence Advisors 1984), many function poorly and fail. An aid must be carefully selected with regard to the individual's degree, type and pattern of incontinence, local anatomy, physical and mental abilities, personal preference, washing or disposal facilities, and cost. No one aid will suit everyone and a range should be provided (Malone-Lee et al 1983). The nurse must be the patient's advocate in this and be prepared to make a case for the supply of the most appropriate items.

Body-worn pads and pants

Most incontinent women, and some men, use a disposable, absorbent pad held in place by pants to collect urine or faeces. Sanitary towels are the most commonly used, but will not cope with any but minimal leakage. Plastic pants are undignified, uncomfortable and can cause considerable skin problems and should not be in routine use. The first alternative to plastic pants was the marsupial pants, with 'one-way' material and a waterproof pocket for the pad. These remain popular, especially in male and female styles. They are unsuitable for faecal incontinence, can be difficult for the manually disabled to use and many people do not like the idea of wetting their pants directly. Other pads are plastic-backed and held in place with stretch pants. All pads are only as good as the quality of their constituents and none will last indefinitely. Gaining in popularity are the all-night body pads and all-in-one diaper systems (similar to babies' disposable nappies). Their use has not yet been evaluated.

Male appliances

Some men are able to use a penile sheath or an appliance in preference to a pad. A retracted penis or poor manual dexterity make their use difficult. A penile sheath should be carefully selected for appropriate size and is most satisfactory if held in position with a double-sided adhesive strip and connected to a leg-bag. Appliances (e.g. pubic pressure urinals) should always be fitted by an experienced appliance fitter.

Bed and chair protection

Bedpads or underpads are the most commonly used incontinence aid in the Health Service. Ramsbottom (1980) has reviewed the literature on their use and found no clear criteria or body of nursing knowledge regarding their uses. In clinical observation she found that many disintegrated, adhered to the skin or leaked, and in 54% of instances more than one was used, thereby cancelling any cost advantages. Nurses were found to put up with poor performance of aids and 'make do' with poor quality and quantity of supplies, having no channel of communication to express dissatisfaction. Bedpads do have their uses but are often expected, quite unrealistically, to cope with all incontinence needs. Washable bedsheets with a stay-dry surface have proved to be comfortable, popular and cost-effective (Smith 1979), but in some instances

laundry provision is inadequate to cope with them.

Nurses must consider more carefully the use of bed and chair protection, possibly refocusing care from protection of the environment to protection of the patient.

Indwelling catheters and the elderly

Generally, the use of an indwelling catheter should be seen very much as a 'last resort' when all other methods of managing micturition have been tried and failed. Widespread, indiscriminate use of catheters has fallen into disrepute, as has their use solely for nursing convenience. A move away from catheters can be shown to benefit even severely incontinent patients in many instances (e.g. Brandberg et al 1980).

The decision to use a catheter should only be made for clear and valid reasons, with a definite goal which can be evaluated, and in full consultation with all concerned, especially the patient. The individual's quality of life should be the prime consideration—will the use of a catheter significantly improve independence, comfort and dignity? For some patients (e.g. someone with severe incontinence which is poorly controlled by an aid) a catheter can be a great benefit, even enabling community rather than hospital care. Each decision should be made on an individual basis and re-evaluated at intervals.

Managing a catheter

Recent research (Kennedy et al 1982, 1983) has highlighted how poorly managed many long-term catheters are. Confused, ignorant management and a lack of knowledge of the principles of catheter drainage were found to be widespread. For example, 30% of nurses said that they would increase catheter size if leaking occurred—the exact opposite of optimal practice. The majority of catheters (57%) were changed before their expected life-span was reached, usually because of blocking or leakage. Only 10% of catheters were not problematic. It was found that smaller catheters were associated with fewer problems and this accords with advice from urologists that small catheters allow drainage of the paraurethral glands and there is therefore less risk of stricture or abscess formation (Blandy 1981). Small (5–10 ml) balloons are also recommended for routine use, but these are not yet widely used in the United Kingdom.

If a patient has to live with a catheter, drainage must be made convenient. For day use, a leg-bag or a bag attached to a waist-belt, garment holder or in a pocket inside trousers or a skirt will hide the urine from public view. Some systems allow direct connection of night bags to the bottom of day bags without breaking the closed system (Kennedy 1984b), which is a benefit in hospital although less vital in the community. The outlet tap should be simple to use and to understand, but many fail to meet these criteria (Kennedy 1983).

Patient teaching and individualised care will overcome many problems. The importance of diet, exercise, fluid intake, personal hygiene and avoiding constipation should be emphasised (Blannin 1982). Sexual function should be discussed, and if the patient is sexually active an alternative to an urethral catheter considered. Sometimes the patient or a partner may be taught to remove and replace the catheter, thus increasing independence. Individual solutions can often be reached for problems (Kennedy 1984a). Leaking may be caused by too large a catheter or balloon, or by an unstable bladder (which may respond to anticholinergic therapy). Routine washouts should be used only when a catheter is found to block persistently. Infections are inevitable and should only be treated if the patient is symptomatic (Brocklehurst 1977). If a catheter causes repeated problems, its use should be questioned as the patient may be better off without it.

Community services for the incontinent

A variety of services are available for the incontinent person who lives at home. Male sheaths and appliances, catheters, bags and some deodorants and skin-care products are available on prescription from the chemist. District nursing services usually provide a range of absorbent products and waterproof sheeting (e.g. mattress covers), but the quality and quantity of such provision varies greatly between health authorities. Most also provide loan of commodes and hand-held urinals, although this is sometimes left to voluntary organisations such as the Red Cross. District nurses may give help with personal hygiene, bathing and management of catheters and appliances.

Social service departments are usually responsible for aids to daily living, such as walking aids, grab-rails and modifications to the home (e.g. provision of a downstairs lavatory). Some departments employ community physiotherapists and occupational therapists who can suggest a range of aids to independence and teach relatives the easiest way of lifting and transferring if this is necessary. A home help may be able to assist with laundry. Some local authorities also provide a laundry service for incontinent people which collects soiled items and delivers them back clean, and a soiled pad collection service.

Various financial benefits may be obtained. If an individual needs attention or supervision in connection with bodily functions, she may qualify for an attendance allowance. If supplementary benefit is already paid, payments for extra costs (e.g. laundry, wear and tear on clothes) or single payments (e.g. to replace a ruined mattress or furniture) may be claimed. Occasionally the cost of a washing machine or similar item may be obtained from social services or a charitable fund.

THE INCONTINENCE ADVISER

With the recognition of the very positive role of the nurse in managing incontinence, the concept of the nurse specialist has grown. In 1977 the Chief Nursing Officer of the Department of Health and Social Security (DHSS) suggested that an appropriate nursing officer be identified as a point of reference for the promotion of continence (Friend 1977). In 1982 there were approximately 50 incontinence (or continence) advisors in the United Kingdom (King's Fund 1983). These nurses have a very diverse role—from clinical casework and running incontinence and urodynamics clinics to teaching, research, acting as a resource and information centre, product development and appraisal, and supplies liaison (Norton 1984).

This role has not yet received comprehensive evaluation. The only study which has examined the role of the incontinence advisor did not demonstrate clear clinical or cost advantages (Ramsbottom 1982), but researchers admit considerable methodological problems, and 'improvement' in incontinence is difficult to document (Badger et al 1983). Certainly costs were increased as more people received services. A nursing clinic which offers advice to patients considered 'hopeless' by medical staff achieved continence for 10% of patients (Blannin 1980, Shepherd et al 1982). A similar clinic has been reported in the United States (Brink et al 1983), and it was found that teaching constituted a major demand on time.

Some nurses fear that a nurse specialist will fragment care. Continence is surely the responsibility of every nurse? In an ideal world this would be true, but it does seem at present that many nurses and patients can benefit from the expertise and teaching of an incontinence advisor. Nursing care can move towards its prime goal in this area—problem-free elimination for the patient.

REFERENCES

Association of Continence Advisers 1984 Directory of Aids, 2nd edn. ACA, London
Badger F J, Drummond M F, Isaacs B 1983 Some issues in the clinical, social and economic evaluation of new nursing services. Journal of Advanced Nursing 8: 487–494
Barker P 1979 Nocturnal enuresis: an experimental study involving two behavioural approaches. International Journal of Nursing Studies 16: 319–327
Bass L 1977 More fiber-less constipation. American Journal of Nursing 77(2): 254–255

Battle E H, Hanna C E 1980 Evaluation of a dietary regimen for chronic constipation. Journal of Gerontological Nursing 6: 527–532
Blandy J P 1981 How to catheterise the bladder. British Journal of Hospital Medicine 25(7): 58–60
Blannin J P 1980 Towards a better life. Nursing Mirror 150(12): 31–33
Blannin J P 1982 Catheter management. Nursing Times 78: 438–440
Brandberg A, Seeberg S, Bergstrom G, Nordqvist P 1980 Reducing the number of nosocomical Gram-negative strains by using high absorbing pads as an alternative to indwelling catheters in long-term care. Journal of Hospital Infection 1: 245–250
Brink C, Wells T, Diokno A 1983 A continence clinic for the aged. Journal of Gerontological Nursing 9: 651–655
British Standards Institution 1979 Access for the disabled to buildings. BS 5810
Brocklehurst J C 1977 Urinary infections: not all patients need treatment. Modern Geriatrics 7(3): 33–36
Brocklehurst J C 1978 The large bowel. In: Brocklehurst J C (ed) Textbook of geriatric medicine and gerontology, 2nd edn. Churchill Livingstone, Edinburgh
Brocklehurst J C, Dillane J B 1966 Studies of the female bladder in old age. Gerontologica Clinica 8: 285–319
Brocklehurst J C, Dillane J B, Griffiths L, Fry J 1968 The prevalence and symptomatology of urinary tract infection in an aged population. Gerontologica Clinica 10: 242–253
Clay E C 1978 Incontinence of urine. Nursing Mirror 146(10): 36–38, (11): 23–24
Connell A M, Hilton C, Irvine G, Lennard-Jones J E, Misiewicz J J 1965 Variations of bowel habit in two population samples. British Medical Journal 2: 1095–1099
Exton-Smith A N 1972 Constipation in geriatrics. In: Avery Jones F, Godding E W (eds) Management of constipation. Blackwell, Oxford
Exton-Smith A N 1975 A new technique for measuring the consistency of faeces. Age and Ageing 4: 58–62
Friend P M 1977 Standards of nursing care. Promotion of continence and management of incontinence. CNO(SNC) (77) 1 Department of Health and Social Security, London
Gilleard C J 1981 Incontinence in the hospitalised elderly. Health Bulletin 39: 58–61
Gilleard C, Mitchell R G, Riordan J 1981 Ward orientation training with psychogeriatric patients. Journal of Advanced Nursing 6: 95–98
Godding E W 1972 Therapeutic agents. In: Avery Jones F, Godding E W (eds) Management of constipation. Blackwell, Oxford
Grosicki J P 1968 Effect of operant conditioning on modification of incontinence in neuropsychiatric geriatric patients. Nursing Research 17: 304–311
Harrison S 1975 Physiotherapy in the treatment of stress incontinence. Nursing Mirror 141: 52–53
Hartie A, Black D 1975 A dry bed is the objective. Nursing Times 71: 1874–1876
Kennedy A 1983 Long-term catheterisation. Nursing Times 79(17): 41–43
Kennedy A 1984a Catheters in the community. Nursing Times Community Outlook 80(6): 51–55

Kennedy A 1984b Drainage system on trial. Nursing Mirror 158: 19–20

Kennedy A, Brocklehurst J C 1982 The nursing management of patients with long-term indwelling catheters. Journal of Advanced Nursing 7: 411–417

Kennedy A, Brocklehurst J C, Lye M D W 1983 Factors related to the problems of long-term catheterisation. Journal of Advanced Nursing 8: 207–212

King M R 1979 A study of incontinence in a psychiatric hospital. Nursing Times 75: 1133–1135

King M R 1980 Treatment of incontinence. Nursing Times 76: 1006–1010

King's Fund Project Paper 1983 Action on incontinence. King's Fund Centre, London

Lepine A, Renaut R K, Stewart I D 1979 The incidence and management of incontinence in a home for the elderly. Health and Social Service Journal 89: E9-12

McLaren S M, McPherson F M, Sinclair F, Ballinger B R 1981 Prevalence and severity of incontinence among hospitalised, female psychogeriatric patients. Health Bulletin 39: 157–161

Malone-Lee J, McCreery M, Exton-Smith A N 1983 A community study of the performance of incontinence garments. Department of Health and Social Security, London

Masterton G, Holloway E M, Timbury G C 1980 The prevalence of incontinence in local authority homes for the elderly. Health Bulletin 38: 62–64

Millard P H 1979 The promotion of continence. Health Trends 11: 27–28

Milne J S, Williamson J, Maule M M, Wallace E T 1972 Urinary symptoms in older people. Modern Geriatrics May: 198–212

Norton C S 1984 The role of the continence adviser. Nursing Mirror 158: in press

Norton D, McLaren R, Exton-Smith A N 1962 An investigation of geriatric nursing problems in hospital. National Corporation for the Care of Old People, London

Parks A G 1980 Faecal incontinence. In: Mandelstam D (ed) Incontinence and its management. Croom Helm, London

Pollman J W, Morris J J, Rose P N 1978 Is fiber the answer to constipation problems in elderly people? A review of the literature. International Journal of Nursing Studies 15: 107–114

Ramsbottom F J 1980 toileting and changing elderly patients in hospital. Department of Geriatric Medicine, University of Birmingham

Ramsbotton F J 1982 Is advice really cheap? Journal of Community Nursing 5(11): 9–16

Reid E A 1974 Incontinence and nursing practice. M. Phil. Thesis, University of Edinburgh

Schwartz D R 1977 Personal point of view. Health Bulletin 35: 197–204

Scottish Home and Health Department 1970 Geriatric accommodation report. SHHD, Edinburgh. (Mimeographed)

Shepherd A M, Blannin J P, Feneley R C L 1982 Changing attitudes in the management of urinary incontinence—the need for specialist nursing. British Medical Journal 284: 645–646

Smith B 1979 A dry bed—and save on costs. Nursing Mirror 318: 26–29

Stanton S L, Cardozo L D 1980 Surgical treatment of incontinence in elderly women. Surgery 150: 555–557

Storrs A 1982 What is care? British Journal of Geriatric Nursing 1(4): 12–14

Thomas T M, Plymat K R, Blannin J, Meade T W 1980 Prevalence of urinary incontinence. British Medical Journal 281: 1243–1245

Turner R K 1980 A behavioural approach to the management of incontinence in the elderly. In: Mandelstam D (ed) Incontinence and its management. Croom Helm, London

Vetter N J, Jones D A, Victor C R 1981 Urinary incontinence in the elderly at home. Lancet 4: 1275–1277

Volpe A, Kastenbaum R 1967 Beer and TLC. American Journal of Nursing 67: 100–103

Wells T J 1980 Problems in geriatric nursing care. Churchill Livingstone, Edinburgh

Willington F L, Yarnell J W G, Sweetman P M 1981 Cleansing incontinent patients. Journal of Advanced Nursing 6: 107–109

Wright L 1974 Bowel function in hospital patients. Royal College of Nursing, London

Yarnell J W G, St Leger A S 1979 The prevalence, severity and factors associated with urinary incontinence in a random sample of the elderly. Age and Ageing 8: 81–85

M. F. Green

13

Maintaining body temperature

Good health depends on the normal metabolic functioning of tissues, cells, and intracellular mechanisms. The maintenance of efficient human metabolism requires that the human body—core and periphery—is kept at or very near 37°C (98.4°F). This applies to normal and premature babies, to children and teenagers, young adults, and to middle-aged and elderly people.

A substantial downward deviation of the deep body temperature may be caused by age-related defects of thermal perception and thermo-regulation, especially in the very young and very old, by life-threatening disease, by drugs and alcohol, by cold, wet and windy environmental conditions, or by any combination of these factors.

Whatever the cause(s) of the lowered body temperature it will itself lead to functional inefficiency of the body generally, and impairment of the normal functioning of certain systems, particularly the vital organs in the core—the brain, heart and lungs. Human beings are homeothermic and have to be kept homeostatically warm. They are not poikilothermic, like snakes or fishes, that can function adequately in and recover from relatively wide extremes of environmental and body temperature. The medically defined hypothermia cut-off point, 95°F, which conveniently converts to the round figure of 35°C, reflects a substantial pathological deviation from the norm. It is arbitrary, however, since some people (especially those with impaired thermoregulation and/or significant disease of the vital organs) may become ill and could even die with core temperatures just above 35°C, or during rewarming. Conversely, the bodies of previously healthy individuals may continue to function adequately for some time even below 35°C.

A drop in body temperature may indicate severe, possibly irreversible terminal illness, e.g. carcinomatosis. This drop reflects either an inexorable decline of body function, or potenitally reversible disease, or avoidable environmental and social problems. In old people a drop in body temperature rather than a fever may be their response to infection, and this may suggest a worse prognosis. Pyrexia also reflects an abnormal state with impaired bodily function. The febrile state is usually due to 'toxins' (e.g. pyrogens) produced by leucocyte and monocyte and antibody reaction to infective agents, or by inflammation, or malignant disease and drug side-effects, or excessively hot weather. Fever is a response to primary disease, is not protective, and may be harmful by impairing normal body responses and repair and healing processes. Dehydration, mental confusion, respiratory and cardiac dysfunction may develop with a raised temperature and mirror the bodily dysfunction seen with hypothermia.

METHODS OF TAKING TEMPERATURES

The mercury column/bulb glass thermometer remains the universally accepted simple, cheap and reasonably reliable method of taking patients' temperatures. Unfortunately, a raised temperature—fever—is the abnormality for which doctors, nurses and patients tend to use a thermometer. The thermometer usually used in clinical practice is calibrated to reveal pyrexia, with a lower limit of 35°C (95°F), through the normal average temperature of 37°C (98.4°F) to 40°C (104°F). Although temperatures below 37°C are likely to reflect some impairment of organ function and an increased risk of hypothermia developing, the accuracy of both the thermometer and the

observer's reading of the mercury column is questionable in the 35–36°C (95–96.8°F) range. These thermometers cannot diagnose hypothermia even when used to take a core reading, e.g. rectally. It is important to remember that a warm drink may falsely raise an otherwise abnormally low oral temperature for a considerable time.

Hypothermia is defined as a core/deep body temperature below 35°C (95°F), which means that the vital organs in the deeper part of the body are clearly below the physiologically normal functional temperature of 37°C (98.4°F). It is important to realise that that the critical diagnostic feature is lowered core temperature, not just a low peripheral temperature of the skin, or in the axilla or mouth, even when a low reading thermometer does reveal a peripheral temperature below 35°C. The low reading thermometer should have a range extending down to at least 25°C (77°F), to ensure accuracy and easy reading below 35°C (Fig. 13.1). The need to check the core temperature to see if the vital organs are abnormally chilled may be prompted by the clinical situation. For example, of an elderly person with a stroke found lying on the floor in a cold room several hours after falling, of

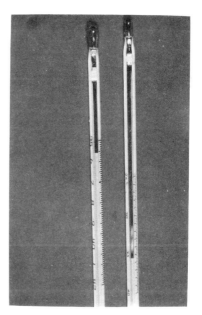

Fig. 13.1 Normal and low reading thermometers.

climbers or swimmers exposed to water, wind and cold weather, or of premature babies in cold rooms. However, hypothermia may develop in old people and young babies, when other more obvious clinical problems dominate the situation (e:g. a fracture) or because of unsuspected thermoregulatory dysfunction.

Therefore, ordinary temperature taking in the mouth or axilla of any ill old person should be carried out with a low reading thermometer. If this reveals a lowered peripheral temperature, especially below 35°C (95°F), then it should be obligatory to check the core temperature for hypothermia, again using a low reading thermometer. It is customary in clinical practice to take the rectal temperature as the reflection of core temperature when checking for hypothermia, preferably leaving the thermometer in place for several minutes. A Uritemp technique has been developed for research surveys which uses a low reading thermometer in a plastic funnel, to measure the temperature of freshly voided urine as a reflection of core temperature (Fig. 13.2). This method of taking the deep body temperature is more acceptable in the research context and is accurate as it is likely to be within 0.1°C (0.2°F) of a rectal reading.

Electrical thermocouples (thermistors) are used in research surveys to measure skin and core temperatures; for instance, the latter is taken by using a thermistor placed on the skin of the inner part of the ear canal. These thermistors are lightweight and can be used with ambulant subjects, and to measure temperature changes whilst 'stressing' the subject in warm and cold environments.

Larger scientific or domestic thermometers are available to mount on a wall, in living rooms, working rooms or bedrooms (Fig. 13.3). These may measure only the ambient temperature (immediate environmental temperature) in the room. More sophisticated thermometers can be used to record the maximum and minimum environmental temperatures during any study period (Fig. 13.4). The humidity of the environment is an imporant factor in temperature control and personal comfort. A wet and windy environment is likely to chill an ill or predisposed person even more, especially when they have thermoregulatory dysfunction. A whirling hygrometer is used to record the wet and dry bulb temperatures of the environment (Fig. 13.5).

Environmental temperatures

Except in very hot weather, rare in temperate countries, humans are surrounded by an environment cooler than themselves. The temperature of the environment varies:

1. With the time of day. The circadian or nyctohemeral rhythm of environmental temperature, being lowest during the night and early morning, is reflected in a similar circadian rhythm in humans. Their core temperature may be 0.5 to 1.0°C (0.9° to 1.8°F) lower at 6 to 7 a.m. than at mid-day or during the afternoon.

2. With the weather. It is lower during autumn and winter months, from October to March, in the northern hemisphere, and during wet and windy weather.

3. With the immediate and environmental temperature in rooms and buildings. Bedrooms, rooms at the top of houses and blocks of flats, and in badly built, badly glazed and poorly insulated dwellings tend to be coldest. Old people often live in cold accommodation and this may be aggravated because of poverty, faulty heating systems, fuel strikes or fuel

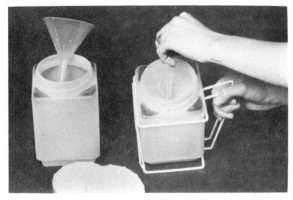

Fig. 13.2 The Uritemp apparatus.

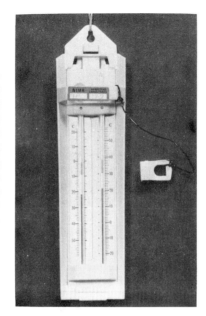

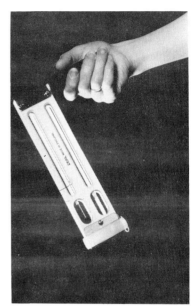

Fig. 13.3 A wall thermometer.

Fig. 13.4 A max/min thermometer.

Fig. 13.5 A whirling hygrometer.

disconnections by Electricity and Gas Boards for non-payment of bills.

Hypothermia is clearly a problem of temperate and polar regions rather than the tropics, but it seems to be a particular problem in some temperate countries rather than others. This may be due to differences in humidity and wind conditions as well as low environmental temperatures in the winter period. If these factors are combined with poor social circumstances, thermally inefficient housing and social isolation, hypothermia is even more likely. This may explain why it is such a problem for the elderly in Britain compared with Canada, North America and most Scandinavian countries, where very low environmental temperatures do occur.

The other side of the same coin of ill health caused by abnormal environmental temperatures is the increased risk of illness and death in very hot weather in temperate and tropical countries. Again, elderly people are particularly at risk as they may have pre-existing diseases (e.g. uraemia) or thermoregulatory dysfunction, and they may deteriorate insidi-

ously due to worsening renal function, dehydration and electrolyte imbalance.

CONTROL OF HUMAN BODY TEMPERATURE

Normal thermoregulation

The maintenance of a normal core temperature depends on the balance between heat generated and heat lost. Metabolism generates heat and is controlled by a complex pattern of central nervous and endocrine (mainly thyroidal) factors and, if necessary, by shivering. An adequate intake of calories, rather than hot foods specifically, is necessary and subnutrition is a potent aetiological factor in hypothermia.

The sensory receptors of environmental temperature and of a person's thermal comfort are in the skin and are linked to the hypothalamic thermostat temperature controller. In cold, uncomfortable conditions the normal response is: to decrease blood flow in the skin by vasoconstriction, stop sweating and start shivering; and to increase heat production, partly by increased pituitary secretion of thyroid-stimulating hormone (TSH). Conversely, in hot conditions the normal response is to: vasodilate blood vessels in the skin, increase sweating and respiration; and decrease TSH secretion.

Babies, young children and small thin adults are more susceptible to cold, wet environments, even if they have no intrinsic thermoregulatory abnormality and no co-existent disease. This is because they have a relatively greater surface area to lose heat from, compared to their body mass. The surface area of neonates is about 15% of adults compared with a body weight which is only 5% of adult figures.

Fat people are more likely to be 'efficient' at conserving their heat core. The elderly tend to lose brown fat which is thought to be a very efficient metabolic tissue and could help generate heat when cold stressed. As a large amount of heat is lost from the head and hands, bald people and anyone with uncovered head and hands are susceptible to cold and wet weather.

It must be remembered that heat loss is not only due to radiation from the skin. Conduction through clothing and into the air, convection increased by the wind, and evaporation increased by wind and wet are also important. Heat is also lost in expired air, in faeces and in urine. Urine loss is important especially if the person is incontinent as this leads to evaporation loss, as well as simple voiding loss. Most people over 65 years of age get up once or twice at night to micturate (see Ch. 12).

Even when the skin/peripheral temperature drops to below 34°C (93.2°F) in cold exposed homes, the core temperature is usually maintained above 36.5°C (97.7°F) for some considerable time. This observation also applies to elderly people.

Abnormal thermoregulation

Temperature perception and discrimination, comfort awareness, hypothalamic thermostat sensitivity and vasomotor response, and circadian rhythm are all increasingly likely to become impaired with advancing age. These defects may be due to senescent 'ageing' or to more specific problems such as cerebrovascular disease or hypothyroidism. Cold old people tend to be the least aware of cold discomfort and this must surely identify them as a serious at risk group (Fox et al 1973a). Of course, it is important to remember that not all old people have homeostatic failure, nor do they have any or many other diseases or are taking toxic drugs. Healthy people of any age may develop hypothermia as a primary event if exposed to cold conditions, e.g. young babies in cold bedrooms, sailors immersed in cold water, or previously fit old people immobilised on the floor of a cold room or outside the house after a fall.

However, 10% of a group of 2000 old people over 65 years studied in winter months did show evidence of thermoregulatory dysfunction as judged by an abnormal core to periphery temperature gradient (Fox et al 1973a). Heat loss due to defective vasomotor, sweating and shivering response continued even when the core temperature of these elderly people was already low at 35 to 35.5°C (95° to 95.9°F), i.e. just above the rather arbitrary discriminant hypothermia temperature. The group also often showed evidence of defective postural control of blood pressure with a significant drop from the lying or sitting to the standing positions. This suggests widespread autonomic dysfunction. The abnormal defective responses were more marked when cold stressed, though a significant group also showed similar defective responses to warmth stressing. The abnormalities became more marked as these subjects aged.

The abnormal temperature gradient in the 'low' pre-hypothermic group is illustrated in Figure 13.6, and the homeostatic abnormalities affecting vasoconstriction, sweating and blood pressure control in the normal and low group in Table 13.1.

There are four important points to be made in explaining the 'onion-skin' illustration (Fig. 13.6).

1. It attempts to illustrate the complex interplay of age, medical, social, anatomical and physiological factors which influence the

Table 13.1 Abnormalities of blood flow response, sweating and postural control of blood pressure. *Source: Fox et al (1973b)*

	'Normal' group (n = 93)	'Low' group (n = 12)
No abnormality	26	1
1 abnormality	32	2
2 abnormalities	31	5
3 abnormalities	4	4

normal maintenance of body temperature and the normal temperature gradient between core and periphery.

2. It compares a 'pre-hypothermia' group of old people with those with normal core temperatures. The pre-hypothermia group had core temperatures between 35° and 35.5°C (95 to 95.9°F). The temperature gradient findings suggest that the pre-hypothermia group continue to lose heat from their periphery despite a lowered deep body temperature. Normally a lowered peripheral temperature would prompt a reduction in skin blood-flow,

sweating, and the maintenance of a gradient between the core and periphery, which reflect the body's attempt to maintain the core temperature at all costs.

3. It has already been indicated that the point which defines hypothermia of 35°C (95°F) is arbitrary. The finding that 10% of older people living in their own homes had deep body temperatures just above the hypothermia level suggests that they were particularly likely to be tipped into actual hypothermia with little or no further pathological or environmental 'insult'.

4. Analysis of the various medical and social correlates suggests that advanced age is a risk factor of both pre-hypothermia and hypothermia.

It has been suggested that similar factors could be operating in small babies, especially those described as premature on the grounds of short gestation or low birth weight (Cross 1978). They too may have defective thermoregulation as well as the problem of relatively large surface area to body mass.

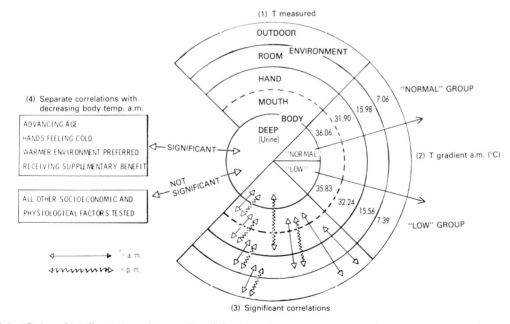

Fig. 13.6 'Onion skin' illustration of 'normal' and 'low' core temperature groups showing core to periphery gradients.

Source: Fox et al (1973b) Reproduced by permission of the authors of the article and the editor of the British Medical Journal.

LOWERED BODY TEMPERATURE

The lower environmental temperature during winter months in Britain and the relatively high humidity, with the rather poor and lonely social circumstances of many of our elderly population, and our generally thermally inefficient housing and insulation (especially that occupied by older people) all conspire to put the elderly population at the greatest risk of developing hypothermia. They may also have coexistent diseases and/or be taking drugs that predispose to or precipitate hypothermia, and/or have age-related thermoregulatory dysfunction. Hypothermia secondary to other problems, or arising as part of multiple pathology, is more likely to occur than primary hypothermia on its own. This situation is even more likely to occur in the 75+ years age group than in the general pensioner population.

What are the facts about the incidence and prevalence of hypothermia? Neonatal hypothermia diminished after the Royal College of Physicians report of 1966, due mainly to increased appreciation of the problem and the provision of more and better equipped special baby units with incubators. That report calculated that about 9000 hypothermic patients were admitted to hospital in the winter months. Even since the report of Fox et al (1973b) drawing attention to the very substantial 'low' core temperature group—10% of people aged over 65 years at home—only about 300 or 400 deaths a year are ascribed to hypothermia. A survey of all hopital admissions of the over 65s to two London Teaching Hospitals in winter months suggested that about 3.6% were suffering from hypothermia, usually with other pathology (Goldman et al 1977). These two surveys do suggest that the hypothermia death certificate figures are a serious underestimate.

Increased mortality in winter months compared with the summer suggests that cold and bad weather is likely to have played a major part in the death, whatever is shown on the death certificate. Certificates showing bronchopneumonia, myocardial infarction or heart failure, and stroke, may not be inaccurate but just incomplete. Hypothermia is very difficult to diagnose at autopsy. These diseases may have been present in addition to the hypothermia, may have been caused by it, or may have precipitated the accompanying disease, e.g. a chest infection, heart attack or a stroke.

Winter mortality figures suggest that, for instance, in December 1973 there were almost 46 000 deaths in England and Wales, but less that 200 cases of hypothermia were recorded in that month. Some records only referred to hypothermia as a contributory factor rather than the prime cause of death. There may be 55 000 to 60 000 deaths in the United Kingdom in a bad winter month, with midsummer figures less that 35 000 deaths a month (Fox et al 1973a, b).

Definite superimposed peaks of specifically recorded hypothermia deaths (even allowing for the underestimate of this diagnosis) can be detected after particularly bad weather during winter months (Bull, 1973). This strengthens the conclusion that many deaths recorded as the result of other diseases may be partly or substantially due to hypothermia, since there are also clear peaks of mortality due to pneumonia, ischaemic heart disease and stroke after bad weather. A provocative but perhaps not inaccurate conclusion is that cold-induced deterioration may contribute to more than 500 elderly people dying a week in winter months.

Recognition of hypothermia

As the core temperature drops, the vital organs become progressively functionally defective. Respiration becomes more difficult and is often wheezy and increasingly ineffective in gaseous exchange. Eventually repiratory arrest develops. The victim becomes confused, unable to respond sensibly and to look after herself, then lapses into coma, may have convulsions, and die. There may be tachycardia intially but with an increasingly poor cardiac output, bradycardia develops. Arrhythmias develop, the most serious being asystole or ventricular fibrillation, which cause

Table 13.2 Clinical effects of hypothermia

Core temperature °C	Effects
37	Shivering. Rise in metabolic and
36	respiratory rate. Discomfort
	Pain. Numbness
35	Metabolism decreases
34.5	Respiration decreases
34	Heart rate and blood pressure drop
33	Confusion and amnesia.
	Muscular rigidity
32	Sleepy. Convulsions. Pain-resistant
30	Unconsciousness. Irregular respiration and heart beat. Loss of tendon reflexes. Dilated pupils
28	Respiration stops. Cardiac fibrillation or arrest
17–20	Death, irreversibly

immediate cardiac arrest. In the presence of other diseases, such as chronic bronchitis, dementia, or ischaemic heart disease, the clinical effects may develop earlier, i.e. with relatively mild hypothermia, and cardiorespiratory arrest may be precipitated by cooling in susceptible people even before severe core hypothermia is established. Table 13.2 illustrates the effects of dropping core temperature even in the absence of other pathologies.

In practice, of course, many other diseases are usually present in older people. As already indicated, these may have increased the susceptibility to hypothermia and conversely may themselves deteriorate more rapidly because of the hypothermia. Their clinical features may distract the medical and nursing observer from thinking of and specifically looking for hypothermia. Figure 13.7 illustrates the complex and detailed possible aetiology of hypothermia developing from an imbalance of the heat generated–heat loss equation. Many diseases affecting elderly people and many adverse socioeconomic and environmental factors may add up in a chronic or acute crescendo fashion to induce dangerous core cooling. Infections may lead to a drop in body temperature rather than a pyrexia. Uraemia may impair metabolism, and hypothermia induces deterioration of renal function. Acute pancreatitis may precipitate hypothermia and core cooling may cause pancreatic necrosis.

Another catch is there are often no good clinical clues to prompt the observer to check for hypothermia, apart from the cold environment and the age of the casualty. Obviously, not all old people with cold skin would have abnormally low core temperatures. A very cold abdomen can be an important clinical clue as this is perhaps the only specific indicator of hypothermia. Otherwise the hypothermic victim just looks ill and is often suspected of having myxoedema (Fig. 13.8). Hypothyroidism is a specific cause of hypothermia but not all hypothermic victims have hypothyroidism.

Drugs and hypothermia

Some drugs, specifically the phenothiazines (e.g. chlorpromazine, thioridazine) act centrally on the hypothalamic thermostat. All sedatives, tranquillizers, hypnotics, antidepressants and psychotropic drugs, may contribute to hypothermia because of psychomotor side effects. They may impair mobility and lead to falls. Other drugs that can also predispose to or precipitate hypothermia are those that affect balance and could therefore lead to falls, e.g. drugs causing postural hypotension, such as diuretics, beta blockers and levodopa. Alcohol inhibits self-protection, causes anaesthesia, probably directly affects the central thermostat, induces dangerous vasodilatation and a false feeling of warmth, impairs peripheral sensation of cold and may cause hypoglycaemia.

Environmental influences

Older people's housing, its insulation and the efficiency of the heating systems are all likely to be less good than for younger people. Insufficient heating and poor insulation require correction which is very expensive. Old people are poorer than the population generally and their domestic environment is often very cold. In three quarters of the subjects visited in the 1972 study, reported by Fox et al (1973b), room temperatures were below the minimum recommended for council housing. The recommendation was by no means generous. More than 50% had

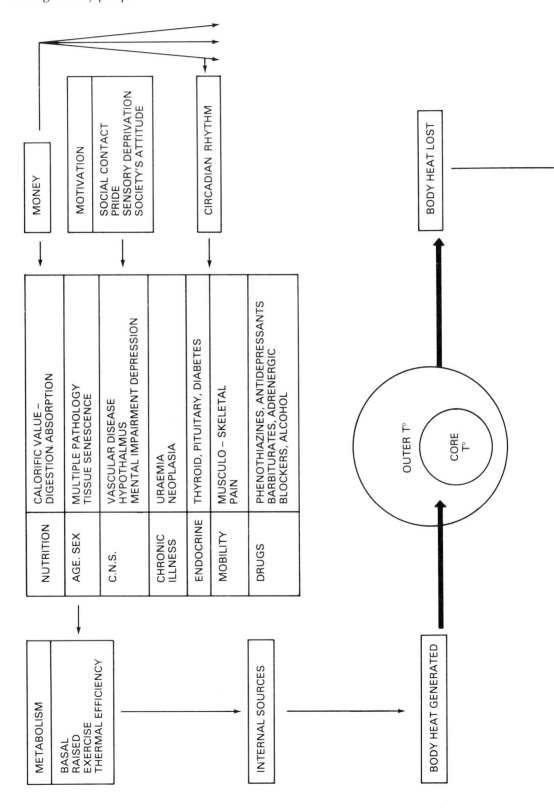

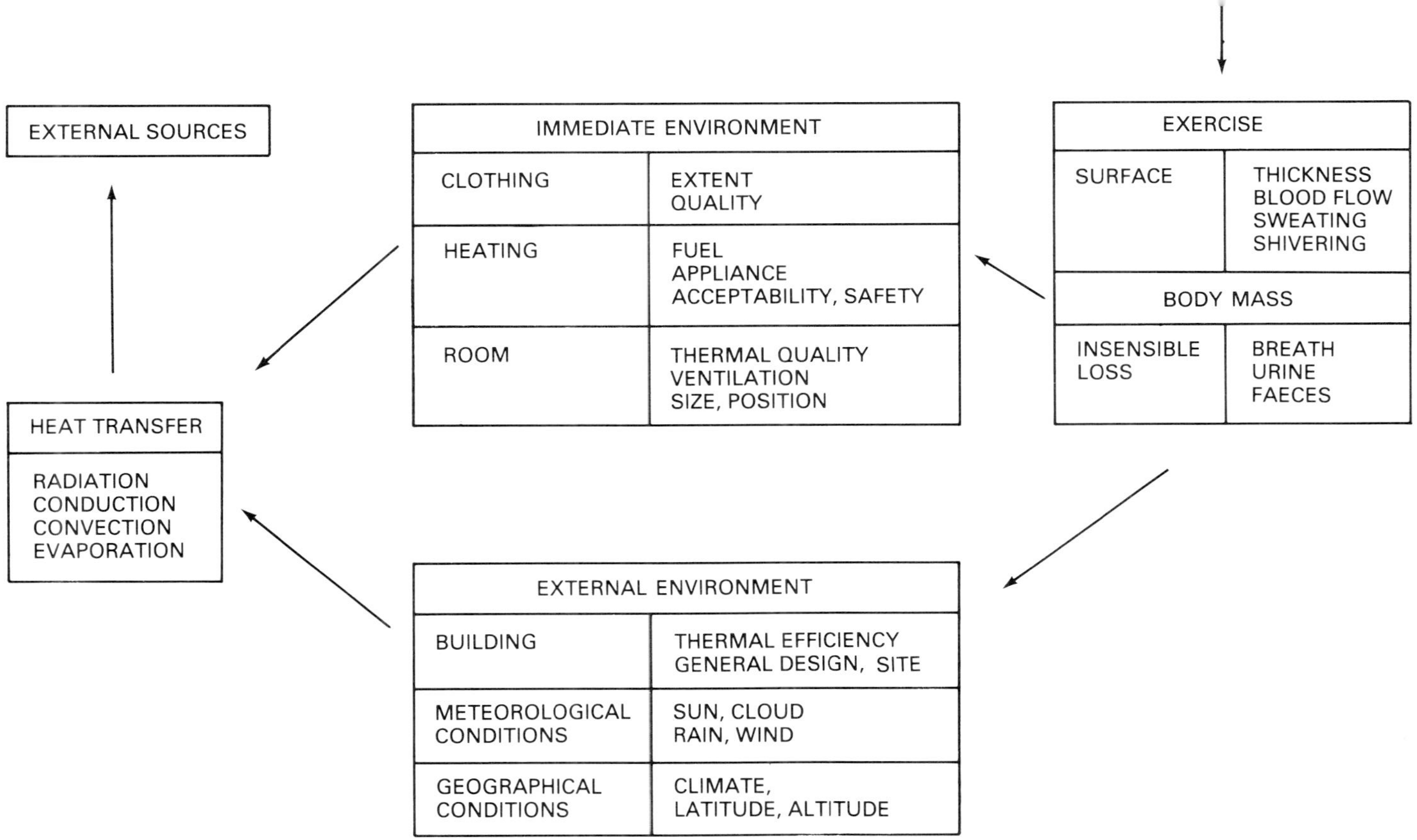

Fig. 13.7 Factors involved in maintenance of body temperature.
Source: Fox et al (1973b) Reproduced by permission of the authors of the article and the editor of the British Medical Journal.

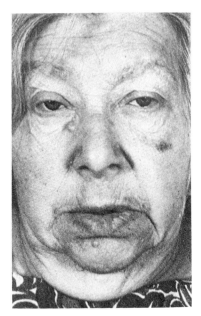

Fig. 13.8 'Hypothermic' casualty.

rooms which were colder than that legally required for offices, shops and railway waiting rooms. In 10% the morning living room temperatures were below 12°C (53.6°F).

Clearly those most at risk are very old, live alone, in cold and draughty, inadequately heated and insulated accommodation, perhaps at the top of tower blocks or in badly maintained houses, are rather poor, suffer from many accumulated pathologies and are taking several drugs, and as a final straw develop thermoregulatory failure. Their bedrooms are cold and their clothes and bedding poor insulators. When cold weather develops or there is a miners' strike or their heating is cut off for non-payment of bills, then hypothermia is a virtually inevitable consequence. Some 9/10ths of old people in cold environments say they do not use more heat because of the cost. Fifty percent of old people at risk of developing hypothermia receive supplementary benefits compared to about a third of those not at risk.

Dickensian conditions still exist. Help the Aged's 'Granny Come Home' (1972) and 'Death in Winter' (undated) and Malcolm Wicks (1978) in 'Old and Cold' have all too clearly outlined the sad socio-economic situation experienced by a minority of old people

in Britain. Indeed, the massive scale of the social problem, the need for a reappraisal of the pension system, and the relative separation between the organisation of social and health services, and the complex medical situation, are probably major factors in the difficulty in stimulating concerted national and local political action to improve the social circumstances of old people in this country.

Aids available

The supplementary benefit system is cumbersome. People of any age have difficulty with administrative bureaucracy and in getting their full rights. One-off payments can be made for new heating equipment, for insulation and even for expensive fuel bills. The Department of Health and Social Security recognised the problem many years ago. Their leaflet, 'Keeping Warm in Winter', published in 1972 was a simple explanation of the problem with constructive suggestions, and their 1983 'Help with Heating Costs' (for people getting supplementary benefit) is a descriptive leaflet about benefits generally and specifically.

Managment of hypothermia

Whether or not other diseases are present, clinical features usually include vasoconstriction with coldness and pallor of the skin, lack of shivering, puffiness of the face, confusion, twitching, slow respiration and pulse, hypotension and cardiac failure, bronchopneumonia, abdominal distension, oliguria and uraemia, with coma and death being inevitable if the dropping core temperature is not reversed.

Existence of other diseases, the age of the patient, the severity of the hypothermia (i.e. how far below 35°C (95°F) it is) and the existence of thermoregulatory defect, will all affect the outcome. Previously fit victims with mild hypothermia, e.g. 34 to 35°C (93.2 to 95°F) core temperatures, may not need admission to hospital. However, in view of the potential seriousness of any core cooling and the possibility of collapse during rewarming, hospital admission should always be considered. General measures:

1. Remove from the cold environment.
2. Minimise continuing heat loss. Space blankets are often recommended for this. These are relatively cheap, non-perishable, highly reflective foil coverings, which are easy to store and available for first-aid. However, if the hypothermic casualty does not start to recover and generate heat the space blanket is only insulating a cold body. The protection from the external temperature provided by space blankets is very little. It might be more sensible to use ordinary blankets or a duvet.
3. Passively rewarm, i.e. do not actively heat the victim with hot-water bottles, electric blankets or heat cradles.
4. Avoid alcohol.
5. Treat coexistent disease appropriately, e.g. heart failure, chest infections, hypothyroidism.
6. Give general nursing care for pressure areas, bladder etc., but do not expose the patient's body more than is absolutely necessary.

The general aim is to allow the body temperature to rise slowly to avoid hypotension, to prevent a drop in the core temperature due to blood flowing to the skin as vasodilatation occurs, and to minimise the chance of too rapid a change in body electrolytes as tissue metabolites pass into the circulation and a diuresis starts to occur. Textbooks often suggest aiming at a rise of the body temperature of about half a degree C (0.9°F) every half hour to an hour, but it is difficult to titrate this accurately in practice. The electrocardiograph should be checked as this may reveal significant arrhythmias and conduction defects. Anti-arrhythmic agents may be indicated.

Additional action accepted by most authorities would include broad-spectrum antibiotics, intravenous fluids, oxygen and thyroxine if specifically indicated, but corticosteroids are not currently popular in the treatment of shocked hypothermic victims.

Although general nursing measures are clearly necessary, excessive handling should be avoided. Urinary catheters and nasogastric tubes should be avoided if possible (except for the comatose patient) because overstimulation may induce dangerous arrhythmias including ventricular fibrillation.

RAISED BODY TEMPERATURE

Older people may react just like younger people by developing fever in response to acute and chronic infections (e.g. of chest and urinary tract), to neoplasia, autoimmune disease and deep vein thrombosis. The common denominator of pneumonia, pyelonephritis or cystitis, subacute bacterial endocarditis, septicaemia, peritonitis, tuberculosis, deep vein thrombosis, inflammatory autoimmune disease, or myocardial infarction, that leads to pyrexia, is thought to be due to pyrogens. These chemicals are released at the site of infection or inflammation and when they circulate around the body they provoke the rise in metabolism and body temperature.

However, the inflammatory response is sometimes impaired or absent in the elderly. There may be little or no neutrophil leucocytosis, and only a slight or no fever. *Hypothermia* may be the response to infections.

Hyperthermia

Infections leading to pyrexia, hot weather and anaesthesia, can be particularly damaging for old people, especially if they have other diseases, or are taking drugs which affect temperature control, or already have some thermoregulatory dysfunction. They may succumb to dehydration, confusion, other organ deterioration (e.g. of the kidney), or to malignant hyperpyrexia.

As with hypothermia it is all too easy to turn a relatively blind eye to the possible deleterious and potentially lethal effect of high environmental or body temperatures in older patients. Even a slight rise in body temperature may reflect a life-threatening deterioration.

SCREENING

Screening programmes and the construction of at-risk registers for the elderly should aim to identify, particularly in the very aged, those with multiple pathology and receiving poly-pharmacy, those unable to care for themselves independently, and the socially isolated, such as those living alone and the recently bereaved. These medical and medico-social markers should be combined with more specific social indicators of risk such as poverty and cold, poor quality housing and social isolation. Checking on room temperatures, especially in the bedroom with a simple cheap static wall thermometer, might identify those most at risk of being in a cold environment, especially as they may not complain of feeling cold. Computerisation offers general practitioners (family doctors) and the primary care team an ideal base for constructing at-risk registers and for prompting constructive preventive action.

Prevention

Screening should identify those most at risk. Action can be taken during the summer to minimise hypothermia by improving insulation and making sure old people have efficient, relatively cheap and easily controlled heating. Every attempt should be made to maintain mobility and ensure social contact, to try and treat diseases which immobilise and destabilise old people, and to avoid phenothiazines and other drugs which impair metabolism and mobility. The provision of wall thermometers has already been mentioned and duvets or low wattage underblankets (that are safe to use even with incontinent patients) are simple to provide and relatively cheap.

There is an urgent need for long-term action to provide better pensions and better provision for supplementary benefits, especially with reference to heating. Ideally, more old people should receive a higher basic pension by right with only a small minority needing supplementary benefits. Perhaps this would happen only if we had a Minister for the Elderly.

Urgent preventive action, such as visiting elderly people known to be at risk, would be necessary when bad weather occurs or acute illness or social crises develop. All doctors and nurses caring for old people should be equipped with, and remember to use, low reading thermometers. Doctors should help to draw public and political attention to the real significance of hypothermia, by identifying it more often as a major specific factor of deaths in winter. There is a general need to provide sufficient aids and adaptations for old people with functional problems, and to provide primary supporting services for the disabled elderly, e.g. home helps, meals-on-wheels, day centres, and living-in help. These general provisions, usually organised by social services departments and volunteer groups, will help to reduce the risk of hypothermia within the general context of improving the quality of life and independent functional ability of old people.

CONCLUSION

Doctors and nurses caring for elderly people should: (1) have a high index of suspicion for abnormally low (and raised) deep body temperatures in old people; (2) have and use low reading thermometers; (3) develop age/sex registers; (4) prompt local and national administrative and political action to improve the financial and social lot of the elderly.

REFERENCES

Bull G M 1973 Meteorological correlates with myocardial and cerebral infarction and respiratory disease. British Journal of Preventive and Social Medicine 27:108
Department of Health and Social Security 1972 Keeping warm in winter. DHSS, London
Department of Health and Social Security 1983 Help with heating costs (for people getting supplementary benefit). DHSS, London
Fox R H, MacGibbon R, Davies L, Woodward P M 1973a Problem of the old and the cold. British Medical Journal 1: 21–24
Fox R H, Woodward P, Exton-Smith A N, Green M F, Donnison D V, Wicks M H 1973b Body temperatures in the elderly: a national study of physiological, social and environmental conditions. British Medical Journal 1: 200–206

Goldman A, Exton-Smith A N, Francis G, O'Brien A 1977 A pilot study of low body temperatures in old people admitted to hospital. Journal of the Royal College of Physicians 11(3):291

Help the Aged 1972 Granny come home. Help the Aged, London

Help the Aged undated Death in winter. Help the Aged, London

Royal College of Physicians 1966 Report of the committee on accidental hypothermia. Royal College of Physicians, London

Wicks M 1978 Old and cold: hypothermia and social policy. Heinemann, London

FURTHER READING

Age Concern 1974 Warm up for winter. Age Concern England

Collins K J 1983 Hypothermia, the facts. Oxford University Press

Health Education Council undated Keeping warm in winter. The Health Education Council, London

Maclean D, Emsilie-Smith D 1977 Accidental hypothermia. Blackwell, Oxford

S. J. Redfern

14

Maintaining healthy skin

THE SKIN

The skin, that most sensitive of organs, is the part of ourselves which is visible to others and which can reflect our emotions, well-being and state of health. The effects of ageing on the skin are regarded, particularly in western societies, as negative, unwanted and to be avoided as far as possible. A tremendous amount of time and money is spent on skin and hair in an attempt to retain one's youthful appearance for as long as possible.

Normal ageing results in changes to the four significant functions of the skin: protection, heat regulation, conveying sensation and body image (see Ch. 3 for further discussion of physiological changes with age). All of these changes may affect an elderly person's comfort and the extent to which (s)he interacts with the environment. If (s)he also suffers from a skin disorder, then the effects of that, together with the perceived negative consequences of an ageing skin, may cause the old person to withdraw from public view completely.

Assessment of the skin

A careful assessment of the skin can give the nurse clues about a patient's emotional state and lifestyle as well as about her state of health. Physical assessment should include observation of:

Moisture—dry, oily, sweaty, discharge
(e.g. vaginal)

Texture—smooth, rough

Temperature—difference between trunk and extremities

Colour and areas of discolouration (e.g. bruising, pigmentation)

Thickness and turgor, wrinkles

Oedema

Blemishes—scars, rashes, soreness

Infestation—head lice, body lice, scabies

Areas of discontinuity—blisters, cuts, ulcers, pressure sores.

Skin lesions are common in elderly people and observation should be made of their location, their structural characteristics, their size, colour and grouping (e.g. in tissue folds, following nerve pathways). Skin lesions can be classified into primary and secondary categories (Carnevali and Patrick 1979). Primary skin lesions include non-elevated macules (such as drug rashes, petechiae, senile purpura, freckles), elevated papules, nodules and tumours (such as senile warts, neurofibromas, psoriasis, insect bites, basal cell carcinomas), and elevated fluid-filled vesicles (such as blisters, second degree burns, infected pimples and boils).

Secondary skin lesions can be crusts from serum, blood or pus (such as impetigo), scales (as in psoriasis, exfoliative dermatitis), lichenification from excessive scratching (as in atopic dermatitis), erosion (as in syphilitic chancre), ulcers (stasis or varicose ulcers, pressure sores), scars (keloid or hypertrophied scarring), and atrophy.

Nursing management

Nursing management of the elderly person's skin should be based on the nursing history and assessment. The aims of nursing care are to help the patient prevent skin problems, to maintain a maximum level of skin function and structure and to promote return to a healthy skin state. The common problems of elderly people with skin disorders are:

1. Discomfort from pruritis, pain, dryness, extremes in temperature, trauma.
2. A low self-concept of body image related

to perceived or actual disfigurement.

3. Disruption of lifestyle as a result of the need for treatment, and dependency on others for assistance with treatment and coping with activities of living.
4. Systemic disturbance, such as fatigue, sleep loss, fluid loss.
5. Potential for developing complications such as infection, skin breakdown, depression. The likelihood of multiple pathology of the frail elderly, coupled with their slower recovery rates in comparison to younger people, mean that their tolerance for additional stress will be low and they may be unable to resist further complications.

Skin discomfort

Generalised pruritis can result from oozing, weeping lesions such as eczema, pemphigus and localised excoriations (e.g. pruritis vulvae, pruritis ani), or it may indicate systemic disorders such as kidney disturbance, diabetes, anaemia, polycythaemia or barbiturate withdrawal. Such conditions require specific medical treatment, but if the main problem is pruritis resulting from dry skin, the nurse can do much to help the patient minimise discomfort. For example, soap removes protective oils and increases skin dryness (see Torrance 1983) and so should be used on axillary and genital areas only. A daily tub bath is unnecessary and water for washing should not be too hot. A non-perfumed emollient containing lanolin applied after washing prevents loss of moisture from the skin. Cotton underclothes are more comfortable to the skin than synthetics. The ambient humidity of living rooms can be increased with humidifiers to prevent skin dryness.

Discomfort also results from the relative inability of elderly people to cope with extremes in temperature (see Ch. 13, Maintaining Body Temperature). Action can be taken to promote optimum blood flow to the skin to maintain body temperature by attending to clothing, bedclothes and electric blankets, ambient temperature, avoiding the 'wind/chill factor' or excessive heat, adequate nourishment, fluids and exercise, and avoiding certain sedatives and tranquillisers (e.g. phenothiazine derivatives) that depress cerebral function and circulation and increase the sensation of cold.

The elderly person has thin, fragile, inelastic skin which is susceptible to trauma and bacterial invasion. The nurse can raise the person's awareness of potential problems and can encourage actions to prevent trauma, for example:

1. Wearing protective clothing such as gloves for dishwashing and gardening.
2. Padding exposed body surfaces such as knees when gardening, using thimbles when sewing.
3. Avoiding direct contact with extreme heat or cold, such as hot water bottles, fires radiators, frozen foods.
4. Avoiding tight clothing which can restrict circulation, such as tight waistbands, tight stockings or socks.
5. Keeping skin abrasions clean and exposed to air to allow drying, unless a dressing of some kind is necessary.

Low self-concept

Skin disorders can be unsightly and from ancient times have carried the stigma of physical and moral uncleanliness with subsequent self-rejection, feelings of guilt and unworthiness. Responses like these can increase the stress which underlies the condition and its severity might increase, and response to treatment decrease. Possible outcomes to such responses are raised anxiety and depression and insomnia.

Sensitive nursing care can be instrumental in enhancing a patient's self-esteem by, for example, touching the affected skin without wearing gloves (unless contraindicated), by looking at the patient without distaste or disgust, by talking with and listening to the patient and her family and friends, and by explaining to the patient and family the nature of the disorder, clarifying misconceptions, and

encouraging them to help with the care required.

Disruption of lifestyle

Skin disorders can be extremely long lasting, debilitating and the focus of a patient's life if the treatments are time-consuming. The manifestations of the disease (e.g. pruritis, oozing, pain, depression, withdrawal), the treatments required (baths, lotions, creams, dressings), the systemic responses which may occur as a result of the disease or the treatment, and the effects of other disabilities of the old person (such as arthritis, immobility, loss of sight), all add to the likelihood of a way of life which is disrupted and which focuses on the skin complaint. The nurse can do much to encourage the old person to continue as far as possible with previous activities and social contacts, and to avoid isolation.

Care of the mouth

Mouth-care procedures for patients in hospital have remained virtually unchanged for over 30 years, even though the swabbing procedure is ineffective and comfort is not maintained or improved (Howarth 1977). Adequate nutrition and hydration and appropriate astringent and antibacterial mouth-washes are the most effective means of keeping the mouth clean, moist and healthy. It is the person who is reluctant to eat and drink who becomes dehydrated and develops a dry, encrusted and dirty mouth rather than the unconscious patient. Such reluctant patients are likely to be found in geriatric wards and old people's homes.

Sodium bicarbonate is an effective cleaning agent for encrusted mouths, but Howarth reported that patients find it unpleasant and so it should be used sparingly. Glycothymoline gives temporary refreshment only. Howarth found that glycerine, or glycerol, was used regularly for lubricating the lips, but although early nursing textbooks gave warning of its astringent properties, no mention of dilution appeared in any procedure sheet or later textbook which she consulted. As she pointed out, since cosmetics firms use 20% glycerol for moisturising creams and 40% for astringent lotions, it would be wise for nurses to do the same or to abandon glycerol for something less damaging, such as lanolin.

As for mouth-cleaning tools, swabs wrapped around forceps are frequently used, but their continued use on the grounds of ease, effectiveness and cost is not justified (Harris, 1980). Harris found that nurses accepted the foam stick applicator and sometimes a swabbed finger was useful, but she concluded that a child's small-headed toothbrush was the most effective.

Since these two studies, the literature has been reviewed by Gibbons (1983), a dentist, and he prescribed the following regime for patients requiring mouth care:

1. A child's small-headed toothbrush with either fluoride toothpaste or chlorhexidine gel, which is effective in inhibiting the development of dental plaque and gingivitis. Harris (1980) recommended an electric toothbrush, each patient being provided with a personal brush head. Interden gum massagers and dental floss should be much more in evidence (Speedie 1983).
2. Sodium bicarbonate solution for encrusted mouths to break down debris and create an alkaline environment.
3. Chlorhexidine mouth-washes for preventing plaque and gingivitis.
4. Vaseline for the lips, which is soothing and lasts longer than other materials.
5. Whole mouth brushing which should include the teeth, gums, palate and tongue and so is suitable for edentulous patients. Since over 80% of the population over 75 years do not have their own teeth (Sofaer 1979), nurses should encourage patients to brush their gums as much as they do their dentures.

This regime is based on research findings, is more effective than traditional mouth care using swabbing techniques, and, as Gibbons observed, is cheaper than the packs issued by the hospital sterile supply departments. Yet the traditional practice remains.

PRESSURE SORES

Although pressure sores (decubitus ulcers) have been a constant plague for the debilitated and chronically ill since the beginning of recorded history (Bennett 1983a), the problem we now face is a relatively new one. With increasing numbers surviving into extreme old age, and with improvements in medical care which enable people to survive the multiple pathology and serious illnesses of old age, the number of those at risk of pressure sores has increased. The costs of a pressure sore to the patient are incalculable and the cost to the National Health Service is staggering. Fernie (1973) estimated this to be £60 million per year, and Scales et al (1982) suggest that an excess of £150 million is more realistic today.

The extent of the problem: pressure sore prevalence

Comparison between the prevalence studies which have been published is difficult because of the different populations sampled and methods used. A Danish study (Peterson and Bittmann 1971) showed a prevalence rate of 43 people with sores per 100 000 of the general population, and rates for patient samples ranged from 1.5% to 94% depending on type and location of patient (Torrance 1983) and definition of sore. In a one-day survey of two Scottish Health Board areas (Jordan and Barbenel 1983), the prevalence rates in the hospital and community patient population were 8.8% and 9.4% respectively. More recently, a survey in 132 hospitals in four health regions in England reported 961 patients with pressure sores, a prevalence rate of 6.7% (David et al 1983).

What is clear is the association of pressure sores with age, with two thirds or more of patients with sores being over 70 years. Other related factors are level of consciousness, immobility, incontinence and medical condition. Nervous system and cardiovascular diseases, and neoplasms are commonly related to higher pressure sore incidence. It is in the geriatric and orthopaedic wards where the vulnerable patient, presenting with a number of these interrelated contributing factors, is likely to be found.

Location and classification of pressure sores

Twenty-two unique types of sore were located on 17 body sites by David et al (1983), but over half the sores were found in the pelvic region and over a quarter on the lower extremities, notably the heels (David et al 1983, Torrance 1983).

Various classifications of pressure sore type have been suggested (Torrance 1983), but the type 1 and type 2 distinction described by Barton and Barton (1981) is widely used. A type 1 sore occurs when sustained pressure causes superficial blistering, and if pressure is unrelieved, it spreads into the deeper tissues to form a deep ulcer. The local blood vessels become occluded with erythrocytes and the endothelial cells of the vessels swell but remain intact. In the case of the type 2 sore, damage starts in the deeper tissues and spreads up to the skin surface. The blood vessels are occluded with platelets and the vessels' endothelial cells become separated and damaged (Bennett 1983a). When skin breakdown is first seen, deep tissue damage has occurred for some time and a deep ulcer is inevitable. Either type of sore usually occurs over bony prominences where there is little opportunity for pressure to be dissipated through fatty tissues. The Bartons have also described a third type of sore, the inactive or indolent sore, which is unlikely to heal and normally occurs in dying patients.

The type 1 sore shows a temperature difference of more than 2.5°C between the ulcer margin and adjacent healthy tissue, whereas the type 2 sore shows a smaller temperature difference (about 1°C) and is much slower to heal. The totally inactive sore is cold and there is no or very little temperature difference between the sore margin and surrounding skin.

Pressure sores are usually classified into five grades or stages (Bennett 1983a):

Grade 1a Blanching erythema. Reactive hyperaemia causes a distinct erythema after pressure is released. Light finger pressure will cause blanching of this erythema, indicating that the microcirculation is intact.

1b Non-blanching erythema. The erythema remains when light pressure is applied, indicating a degree of microcirculatory disruption and inflammation.

Grade 2 Superficial damage—epidermal blister.

Grade 3 Dermal ulcer—whole skin thickness including necrosis and eschar.

Grade 4 The lesion extends into the subcutaneous fat.

Grade 5a Involvement of deeper soft tissues.

5b Involvement of bone and/or joints.

This classification cannot indicate whether the sore is deteriorating or showing signs of healing. David et al (1983) attempted to overcome this problem by recording the presence of granulation tissue, scar tissue, scab formation, necrotic material and purulent smell. The more knowledgeable the nurse is about the underlying pathology and predisposing factors contributing to pressure sores, the more likely will (s)he plan effective preventive and treatment regimes.

Causes and predisposing factors in pressure sore development

The factors which contribute to the development of pressure sores are numerous and interactive, and although direct pressure is one of the most important, not every patient exposed to pressure will develop a sore. The healthy person can lie immobile for several hours without injury, yet a susceptible patient can develop a sore within an hour. This is because the susceptible patient is victim to several predisposing factors which together render him or her extremely vulnerable.

Direct pressure compresses tissues and if it is greater than the mean capillary pressure (20–25 mmHg), then the capillaries in this region are occluded and the tissues they supply are deprived of blood and the oxygen and nutrients it carries. If the pressure is prolonged for more than about two hours, then a pressure sore will develop in the susceptible patient, although some patients, notably paraplegics, can develop sores in less than two hours. Complications of pressure are shear and friction forces which can occur when the patient slides down the bed or is dragged up it. Shearing forces cause local vessels to be obliterated, kinked and ruptured, so forming thromboses and destroying the microcirculation, as occurs in the type 2 sore.

The predisposing factors which increase a patient's vulnerability to pressure sores are often divided into intrinsic and extrinsic factors.

Intrinsic factors

Body type. The bonier body is more susceptible to pressure sores, but the obese immobile patient who is difficult to lift is vulnerable to shearing forces and friction.

Immobility. Normally, excessive pressure causes discomfort and a spontaneous change of posture even during sleep. A healthy person changes position once every 15 minutes or so during sleep, and a reduction in the number of spontaneous body movements during sleep is directly related to an increase in the incidence of pressure sores (Exton-Smith and Sherwin 1961). Therefore, any condition which reduces mobility or the sensation of pain, such as paralysis, anaesthesia, clouding of consciousness, sedation, mental apathy or very poor physical condition, can contribute to sores.

Nutritional state. Malnutrition may be more common in institutionalised patients than is realised and increases susceptibility to pressure sores through devitalisation of tissues. The nutrients particularly important for the prevention of pressure sores are protein and amino acids, ascorbic acid and zinc (Torrance 1983). A negative nitrogen balance is associated with oedema and this renders the patient extremely susceptible to pressure sores.

Incontinence. Norton et al (1962) found that 38% of incontinent patients developed pressure sores compared with 7% who were continent. The exact nature of the relationship between pressure sores and incontinence is not clear, but wet skin or clothing and bedding can cause maceration of the skin and damage from friction on movement. It is likely that the incontinent patient is susceptible to pressure sores because of other factors such as immobility and neurological disease.

Infection. Pyrexia produces an increase in metabolic rate and demand for oxygen which will endanger existing ischaemic areas. Bacteria further increase the demand on local metabolism for their own requirements and those of the body's defence mechanisms. And severe infection weakens the body's reserves by causing nutritional disturbance (Torrance 1983).

Anaemia and vascular disease. A reduction in the threshold level of pressure which tissues can withstand will occur with any condition which decreases the quality or quantity of blood reaching those tissues, and pressure injury is more likely. Thus cardiac disorders, anaemia, peripheral vascular disease and arterioscleriotic disease are important predisposing factors in pressure sore development.

Neurological disease. Whether it is the disease itself or the consequent lack of sensation and mobility of patients with such conditions as paraplegia, multiple sclerosis and cerebrovascular accidents, their susceptibility to pressure sores is well known. Other intrinsic factors are age and illness of any kind. Ageing skin loses its elasticity, subcutaneous fat and some muscle atrophy occurs. Furthermore, because of the likelihood of multiple pathology, the elderly are particularly at risk, for example, those with diabetes mellitus, rheumatic disease, orthopaedic conditions, muscular wasting diseases, burns and renal disease (Torrance 1983).

Extrinsic factors

Skin hygiene. The traditional practice of washing patients' pressure areas every two hours as a matter of course is, fortunately, out of favour. Although frequent washing of the incontinent patient is necessary, overzealous use of soap and water can be harmful because protective oils are lost, the skin pH is altered, and dehydration occurs (Lowthian 1982, Torrance 1983).

Massage. Vigorous skin massage is another traditional practice which can be dangerous to vulnerable tissues, particularly where non-blanching erythemia suggests existing early damage (Barbenel et al 1983, Torrance 1983). Dyson (1978) reported a reduction of 38% in the incidence of pressure sores in a group of elderly patients who were not rubbed, compared with a group who received the usual pressure area massage. Post-mortem examination of tissues from the massaged group showed extensive damage compared with virtually none in the non-rubbed group.

Patient positioning, lifting and bedmaking. Patient positioning, lifting and bedmaking can contribute to pressure sore development if done incorrectly so that damage from pressure, friction and shear forces occur. These forces are particularly hazardous for the patient sitting up in bed, and tight bedding can completely restrict the movement of the debilitated patient.

Drugs. Any drug which decreases sensation or mobility can increase the likelihood of pressure sores. Thus, sedatives, transquillisers, opiates and alcohol should be used with care. Prolonged use of oral steroids and anti-inflammatory drugs should be avoided because they delay the healing process.

The patient support system. The support system, be it a bed, chair, operating table or theatre or casualty trolley, can contribute to pressure sore development in two ways: its inability to distribute or relieve pressure on the body and its effect on the interface between skin and support surface. A hard surface increases areas of high pressure such as on the sacrum and heels, and the mattress or cushion cover can be so tight as to cause a hammock effect which increases the load on the tissues. This can be reduced by ensuring that the mattress or cushion moulds round the body yet is sufficiently thick to avoid 'grounding', where the body is not kept clear of the bed or chair base.

A soft surface is more likely than a hard one to distribute pressure evenly and reduce pressure sufficiently to avoid tissue distortion, but if the support is one of uniaxial rather than triaxial or hydrostatic loading, then tissue distortion can occur (Torrance 1983). Uniaxial, or one-directional pressure on the tissues causes stretching and compression of the blood vessels, whereas triaxial loading directs pressure on the tissues in three directions simultaneously, so avoiding damage to vessels.

The ordinary foam mattress of the hospital bed does not provide triaxial support, it is often too thin to prevent grounding, and the mattress cover may be too tight to avoid pressure from hammocking. In addition, the waterproof material of the cover and of pillows and drawsheets may have adverse effects on the skin, causing heat retention, high skin humidity and sweating. Thus the patient will be both uncomfortable and at risk of developing a pressure sore.

Assessment of the patient at risk

The nursing assessment of any elderly patient should include a pressure sore risk assessment. The continuing dwindling of resources in the National Health Service makes it increasingly important for nurses to know with confidence which patients are at risk and where the resources should be focused. Assessment of risk can be done very easily by nurses using one of the rating scales available. The most well-known, the pressure sore risk rating scale (Norton scale) (Fig. 14.1), was developed by Norton and her colleagues (1962) over 20 years ago, and has only recently

A		B		C		D		E	
Physical condition		Mental condition		Activity		Mobility		Incontinent	
Good	4	Alert	4	Ambulant	4	Full	4	Not	4
Fair	3	Apathetic	3	Walk/help	3	Slightly limited	3	Occasionally	3
Poor	2	Confused	2	Chairbound	2	Very limited	2	Usually/urine	2
Very bad	1	Stuporous	1	Bedfast	1	Immobile	1	Doubly	1

Instructions for use
1. Score patient (1–4) under each heading (A–E), and total the scores.
2. A score of 14 or less indicates the patient is at risk and preventive care is necessary.
3. When sacral oedema is present the patient might be at risk even with a high score.
4. Assess the patient regulary.

Source: Doreen Norton, Rhoda McLaren and A.N. Exton-Smith, An *Investigation of Geriatric Nursing Problems in Hospital*, London, National Corporation for the Care of Old People, 1962 (reprinted by Churchill Livingstone, Edinburgh, 1975). Reproduced by permission of NCCOP.

Fig. 14.1 The pressure sore risk rating scale (Norton scale). *Source: Norton D, McLaren R, Exton-Smith A N 1962. Reproduced by permission of NCCOP.*

begun to be used by practising nurses.

There is some evidence that the Norton scale is a reasonably valid predictor of patients at risk (Roberts and Goldstone 1979, Goldstone and Goldstone 1982), but it does not take into account other factors known to be significant in pressure sore development, such as nutritional status, body build and certain diseases.

The Knoll scale (Fig. 14.2) is more detailed but also simple to use. This takes into account oral nutritional and fluid intake and predisposing diseases (diabetes, neuropathies, vascular diseases, anaemias) as well as general state of health, mental status, activity, mobility and incontinence. It also weights certain factors by doubling the score of patients with high (i.e. at risk) scores on certain factors. The scoring system is the reverse of that for the Norton scale, so that high scores (above 12) indicate at risk. In a comparison of elderly patients' at risk scores using the Norton and Knoll scales, we found a correlation of -0.86 ($n = 85$) which suggests quite a high level of interscale agreement.

The Royal National Orthopaedic Hospital at Stanmore, Middlesex, has recently developed the pressure sore prediction score which is

PARAMETERS	0	1	2	3	Score
General state of health	Good	Fair	Poor	Moribund	———
Mental Status	Alert	Lethargic	Semi-comatose	Comatose	———
			Count these conditions as double		
Activity	Ambulatory	Needs help	Chairfast	Bedfast	———
Mobility	Full	Limited	Very limited	Immobile	———
Incontinence	None	Occasional	Usually of urine	Total of urine and faeces	———
Oral nutrition intake	Good	Fair	Poor	None	———
Oral fluid intake	Good	Fair	Poor	None	———
Predisposing diseases (Diabetes, neuropathies, vascular disease, anaemias)	Absent	Slight	Moderate	Severe	———

The higher the score the greater is the potential to develop decubitus ulcers.
Patients with scores above (12) should be considered at risk.

Fig. 14.2 The Knoll scale for liability to pressure sores. *Reproduced by permission of Knoll Pharmaceutical Co., New Jersey.*

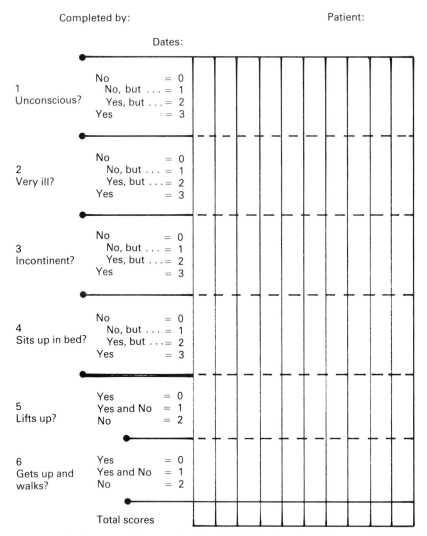

Fig. 14.3 Pressure sore prediction score. *Source: Lowthian P T 1983. Reproduced by permission of Macmillan.*

claimed to be simple and relatively objective (Lowthian 1983). The patient is assessed on six dimensions (see Fig. 14.3), and intermediate category assessments are allowed which do not depend on the nurse's understanding of unfamiliar terms (like stuporous), yet enable her to use clinical judgment. Preliminary research with the scale has shown a close association between risk score and development or deterioration of sores.

A more sophisticated technique for pressure sore risk assessment is thermography or radiometry which can detect temperature differences in the tissues and can identify damaged (i.e. relatively avascular) tissue before anything is noticeable clinically. A portable instrument was developed and tested by Newman and Davis (1981) and shown to give a precise and reliable indication of early tissue damage. Its use could be justified in clinical areas containing a high proportion of vulnerable patients.

Ultrasound has also been used to detect early tissue damage, for example at the Stoke Mandeville spinal injuries unit. No doubt more sophisticated techniques will continue to appear, but nurses should use one of the existing rating scales which are simple and relatively unambiguous.

Preventing pressure sores

Preventing pressure sores for the patient at risk is a responsibility for all members of the care team and particularly the nursing staff who have the most contact with the patient. Relieving pressure on the patient is one of the fundamental aims of prevention and this applies as much to chairbound as to bedbound patients. In fact, the totally helpless chairbound patient might be at greater risk than the same patient in bed because body weight is not distributed over such a large area, and preventive measures are not applied so rigorously. Jordan and Barbenel (1983) found that 29% of totally helpless chairbound patients had pressure sores compared with 9% of totally helpless bedbound patients.

Pressure-relieving or automatic turning beds remove the need for manual turning, but if these are not available or not indicated then the patient or nurse must take on the responsibility. Two hourly pressure relief is the usual practice for patients at risk but individual needs vary. Lowthian's (1979) 24-hour turning clock is a simple aid which can be adjusted to the patient's needs and reduce the possibility of the care being forgotten (Fig. 14.4). It is also suitable for the chairbound patient who can be taught to shift position and do regular push-ups in the chair every 15 minutes or so. The obese hemiplegic patient may not, however, be able to do push-ups, and should regularly be helped to stand and gain balance, or be taken for frequent walks to relieve pressure areas.

Careful positioning of the body and limbs is important to prevent contractions and pressure sores where bony prominences touch each other. Judicious use of pillows and back supports can help and bed cradles relieve the weight of bedclothes and footrests the shear forces of 'forward slide'. Patients should be taught the dangers of pressure and to manage

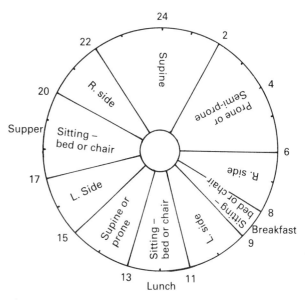

Fig. 14.4 Twentyfour-hour 'turning clock' for a mainly bedfast patient at risk of pressure sores. *After Lowthian 1979.*

their own pressure relief regime as far as possible.

Nurses should be taught correct lifting techniques which ensure patients are lifted clear of the support surface. The shoulder lift is advocated for heavy patients (Scholey 1982) and is less backbreaking for the nurse than the standard lift, yet in our experience, it is used less frequently.

A healthy nutritional state is essenital for pressure sore prevention, and the elderly are more at risk from malnutrition than many other patient groups. There is evidence that a diet adequate in fluid, protein, iron, vitamin C and zinc sulphate is necessary to prevent tissue damage and promote healing (Abbott et al 1968, Moolton 1972, Taylor et al 1974, Guttman 1976).

Bearing in mind the dangers mentioned earlier of excessive washing of skin and vigorous massage of pressure areas, skin should be kept clean and dry, and massage avoided. The value of most of the topical applications used in the prevention of pressure sores is doubtful and astringents such as methylated spirit, alcohol and witch hazel can be harmful (Torrance 1983). Dry skins which have lost their natural oils will benefit from the application of oil-based creams, and barrier creams containing silicone or zinc, can help prevent skin maceration of incontinent patients.

Preventing pressure sores involves attending to all those risk factors mentioned earlier which may be present. Without appropriate medical treatment of anaemia, cardiovascular, peripheral vascular and neurological conditions, and without recognition of the contribution of certain drugs to the development of pressure sores, the preventive nursing care outlined here will achieve little success.

Patient support systems in preventing pressure sores

The ideal support system for the susceptible patient should fulfil the following requirements (Torrance 1983, p 29–30) and be comfortable for the patient:

1. Distribute pressure evenly to avoid tissue distortion and disruption of the micro-circulation, or
2. provide frequent relief of pressure by varying the areas under pressure.
3. Minimise friction and shearing forces.
4. Provide a comfortable ventilated interface environment.
5. Be acceptable to the patient and not restrict movement.
6. Not impede nursing procedures.
7. Be easy to lift patients on and off.
8. Be readily adaptable for external cardiac massage.
9. Easily maintained and cleaned.
10. Realistically priced.

No support system available fulfils all the requirements. The effective ones are complicated to use and extremely expensive. Torrance (1983) has classified the numerous support systems available into four types: those which alternate the area of the body under pressure; those which reduce and distribute pressure evenly (moulding devices); those which assist or simulate normal move-

ment and turning; those which protect specific body areas. Space precludes more than a brief discussion of each category but the interested reader is referred to Torrance's comprehensive chapter.

Devices which alternate the area of the body under pressure. The alternate pressure mattress (APM), or ripple mattress, is one with which all nurses are familiar and which operates by exerting intermittent high pressure on the body so that no part of the body is continuously under high pressure. The original small-cell APM has been shown to be ineffective in preventing pressure sores, but the large-cell APM is effective if it is working properly and used in conjunction with a regular turning regime (Bliss et al 1967). It is often the case that APMs are incorrectly installed or are faulty, and even though the red warning light is on, no action is taken by the nurses. This can be extremely dangerous for the patient.

Other types of APM are available, some with longitudinal cells or 'bubble' pads, but the only one which will be mentioned here is the Pegasus air wave system (Dermalex Co. Ltd). This is similar in principle to the ripple mattress except that there are two layers of air cells and every third cell is deflated in turn. The mattress is ventilated by pinholes through which air passes and is dispersed around the patient through a washable wool fleece placed on top of the mattress. The air wave system (AWS) has been shown to be more effective than the large-cell APM in preventing pressure sores and reducing the severity of existing sores (Exton-Smith et al 1982). The AWS did not break down during the trial, whereas the Ripple mattresses did on several occasions.

Pillows or foam blocks can be placed strategically on an ordinary mattress so that there are gaps at pressure points. This can be effective if used with regular turning, but pressure and shear stresses are relatively high either side of each gap.

Devices which reduce and distribute pressure evenly. These surfaces mould themselves to the body contours so reducing any points of high pressure. They tend to be fairly sophisticated devices which must have sufficient volume to displace the patient's weight without 'grounding', and have an enveloping membrane which is not so tight that it causes hammocking. They also aim to provide triaxial rather than uniaxial loading so avoiding tissue distortion.

Examples of these systems are cut foam mattresses, water beds which achieve true flotation, the air-fluidised bed (Astec Environmental Systems Ltd), the low air loss bed system (Mediscus Products Ltd), the Simpson-Edinburgh low pressure air bed (Robert Kellie and Son Ltd.), bead pillow mattresses, sawdust and sand beds and the plaster bed. Torrance (1983) provides a comprehensive list of products related to pressure sores and their manufacturers. Many of these beds have been subjected to fairly rigorous research trials and found to be effective in preventing and treating pressure sores (Kenedi et al 1976), but the most efficient systems tend to be complicated, cumbersome and expensive. The cost, however, pales to insignificance if it is compared with the cost to the patient and to the National Health Service of treating pressure sores.

A fairly new mattress, the Stanmore Vaperm patient support system, has been developed at the Royal National Orthopaedic Hospital, Stanmore (Lowthian 1983, Scales et al 1982) and is a cheaper alternative to the low air loss bed system also developed there. It consists of five densities of fatigue-resistant polyurethane foam and has pressure-relieving channels inside the foam at vulnerable body sites like the sacrum and heels. Pilot trials suggest that it is effective in preventing pressure sores and in providing a compatible dry microclimate between the skin and mattress because the covering material is waterproof but permeable to water vapour.

Marshall and Overstall (1983) compared seven locally available beds by measuring interface pressures of each with healthy volunteers as subjects. On the grounds of efficient pressure distribution and cost the authors recommended the Nuclea foam mattress over the standard foam mattress, the Talley ripple mattress, two water-beds, the Mecabed net suspension bed and the Spenco Silicore padding mattress. The Nuclea foam mattress is a relatively cheap system which combines the properties of water and foam.

Devices which assist or simulate normal movement and turning. The main feature of these systems is that they help the nurse or patient to relieve pressure by assisted turning. Simple devices are the overhead handgrip, handblocks for the patient to lift herself clear of the bed, and the rope ladder fixed to the end of the bed with which the patient can pull herself forward. Other systems assist turning with manual, electric or automatic controls. The Co-Ro constant turning bed automatically turns the patient from side to side 15 times an hour. The Egerton tilting and turning bed and the Stryker Circo-electric bed have attendant-controlled electric motors which assist in turning. Net suspension beds (Mecabed, Egerton) are open-mesh nylon hammocks in which the patient can be turned very easily by one nurse operating two handles.

Devices which protect specific body areas. These devices include pads, fleeces, cushions and heel, elbow and sacral protectors. Natural and artificial fleeces are extremely popular, they are soft and comfortable and keep the skin dry. They are not, however, very effective in relieving pressure and avoiding tissue distortion and they can have very high friction values (Lowthian 1983). Laundering was a problem with early models but modern fleeces wash well as long as the manufacturers' instructions are followed. In a comparison of 11 natural and synthetic fleeces, Denne (1983) found the synthetic fleece Mullipel to be the best in terms of accommodation depth, laundering and degree of matting. However, in an earlier study, Denne (1979) concluded that natural fleeces were more effective than synthetics in reducing friction and in keeping the skin dry: and so the decision on what to buy is not easy.

Numerous pads and cushions are on the market, such as foam, Silicore, bead, gel, water, air alternating pressure cushions and mixtures (e.g. gel or water and foam). It is important that the cushion is fitted to the patient and chair or wheelchair in which it will be used. The occupational therapy department in hospitals can give nurses and patients advice on wheelchair adaptation and maintenance, and a comprehensive book has been published by the Royal Association for Disability and Rehabilitation (RADAR) on choosing the best wheelchair cushion to suit individual needs (Jay 1983). Most cushions are unable to relieve pressure to such an extent that manual pressure relief is unnecessary, and the cushion cover may reduce the efficiency of the cushion's pressure distribution properties. Thus pressure relief is still necessary by patients doing regular push-ups or being helped to stand and walk where possible.

There are a number of sacral, elbow and heel protectors available made of foam, gel, air padding and bandages. It is unlikely that these make a great contribution to the prevention of pressure sores, and some may be harmful by restricting the blood supply, such as the heel 'doughnut' made from bandages (Lowthian 1983). There is no doubt that with high quality nursing care more pressure sores can be prevented. The bewildering array of aids on the market for preventing and treating pressure sores makes choosing what is best in terms of cost and effectiveness very difficult. More valid evaluative research is required and should be used by the health team to make an informed choice on what to buy. So often a bulk order for a piece of equipment is continued unquestioningly without thought for new developments which may be cheaper and more effective. The ubiquitous ripple mattress is a case in point.

Very few of the aids available remove totally the need for continued preventive care by nurses. Most, at best, reduce the frequency with which pressure relief is required, and if nurses do not appreciate the principles on which the device works and its limitations, then the patient is in considerable danger.

The management of pressure sores

Meticulous attention to preventive care, both systemic and local, can avoid the development of pressure sores for most patients. However, in the case of inactive sores, which almost always occur in the terminally ill, nothing will be effective, and nursing care should focus on the promotion of comfort even if this means that the patient lies or sits directly on the sore.

Management of the patient with pressure sores must focus on pressure relief, removing and avoiding predisposing factors, and wound care. Relief of pressure has been discussed in some detail already, and general management should focus on the predisposing factors mentioned earlier. For example, the medical condition of the patient should be stabilised, anaemia treated with blood transfusion if severe, oedema removed with diuretics, systemic infection treated with antibiotics, and incontinence investigated and treated. A balanced fluid and nutritional intake is essential, with supplements of protein, vitamin C, iron and zinc where necessary. Drugs should be prescribed cautiously and if possible, those known to delay healing, such as corticosteroids and anti-inflammatory drugs avoided.

Assessment of pressure sores

It is impossible to judge the rate of healing or deterioration of a wound or the effectiveness of local treatments without an assessment of the size and severity of the sore. The difficulty in finding a valid method of measuring sore size and healing rate has dogged many researchers who have attempted to evaluate local treatments. Techniques used include measurement of wound diameter, tracing the sore outline on transparent film, photographing the sore against a centimetre measure, or using thermography. These measures cannot document changes in wound volume or in the general state of the wound (degree of smell, pus, inflammation, necrosis, etc.). Some researchers have attempted to solve this by developing complex rating scales or calculating 'healing indices', which, for example, measure wound size in relation to days of healing. Others have measured wound volume with dental impression-making material, or the Silastic foam dressing (Dow Corning Ltd) used to dress deep, granulating wounds. The nurse needs a simple, easy to use, assessment technique which is reasonably valid. The sore outline traced on transparent film provides a useful guide to healing if done regularly (say, weekly) and filed in sequence in the patient's notes.

Wound healing

Intense cellular and biochemical activity occur during the process of wound healing in which there are four stages of repair (Westaby 1981a): traumatic inflammation (0–3 days), destructive phase (1–6 days), proliferative phase (3–24 days), maturation phase (24 days–1 year). Two mechanisms which are extremely important to the process of healing are contraction and epithelialisation (Westaby 1981b). Large sores can be closed by contraction and, as skin elasticity is retained, the result functionally and cosmetically is good. Epithelialisation occurs in conjunction with contraction. Hair follicles and the wound margins provide the main sources of epidermal regeneration, and in shallow wounds which contain viable hair follicles, migration of epidermal cells across the wound surface can occur fairly rapidly. Winter (1976) demonstrated that it takes seven days to bridge the gap between two hair follicles. For deeper wounds, healing is much slower because the sources of epidermal regeneration, other than the wound margins, are lost.

Epithelialisation occurs over living tissue and travels under any scab that has formed. It is now established (Winter 1976) that epithelialisation is much faster if it occurs in a moist, oxygenated environment compared with the dehydration which accompanies scab formation. This has important implications for choice of wound dressing materials. Winter found that 100% epidermal regeneration occurred two to three times faster with wounds covered with an occlusive, oxygen-permeable dressing, such as Op-site (Smith and Nephew Ltd) or Lyofoam (Ultra Laboratories Ltd) compared with wounds covered with a conventional dry dressing.

Debriding and cleaning wounds

There is a bewildering number of substances available to put on pressure sores, yet very few have been tested systematically for their contribution to wound healing. Debriding a pressure sore of all necrotic tissue is necessary before healing can begin, and surgical, chemical or enzymatic debridement is used. The quickest method is to debride and clean the wound surgically under a general anaesthetic which often precedes wound closure by skin or muscle flap graft. This technique tends to be used only for large pressure sores which have not responded to other treatments, but a certain amount of debriding of necrotic tissue can be done by the nurse with scissors.

The chemical debriding agents in frequent use in the United Kingdom are the hypochlorite solutions (Eusol, Milton), hydrogen peroxide and creams such as Aserbine (Beecham Research Laboratories) and Malatex (Norton and Co. Ltd). Eusol is used extensively in the National Health Service and, although it is considered to be an effective debriding agent of necrotic tissue, it acts also on healthy granulation tissue, impeding growth and causing pain. Barton and Barton (1981) have suggested, from case study material, that with infected pressure sores, Eusol may cause the release of endotoxins into the blood stream which could lead to renal failure. Although further evidence is required, nurses should be careful to use Eusol only on necrotic tissue and to stop its use when debriding is complete.

Proteolytic enzymes which liquify and debride necrotic wounds are apparently more extensively used in the United States than in Britain. Varidase Topical (Lederle Laboratories) is becoming popular in this country, and it desloughs the wound without damaging healthy tissue (Torrance 1983). Varidase can be either applied directly to the wound or as a soaked gauze pack. It can also be injected under a scab or the scab can be scored with a scalpel until oozing occurs and a Varidase-soaked gauze dressing applied.

There is some evidence for the effectiveness of Varidase, and nurses should persist with its use, because the sore may initially appear to enlarge due to the removal of slough. Signs of healing will not be apparent for several days.

Dextranomer beads (Debrisan, Pharmacia Ltd) are porous and hydrophilic and absorb fluid from the surface of moist, suppurating wounds so acting as an effective cleansing agent. They absorb any bacteria in the wound exudate and allow tissue granulation to occur in a moist environment. Debrisan dressings should be changed at the point of bead saturation, and care should be taken to remove all used beads before applying more. There is considerable evidence for the effectiveness of Debrisan (Torrance 1983), but it should be used only on moist exuding wounds. If used inappropriately, it is a waste of money. The more usual methods of removing bacteria from pressure sores are by mechanical cleaning and application of a topical antiseptic. Mechanical cleaning is usually done by swab and forceps or gloves, or by irrigating the wound. Antiseptic lotions and creams, such as cetrimide, chlorhexidine and povidone-iodine, are frequently used on infected pressure sores. There are few acceptable guidelines on what nurses should use, but Barton and Barton (1981) favour povidone-iodine on superficial wounds and the cetrimide cream, Cetavlex (ICI Ltd) in deep sores. Very little valid research is available to assist the nurse in her choice of preparation, and on the whole, the decision is based on the nurse's or doctor's preference.

Wound dressings

Turner (1982) lists the criteria necessary for the optimum dressing:

1. To maintain high humidity between the wound and the dressing
2. To remove excess exudate and toxic compounds
3. To allow gaseous exchange
4. To provide thermal insulation to the wound surface
5. To be impermeable to bacteria
6. To be free from particles and toxic wound contaminants
7. To allow removal without causing trauma during dressing change. (p 43.)

No dressing as yet achieves all these requirements, but some fairly recent products do help in the healing process. Different pressure sores of course require different dressings, but in order to aid healing the dressing should prevent dehydration and contamination. The conventional dry gauze dressing achieves neither; it exposes the wound surface to dehydration so allowing scab formation, and the dressing fibres often become entangled in the scab, resulting in fresh trauma when the dressing is removed. For a healthy person, allowing a fairly superficial wound to become dehydrated presents few problems because healing will occur, but if a dressing is needed at all, a non-adhesive one would be wise.

With a debilitated elderly person, healing may be prolonged and nurses should take action to reduce discomfort to a minimum. In this case, a fairly shallow wound should be covered with a dressing which prevents dehydration such as Op-Site. This occlusive oxygen-permeable adhesive polyurethane membrane creates a moist wound environment, allows passage of oxygen, carbon dioxide and water vapour, and prevents entry of water, bacteria and viruses. No dehydration occurs and so no scab is formed, which enables rapid migration of epidermal cells across the wound surface. After cleaning and debriding if necessary, the shallow wound should be covered by Op-Site, or equivalent, and left undisturbed until healing is complete, unless clinical signs of infection occur. Eventually, the dressing will slough off during washing. Nurses often find it difficult to leave it alone because wound exudate collects under the membrane and may look contaminated. If the membrane bulges with exudate this can be aspirated through the dressing with a needle and syringe, and the puncture site covered with another piece of Op-Site. Op-Site is the best known of the semipermeable dressings in the United Kingdom but others now exist, e.g. Tegaderm (3M PLC).

The semipermeable dressings now available are gradually replacing the non-adhesive paraffin impregnated dressings (Tulle Gras, Jelonet, Sofratulle). These do retain a moist environment until they dry out, and they are usually covered with a gauze dressing which can become incorporated into the wound. They have the same disadvantages as dry gauze dressings unless they are changed frequently before they dry out.

The deeper pressure sore presents a different problem because it will almost certainly be infected (unless it has been surgically debrided) and will require regular cleaning and debriding. Dehydration of a deep wound which has dermal as well as epidermal damage is a much more serious problem than for shallow wounds because an already impoverished environment for healing is damaged further. Dehydration destroys the remnants of any hair follicles left, so removing all sources of epidermal regeneration except the wound edges. Furthermore, if a deep sore has been surgically or chemically debrided and then left with a dry dressing or one which dries out rapidly, then newly exposed healthy tissue and its vasculature die, and granulation cannot occur.

There does not seem to be a single best dressing material for the deeper sore, except of course, skin in the form of grafts or flaps. These are usually applied after surgical debridement, which is an effective but relatively rare choice of treatment for elderly patients with deep pressure sores. There are some semipermeable dressing materials with a hydrophilic surface and foam backing which absorb exudate, such as Lyofoam (Ultra Laboratories Ltd), and Synthaderm (Armour Pharmaceutical Co. Ltd). These provide a moist wound environment, and require changing frequently when wound exudate is profuse and contaminated. In fact, the manufacturers suggest two layers of Lyofoam on deep sores. If exudate is extremely excessive, highly absorbent cotton wool and gauze pads could be placed over the semipermeable dressing so that a moist environment is retained. As with Op-Site, nurses should persist with these hydrophilic foam dressings, even if the wound looks messy and macerated. This is normal and it is only after about six days that a dramatic improvement will be seen.

The technique for deep sores favoured by the Bartons (1981) is to irrigate the wound with saline and debride with scissors, fill the cavity with Cetavlex (Cetrimide) cream (ICI Ltd), cover with a Melolin dressing (Smith and Nephew Ltd) and secure with Micropore tape. They recommend that the dressing is changed two or three times weekly.

Other treatments

Many treatments continue to be used on pressure sores by nurses even though their effectiveness is uncertain or known to be nil. Insulin, egg white and oxygen and numerous creams, ointments and sprays have not, generally, been shown to be effective, although there is some evidence that hyperbaric oxygen accelerates healing (Torrance 1983). Some creams which have a specific debriding (Aserbine, Malatex) or antiseptic (Cetavlex, povidone-iodine) function may be effective, but certain ointments such as the vaseline found in tulle gras dressings can provide a totally occlusive dressing which prevents the passage of essential oxygen to the wound surface and delays healing (Winter 1976). Ice, vibration, electrotherapy, infrared and ultraviolet irradiation and ultrasound are used in the treatment of pressure sores, particularly by physiotherapists. Each has been claimed to be effective, and the evidence for ultrasound in both cleaning sores and stimulating healing seems to be quite substantial (Torrance 1983).

Evaluation

The bewildering variety of products available which purport to assist in the prevention or healing of pressure sores means that evaluating the treatment and care given to each patient as well as systematic product evaluation with valid research studies is essential. Evaluating the effects of nursing care and treatment is not something which comes naturally to many nurses. But evaluation need not be difficult as long as an effective assessment of the patient's problems is made before treatment begins, using measurement where possible. Assessment of the extent to which the patient is at risk of developing pressure sores should include use of one of the rating scales mentioned earlier and knowledge of the intrinsic and extrinsic factors known to contribute. The effects of treatment should be evaluated at regular intervals by repeated assessment which are compared with the initial baseline assessment. A similar assessment is required for the patient who has a pressure sore, together with some kind of measurement of the sore size before treatment and at regular intervals during treatment.

Pressure sores are wounds which have a complex aetiology and pathology. It follows that their prevention and treatment are also complex and cannot be the sole responsibility of any one health professional. Adequate assessment, care and evaluation requires a team effort which includes the patient.

Improving the basic education of nurses, doctors and paramedical staff would expand their knowledge of preventive and treatment practices, but knowledge continues to increase with new research and development, and it is difficult for practising nurses and doctors to keep up to date. A pressure sore team, consisting of doctors, nurses, physiotherapists, etc. with particular interest and knowledge could provide assistance and a monitoring role. Or a clinical nurse specialist in pressure sore care might be a solution, such as the nursing officer for tissue viability described by Dowding (1983). Specialists like these could be instrumental in promoting sound practice and disseminating new information to nurses and others, and in redrafting and up-dating procedure manuals.

The increase of very old, frail people is continuing and therefore the number of patients at risk from pressure sores is rising. In these days of dwindling resources, prevention is much cheaper than cure, as well as being more effective and acceptable to patients. In order for patients to receive high quality care, nurses and their colleagues must expand their knowledge and incorporate the results of valid research into their planned individualised patient care.

REFERENCES

Abbott D F, Exton-Smith A N, Millard P H, Temperly T M 1968 Zinc sulphate and bedsores. (Letter.) British Medical Journal 2:763
Barbenel J C, Forbes C D, Lowe G D O (eds) 1983 Pressure sores. Macmillan, London
Barton A, Barton M 1981 The management and prevention of pressure sores. Faber, London
Bennett G C J 1983a Pressure sores revisited. Geriatric Medicine 13(5): 415–418
Bennett G C J 1983b Treating pressure sores. Geriatric Medicine 13(6): 493–494
Bliss M, McLaren R, Exton-Smith A N 1967 Preventing pressure sores in hospital: controlled trial of a large-celled ripple mattress. British Medical Journal 1: 394–397
Carnevali D, Patrick M L 1979 Nursing management for the elderly. Lippincott, Philadelphia
David J A, Chapman R G, Chapman E J, Lockett B 1983 An investigation of the current methods used in nursing for the care of patients with established pressure sores. Nursing Practice Research Unit, Northwick Park Hospital and Clinical Research Centre, Harrow, Middlesex
Denne W A 1979 An objective assessment of the sheepskins used for decubitus sore prophylaxis. Rheumatology and Rehabilitation 18: 23–29
Denne W A 1983 Prevention of pressure sores: a study of the mechanical properties of fleeces. Nursing Focus May/June: 8–9
Dowding C 1983 Tissue viability nurse—a new post. Nursing Times 79(24): 61–64
Dyson R 1978 Bedsores—the injuries hospital staff inflict on patients. Nursing Mirror 146(24): 30–32
Exton-Smith A N, Sherwin R W 1961 Prevention of pressure sores: significance of spontaneous bodily movements. Lancet 2: 1124–1126
Exton-Smith A N, Wedgewood J, Overstall P W, Wallace G 1982 Use of the 'air wave system' to prevent pressure sores in hospital. Lancet 1: 1288–1290
Fernie G R 1973 Biochemical aspects of the aetiology of

decubitus ulcers on human patients. Unpublished PhD Thesis, University of Strathclyde, Glasgow

Gibbons D E 1983 Mouth care procedures. Nursing Times 79(7):30

Goldstone L A, Goldstone J 1982 The Norton score: an early warning of pressure sores? Journal of Advanced Nursing 7(5): 419–426

Guttman L 1976 The prevention and treatment of pressure sores. In: Kenedi R M, Cowden J M, Scales J T (eds) Bedsore biomechanics. Macmillan, London p 153–160

Harris M D 1980 Tools for mouth care. Nursing Times 76:305, 340–342

Howarth H 1977 Mouth care procedures for the very ill. Nursing Times 73(10): 354

Jay P 1983 Choosing the best wheelchair cushion: for your needs, your chair and your life style. Royal Association for Disability and Rehabilitation, London

Jordan M M and Barbenel J C 1983 Pressure sore prevalence. In: Barbenel J C, Forbes C D, Lowe G D O (eds) Pressure sores. Macmillan, London

Kenedi R M, Cowden J M, Scales J T (eds) 1976 Bedsore biomechanics. Macmillan, London

Lowthian P T 1979 Turning clocks system to prevent pressure sores. Nursing Mirror 148(21): 30–31

Lowthian P T 1982 A review of pressure sore pathogenesis. Nursing Times 78(3): 117–121

Lowthian P T 1983 Nursing aspects of pressure sore prevention. In: Barbenel J C, Forbes C D, Lowe G D O (eds) Pressure sores. Macmillan, London

Marshall M, Overstall P 1983 Mattresses to prevent pressure sores. Nursing Times 79(24): 54–59

Moolton S E 1972 Bedsores in the chronically ill patient. Archives of Physical Medicine and Rehabilitation 53: 430–438

Newman P, Davis N H 1981 Thermography as a predictor of sacral pressure sores. Age and Ageing 10: 14–18

Norton D, McLaren R, Exton-Smith A N 1962 An investigation of geriatric nursing problems in hospital. Re-issued 1975. Churchill Livingstone, Edinburgh

Peterson N C, Bittmann J 1971 The epidemiology of pressure sores. Scandinavian Journal of Plastic and Reconstructive Surgery 5: 62–66

Roberts B V, Goldstone L A 1979 A survey of pressure sores in the over sixties on two orthopaedic wards. International Journal of Nursing Studies 16(4): 355–364

Scales J T, Lowthian P T, Poole A G, Ludman W R 1982 'Vaperm' patient-support system: a new general purpose hospital mattress. Lancet 2: 1150–1152

Scholey M 1982 The shoulder lift. Nursing Times 78(11): 506–507

Sofaer B 1979 The loss of dentures in hospital. Nursing Times Occasional Paper. 75(21): 85–88

Speedie G 1983 Nursology of mouth care: preventing comforting and seeking activities related to mouth care. Journal of Advanced Nursing 8(1): 33–40

Taylor T V, Rimmer S, Day B, Butcher J, Dymock I W 1974 Ascorbic acid supplementation in the treatment of pressure sores. Lancet 2: 544–546

Torrance C 1983 Pressure sores: aetiology, treatment and prevention. Croom-Helm, London

Turner T 1982 Which dressing and why—1. Wound care series no.11 Nursing Times 78(29): 41–44

Westaby S 1981a Healing: the normal mechanism—1. Wound care series no.3 Nursing Times 77(47): 9–12

Westaby S 1981b Healing: the normal mechanism—2. Wound care series no.4 Nursing Times 77(51): 13–16

Winter G 1976 Some factors affecting skin and wound healing. In: Kenedi R M, Cowden J M, Scales J T (eds) Bed-sore biomechanics. Macmillan, London, p 47–54

15

M. Fordham

Sleep and rest

Fond words have oft been spoken of thee, sleep!
And thou hast had thy store of tenderest names;
The very sweetest words that fancy frames
When thankfulness of heart is strong and deep!
Dear bosom child we call thee, that dost steep
In rich reward all suffering, balm that tames
All anguish, saint that evil thoughts and aims
Takest away, and into souls dost creep
Like a breeze from heaven. Shall I alone,
I surely not a man ungently made,
Call thee worst tyrant by which flesh is crost?
Perverse, self-willed to own and to disown,
Mere slave of them who never for thee prayed,
Still last to come where thou are wanted most!

William Wordsworth

INTRODUCTION

Sleep is a state of reduced responsiveness (or increased threshold) to external stimuli. In other words it is an altered state of consciousness from which a person can be aroused if the stimulus is sufficient. It is the inactive part of the circadian sleep-wake cycle, and is characterised by particular electro-encephalographic patterns and by lowering of the metabolic rate. Healthy adults move their position 30–40 times per night.

Although sleep is a normal state, it can be difficult to distinguish from abnormal states of stupor or coma, and sleep can be deliberately simulated. It is not uncommon for nurses who are caring for the sick and elderly to be faced with the problem of distinguishing between normal sleep, incipient stupor, and feigned sleep. Indeed, if concern for the well-being of an elderly person is great, and doubt exists about the nature of his or her unresponsiveness, we almost reflexly resort to vocal or tactile stimuli to test the state of affairs—much to the annoyance of the 'sleeper'. However, sleep is a potentially dangerous (life threatening) state for some people, and the most common time of death is between 04.00 and 07.00 hours.

Nurses have informally gleaned a wealth of information about the sleeping patterns of the elderly. We have observed the sick and frail elderly and to a lesser extent the healthy elderly in hospital and Homes. However, until the last few years we have had little scientific knowledge to back our hunches or inform our biases. Yet next to the elderly persons themselves we have the greatest vested interest in understanding the sleep of the elderly. Firstly because our aim is to promote the optimal functioning of the elderly folk in our care and secondly because their sleep–wake pattern could have important implications for the 24-hour nursing workload and therefore for the way in which we choose to deploy the limited number of staff available in most geriatric nursing environments.

There are a number of beliefs about sleep which we and elderly persons are likely to hold. Some are philosophical and open to debate and others are scientific hypotheses which are open to testing by research. If we are to provide optimal care for the elderly we need to examine the state of knowledge and our own beliefs and biases. The philosophical debate as to why or whether sleep is needed by humans rumbles on. Is sleep merely a hangover from evolutionary times when it was dangerous to move in the dark because of the risk of predators? Is it an essential means of energy conservation? Is sleep necessary for restitution of brain and body function? Individuals vary in their apparent need for sleep. Some people claim to and actually take very little sleep, others sleep longer than the normal 7–9 hours per day. However, the vast majority become concerned if they fail to sleep as long as is normal for them.

Two major propositions about sleep underly the discussion in the remainder of this chapter. Efficient functioning of elderly people when they are awake is fundamentally dependent upon (1) the quality and quantity of their sleep and (2) the pattern of their sleep–wake circadian rhythm. It is not possible to understand the particular problems of sleep in the elderly without examining the general state of knowledge about sleep.

NORMAL ADULT SLEEP

Most research on sleep has used young healthy adults as subjects. The physiological functioning of the brain, muscles, cardiac, respiratory and reproductive systems during sleep have been recorded, as well as the effects of total and selective sleep deprivation. Reviews of this research can be found in Colquhoun (1971, 1972) and Minors and Waterhouse (1981). Monitoring of sleep classically uses scalp electrodes to measure electroencephelographic (EEG) and electro-occulographic (EOG) changes, plus body electrodes and thermisters to record muscle (electromyographic), respiratory, cardiovascular and temperature changes. Hormone, electrolyte and other chemical levels in the blood can be monitored by the use of venous catheterisation. The print-outs of this monitoring are termed polygraphic records.

Sleep stages

Findings from this monitoring of sleep have led to the distinction of two major types of sleep, orthodox and paradoxical, defined by the EEG and EOG pattern. Sleep begins at stage 0, resting with eyes shut, and with alpha rhythms (8–12 cycles per second) on EEG. This is followed by orthodox, or non-REM (rapid eye movement), sleep which has four stages. As a person passes from stage 1 to stage 4 EEG rhythms become progressively slower, until large slow waves 0.5–3 cycles per second and 5–10 times the amplitude of wakefulness occur. Stage 1 has characteristic waveforms called 'sleep spindles' and 'K complexes'. Stages 3 and 4 slow waves are called delta waves and these stages are referred to as slow wave sleep (SWS). The person becomes more deeply asleep as they pass from stage 1 to stage 4. Paradoxical, or REM, sleep occurs from time to time. This is a qualitatively different type of sleep in which the EEG appears similar to that of wakefulness (low voltage desynchronised). Rapid eye movements occur beneath closed lids and skeletal muscle tone is lost.

The distinction between orthodox and paradoxical sleep is important. It becomes progressively more difficult to arouse someone as they pass from stage 1 to stage 4, but even more difficult to awaken them during paradoxical sleep, when skeletal muscles are functionally paralysed. The main differences between these types of sleep are summarised in Table 15.1.

A major hypothesis is that both types of sleep are needed for restitution of body and brain function. It can be seen from Table 15.1 that orthodox sleep seems to be dominated by the activity of the parasympathetic nervous system. As growth hormone levels are high it

has been suggested that anabolic processes of growth and tissue repair occur optimally during this stage (Beck et al 1975). Some of the evidence supports this view, although Horne (1980) disputes this hypothesis as he says that the peak in human 'growth hormone found during non-REM sleep' (Takahashi et al 1968) may not facilitate optimum protein synthesis and mitosis since nutrient levels may be low during night-time fasting. A potential danger to life may result from the lowered metabolic rate and hypothermia during SWS.

Paradoxical sleep, on the other hand, appears to be dominated by sympathetic nervous system activity. Indeed, cardiac output, heart rate and blood pressure can surpass waking levels, and angina and ventricular arrhythmias can occur during this stage. Respiration may mimim Cheyne-Stokes patterns, and apnoeic attacks may occur (Guilleminault and Dement 1978). However, it is a stage of sleep thought to be crucial to the maintenance of mental–emotional equilibrium.

In a typical night it has been found that adults pass through a complete cycle of stages approximately every 90 minutes, or 4–6 times per night. One complete cycle is illustrated in

Table 15.1 Types of sleep. *Adapted from Kogeorgos, 1980*

	Non-REM Orthodox	REM Paradoxical
Electroencephelogram (EEG)	Slow waves, 0.5–3 cycles/second plus sleep spindles and K complexes	Low voltage, desychronised waves
Eye movement Electrooculogram (EOG)	Absent, or slow rolling	Rapid eye movements
Muscle tone	Reduced	Abolished
Heart and respiratory rate Blood pressure Metabolic rate	Steady, regular, slow Lowered Lowered	Increased, irregular Raised Raised, relative to non-REM
Penile erection Vaginal blood flow	Rarely Lowered	Yes Increased
Growth hormone	Increased	No change
Dreaming	Infrequent	Frequent, vivid
Response to external stimuli	Reduced as pass from stage 1 to stage 4	Less responsive than stage 4. Very difficult to awaken

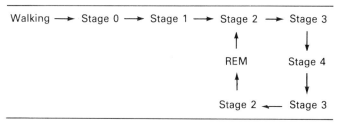

Fig. 15.1 Sleep cycle. *Sanford 1982.*

Figure 15.1. The length of time spent in each stage during the night differs such that more orthodox sleep occurs in the early part of the night and more paradoxical sleep in the early morning.

SLEEP OF THE ELDERLY

Sleep length and sleep cycles

So far we have been discussing the sleep of adults in general. Does the sleep of the healthy elderly person differ? Is it normal for the elderly to sleep less well at night than younger adults?

Questionnaire survey findings support the view that the elderly are generally dissatisfied with their sleep and indeed the use of sedative-hynotic medication appears to increase with age. McGhie and Russell (1962) conducted a survey of 2466 subjects in Britain of all age groups. They found that there was a significant increase in the proportion of people over 65 years who claimed to sleep less than five hours per night. Twenty to 30% of the elderly reported frequent night awakenings, 15% waking before 5.00 a.m. and 25% of men over 65 years and 40% of women over 45 years described themselves as light sleepers. In this and similar studies complaints of sleeping difficulties tended to be higher for females than males. However, when objective measurements of sleep are taken, many research studies have found that elderly men have more disturbed sleep than elderly women (Dement et al 1982a, Webb 1982). Coleman et al (1981) monitored the sleep of 83 people aged over 60 years and compared their sleep with that of 423 younger adults. They

found that the total amount of sleep was less for the elderly although the number of daytime naps increased. The elderly were more frequently awake and awake for longer periods during the night after the initial sleep onset. Webb and Swinbourne (1971) observed 19 people aged 66–96 years over 24 hours and found that although they spent 11–12 hours in bed they only averaged 8.5 hours sleep, including daytime naps. Their findings suggest that the sleep of the elderly is not less than that of younger people but is more variable in distribution throughout the 24 hours.

So although some early studies such as Feinberg (1968) state that the total sleep time declines with age, many more recent studies report that the amount of sleep per 24 hours and the need for sleep does not decrease with age. Dement et al (1982b) state categorically that 'fragmented sleep in persons of advanced years is not the result of decreased sleep need' (p. 31). According to Dement et al (1982b) great individual variability in sleep has been found and significant ageing trends rarely demonstrated. As with other age groups individuals cannot automatically be assumed to follow the general trend. On the whole, however, it seems that the elderly spend more time lying in bed at night without attempting to sleep, and more time unsuccessfully trying to sleep than younger folk. They also spend more time in bed in the daytime resting or napping, but their total sleep time is not usually significantly increased compared with the young.

The major changes in sleep stages with age are summarised in Table 15.2. There is an increase in light sleep and decrease in deep sleep stages 3 and 4. The relative amount of paradoxical or REM sleep is found to persist

Table 15.2 Sleep pattern and age. *Adapted from Feinberg 1968*

	REM	Stage 1	Stage 2	Stages 3 and 4	Total
Infant —Newborn —1 Year	50% 20–30%				14–18 hours
Young, active, healthy adult	25%	5–10%	50%	15–20%	6–9 hours
Elderly	20–25% (Decline associated with impaired intellectual functioning)	Increased	Unchanged	Decreased	Total unchanged but fragmented

until extreme old age, although a decline in the proportion of REM sleep seems to correlate with reduced intellectual functioning and organic brain syndrome. Many studies of REM sleep have shown that there is a change in the circadian rhythm such that REM sleep is more evenly distributed throughout the night than in younger adults.

The relationship between night-time sleep and daytime behaviours

According to Dement et al (1982b), and in agreement with common belief, 'it is axiomatic that there is a relationship between sleep at night and the way we feel during the day' (p 30)

Most of us have felt the general effects of lack of sleep, including tiredness, headache or sensation of a tight band around the head, eye problems, such as 'prickling' or heavy lids, lack of muscle co-ordination, maybe even affecting speech (dysarthria) decreased facial expression and difficulty in maintaining attention. However, many of the symptoms attributed to lack of sleep in young folk are labelled as part of the ageing process in the elderly. Amongst these, Dement et al (1982b) include 'losses of abilities to perform highly skilled tasks in a rapid fashion, to resist fatigue, to maintain physical stamina, to unlearn or discard old techniques, and to apply the rapid judgment needed in changing and emergency situations.' (p 30)

Only those studies which cover the whole 24 hours can elucidate the relationship between night-time sleep and daytime naps. Many sleep researchers support the view that the daytime sleepiness of the elderly is the direct consequence of night-time sleep deprivation. Johns (1975) found that not only did the amount of time awake after initial sleep onset increase with age, but that night-time wakefulness was associated with increasing amounts of sleep during the day. His conclusion was that daytime naps were compensating for broken night-time sleep.

Some studies have used a standard measure of daytime sleepiness termed 'sleep latency'. This is the speed of falling to sleep as measured by EEG polygraphic recordings. This sleep latency can be measured at any time of the day or night and is a more valid and reliable measure of sleepiness than naturally occurring naps. Measurement is precise and objective, and the opportunity and environment for sleeping is controlled. In a study of healthy, elderly subjects who were in bed for 10 hours per night, seriously fragmented and interrupted sleep was found (Carskadon et al 1982). About 60% of the subjects had more than 100 brief or prolonged arousals during the night's sleep. The number of brief arousals per hour of nocturnal sleep was predictive of daytime sleepiness, as measured by sleep latencies. The sleep latency scores suggested that a substantial number of elderly persons are pathologically sleepy in the daytime even when they do not complain of sleep problems.

CAUSES OF SLEEP PROBLEMS IN THE ELDERLY

If we aim to promote sleep in the elderly we need to examine all possible causes for sleep abnormalities. We stand little chance of making logical decisions or taking helpful action unless we attempt to answer the following question: Are elderly people who appear sleepy, inattentive, uncoordinated and resistant to change, suffering from the inevitable effects of ageing, sleep deprivation, drug intoxication or specific disease?

Biological rhythms, ageing and sleep

Disorders of the sleep–wake schedule are said to occur if either this rhythm is out of phase with other internal rhythms or with society's expectations of sleep–wake time.

One view of the ageing process is that it is characterised by the disorganisation of biological rhythms. The sleep–wake activity pattern is a circadian rhythm (around a day) but all bodily functions display rhythmicity with peaks and troughs occurring at intervals of seconds, minutes, hours, days, months or years. Health and well-being is dependent upon these rhythms being synchronised with one another, and this synchronisation is affected not only by internal events but also by external cyclic inputs (Zeitgebers) such as light–dark and socially determined rest activity cycles and eating times (Reinberg 1966). The regular alternation of sleep–wakefulness is regarded as a fundamental biological rhythm which in normal circumstances is able to entrain (synchronise) other circadian rhythms.

Samis and Capobianco (1978) in a book on ageing and biological rhythms stated in their introduction:

Senescent deterioration in form and function may be due, at least in part, to alterations in an organism's ordering among processes in time, with the result that the organism's adaptive capacity and vigor decreases and consequently its probability of death increases. If with advancing age, the circadian temporal organisation of an organism becomes altered, either by becoming more rigid and consequently less amenable to adaptive changes, or becomes disorganised in time, the consequences could have a profound influence on vigor and adaptive capability.

Shock (1977) suggests that internal desynchronisation may be part of the general breakdown of regulatory mechanisms accompanying normal ageing. One interesting hypothesis put forward by Winget et al (1972) suggests that prolonged bed-rest may cause desynchronisation of circadian rhythms. Dement et al (1982a) speculate that postural change alone—presumably prolonged lying—may in itself cause some of the changes in rhythms found in the elderly.

It is obvious that the sleep–wake circadian rhythm of some elderly people remains virtually unaltered with age. But other elderly people have grossly changed patterns of sleeping. There are two main theories put forward to explain this change. One that the sleep pattern of the elderly is a reversal of day and night (Armstrong-Esther and Hawkins 1982). The other that the elderly revert to the childhood pattern of multiple sleeping time in 24 hours. Further research is needed to test these hypotheses, but as social cues are extremely important in maintaining a 24-hour rhythm of sleep–waking, all sorts of bizarre sleep–wake cycles can and do occur in the elderly. Winfree (1982) stated that 'some sightless individuals, some recluses and some older people living indoors with little social contact, sometimes retire and rise later and later every day like the tides—eventually pursuing their solitary interests by night and sleeping by day, 180° out of phase with surrounding society; they drift still later into synchrony again after another two weeks or so' (p R200). Isolation studies have demonstrated clearly that bereft of time cues, internal desynchronisation occurs in about one fifth of young people, but in all older people.

When we first meet such elderly isolated

folk they could be in any phase of their disrupted or drifting sleep–wake pattern, including a reversal of day and night. Many elderly living with their families, or communally in hospital or Homes, seem to shift their sleep rhythms to earlier times, being drowsy in the evening and 'larks' in the morning. A breakdown in the biophasic pattern of sleep and wakefulness and a return to the polyphasic alternations of infancy are well documented (Webb 1982). It should be noted that the elderly do not follow infancy patterns in all respects. They do not return to sleeping 14–18 hours per day, nor does the high proportion of REM sleep found in infancy return.

The picture of changes of other circadian rhythms with age is not fully explored, but alteration in urinary electrolytes (Lobban and Tredre 1964) and cortisol (Serio et al 1970) rhythms have been documented. A reduction in the peak of growth hormone as stages 3 and 4 sleep are reduced, has been found. The latter finding suggests that night-time sleep may be less restorative to body tissues in the aged than the young. One interesting finding by Wessler et al (1976) was that institutionalised elderly patients had a high order of circadian regularity and synchronisation, and they concluded that the strict institutional regime was probably beneficial. There is some anecdotal evidence that a regular lifestyle plays a part in longevity and health. However, we should perhaps be wary of abruptly imposing a particular regime of sleep–wake on the elderly, as their cycles are likely to be less adaptable and more easily disrupted than those of younger people (Preston 1973) and they need time to adapt to an unfamiliar regime. It may well take a couple of weeks or even months to nudge them into synchrony. Settling them for sleep one hour later each 24 hours would be a logical ploy to try. Forcible walking or awakening such elderly persons from daytime sleep would be both cruel and unlikely to achieve the aim of restoring a normal sleep–wake pattern. This is not to deny that some elderly folk nod off by day with sheer boredom. A routine of daytime activities

including both physical and mental stimulation undoubtedly helps to maintain a healthy normal sleep–wake schedule for those whose rhythms are in synchrony, but abruptly enforced daytime activity will not help either the sleep deprived or the desynchronised elderly person.

Sleep deprivation

Sleep deprivation has been studied in young rather than elderly adults. The effects of total sleep deprivation on performance and mood can be dramatic. Apart from the tendency to fall asleep and perform simple well-learned tasks, such as walking, in a semi-automatic way, subjects tend to become irritable, disoriented, with slurred speech, even deluded, paranoid and hallucinated. An apparently analogous phenomenon in sleep-deprived seriously ill patients has been described as the intensive care syndrome (Helton et al 1980, Sanford 1982). Williams et al (1967) selectively deprived healthy subjects of different stages of sleep. Those who were prevented from having orthodox sleep complained of physical discomfort and were withdrawn and concerned over vague physical complaints or changes in body feeling. Those who were deprived of paradoxical sleep became anxious, insecure, withdrawn and some showed signs of confusion.

It seems possible, if not probable, that many of the complaints and problems of the elderly could be a result of sleep deprivation. Some elderly people including the healthy may lack all stages of sleep. Others, especially those taking hypnotic drugs and those with organic brain syndrome, may lack paradoxical sleep. The elderly in particular risk losing out on sleep length when their time in bed is constrained if night-time sleep efficiency (time in bed/total sleep time) is reduced.

The finding that many healthy old people spend much of their sleeping time in light stages of sleep from which they awaken either momentarily or for long periods, certainly suggests that unless daytime naps are obtained many of them lack sleep. It is not uncommon for night nurses and elderly patients to give very different accounts of the amount of sleep obtained. We should perhaps take heed of the finding that as many as 100 transient arousals per night (10 seconds or less) showed up on polygraphic records of 60% of healthy elderly people. Many or all of the brief arousals would not be visible to the observer.

Environmental causes of sleep disturbance

There are a number of aspects of the environment in which we care for the elderly which may increase their sleep disturbance and deprivation.

Hospital or institutional admission

Research on the effect of hospitalisation on the sleep of the elderly has compared institutional and home sleeping patterns. Pacini and Fitzpatrick (1982) investigated the sleep of 38 elderly people (average age 69 years) half at home and half during the first seven days of admission to medical/surgical wards. The hospitalised patients did not undergo surgery and were mainly cared for in private or semi-private rooms. The findings from self-kept sleep charts and sleep pattern questionnaires were that nocturnal sleep time was reportedly shorter in hospital. This was attributed to being woken for recording of vital signs, medication or venesection. More daytime sleep occurred in the hospitalised and they went to bed and were awakened earlier. However, the reported levels of anxiety, provoked by new medication and conern about impending investigations and discharge dates were higher in hospital and health and fatigue status was lower. So poor nocturnal sleep was not attributed solely or even primarily to the hospital environment, but to a significant extent to the status and anxiety levels of the person admitted. People in long-term institutional care, on the other hand, may adapt to the pattern of life and sleep well, especially if they are neither acutely sick nor insecure. As mentioned earlier, Wessler et al

(1976) thought the strict institutional regime beneficial.

Many environmental factors, including boredom, social isolation, and physical confinement, are likely to result in excessive sleepiness, whereas heat, cold, light, movement and noise are liable to disturb sleep.

Noise effects on sleep

Auditory threshold awakening from stage 4 (deep) sleep has been found to be lower in the elderly so that they are more easily aroused from sleep than younger people (Roth et al 1972). Gress et al (1981) observed the nocturnal behaviour of 11 elderly (60–97 years) persons in an institution between 11 p.m. and 7 a.m. on three nights. Their main findings were that sounds seemed to be amplified at night. Loud conversation, laughter and careless handling of supplies and equipment were observed to disturb some patients. Three subjects slept solidly each night, but the remainder were awake or up at least once. 4 a.m. seemed to be the only hour at which all patients were in bed on all three nights, and 2 a.m. was the most wakeful time.

Ogilvie (1980) compared the noise levels in a nightingale ward and a cubicle race-track ward. The patients were elderly. The nightingale ward was noisier than the cubicle but in both wards noise levels at night were comparable to 'a living room by day', and the average of noise levels on both wards consistently exceeded the recommended level of 35 decibels (dB(A)) for a bedroom at night often by as much as 15 dB. People—staff and patients—were the most frequent source of noise, but the loudest noises came from equipment such as telephones, trolleys, doors.

Confused patients and conversations with the hard of hearing can pose considerable problems when attempting to reduce noise at night. Indeed, increasingly high dosages of sedatives are sometimes requested for noisy patients in the hope that this will allow the other patients to sleep at night and reduce the night nurses' stress levels. This is an understandable reaction, but other solutions and detailed assessment by both nurses and doctors should be undertaken before 'stoning' the apparently demented even further out of their minds. Can the physical condition of the patient be improved such that they are less liable to nocturnal confusion? Would a reduction in sedation be more efficacious than an increase? If the noisy patient's behaviour is intractable, what is the bed position in which they will cause least disruption? Should more staff be on night duty so that such persons can be 'specialed'? Where an institution has many such night-awake and noisy patients, should we have a special ward for them (Armstrong Esther and Hawkins 1982)?

Night staff are not alone in shouldering the responsibility for reducing noise and other environmental irritants at night—although it is axiomatic that they should be vigilant about their own noise making. Footfall, talking, and nursing procedures should be as quiet as possible and we should remember that being out of sight, in the kitchen, duty room or office does not make noise 'out of sound'. However, the day staff have infinitely more resources available to them than the night staff. Oiling door hinges and trolley wheels, fixing windows, lights, heating, etc. can be accomplished by day. The services of administrators, carpenters and electricians may all need to be used to reduce the problem. It would not be beyond our wit to identify the major noise sources in our area and remove or reduce many of them. Patients themselves would readily supply a list of disturbances for us, as Sue Hopkins did (1980).

Dietary effect on sleep

Dietary habits seem to be important determinants of sleep patterns. People who are gaining weight tend to sleep more and have a higher proportion of REM or paradoxical sleep, whereas those losing weight and anorexic persons sleep less and have disturbed sleep. An article by Beecham Foods Nutrition Information Centre (1978) discussed 'How Diet Affects our Sleep?' This article reviewed research on the complex effects on sleep of amino acids such as tryptophane and levels of the brain transmitter serotonin. Serotonin is known to have effects upon mood regulation, pain sensitivity and sleep.

Horlicks was for a long time advertised as promoting sleep. In one study, sleep following Horlicks was found to be less interrupted than sleep following either hot milk or a soya and egg drink. However, it would seem that the continuance of a person's normal eating habits is more crucial than any particular food or drink. Volunteers in another study were either given a food drink or an inert capsule at bedtime. 'The subjects who normally took a bedtime snack slept better after the food drink, while those who usually had no food in the late evening slept better after the placebo' (p 35). This suggests that it is important in promoting good sleep to provide nourishment at the time the elderly person would usually take it and not assume that everyone should have the same regime. It is probable that the supper meal is too early for many people both in hospital and in institutional care. We may need to provide snacks later in the evening and ones which are similar to those which the person would take at home.

Research on sleep following coffee found sleep to be disturbed within the first three hours and slow wave (orthodox) sleep reduced, although the total length of sleep was unchanged. More than 10 cups of caffeine beverages per day results in dependence and tolerance. Early morning drowsiness owing to caffeine withdrawal and the obligatory cup of coffee to wake up is a widespread phenomenon for all age groups, including the elderly. The sleep disrupting effect of caffeine greatly increases with age (Karacan et al 1976). Adam (1980) states that two cups of coffee at bedtime cause very disturbed sleep in the elderly.

Anxiety and sleep

Any acute emotional arousal or conflict caused by a loss or perceived threat can result in brief periods of sleep disturbance. Causes include bereavement of person or places, abrupt change in lifestyle such as illness, hospital or institutional admission or discharge, and intense positive feeling such as may result from the birth of a grandchild, or the security of being cared for after a struggle to manage alone.

The majority of people respond with difficulty in falling asleep, intermittent awakening during the night and early morning arousal. They may lose a substantial amount of sleep but are not truly sleepy by day, feeling fatigued, aching and 'washed out' but unable to nap. Some people respond with excessive difficulty in remaining awake, tending to stay in bed longer than usual and returning to bed frequently during the day to nap.

Both reactions to stress can be adaptive. The first maintains vigilance to cope with the new situation, the second conserves energy. They represent different coping styles which are likely to be typical of the individual. After a few weeks the emotional reaction resolves and sleep returns to normal. As the lives of many elderly people are strewn with major and minor losses and threats, we should expect to see these sleep disruptions fairly frequently.

More persistent periods of sleep disturbance may arise from chronic tension-anxiety states. Sleep disturbance seems to be conditioned to chronic anxiety and the sleep problem and tension mutually reinforce one another. Such elderly people may stay in bed longer in an effort to resume sleep and try to nap with little success. High muscle tension may result in complaints of back and headache and pulse rates may be fast. They may complain of worried thoughts and anxious dreams, exhibit restless vigilant behaviour, and regard tension as normal for themselves. Sometimes these people sleep better in a new or strange environment which has no conditioned associations with the sleep problems. Changing factors such as smells, furniture and bedroom routines may help. Other people are conditioned to internal factors and 'trying to fall asleep' results in central nervous system arousal. These people fall asleep when doing such things as reading, watching television, etc. but become fully alert when lying in bed trying to sleep. Less commonly, the persistent tension results in chronic weariness and excessive sleeping, bed-rest and napping. Such fatigue prone patients learn to 'take to bed'. The term 'neurasthenia' has been applied to such people. They are liable to develop a disorder of their sleep–wake circadian rhythm. They may be in a state of chronic despair or mild depression and concerned about somatic illnesses and symptoms. Their sleep problem is sometimes further confounded by taking sedatives for 'nerves'.

Drugs associated with sleep disorders

Most CNS stimulants and depressants have a more dramatic effect on functioning of the elderly and so are more disturbing to their sleep patterns, according to Coleman et al (1981). The effects of these drugs are well documented and are summarised below:

Central nervous system (CNS) depressants

Sedatives, hypnotics, tranquillisers, anticonvulsants, antihypertensives, antidepressants, antihistamines, beta adrenergic blockers, alcohol.

Sustained use. Elderly people in particular are liable to develop excessive somnolence when these drugs are used therapeutically in moderate to high doses. In addition to sleepiness they feel groggy, depressed, unstable, shaky, agitated and may even have episodes of amnesia or paranoia. Use of large bedtime doses may result in alveolar hypoventilation.

Tolerance and withdrawal. With sustained use CNS depressants become ineffective in inducing sleep leading to physical and psychological dependence, increasing dosage, plus intermittant attempts to reduce or withdraw the drugs. The person who has become tolerant to sedatives—including barbiturates and non-barbiturates such as glutethamide, chloral hydrate, methaqualone, antihistamines, bromides, benzodiazepines and alcohol—develops long (more than five minutes) and frequent periods of wakening from sleep, especially during the second half of the night. The time to fall asleep also gets longer as the person becomes used to the drug. If the drug is omitted sleep latency may be several hours. Residual (hangover) effects during the day include sluggishness, poor co-ordination, ataxia, slurred speech, visual problems, and in the late afternoon restlessness and nervousness. Gradual withdrawal from sedatives results in an improvement in sleep for many people, though after long habituation the individual may not return to an absolutely normal sleep pattern. Rapid reduction or abrupt withdrawal of CNS depressants, almost completely disrupts sleep. REM sleep is suppressed by these drugs and REM rebound can precipitate terrifying nightmare attacks. Withdrawal symptoms of nausea, muscle tension, aches, restlessness and nervousness are likely to occur in the succeeding days and sleep-related myoclonus may appear. Most alcoholics return to a normal sleep pattern 10–14 days after drinking ends.

CNS stimulants

Amphetamines, methylphenidate, sympathomimetic drugs, analeptics, caffeine. Apart from drug abusers, the majority of stimulants are prescribed to treat medical conditions, e.g. appetite suppressant drugs for weight reduction, sympathomimetic drugs for asthma and chronic obstructive airway disease, analeptics for mood elevation of the depressed, stimulants for patients with somnolence especially narcolepsy.

Sleep onset is delayed and total sleep time declines. To overcome the resultant daytime sleepiness more stimulants may then be taken. Sudden episodes of sleepiness by day—the 'crash' of the stimulant-dependent individual—occurs from time to time. The person may also be anxious and irritable, have difficulty concentrating and even become severely depressed and suicidal.

Sustained use or withdrawal from other drugs

Many drugs interfere with sleep. Two lists are particularly mentioned in the classification of sleep disorders, some of which are recognised for their psychotropic action, others not.

Group 1. Antimetabolites and other cancer chemotherapeutic agents, thyroid preparation and anticonvulsants such as phenytoin, monoamine oxidase inhibitors (MAOI), adrenocorticotrophic hormone (ACTH), alpha-methyl-dopa, propranolol and many others. Sleep onset is delayed by the drugs in group 1, and they also result in interrupted sleep and early awakening. The severity of the effect depends on the drug dosage.

Group 2 includes diazepam, the major tranquillizers, sedating tricyclics and sometimes MAOI, marijuana, cocaine, phencyclidene, opiates and even aspirin-containing drugs. Sleep is improved during the use of group 2 drugs, but sleep disturbance occurs during withdrawal in the same way as withdrawal from other CNS depressants.

Illness and sleep disturbance

The majority of illnesses result in sleep disruption and further confound the sleep problems of the elderly. The sleep problem will only improve when the underlying medical condition is alleviated or cured.

Psychiatric illnesses

Psychiatric disorders which are associated with sleep problems include phobic, obsessive-compulsive and other neurotic disorders. Patients with psychotic depression generally fall asleep readily, but have difficulty in maintaining sleep and wake early in the morning feeling fatigued, achy and 'washed out'. Patients in the depressed phase of manic-depressive psychosis and those with mild depressive disorders tend to be excessively sleepy by day. Mania or hypomania results in ·difficulty in falling asleep and short sleep time.

Such people may wake refreshed after as little as two or four hours sleep. It should be noted that the more elderly the patient with depression the greater the sleep loss in the second half of the night. Schizophrenia and schizoaffective disorders can result in partial or complete inversion of the day–night sleep cycle, and extreme agitation in the first half of the night. The extent of sleep disruption will depend on the severity of the illness.

Physical pathologies

Conditions of the central nervous system are particularly liable to disrupt the quantity and quality of sleep. Many cause pain, parasthesia and abnormal movements. Some fundamentally alter the state of consciousness.

Lesions of the brainstem and hypothalamus and cerebral atrophy may disrupt sleep onset and maintenance, whether they are due to neoplasms, vascular disorders, CNS infections, trauma, toxicity or degenerative changes. Roffwarg (1979) states: 'The confusional pattern at night in patients with organic mental disorders should be differentiated from the very brief episodes of nocturnal confusion often experienced by elderly patients subject to a new environment. However, it is not known to what extent degenerative changes in the CNS are responsible for symptoms of insomnia in otherwise apparently normal elderly people' (p 47).

Daytime somnolence is associated with many CNS pathologies. Raised intracranial pressure from any cause, including tumours (especially those of the pineal and posterior hypothalamus and any which impinge on the third ventricle), subdural and subarachnoid haemorrhage and hydrocephalus, all cause hypersomnolence. Severe daytime somnolence may develop gradually 6–18 months following head injury. Many toxic and infectious conditions result in excessive sleepiness whether fungal, viral or bacterial, including neurosyphilis, encephalitis lethargica and trypanosomiasis.

Brain surgery for intractable pain, Parkinsonism and psychiatric disorders sometimes produce abnormal sleep patterns and somnolence. Peripheral nerve and muscular diseases such as peripheral neuritis, fibrositis and myotonic dystrophies are also catalogued as causes of sleep disruption.

Almost all major endocrine and metabolic diseases result in sleep disruption and/or excessive daytime sleepiness, including Addison's disease, Cushing's syndrome, diabetes mellitus and hypoglycaemia, hyper- and hypothyroidism. Renal failure and uraemia result in excessive sleepiness. Hepatic failure is often accompanied by nocturnal delirium. Gastrointestinal disease, especially ulceration and sleep-related dyspepsia interfere with sleep.

Poor cardiac and respiratory function tends to deteriorate further during sleep resulting in angina, palpitations, cardiac arrhythmias, myocardial incompetence, coronary artery insufficiency, nocturnal dyspnoea and hyperpnoea, and worsening of Cheyne-Stokes respirations. The incidence of asthmatic attacks is highest at about four hours before the mid-point of the subject's nocturnal sleep span. Respiratory impairment during sleep can be a major problem for the elderly.

Sleep apnoea (Sleep-related cessation of breathing)

This may be either central (CNS) apnoea in which no respiratory effort occurs or upper airway obstructive apnoea in which respiratory snoring increases until a loud choking inspiratory gasp occurs when the patient's respiratory effort overcomes the occlusion, or a mixture of both. Respiration is normal during the waking state. More than 100 apnoeic attacks may occur per night. Although sleep apnoea syndrome may occur at any age the frequency seems to be high in elderly people over 60 years. The ratio of men to women is 30:1.

In most cases no anatomical defect is apparent, though sleep apnoea syndrome especially of the obstructive variety, tends to be associated with a short thick neck with or without obesity. Acromegaly, hypothyroidism and nasal polyps may cause secondary mechanical airway problems. Forty per cent of people with this syndrome have hypertension and the severely affected may have heart failure consequent to sleep apnoea.

Those suffering from sleep apnoea usually fall asleep quickly, but waken several times during the night, sometimes gasping for air or with a sensation of choking and anxiety. The obstructive apnoeic patient, although noisy and exceedingly restless during attempts to breathe may be totally unaware of the difficulty which has awakened him from sleep. Sufferers do not become fully awake every time an apnoeic attack occurs, even though they repeatedly become hypoxic and hypercapnoeic. Cardiac arrhythmias occur and the obstructive apnoeic is particularly at risk of sudden death during sleep as a consequence. Excessive daytime sleepiness is the major complaint of obstructive or upper airway sleep apnoea. Many patients have headaches and a degree of disorientation on waking, and some have drenching night sweats.

Drug treatment and even weight reduction are not always effective though Tirlapur and Mir (1982) advocate weight loss for the obese patient. According to Parkes (1981) surgery for obstructive apnoea can be highly effective in relieving the problem, including tonsilectomy and thyroidectomy where relevant—and tracheostomy may be accepted as a permanent cure by some sufferers.

Alveolor hypoventilation

Tidal volume decreases during sleep resulting in hypercapnia and hypoxaemia, without apnoeic attacks. There is a failure of ventilation to respond to chemical control. Causes in adults include massive obesity, chronic obstructive pulmonary disease, scoliosis, cordotomy and neurological lesions of respiratory control centres, poliomyelitis, myotonic dystrophy and narcolepsy.

Nocturnal sleep is disturbed for those who have actual or potential signs of daytime alveolar hypoventilation. Some complain primarily of sleep disturbance, others primarily of daytime sleepiness. An important finding by Calverley et al (1982) was that of patients with chronic obstructive airways disease, 'blue bloaters' who have daytime hypoxaemia and hypercapnia have significantly more hypoxaemic episodes during sleep than 'pink puffers'. Giving continuous oxygen (O_2) at night reduced the number of hypoxaemic episodes and increased the amount of deep orthodox sleep. Wakefulness was reduced so that the sleep of 'blue bloaters' taking O_2 was similar to healthy normal people.

Sleep-related leg movements

These symptoms are predominantly seen in middle-aged and elderly persons. Nocturnal myoclonus involves repetitive and highly stereotyped leg muscle jerks, occurring about every 20–40 seconds for a few minutes or an hour in episodes of 30 or more jerks. The contraction always consists of extension of the big toe plus partial flexion of the ankle, knee and sometimes hip. These movements only occur during sleep, and are always followed by partial arousal or awakening. The jerks are not linked with whole body movements and are often not visible to the observer nor consciously perceived by the sleeper, but recorded by electromyography (EMG). People with nocturnal myoclonus complain of frequent nocturnal awakening, unrefreshed sleep and daytime sleepiness. The incidence of leg cramps, disruption of bedclothes and falling out of bed is generally higher than in the rest of the population.

'Restless leg' syndrome

This is an extremely disagreeable deep sensation of creeping inside the calves whenever sitting or lying down, resulting in an almost irresistable urge to move the legs. The aetiology is unknown, though inadequate circulation, motor neurone disease or inheritance may be implicated. Almost all patients with 'restless leg' syndrome also have nocturnal myoclonus, though not vice versa. It results in difficulty in maintaining unbroken sleep periods, with consequent complaints of insomnia by night and somnolence by day. The 'restless leg' syndrome becomes more severe with age and is exacerbated by sleep deprivation. Some people can gain relief by vigorous leg exercises.

Parasomnias (undesirable physical phenomena associated with sleep) may be exhibited by the old as well as the young. Sleep walking in the elderly is more likely to be due to psychomotor epilepsy, fugue states or sleep drunkenness than to true somnambulism. Nightmares are more prevalent at times of emotional stress and during REM rebound from drug withdrawal. Elderly persons with sleep-related inadequacy in swallowing saliva are at risk of respiratory aspiration, and sleep-related gastrointestinal reflux may result in oesophageal stricture or aspiration pneumonia. The primary sleep disorders such as narcolepsy and idiopathic CNS hypersomnolence persist into old age, so may be occasionally seen. The habitual long and short sleepers will also continue this pattern into old age.

Conclusions

Sleep research has gone a long way to helping us understand the sleep problems of the elderly. We can use this knowledge to assess, care for, teach and sympathise with the people in our charge. It may help us and the elderly people to overthrow the prejudice that 'sleeping by day is a sin'.

Most current sleep researchers consider elderly folk to need the same amount of sleep as younger people and to be at risk of becoming seriously sleep-deprived if they are not given lengthened opportunities to sleep compared with the young. All seem to agree that the potential causes of insomnia increase in old age, that the primary sleep abnormalities do not remit, secondary sleep abnormalities increase and that hypnotic overuse is endemic in the elderly population with all its deletrious side-effects.

The most common causes of awakening reported by sleep observers of the elderly are sleep apnoea, nocturnal myoclonus (Carskadon et al 1982), physical discomfort especially distended bladder and urinary urgency (Webb and Swinbourne 1971), pain, 'restless legs' and dyspnoea.

According to Roffwarg (1979) the most common causes of sleep disturbance for adults include 'chronic pain (especially due to rheumatism and arthritis), nocturnal dyspnoea, nocturnal discomfort from pruritis, peripheral neuritis, enforced positions, strangury, dyspepsia, cerebral degeneration, abnormal movements, secondary disturbance of the circadian sleep–wake cycle and the environmental factors associated with hospitalisation' (p 49).

The most important and consistent finding of sleep problems for the elderly is the number and length of periods of awakening after sleep has started. However, as in all age groups, there are considerable individual differences. Research findings may reveal statistically significant differences between the sleep of the young and the old, but we can never assume that the individual elderly person in our care conforms to a trend. Detailed assessment is essential before we plan our care.

ASSESSMENT OF SLEEP

The initial assessment of sleep or lack of it by both medical and nursing staff relies heavily on the subjective report of the sleeper. Deeper analysis of the sleep problem is possible. Nurses have the inestimable advantage of being present night and day to assess the objective sleep and wake behaviour of individuals, whereas doctors and sleep researchers are able to undertake polygraphic recordings of internal events such as neurological and cardiovascular responses.

There are a number of potential problems which face us when assessing the quantity and quality of patients' sleep. To what extent do the person's subjective complaints about sleep correspond to objective measureable sleep problems? The correspondence is not absolute by any means. From some of the research discussed earlier it is obvious that some elderly people who have no sleep complaints in fact have multiple micro-arousals during their night's sleep and spend much of their sleep in light stages of sleep. Micro-apnoeic arousals and even nocturnal myoclonic attacks will not generally be visible even to the most observant night nurse, but the aftermath of daytime sleepiness and complaints of poor sleeping will be genuine. On the other hand, some elderly (and younger) people who complain of poor sleep do not exhibit EEG abnormalities when monitored in sleep laboratories.

An important distinction needs to be made between the person who is fatigued but tense and although longing to sleep is rarely able to do so, and the person who is tired and suffering from sleep deprivation who if given the opportunity will be able to make up the sleep lack by spending a longer time in bed at night and taking daytime naps. Severely sleep-deprived persons will eventually fall asleep whatever the surrounding activities, whereas the fatigued tense person is likely to be vigilant of all that is happening.

What about the person whose circadian rhythms are out of phase with surrounding society—wanting and able to sleep for long periods by day and having difficulty in sleeping by night? A detailed assessment of their sleep–wake patterns and social responses over the weeks before we meet them, plus a 24-hour diary of sleeping needs to be kept day after day before we can be certain of this diagnosis. We should not expect to be able to reverse the situation 'overnight'. We should obviously be wary of dismissing complaints about poor night-time sleep. Apart from any other consideration it is important that the

Table 15.3 Measurement tools for assessing sleep

Objective
1. Polygraphic recordings, EEG, EOG, EMG, HR, RR, T Oxygen levels in blood or ear oxymetry
2. Movement—pressure transducers on bed —accelerometers on arms/legs
3. Observation of sleep–wake timing and behaviour using sleep charts

Subjective
1. Self-report or questionnaire, or sleep diaries

Assessment of fatigue and hypnotic drugs
1. Choice reaction time and critical flicker fusion threshold
2. Observation of person's behaviour and appearance
3. Rating scales of subjective feelings and questionnaires

elderly person feels they have slept well, that we are willing to listen and do all in our power to provide an environment in which they have the opportunity to sleep. Table 15.3 illustrates some of the methods of sleep assessment used by researchers.

When caring for the elderly, nurses are usually confined to observations of patients' sleeping and waking behaviours and subjective reporting by the elderly person and his/her relatives. The areas which need to be assessed by the nurse or carer and the type of questions which can be used are shown in the following assessment of sleep.

Sleep assessment format

> Name
> Age
> Sex
> Medical diagnosis
> Investigations
> Admission
> Discharge.

Major areas to be assessed

1. Normal pattern of sleep in health.
   Sleep pattern during periods of stress in life.
   Current sleep pattern—including day and night:
   (a) night and day nurse's (carer's) report of sleep pattern plus possible causes of sleep problems;

(b) patient's opinion of cause of problems and patient's views of what would solve the problems.

If elderly person, relative or carer, identify a sleep problem then the following areas should be assessed in depth:

2. Drugs, especially narcotics, hypnotics, stimulants and sympathomimetics.
3. Nutritional status especially hyperphagia, anorexia, starvation, gaining or losing weight.
4. Normal eating and drinking habits. Special diets, recent changes, pre-sleeping food and drink.
5. Emotional state such as anxiety or depression, plus possible causes.
6. Daytime and night-time symptoms—awake and asleep, e.g. pain, discomfort, nocturia, incontinence, cough, dyspnoea, night sweats, snoring, disorientation.
7. Waking activities. Postural or other constraint on movement.
8. Sleeping environment—ward, institution, home, especially noise, light, cold, nursing/medical procedures interrupting sleep.

Sleep questionnaires (Malasanos et al 1977)

Using a selection of the following items will give the nurse comprehensive information about a patient's sleep pattern and problems.
(a) Normal pattern
(b) Since admission/illness

1. How well do you normally/recently sleep?
2. What time do you usually/recently go to bed? Prepare to sleep?
3. Do you fall asleep right away—normally/recently? *or* How long does it take you to fall asleep?
4. Do you wake up in the night?
5. What wakes you once you have fallen asleep?
6. What (if anything) helps you get back to sleep?
7. What time do you normally/recently wake in the morning?

8. Do you normally take naps in the day? If yes—when, for how long?
9. How do you feel (?rested) when you wake up?
10. Do you dream at night?
11. Has anyone ever told you that you:
—grind your teeth at night
—walk or talk
—snore?
12. How much sleep do you think you should have to stay healthy?
13. Have you had any worries recently?
14. What activity/work do you normally do in the daytime?
15. What do you normally do in the hour or so before night-time sleep—watch television, read, bath?
Preparation for sleep:
1. What do you do just before going to bed to sleep
— lock up house, let cat out, wash face, clean teeth, say prayers?
2. Do you eat before going to sleep? If Yes—what?
3. Do you drink before going to sleep? If Yes—what?
4. Do you take any medicines to help you sleep?
5. Are you taking any other medicines at all?
Sleeping environment:
1. Do you need special bedding to help you sleep?
2. How many pillows do you use?
3. Do you sleep with lights on/off?
4. Does a light bother you?
5. Do you need absolute quietness to sleep?
6. Do noises keep you awake, or wake you up?
7. Do you need the bedroom cold/warm to sleep?
8. Do you sleep with the window open at night?

Pre-sleep tiredness questionnaire (Porter and Horne 1981):

1. Do you feel you have gone to bed—too early, at the right time, too late?

2. Has your day been—enjoyable, normal, upsetting?
3. Have you fallen asleep during the day? If Yes, when and for how long?
4. How sleepy have you felt in the last ¼ hour?

|————————————————————————|

Alert   Sleep onset soon

5. How tired have you felt in the last ¼ hour?

|————————————————————————|

Not tired   Very tired

Post-sleep questionnaire:
1. At what time did you:
   (a) fall asleep last night?
   (b) wake up this morning?
   (c) get out of bed this morning?
2. Which of the following phrases do you consider best describes the quality of your sleep last night?

|————+————+————+————|

Much	Better	Normal	Worse	Much
better	than		than	worse
than	normal		normal	than
normal				normal

3. If you did not sleep well, please give reasons, if any, e.g. cramp, noise, not tired, hungry, full bladder.
4. What woke you this morning, e.g. alarm, person, light, bladder?
5. If you could, would you have liked to have slept longer this morning?

Assessment of sedative giving/withdrawal:
1. Leeds sleep evaluation questionnaire (Hindmarch 1980)
   (a) Ease of getting to sleep

   Extremely difficult ————— Extremely easy

   (b) Ease of awakening

   Extremely difficult ————— Extremely easy

   (c) Quality of sleep

   Excellent ————— Extremely poor

   (d) Extent of 'hangover' following awakening
   Severe —————None
2. The following words produced a significant difference in response between those who had received diazepam and those who had received a placebo (Weber et al 1975). Those on diazepam were more likely to

mark the line close to the right-hand (sleepy) words.

Strong	—————	Weak
Refreshed	—————	Tired
Energetic	—————	Lazy
Vigorous	—————	Exhausted
Awake	—————	Sleepy
Stimulated	—————	Sedated
Efficient	—————	Inefficient
Attentive	—————	Distracted
Able to concentrate	—————	Unable to concentrate

Patient goals/objectives regarding sleep

1. The elderly person will sleep at the normal times and for the normal length for him/her.
2. The elderly person will have undisturbed sleep at night.
3. The elderly person will have rest-time during the day.
4. The elderly person will feel and appear rested.
5. The elderly person will understand the use of sedatives and analgesics.
6. The elderly person will be able to plan his/her return to a healthy sleep–wake activity pattern.

The exact goals and the priority for intervention will depend upon the findings of the assessment.

Nursing intervention to promote sleep

1. Management of environment, e.g. position of beds, oiling door hinges and trolley wheels, ventilation, lighting, reduction of staff noise at night.
2. Planning 24-hour sleep–activity patterns suitable for the individual.
3. Helping patient to achieve pre-sleep rituals as near as possible to his/her normal pattern.
4. Provision of nutrition and fluids at times normal for that patient.
5. Organisation of nursing, medical and other intervention to give patient undisturbed periods of time (90 minutes

at least for one complete sleep cycle).

6. Relief of physical symptoms which interrupt sleep, e.g. pain, frequency, dyspnoea, cough.
7. Discussion and relief of psychological distress.
8. Review of the dosages and effects of sedatives and stimulants.
9. Patient teaching regarding sleep habits.
10. Treatment of any underlying medical/surgical condition.

The area of intervention over which nurses have most control are the sleeping environment and nursing interruptions of sleep. However, the total management of factors likely to disrupt sleep patterns requires discussion, decisions and action to be undertaken jointly by nurses, medical, paramedical and administrative staff, as well as help from engineers and porters.

Reassessment or ongoing assessment of sleep

This requires the repeated assessment of all the factors which were originally assessed.

The primary question which is being asked in reassessment is: Have the patient's goals been achieved or not? If not, why not? Have we or the patient failed to carry out the planned intervention?

Were the goals unrealistic? For example, we and the patient may have to accept disturbed night sleep as an intractable problem if the patient has irreversible CNS pathology. Were we trying to push the elderly person into a pattern of sleep which suited our needs rather than hers?

Finally, a word on loneliness

Could we be more adventurous and enable institutional care to be more like home; where possible, allowing family members to settle their elderly for the night, and spouses (or partners) to sleep together if they wish?

Many elderly folk have had the physical comfort and warmth of a spouse in their bed for decades and either owing to bereavement or to hospital or institutional admission or both have to face the night in solitude. Some have substituted their pets as bed companions whilst at home. Others may be in a state of mental regression in which they long once more to hold their children and babies in their arms or even to be held again in their own mother's arms. Goodman, a poet in her seventies, wrote of the need to be mothered:

Sleeping pills
> The light within me clicks
> Who put out the light?
>
> It is dark
> I am alone, afraid,
> Mother, Mother,
> I can't sleep.
>
> My mother does not come,
> My mother is dead.
>
> One pill,
> Two pills,
> Three pills,
> Mother me, pills.

Night nurses often have a closer relationship with wakeful patients than day nurses. The comfort of a person who will listen to the troubles and anxieties at the end of the day and give a loving touch or hug may be the best tranquilliser in the world.

REFERENCES

Adam K 1980 A time for rest and a time for play. Nursing Mirror 150(10): 17–18
Armstrong-Esther C A, Hawkins S C H 1982 Day for night. Circadian rhythms in the elderly. Nursing Times 78(30): 1263–6
Beck U, Brezinova V, Hunter W et al 1975 Plasma growth hormone and slow wave sleep increase after interruption of sleep. Journal of Clinical Endocrinology and Metabolism 40(5): 812–815
Beecham Foods Nutrition Information Centre 1978 How diet affects sleep. Nursing Mirror 147(20): 32–35
Calverley P M A, Brezinova V, Douglas N J, Catterall J R, Fenley D C 1982 The effects of oxygenation on sleep quality in chronic bronchitis and emphysema. American Review of Respiratory Disease 126(2): 206–210
Carskadon M A, Van den Hoed J, Dement W C 1982 Insomnia and sleep disturbances in the aged. Sleep and daytime sleepiness in the elderly. Journal of Geriatric Psychiatry 13(2): 135–151

Coleman R, Miles S L, Guilleminault C 1981 Sleep–wake disorders in the elderly: a polysomnographic analysis. Journal of the American Geriatric Society 29: 289–296

Colquhoun W P (ed) 1971 Biological rhythms and human performance. Academic Press, New York

Colquhoun W P (ed) 1972 Aspects of human efficiency: diurnal rhythm and sleep loss. English University Press

Dement W C, Miles L E Carskadon M A 1982a Changes in the sleep and waking EEG's of non-demented and demented elderly subjects. Journal of the American Geriatric Society 30(2): 86–93

Dement W C, Miles L E, Carskadon M A 1982b 'White Paper' on sleep and ageing. American Geriatric Society Journal 30(1): 25–50

Feinberg G I 1968 The ontogenesis of human sleep and the relationship of sleep variables to intellectual function in the aged. Comprehensive Psychiatry 9: 138–147

Gress L D, Bahr R T, Hassanein R S 1981 Nocturnal behaviour of selected institutionalised adults. Journal of Gerontological Nursing 7(2): 86–92

Guilleminault C, Dement W C 1978 Sleep apnoea syndromes and related sleep disorders. In: Williams R L, Karacan I (eds) Sleep disorders: diagnosis and treatment. Wiley, New York, p 9–28

Helton M C, Gordon S H, Nunnery S L 1980 The correlation between sleep deprivation and the intensive care syndrome. Heart and Lung 9: 465–468

Hindmarch I 1980 Calling time on hypnotic drugs. Nursing Mirror 150(11): 37–38

Hopkins S 1980 Silent night? In: Redfern S J, Fordham M (eds) Nursing 20 Sleep and Comfort 870–873

Horne J A 1980 Sleep and body restitution. Experientia 36: 11–13

Johns M 1975 Factor analysis of subjectively reported sleep habits and the nature of insomnia. Psychological Medicine 5:83

Karacan I, Thornby J I, Anch A M et al 1976 Dose response effects of coffee on the sleep of normal middle aged men. Sleep Research 5:71

Koreorgos J 1980 Sleep and sleep disorders. Practitioner 224: 717–721

Lobban M, Tredre B 1964 Diurnal rhythms of renal excretion and of body temperature in aged subjects. Journal of Physiology 170:29

McGhie A, Russell S 1962 The subjective assessment of normal sleep patterns. Journal of Mental Science 108:642

Malasanos L, Barkauska V, Moss M, Stoltenberg-Allen K 1977 Health Assessment. Mosby, St Louis

Minors D S, Waterhouse J M 1981 Circadian rhythms and the human. Wright, Bristol

Ogilvie A J 1980 Sources and levels of noises on the wards at night. Nursing Times 76(31): 1363–1366

Pacini C M, Fitzpatrick J 1982 Sleep patterns of hospitalised and non-hospitalised aged individuals. Journal of Gerontological Nursing 8(6): 327–332

Parkes J D 1981 Day-time drowsiness. The Lancet 2: 1213–1218

Porter J M, Horne J A 1981 Exercise and sleep behaviour: a questionnaire approach. Ergonomics 24(7): 511–521

Preston F 1973 Further sleep problems in airline pilots on world-wide schedules. Aerospace Medicine 44:775

Reinberg A 1966 Circadian rhythms. (Letter.) Journal of the American Medical Association 196:108

Roffwarg H P (ed) 1979 Diagnostic classification of sleep and arousal disorders. Sleep 2(1): 1–137

Roth T, Kramer M, Trinder J 1972 The effects of noise during sleep on the sleep patterns of different age groups. Canadian Psychiatric Association 17: 197–201

Samis H V, Capobianco S 1978 Ageing and biological rhythms. Advances in Experimental Medicine and Biology 108. Plenum Press, New York

Sanford S 1982 Sleep and its implications for intensive care nursing. International Intensive Care Nursing Conference. Proceedings p 73–77

Serio M, Romano M, DeMagistris L et al 1970 The circadian rhythm of plasma cortisol in subjects over 70 years of age. Journal of Gerontology 25:95

Shock N 1977 Biological theories of ageing In: Birren J, Schaie K (eds) Handbook of the psychology of ageing. Van Nostrand Reinhold, New York

Takahashi Y, Kipris D M, Daughaday W H 1968 Growth hormone secretion during sleep. Journal of Clinical Investigation 47:2079

Tirlapur V G, Mir M A 1982. (Letter.) Lancet 1: 163–164

Webb W B 1982 Sleep in older persons: sleep structures in 50 to 60 year old men and women. Journal of Gerontology 37: 581–586

Webb W B, Swinburne H 1971 An observational study of sleep of the aged. Perceptual Motor Skills 32: 895–898

Weber A, Jermini C, Grandjean E P 1975 Relationship between objective and subjective assessment of experimentally induced fatigue. Ergonomics 18: 151–156

Wessler R, Rubin M, Sollberger A 1976 Circadian rhythm of activity and sleep-wakefulness in elderly institutionalised patients. Journal of Interdisciplinary Cycle Research 7:333

Williams R, Agnew H, Webb W 1967 Effects of prolonged stage 4 and 1-REM sleep deprivation EEG task performance and psychologic responses. US School of Aerospace Medicine Report

Winfree A T 1982 Circadian timing of sleepiness in man and woman. American Journal of Physiology 243(3): 193–204R

Winget C, Vernikos-Danellis J, Cronin S 1972 Circadian rhythm asynchrony in man during hypokinesis. Journal of Applied Physiology 33:640

16

C. Webb

Expressing sexuality

WHAT IS SEXUALITY?

Sexuality is much more than physical acts of sex. It encompasses 'the quality of being human, all that we are as men and women . . . encompassing the most intimate feelings and deepest longings of the heart to find meaningful relationships' (Hogan 1980, p. 3). Sexuality and sensuality go to make up our self-concept and how we see ourselves and are seen by others. Our sexual self-concept, like all other parts of our personality, is a social phenomenon. We learn through living in a culture what are its expected and approved forms of behaviour, and if we do not live up to these norms we may experience guilt and feelings of inadequacy.

SEXUALITY IN WESTERN SOCIETIES

Myths and stereotypes

Sexuality in western societies is tied to youth and physical attractiveness, and media portrayals of beautiful young women and handsome young men are bombarded at us virtually 24 hours a day in advertisements on television, in public transport, on billboards and in magazines. Feminine delicate features and slim bodies or masculine rugged, sporty leanness are what we are urged to strive for. No advertising executive would dream of using images of elderly people with thinning, receding, greying hair and sagging breasts or abdomens to create an image of beauty and desirability. Mellowed, comfortable pictures of older people may sell thermal underwear or storage heaters, but there is nothing sexual or sensual about these. Very much to the contrary, older people are generally assumed to be sexless. Libido and sexual needs are thought to decline along with loss of the culturally valued outer signs of beauty or handsomeness, and at the same time sexual capacity fades too. Social usefulness is defined for men by productiveness at work and retirement from work may be associated in people's minds with retirement from sexual life as well (Kuhn 1976). For women the menopause is widely believed to herald this sexless, useless phase. People are declared obsolescent and cast aside as if they were a worn-out washing machine or broken-down car. This social devaluation is further signified and realised in the form of low old-age pensions.

Double discrimination

Even within this discrimination against elderly people there is yet further discrimination. Men who still show signs of sexual activity are labelled 'dirty old men', but there is a 'good public relations' side to this (Sontag 1978). Men are supposed to maintain their 'manhood' for longer than women, and society lends approval and even celebrity to those who father children at an advanced age. Charlie Chaplin and Pablo Picasso were two of these famous fathers. But there are no lauded 'dirty old women'. Signs of wanting a sexual relationship, 'flirting', and dressing like lamb when one is really mutton are viewed as unseemly and distasteful or even disgusting in a woman. Older men may be described as handsome but older women are never beautiful (de Beauvoir 1973, Sontag 1978).

Balding in men is often said to be a sign of increasing virility, and greying hair denotes a distinguished man. Women's thinning hair is never seen as enviable, however, and certainly not as an indication of increased sexuality. Rather, women often colour rinse their greying hair to make it more 'attractive'. It is

noteworthy that the English language has no parallel term for virility to describe high levels of sexuality in women—the phenomenon is not supposed to exist and so a name is not needed (Webb 1983).

The bad faith involved in these two sets of double standards for the old and young and for women and men (Sontag 1978) is further evidenced in jokes. A Dr Palmore has studied jokes related to ageing and sexuality and found that in general they reveal a hostile and negative view of ageing. However, jokes about women were negative in 77% of cases while this was true of only 51% of jokes about men (Puner 1974). Other cultural myths about sexuality in old age promote ideas that it is acceptable for older men to marry younger women. Indeed this is a cause for congratulation and envy of the man. Older women should not marry younger men, and such an act on the part of the woman would lead to accusations of cradle-snatching as well as to doubts about the motives or psychosexual adjustment of the man (Kuhn 1976). Marriage or remarriage by old people is generally frowned upon, and Trimmer (1978) considers this to be due to links between sexuality and procreation in our culture. Thus once procreation is no longer possible all sexual activity should cease.

These myths and stereotypes act as self-fulfilling prophecies for the elderly (Kuhn 1976). They are told that they are sexually unattractive, unwanted and useless and this information rebounds on their self-concept and adds to their negative self-view (Weg 1983). As a result, when they experience sexual urges they think these are abnormal and feelings of guilt, shame and embarrassment ensue.

The experts' prejudices

Even among the 'experts' there are prejudices to be found. Sexual relations may be discussed in textbooks only in terms of marital relations, implying that there is no place for sex unless people are married. Masturbation may be seen as acceptable in the absence of a marital partner but not as an activity which anyone might partake of by choice , as in the articles written by Costello (1975) and Puner (1974). Scully and Bart discovered in 1973 that few of the findings of Masters and Johnson's famous and extensive studies of sexual behaviour had worked their way through into current textbooks in the space of 10 years since their publication. They found a widespread belief among medical writers in the 'normality' of vaginal orgasm and little reference to clitoral orgasm. Today, over 10 years later still, the same observations can be made of the literature on ageing and sexuality. The clitoris and its function are rarely mentioned, and marital sex is used as the standard for discussion of other forms, which are only of importance in the absence of a marital partner. This confirms a view of vaginal intercourse as the norm for women and the only way for men to achieve sexual satisfaction. Homosexuality and bisexuality are rarely discussed.

Sex can be good for you

After all this pessimism and simple inaccuracy it is a refreshing relief to learn that sex is good for elderly people. In a study of 70-year-old women and men in Sweden, Persson (1980) found that men who continued to have sexual intercourse slept better, had better mental activity and a more positive attitude towards sexual activity in the elderly. Similarly, women who continued to have sexual intercourse retained their former levels of emotional stability, had low levels of anxiety, had better mental health, felt generally more healthy and had a positive attitude towards sexual activity in the elderly.

Sexual activity has been said to help arthritis, reduce physical and psychological tensions and promote a good physical condition (Butler and Lewis 1973, quoted in Robinson 1983 and Kuhn 1976). Taking the wider concept of sexuality, too, the value of continuing to take account of this dimension of humanity into old age is sympathetically expressed by Weg (1983) when she says, 'The intimacy and warmth often associated with

sexual expression have significance beyond the pleasurable release of sexual tension—an important assertion and commitment of self and a reaffirmation of the connection with life itself' (p. 45).

On that positive note, myths and stereotypes will be left behind in order to consider the realities of sexuality and the elderly.

SEXUALITY AND THE ELDERLY

Physiological aspects

Physiological changes occurring with ageing have a relatively small part to play in sexual function.

In older women, vaginal lubrication is slower, vaginal expansion and contraction of the uterus are depressed, the labia are no longer elevated and the fat under the mons veneris is much reduced. The clitoris remains relatively unaltered but low levels of oestrogen may cause vaginal soreness, painful clitoral stimulation and uterine spasms during orgasm (Berman and Lief 1976, Trimmer 1978, Masters and Johnson 1981). Women remain capable of multiple orgasms and may experience an increase in sexual desire after the menopause, when androgens are minimally opposed by oestrogens (Weg 1983) and fear of unwanted pregnancy is gone (Puner 1974).

Masters and Johnson (1981) report that men over the age of 60 years take longer to achieve full penile engorgement, and may have a decrease in expulsive pressure and a reduction in the volume of ejaculatory fluid expelled. Also, although levels of sexual interest may remain, the subjective desire for ejaculation may be reduced. Erection is more rapidly lost after ejaculation than in the earlier years. Men may be affected by 'performance anxiety' if they are unaware that these changes are normal and do not herald the termination of sexual activity. Women, too, may feel threatened if their partners do not ejaculate (Hendricks and Hendricks 1978).

Contrary to popular mythology, both elderly women and men report that it is factors in the male which usually lead to the cessation of sexual activity, and not disinterest on the part of the female (Hendricks and Hendricks 1978). The most common of these male factors are illness, lack of interest, and inability to have an erection (impotence). Berman and Lief (1976) also consider lack of knowledge about normal sexual function and a poor marital relationship to be important influences. There is wide agreement that psychosocial factors have a much greater impact on sexuality in the elderly than physiological factors (Hendricks and Hendricks 1978, Sontag 1978, Masters and Johnson 1981, Corby and Zarit 1983, Weg 1983).

Psychosocial aspects

Past sexuality is the best predictor of levels of sexual activity in the elderly (Persson 1980, Masters and Johnson 1981). People who are at present in the elderly age groups were brought up as young people in a period of strict religious, Victorian or Edwardian morality (Comfort 1977). They were taught that sex was an activity to be confined to the marital relationship and for purposes of procreation, at least for women. Thus sex outside marriage and sexual activity for simple pleasure, such as after the menopause or by masturbation, were sinful (Kuhn 1976, Weg 1983).

Women's tendency to live longer than men and therefore to be left without a marital partner, the earlier decline in sexual function in men already noted, and the cultural prescription that men should take the initiative in sexual relations make women's position more unsatisfactory. Nevertheless, studies report that increasing numbers of women in the 50 to 70 age group masturbate, suggesting that social mores are becoming more flexible (Hendricks and Hendricks 1978).

Single elderly people face particular problems according to Corby and Zarit (1983) because they are not thought to have a legitimate right or need for sexual privacy, whether at home or in institutions. Frequently, sexual expression is discouraged in institutions by the physical segregation of the sexes, and this may be because of fears of 'inappropriate' sexual behaviour or of complaints from relatives who find the elderly person's sexuality anxiety-provoking. Corby and Zarit report on a study by Silverstone and Wynter in 1975 in which a 'heterosexual living space' was introduced in an institution. Better social adjustment followed, seen for example in improved grooming and less swearing by men, greater use of privacy by closing doors when dressing, and overt sexual contacts.

Homosexuality in relation to the elderly has been little studied, but the problems faced by older homosexual women and men are probably little different from those of heterosexuals, in that the major one is finding suitable partners (Weg 1983). Homosexual men may be damaged by similar stereotypes to those applied to heterosexuals because generalisations are usually based on a youth-oriented perspective and the assumption that all homosexual men are alike. For older lesbians life may be easier because the number of eligible partners may be larger and because of a commitment to longer-term relationships (Weg 1983).

Psychosocial factors, then, play a greater role in influencing sexuality and sexual function in the elderly—as indeed they do at other stages of adult life. Availability of a suitable partner, physical health, past sexual activity and living accommodation are among the strongest factors involved. For women, continuing sexual activity is positively related to a warm and socially approved relationship with a male while for men boredom, fatigue, illness, overindulgence in food and drink, and fear of performance failure are reported to inhibit satisfactory sexual activity (George and Weiler 1981). Above all, it should be emphasised, to quote Weg again, that 'there is no one way to love or to be loved; there is no one liaison that is superior to another. No one lifestyle in single-hood or marriage, heterosexual or homosexual, will suit all persons. Self-pleasuring, homosexuality, bisexuality, celibacy and heterosexuality are all in the human repertoire' (Weg 1983, p. 76)

Ill health, disability and sexuality

Any illness or disability can disturb a person's self-concept, and the sexual self-concept is no exception (Weinberg 1982). General bodily disturbances, weakness, tiredness and malaise occur to varying degrees in all illnesses. The result is that there is less energy for investing in self-care, clothing, appearance, and for home, leisure, social and sexual activities. This leads to a rebound effect on self-esteem, energy levels fall further, and the vicious circle goes round again. In relation to sexuality, a further complication arises because it is known that the elderly are less likely than younger people to restart sexual activity after a period of cessation, such as a break due to illness (Berman and Lief 1976). Over and above these generalised effects, each illness or disability has its own unique repercussions for sexuality, in the broad sense of the term. Certain medical conditions and physiological changes are more common among the elderly than in the rest of the population and, although there is not space to go into detail about every possible condition, some important effects on the main body systems will be outlined.

Cardiovascular conditions, especially myocardial infarctions, are a great source of anxiety in relation to sex, especially for men. Hendricks and Hendricks (1978) state that 'actually sex requires no more exertion than taking a brisk walk or climbing a flight of stairs' (p. 69), and Comfort agrees that 'sex is a highly undangerous activity. Stopping it unwillingly is far more dangerous than a little exertion' (Comfort 1977, p. 193). Sudden death during or after intercourse is rare and the benefits of intercourse, including a sense of well-being, less depression, gentle exercise, and reduction of tension outweigh the risks (Weg 1983).

Respiratory disorders can cause shortness of breath, cough, recurrent infections, chest deformity and orthopnoea, with obvious implications for sexual acts and perhaps less obvious ones for the sexual self-concept. Inability to perform sexual activity without breathlessness will lead to feelings of inadequacy. Coughing and expectoration of large amounts of purulent sputum or being unable to adopt certain positions will cause embarrassment, if they do not make sexual intercourse impossible.

Musculoskeletal conditions and changes associated with ageing may cause weakness, limitation of movement, deformity and pain. Chronic pain such as that of arthritis can be extremely depressing and debilitating, and lead on to loss of interest in sex as well as decreased possibilities of performing satisfying sexual acts. On the positive side, sexual activity increases adrenal corticoid production, which may relieve arthritic symptoms (Weg 1983).

Nervous system changes in old age may affect perception and sensation, and thereby inhibit sexual response. Eyesight, hearing and touch all play a part in sensuality as well as in actual sex acts. More spectacularly a stroke with its possible paralysis, loss of speech and continence, loss of independence and perhaps depression will have potentially devastating effects on all aspects of life, including sensuality and sexuality. Parkinson's disease too may have a very damaging outcome for self-confidence and self-concept, so that the sufferer feels sexually undesirable.

Common endocrine disorders occurring in old age are hypothyroidism and diabetes mellitus. People with hypothyroidism may be lethargic and lacking in interest in themselves, their surroundings and others, and may gain weight and lose hair. These may make them feel unattractive to others, which will further decrease the likelihood of partaking in sexual activities. Diabetes mellitus can cause specific complications both for women and men. For women, vaginal lubrication is delayed and scant even when oestrogen levels are adequate. There is therefore an increased susceptibility to vaginal soreness and infection, which is a disincentive to sexual activity. For men, retrograde and/or premature ejaculation may occur and as many as 50% of sufferers cannot have an erection. The cause may be changes in the arterial bed or neuropathy, but no satisfactory treatment has been found (Weg 1983). The multiple complications of diabetes, including cardiovascular disease, renal damage and neuropathy also have effects on sexuality and sexual function.

Genito-urinary conditions in women and men have perhaps the most obvious link with sexual activity and sexuality. Men widely believe that prostatectomy means the end of sexual activity but this is not so in the majority of cases. Suprapublic and perineal operations lead to impotence more commonly than transurethral resection, but with the latter retrograde ejaculation may be distressing (Weg 1983). Comfort (1977) recommends all men to discuss sexual activity specifically with their surgeon prior to prostatectomy and make it clear if they wish to continue to have intercourse afterwards. Incontinence, urinary infections and atrophic vaginitis involve local pain or discomfort which may inhibit feelings and responses as well as making the person feel unclean or unattractive.

Cessation of sexual activity has been attributed to ill-health, particularly by men, but illness and disability do not necessarily mean that an active sex life is impossible or that sensuality and sexuality are compromised. Self-concept and confidence may be low and the sufferer may fear rejection, but desires and feelings continue (Costello 1975, Hogan 1980, Weg 1983). Reference has already been made to the effect that institutionalisation, including hospitalisation, may have on clients' or patients' opportunities for sexual expression. The role of the nurse in minimising these disturbances and promoting healthy sexuality will be discussed in the concluding sections, after considering some aspects of the treatment of illness.

Treatments and sexuality

People sometimes joke about the treatment being worse than the disease, but with regard to sexuality this may be no joke: it can be the devastating truth. Any surgical operation, for example, causes temporary disturbance of health which can also disrupt sexual activity. Particular operations, however, can have permanently destructive effects because they change the body image and the person's self-concept as an intact and sexually desirable being. Mastectomy, amputation and stoma formation are instances of this (Webb 1982) but other operations can in a less visible way have a similar effect, as Wilson-Barnett found with coronary surgery (Wilson-Barnett 1981).

Many drugs, both social and medically prescribed, affect sexual function, either as part of their desired mode of action or by causing debilitating side-effects. An example of a social drug which compromises sexual activity is alcohol, which has a depressant effect on the central nervous system with resulting impotence. Cigarettes cause respiratory illnesses and dysfunction as well as a halitosis which hardly adds to sexual appeal. As a Health Education Council poster says, 'Kiss a non-smoker and taste the difference!'

Narcotics, tranquillisers, sedatives and anxiolytic drugs depress the central nervous system and suppress libido. Numerous anti-hypertensive drugs such as chlorothiazide, hydrallazine and methyldopa have the same effect, and tricyclic and monoamine oxidase inhibitor antidepressants can cause impotence. Other common drugs occasionally reported to have adverse effects on sexuality include cimetidine, which can cause impotence and gynaecomastia, and propranolol, which can lead to impotence (Hogan 1980, Weinberg 1982, Weg 1983).

The situations described in the two previous sections on ill-health, disability and treatments assume even greater importance when it is remembered that elderly people may be experiencing multiple pathology and concomitant multiple medications and treatments. Nurses can do much to help patients and clients in these circumstances to express their sexuality in the way they themselves choose as most appropriate. Weinberg (1982) proposes that nurses should function as educators and advocates in relation to sexuality and the needs of the elderly, and these two roles will be discussed in the concluding sections.

ROLES FOR NURSES

Nurses as educators

The primary need of elderly people is for information regarding sexuality. Myths and stereotypes need to be stripped of their credibility and replaced with accurate information about sexual functioning and sexuality. Knowledge of how anatomy and physiology evolve with ageing would do much to dispel anxieties and shame in an age group which often feels that its sexual feelings are manifestations of over-sexuality or sinfulness (Burnside 1976, Renshaw 1981). Sexuality and sensuality should be tactfully raised when taking a nursing history, and this also provides the first opportunity for education about normal functioning. Subsequently, when carrying out nursing care or working with clients, nurses should be alert to cues pointing to covert requests for information or to knowledge deficits, and should discuss these in an open, accepting and informative style. In this way elderly people can come to accept and feel comfortable with their own thoughts, feelings, fantasies and urges. Whether they wish to be sexually active or not they may have insecurities which need to be brought out into the open. This may equally apply to their families, whose own anxieties may cause or add to those of elderly people themselves and nurses can therefore assist by giving information to relatives of elderly people. Comfort (1977) suggests that staff who are unwilling to do this have sexual problems of their own which they are projecting on to elderly people.

It is just as important to take account of sexuality with those who do not wish to be sexually active. Whilst it would be undesirable to upset them by pressing them to behave in ways which others find liberating, sexuality is a much wider matter than sexual acts, as we have discussed. People who are sexually inactive, whether by choice or circumstances, are still sexual beings in this broader sense and have needs which nurses should try to meet (Comfort 1977, Robinson 1983, Weg 1983).

Nurses as advocates

The advocate role includes speaking for patients when they are not able to influence the situation themselves and working to provide services and facilities which they require. Nurses, whether working in clients' homes or institutions, are in a potentially strong position to influence the care elderly people receive and to contribute to meeting their needs in relation to sexuality.

Elderly people in health and illness have the same needs in relation to sexuality as every other adult. Acts of intimacy and warmth, companionship and love, self-respect and the respect of others help to maintain an intact self-concept at this stage of life as at any other. Indeed close friendships may be more important because relationships with family and friends grow fewer as some of them die, and work and social roles are curtailed with retirement and decreased mobility (Weg 1983). Physical appearance and dress are fundamental and highly visible ways of expressing sexuality and individuality. Maintaining a dignified style of dress and presentation is essential to self-respect but this may not be as easy as it used to be for people who have a lower income than during their working lives and cannot so easily get about to make purchases and launder their clothes. Full individually owned clothing, including underwear, with washing facilities should be an obligatory provision. Impaired mobility and eyesight may make it difficult to keep hair clean and groomed. Attractive and comfortable dentures, spectacles and hearing aids are a necessity for the elderly, and functionality is not the only consideration required. Help with keeping up appearance may be needed by elderly people, who will feel that this is not an added refinement or the 'icing on the cake', but is their basic right as human beings.

Privacy, too, is something we all need at times, whether to give an opportunity for quiet thinking, to attend to personal hygiene and grooming, or to carry out sexual acts. When elderly people live with their younger families or in institutions this need is easily forgotten. Doors may be left open routinely and people may enter the room without knocking and waiting for permission to enter. Privacy is virtually absent where a room is shared with another resident or the old person sleeps in a downstairs room which the family uses as a living room during the daytime.

As well as assisting people to satisfy their needs in these respects, nurses may have opportunities to influence medical treatment in relation to sexuality. For example, an elderly woman suffering from atrophic vaginal changes will benefit from using oestrogen cream. The prescription of systemic hormones is more problemmatic because of possible undesired effects including carcinogenesis (Trimmer 1978). An elderly man is unlikely to need such intervention because hormonal insufficiency appears to have little effect on male sexual potency (Finkle 1971). Nurses may be the first to notice that a drug is adversely affecting a patient's sexuality or, through closer knowledge of individual patients or clients, may be able to draw a doctor's attention to the effect an illness or handicap is having in this respect.

CONCLUSION

All nurses cannot and should not be sex therapists. This is a role which requires extensive specialist training (Hogan 1980, Weinberg 1982). But all nurses should be able to identify problems, intervene appropriately by teaching or counselling within the limits of their knowledge, or by referring patients or clients to specialists for help. Our cultural norms and values in the realms of sexuality have changed enormously in this century and particularly in the last 25 years (Robinson 1983). Our future clients and patients are likely to be increasingly assertive of their needs and rights in relation to sexuality. It is our responsibility as professionals to ensure that we are educated and equipped with the knowledge and skills to fulfil our obligations to them.

REFERENCES

Berman E M, and Lief H I 1976 Sex and the aging process. In: Oaks W W, Melchiode G A, Ficher I (eds) Sex and the life cycle. Grune and Stratton, New York

Burnside I M (ed) 1976 Nursing and the aged. McGraw-Hill, New York

Comfort A 1977 A good age. Mitchell Beazley, London

Corby N, Zarit J M 1983 The unmarried in later life. In: Weg R B (ed) Sexuality in the later years. Roles and behavior. Academic Press, New York

Costello M K 1975 Sex, intimacy and aging. American Journal of Nursing 75(8): 1330–1332

De Beauvoir S 1973 The coming of age. Warner Paperback Library, New York

Finkle A L 1971 Sexual function during advancing age. In: Rossman I (ed) Clinical geriatrics. Lippincott, Philadelphia

George L K, Weiler S J 1981 Sexuality in middle and late life. Archives of General Psychiatry 38: 919–923

Hendricks J , Hendricks C D 1978 Sexuality in later life. In: Carver V, Liddiard P (eds) An ageing population. Hodder and Stoughton/The Open University, Sevenoaks, Kent

Hogan R 1980 Human sexuality. A nursing perspective. Appleton-Century-Crofts, New York

Kuhn M E 1976 Sexual myths surrounding the aging. In: Oaks W W, Melchiode G A, Ficher I (eds) Sex and the life cycle. Grune and Stratton, New York

Masters W H, Johnson V E 1981 Sex and the aging process. Journal of the American Geriatrics Society 29(9): 385–390

Persson G 1980 Sexuality in a 70 year old urban population. Journal of Psychosomatic Research 24: 335–342

Puner M 1974 To the good long life. Macmillan/The Open University, London

Renshaw D C 1981 Sexuality in older women? Journal of Clinical Psychiatry 42(1): 3–4

Robinson P K 1983 The sociological perspective. In: Weg R B (ed) Sexuality in the later years. Roles and behavior. Academic Press, New York

Scully D, Bart P 1973 A funny thing happened on the way to the orifice. American Journal of Sociology 78: 1045–1049

Sontag S 1978 The double standard of ageing. In: Carver V, Liddiard P (eds) An ageing population. Hodder and Stoughton/The Open University, Sevenoaks, Kent

Trimmer E 1978 Basic sexual medicine. Heinemann, London

Webb C 1982 Body image and recovery from hysterectomy. In: Wilson-Barnett J, Fordham M (eds) Recovery from illness. Wiley, Chichester

Webb C 1983 Words fail me. Nursing Times Volume 27 (6 July): 62–66

Weg R B (ed) 1983 Sexuality in the later years. Roles and behaviour. Academic Press, New York

Weinberg J S 1982 Sexuality. Human needs and nursing practice. Saunders, Philadelphia

Wilson-Barnett J 1981 Assessment of recovery: with special reference to a study with post-operative cardiac patients. Journal of Advanced Nursing 6: 435–445

17

S. M. Gollop

Pain and discomfort

Pain is a universal human experience which is personal and private. It cannot be fully shared or known for certain by another person (Lewis 1978). Sternbach (1968) defined pain as an abstract concept which refers to (a) a private, personal sensation of mind, (b) a harmful stimulus signalling current or impending tissue damage and (c) a pattern of impulses which operate to protect the organism from harm. Tissue damage or breach of a defence mechanism arouses the autonomic nervous system and such emotions as fear and anxiety, with all the physical consequences of nervous system and hormonal activity. Pain is useful as a protective mechanism, drawing a person's attention to actual or impending damage and motivating that person to seek help. Tissue damage is not the only component of pain and many factors operate to modify both the experience of pain and its expression. Weisenberger (1977) reported the following factors as influencing pain: (1) the circumstances in which it occurs, (2) the individual's socialisation, (3) past experience of pain, (4) the personality and mood of the person in pain, and (5) the significance or meaning of the pain to the person experiencing it. Cohen (1979) describes four types of pain—social, psychological, physical and spiritual, which make up the total pain experience.

THE AGEING PROCESS AND PAIN

Physical changes occur in the central and peripheral nervous system which influence the experience of pain. Timiras and Vernadakis (1972) report these changes as both structural and functional. Lost neurones are not replaced with a consequent reduction in the total number of functioning neurones and therefore a reduction of the number of pathways available for impulses to travel. Changes in the cytoplasm of neurones and supporting cells lead to altered function. Reduced cerebral blood flow and slight hypoxia resulting from a less efficient circulation also alter neuronal functioning. Impaired lung function may increase hypoxia and further impair neuronal efficiency. In the elderly, these changes lead to a reduction in the strength of specific nerve impulses. Fewer neurones and fewer synapses reduce the ability of the brain to 'tune' or refine impulses. Changes in enzyme activity at synapses result in a general slowing down in response to a specific stimulus. This causes an increase in background 'noise' with some neurones generating random impulses while others fail to respond. If specific impulses signalling, for example, pain are weak then there is a tendency for them to merge with the increased background noise of general brain activity and become non-specific. This acts to increase 'noise' even further and can result in the person experiencing mental confusion or an inability to pinpoint the pain.

Changes in the peripheral nervous system include a reduction in the numbers of large fibres in afferent, sensory nerves with a consequent increase in small fibre activity and an increase in the time taken to perceive a stimulus. Afferent conduction velocities seem unchanged. Efferent, motor nerves show a drop in conduction velocity with a selective reduction in fast conducting fibres. Conditions surrounding the neuromuscular junction also influence the response, with poor local circulation or change in local tissue temperature slowing the response still further.

Welford (1980) suggests that the ageing nervous system becomes more prone to overactivity with less efficient homeostatic mechanisms. Schultz (1982) summarises the consequences of ageing of both the central and peripheral nervous system to be a reduced ability to respond to stress. Ageing reduces the sensitivity and responsiveness of tissues to hormones and other substances. Functional changes indicate that when an older person is confronted with new, stress-inducing events they reach higher levels of arousal and require more time to return to baseline. Schultz (1982) considers cognitive changes of older people and reports that any given experience is likely to elicit several related emotional responses at once. Many experiences are important for their emotional content, and long-term memories provide a context against which any new emotion-arousing event is evaluated. Old people are confronted with an increase in new emotional experiences associated with loss, as with loss of spouse or a decrease in physical mobility. Such events are more likely to arouse negative, painful emotions which are immediate and long lasting. New positive events are rarer when evaluated against stored long-term memories. A first grandchild happens once, the arrival of subsequent grandchildren may arouse less strong positive emotions.

Negative mood and depression are found slightly more often in elderly than in young people (Von Knorring et al 1983), and pain is a common symptom for patients with depressive disorders (Merskey and Spear 1967). Von Knorring et al (1983) found that depressed patients with pain were more anxious about their bodies and had more muscular tension than depressed patients who denied pain. Bowers (1968) found in laboratory tests that subjects who were unable to relieve or avoid pain suffered more than those with the facilities to control it. Skevington (1983) studied patients with chronic back pain. She found more depressive symptoms among the pain sufferers than among a matched control group. Frequent depressive symptoms were correlated with intense emotional pain. The depressed subjects believed that they were not to blame for failing to control their pain but also believed that nobody could help them. This set of attitudes she termed 'universal helplessness'.

Elton (1978) found that chronic pain was associated with low self-esteem. The raising of self-esteem was correlated with a reduction in pain. Longino and Kart (1982) studied the effects of activity on life satisfaction of elderly people. They found that informal activity with friends, relatives and neighbours increased life satisfaction. Formal activity in voluntary associations was associated with a decrease in life satisfaction. They found that voluntary associations fostered a social structure which rewarded the healthy, those who had lost fewest loved ones and those who were close to their children. Those who fell short of any of these criteria were termed 'poor dears' and reinforced feelings of low self-esteem and low life satisfaction.

In summary, for the elderly adult pain impulses are less clearly defined and reaction time is slowed but autonomic arousal takes longer to settle to baseline activity. The emotions aroused are more likely to be negative with an increase in the incidence of depression, low self-esteem and feelings of helplessness and loss of control. These points need to be taken into account when nursing an elderly person with pain. They influence the assessment of pain and the choice of intervention to relieve pain. Since chronic pain is associated with depression and low self-esteem, the emotional state of the person is important and suitable strategies are chosen to relieve psychological suffering as well as physical pain.

PAIN ASSESSMENT

McCaffery (1972) suggests the following definition as the nurse's guide to pain assessment: 'Pain is whatever the experiencing person says it is and occurs whenever he says it does.'

Jacox (1979) found that 70% of patients suffering from short-term, long-term or progressive pain did not want to discuss it. They did not want to be seen as complainers or to bother other people who had their own problems. Jacox also found that the majority of patients denied pain at the start of the interview but indicated at least mild discomfort after 10 or 15 minutes of talking. The nurse needs all her interpersonal and communication skills to gain accurate information, especially when assessing an elderly person.

The interview

In the light of Jacox's findings it is suggested that the following information is gathered before pain measurement is attempted. The elderly person is interviewed as a first assessment so that the nurse can gain an accurate picture of what the person is experiencing. The elderly person should be as comfortable as possible with few distractions. To help communication, the person in pain is offered her glasses, hearing aid or dentures, as appropriate. The nurse should sit facing the person in pain. By sitting the nurse conveys that she has time to listen to answers and facing the person enables her lips, eyes and facial expressions to be clearly seen. All this helps to convey to the person in pain that the nurse is interested in the answers to her questions. An older person takes longer to process incoming information and to respond to it, so allow her adequate time to think and to answer. If too little time is allowed for a reply and the question is repeated or even rephrased then the patient can become confused and her response is delayed.

To get a complete picture of the pain experience the following information is gathered by asking open questions.

1. How long have you had the pain?

Some people may have been in pain for months or years, and will have found ways of coping with it. For others, pain may be a recent experience and they may need help to build positive coping strategies. Asking about previous pain experiences will also reveal any opportunity to build coping strategies. Asking how present pain compares with previous experience will help to reveal the person's attitude towards it, for example: 'It's not so bad as when I had a heart attack', or 'It's worse than anything I've ever had before'. Asking what makes the difference between the present and past pain experiences will help to reveal further attitudes or problems. For example, the patient may say, 'I thought I was dying with my heart attack, but I won't die with this', or 'I can't do anything when the pain is bad.'

2. When it starts, how long does it last?

It is important for the nurse to know if the pain lasts minutes or hours. Pain relief methods can be devised to suit the individual. For example, angina may be relieved by rest or only by glyceryl trinitrate.

3. What makes it worse?

Knowledge of aggravating factors allow the nurse to plan her care to avoid those situations whenever possible. Walking will precipitate intermittent claudication or angina. How far the person can walk before having to stop is an indicator of the severity of the underlying condition. It gives an idea of how limited is the mobility of this person. The pain of rheumatoid arthritis may be worst in the morning after a night in bed. Constant chronic pain may be worse in the evening when fatigue has lowered the person's pain tolerance, or it may keep the person awake at night when in a quiet, dark room there is little to distract attention from the pain.

4. What makes it better?

Answers may include information on analgesics from the chemist. Aspirin taken regularly may induce indigestion while codeine-containing compounds may contribute to constipation. Information can be gained about prescribed drugs which relieve pain and are taken regularly. Questions about the effectiveness of such drugs will provide useful information for the doctor who is to prescribe for a person admitted to a hospital or institution. Perhaps a drug is effective only if taken more frequently than prescribed with the risk of accumulation in the body due to delayed metabolism and excretion of drugs in old people (see Chapter 20).

Many people are not consciously aware of their coping strategies or are shy of revealing them. 'What else do you do to make the pain better?' may elicit answers ranging from 'Rest until the angina goes' to 'I keep my knees warm with a flannel bandage'. Perhaps the person moves stiff, aching joints frequently by walking short distances. Counter-irritant creams may be used over painful joints and not being able to use these in hospital may cause the person to become anxious.

'What do you think about to make the pain better?' will help to uncover cognitive coping strategies. Some people can 'lose' themselves in a book or by watching an exciting football match on television. Others may use their imaginations, remembering past scenes or imagining themselves in different surroundings. Some people imagine a scene that makes them feel peaceful, for example, a country walk by a river. They may be shy about sharing their fantasies and need encouragement to do so. The nurse must be non-judgmental in her attitude and support the person by admitting that most people have an active fantasy life. The coping strategies that are positive, relieving pain and promoting health should be encouraged and made part of a care plan.

5. Where is it?

Location of pain can be an important indication of the cause. However, because sensory stimuli to an ageing brain may merge with background brain activity, some elderly people find it difficult to be specific about location of pain. This is particularly true of pain from internal organs. Visceral pain is usually experienced as referred pain, the pain being experienced as located in an area distant from the site of disease but within the area supplied by the stimulated sensory nerve. The person in pain may be vague as to the exact location. Pathy (1967) found that of a sample of elderly patients who had had a recent myocardial infarction only 19% said they had chest pain. Pain is decreased or may be absent in other acute conditions and the nurse must include other physiological as well as psychological measures to monitor the condition of the patient.

Asking the patient to touch the pain or the painful area will help to identify its location. Hunt et al (1977) found differences between the patient's and the nurse's perception of where the pain was located. Using a front and rear view body diagram, patients were asked to shade in all the areas that were painful. When nurses were asked to do the same, they were aware of fewer sites of pain with a more confined distribution. Raiman (1981) describes the London Hospital pain chart (Fig. 17.1) which was developed as a result of the work of Hunt et al (1977). The patient is asked to shade in all painful areas and indicate the intensity of the pain in each area. It may be that pressure is contributing to the total pain experience, and so relieving the pressure will decrease the pain and reduce the need for analgesic drugs.

6. What does it feel like?

Asking the person to describe what they are feeling helps the nurse to understand and share the experience. The words used may indicate the emotional response of the person to pain. Research into the words used to describe clinical pain has revealed that in some instances these words can discriminate between people suffering from specific disorders. Reading et al (1979) were able to discriminate between women attending the gynaecology outpatient department with primary dysmenorrhoea from those with dysmenorrhoea secondary to an intrauterine contraceptive device. Each group of woman used different words to describe their pain. Bourbonnais (1981) found post-operative

patients most frequently used 18 words or phrases to describe their pain, e.g. tender, crushing, squeezing, sharp, burning, sore, aching, gnawing.

7. How bad is it?

The intensity of the pain is important especially for the evaluation of pain relief. This information completes the picture of the pain experience. A visual analogue scale (VAS) or 10 cm line is a useful device which enables the nurse to understand the intensity of the pain experienced by another. Bourbounais' (1981) pain ruler uses a vertical line with 0—no pain at the bottom and 10—uncontrolled pain at the top. The mark 5 is labelled moderate pain while marks 7–9 are labelled extreme pain interfering with activities. The London Hospital pain chart (Fig. 17.1) includes a six-point scale for rating pain intensity.

Using a scale, the nurse can ask: How bad is the pain right now? How bad is the pain at its worst? How intense is the pain after the most effective method of pain relief? Which method is most effective and how long does it take to reduce the pain? These questions provide useful information for care planning.

This interview will take some time during which the person has been asked to focus her attention on her pain experience. For some people this can result in a more acute awareness of pain which may be distressing. Offer analgesics or some method of pain relief after the interview. Reassure the person that such an interview will not be repeated. Frequent monitoring of pain and its relief will take much less time. If pain is severe and has resisted previous attempts at control, then a pain chart is a useful method of assessing pain regularly and is less distressing than the initial interview.

Problem definition

Unless the cause of the pain is known, appropriate interventions are difficult to devise. The problem should be written stating

This chart records where a patient's pain is, and how bad it is, by the nurse asking the patient at regular intervals. Any regular time interval may be chosen; otherwise, if anagesics are given only 'as required', make observations 2-hourly, but if analgesics are being given regularly, make observations with each dose and half-way between each dose.

Using the chart
1 Ask the patient to mark all his or her pains on the body diagram below. Label each site of pain with a letter (i.e. A, B, C etc).
2 At each observation time, ask the patient:
- to assess the pain since the last observation, using the scale above the body diagram. Take each site separately, and enter the number or letter in the appropriate column
- to assess the pain overall since the last observation, using the same scale. Enter in column marked 'All'
- ask for comments and record them
3 Write down any analgesic given since last observation – name, dose, route and time given.
4 Write down your own comments and any other action taken to relieve pain, including nursing care. Use the back of the chart as well, if necessary.

Excruciating	5
Very severe	4
Severe	3
Moderate	2
Just noticeable	1
No pain at all	0
Patient sleeping	S

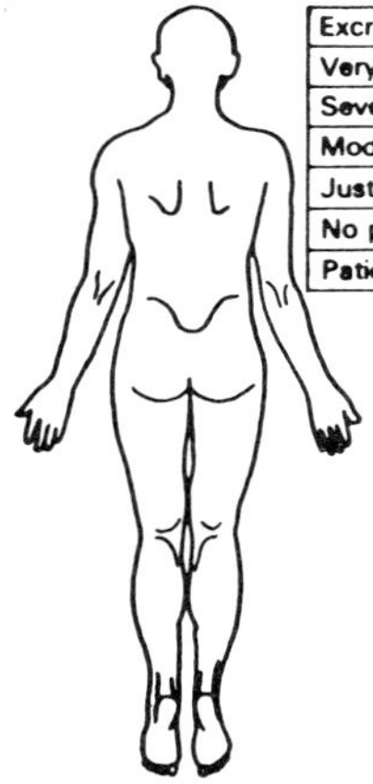

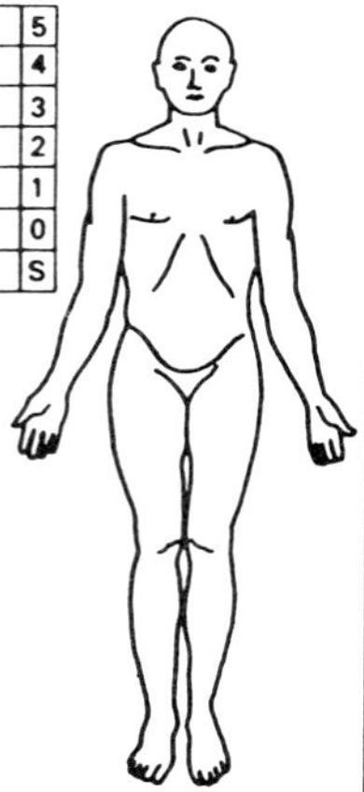

Sheet number

Patient identification label

Date and time	Sites									Analgesic given (name, dose, route and time)	Patient's comment	Comment and action (Nursing care)	Initial
	A	B	C	D	E	F	G	H	All				

Fig. 17.1 The London Hospital pain chart.

Source: Raiman (1981) Reproduced by permission of Jennifer Raiman, The London Hospital, Department of Pharmacology and Therapeutics, and Nursing Journal.

a causal relationship where possible, for example 'Pain in the right hip related to osteoarthrosis, or 'Pain in the thoracic region related to osteoporosis and vertebrae collapse'. Although the medical treatment of osteoarthrosis or osteoporosis is not the responsibility of the nurse, her knowledge of the anatomy, physiology and pathology involved will help her to plan care designed to limit further damage, reduce pain and enable the person to continue to function within the limits imposed by the disorder.

The pain itself may cause other problems, for example a reduction in mobility with consequent danger of damage to pressure areas or the increased risk of a chest infection. In this case, the outcome of pain can be included in the problem statement, for example 'Pain in the right hip related to osteoarthrosis and severely limiting mobility' or 'Limited mobility related to osteoarthrosis and pain in the right hip'. In this way, nursing interventions can be linked together and evaluation of care can be planned in terms of both a reduction in pain and an increase in observed mobility.

CARE PLANNING

Aims of care

Having defined the cause of the pain and its consequences, the aims of care are stated in terms of observable or measurable patient behaviour written within a realistic time frame. If a pain chart is to be used to measure pain control, then the first aim will be that the intensity of the pain is less than it was. The aim of care could be stated as 'The intensity of pain will be three or less using the London Hospital pain chart every 3 hours', or 'The patient will be able to walk to the toilet as necessary with no pain'. Once pain control is established, the aim of care can be that pain relief is maintained and pain is measured at 0–2 on a 10 cm scale.

The nurse's knowledge of drugs and other treatments is important here. If anti-inflammatory drugs are prescribed, the nurse must know how long they will take to be effective. Analgesics may be prescribed at the same time. If the underlying cause of the pain is an inflammatory process then in time the dose and frequency of analgesics should decrease as the inflammation subsides. If depression is a feature of this person's problems then the nurse should know how long antidepressent drugs take to be effective. Some tricyclic antidepressants rely on accumulation of the drug so a delay of 10 days is expected before elevation of mood occurs. If anxiety is a feature of the pain then the aims of care may include the patient's report of feeling less anxious as well as a reduction in a raised pulse rate and blood pressure. As was discussed earlier, an ageing person's central nervous system takes longer to be aroused, but once the homeostatic maintenance of pulse and blood pressure have been stimulated, they take longer to return to baseline functioning. This is of particular importance for elderly people with heart disease or hypertension. Further strain on the heart imposed by anxiety could further impair its function, with consequent alterations in blood flow to the brain, liver and kidneys and deteriorating function of those vital organs. Aims of care concerned with anxiety need a longer time frame before a return to normal activity can be expected.

Care prescriptions

The interventions are chosen to fulfil the aims of care in the light of the problem statement. Nursing care to be carried out should be written clearly and simply so that any person looking after the patient knows exactly what to do. Continuity of care is important so that evaluation of care can be effective. Each nurse should give the same care until its effectiveness has been evaluated. If care is changed before evaluation, then the change cannot be attributed to the care prescribed since it may be due to the change in care. Differences in care given may result in fluctuations in the patient's response to care and any useful intervention will not become apparent.

Chronic pain

This is pain that has been present for months or more. The intensity may be moderate or severe, but its persistent presence has enabled the nervous system to adapt and the physiological, psychological and behavioural manifestations will be less obvious or different from those of acute pain. The pulse rate and blood pressure may not rise with chronic pain and the person's coping strategies may enable them to function in spite of pain.

Musculoskeletal disorders. Osteoarthrosis is a disorder characterised by relapses and remissions. Hooker (1978) reports a study which found that pain and stiffness seemed related to the weather. Patients in a temperature regulated hospital environment could tell if there had been a frost or if it would rain tomorrow. When joints are diseased, then muscular function is also altered. Muscles may go into spasm to protect an eroded joint surface with resulting immobility and reduced circulation impeding both the nutrition and elimination of waste products from the affected parts. Accumulated waste products can contribute to the pain.

Rheumatoid arthritis. This is a systemic illness characterised by remission and relapse. The person in relapse feels ill as well as being in severe pain. The pain is present continuously, reducing to a dull ache in a remission stage. When a person feels ill then tolerance to pain is reduced and previous coping strategies may fail. The return of a relapse with severe pain and general illness may result in depression or confusion, and these symptoms may be the first clues the nurse has that a relapse is in progress.

Parkinson's disease. Although this is a disorder of the central nervous system it results in muscular rigidity and this causes aches and pains. The flow of blood through affected muscles is impaired with resulting reduction in oxygenation and nutrition and impaired elimination of waste products which can cause pain. The muscle spasm causing the rigidity is also a cause of pain.

Stroke. This, too, is a central nervous system disorder, but aches and pain can arise from the resulting hemiplegia. The shoulder joint is anatomically shallow and owes its stability mainly to the large number of muscles which encircle and support it. When the muscles of the shoulder girdle are paralysed, then the stability of the joint is compromised. Any strain on the joint, perhaps related to the handling of the patient during nursing care, can result in subluxation of the joint with the space between the head of the humerus and the glenoid fossa being increased. This puts a strain on the joint capsule, resulting in inflammation and pain. Careful handling of the weakened shoulder joint is essential. All the joints of the paralysed side need to be exercised gently at regular intervals or stiffness of joints occurs. The risk of muscular atrophy increases but when these stiff joints are moved they cause pain. This pain on movement can encourage the patient to remain immobile with resulting delay in possible rehabilitation.

Interventions

Drugs

Although drug treatment is the responsibility of the doctor, the monitoring of the effectiveness of such treatment is often delegated to the nurse. The treatment of hypertension is usually monitored by the nurse's regular recording of blood pressure. The monitoring of the effectiveness of pain relief can be achieved in a similar way, by the regular use of a pain chart until an effective regime is established. The ageing process alters the absorption, distribution, metabolism and elimination of drugs (see Chapter 20). Where analgesics, anti-inflammatory drugs and antidepressant drugs are given to the same person, signs of toxicity or interaction must also be monitored. Any alteration in the level of conscious awareness or the onset of mental confusion in patients taking these drugs warrants a close look at the functioning of all the body systems with particular attention to fluid balance. Some elderly people restrict their fluid intake in order to reduce urination. This can result in a fluid intake that is insufficient to ensure adequate elimination of drugs from the body.

Coping strategies

Patients with past experience of pain may have a variety of ways of coping. During assessment these strategies will have been identified. Copp (1974) reported distraction strategies such as counting tiles on the ceiling or flowers on the curtains, whistling or talking a lot. The most appropriate of these coping strategies can be included among the interventions and the patient encouraged to continue their use.

Distraction

Distraction can be provided by the patient's imagination. Some patients become anxious in anticipation of a procedure. Being turned regularly while in bed can be potentially painful and anxiety provoking for a patient with arthritis or a fracture. Such a person can be helped to find a scene which she finds fascinating and on which she can concentrate during the procedure. The scene should be pleasant and interesting but not anxiety provoking. The patient can practise day-dreaming or concentrating on the scene before the procedure starts. Her conscious attention is held by the scene and unpleasant sensations or anxieties aroused tend to disappear. Distraction does not replace adequate analgesia but can help to make a potentially distressing event more pleasant.

Any sensory input can provide useful distraction from pain. For those with poor concentration the type of distraction may have to change frequently in order to be useful. Watching a favourite television programme can be diverting, while sitting in front of a television for long periods can become boring.

Relaxation

McCaffery (1972) defined relaxation as a state of freedom from anxiety and skeletomuscular tension. The mind and body function as a unit with events affecting one part also affecting the whole. Since an elderly person takes longer to recover from the effects of anxiety, relaxation can aid this recovery. From the literature reported earlier, muscular tension is increased in depressed people reporting pain. The rigidity of Parkinson's disease can also be painful. Learning to relax can help to reduce anxiety and the aches and pains of muscular tension.

Progressive relaxation exercise. Jacobson (1974) stated that anxiety and muscular relaxation produce opposite physiological effects and therefore cannot exist together. Progressive relaxation exercise teaches discriminatory control over skeletal muscle until the subject can produce low levels of tone in major muscle groups. McCaffery (1979) stated that relaxation can reduce potentially painful stimuli by reducing painful muscle contraction. She also found relaxation to be a good way for patients in pain to combat fatigue and unwanted sleepiness. A period of relaxation before visitors arrive can help the patient to maintain relationships with family and friends, which is an important factor in increasing life satisfaction. Gollop (1983) describes in detail the teaching of progressive relaxation exercise. Once learned, this technique is something the patient can do for herself, so regaining some personal control, which is one factor in raising self-esteem. Reduction in muscular tension may alter the blood flow through muscle groups, allowing waste products to be eliminated more easily. Feelings of warmth and well-being have been reported after relaxation. Christoph et al (1978) reported that the physiological response to progressive relaxation will differ from one person to another but there is some indication of a reduction in autonomic arousal with a slower respiratory rate and a drop in pulse rate and blood pressure.

Breathing

Pelletier (1977) reported breathing patterns to

be indications of emotional states. Breathing becomes irregular with anger, faster with anxiety and slow and deep with relaxation. For older people with respiratory disease, increased or irregular respiratory rates may be related to chronic bronchitis or emphysema. A respiratory assessment will be necessary before breathing exercises are taught to assess the implications for the patient of altering the respiratory pattern. When muscular relaxation has been achieved by progressive relaxation exercises, the patient can be told to notice her breathing. Respiration is slowed by relaxation, and passive attention to the deep, slow, ebb and flow of the breath can help to calm the mind by 'letting go' more fully on the passive exhalation. Also muscular relaxation can be increased. The slowness of respiration prevents hyperventilation which must be avoided.

Some people are able to relax by taking slow, deep breaths and relaxing while exhaling. Although this may come only after practice it can be useful when anticipating a distressing event. Slow, rhythmic breathing without relaxation can distract from pain. Breathing to a count of 'In, one, two, three—out, one, two, three' can help to reduce anxiety. Inspiration and exhalation should be slow and easy without a pause. Rapid inhalation and breath holding is to be avoided, as is hyperventilation. Rapid changes in blood gas composition are detrimental to the patient. Rapid, deep breathing can reduce carbon dioxide levels, leaving the patient giddy and nauseated. Breath holding increases muscular tension and alters the flow of blood within the brain and thoracic organs. When combined with relaxation and tailored to the physiological status of an individual, breathing exercises can aid oxygenation of tissues, leaving the patient feeling alert and well.

Guided imagery

This uses a person's ability to imagine pictures, sounds, smells and tactile sensations. Memories or daydreams can take this form. The use of imagery as distraction during distressing procedures has been discussed above. In this context, imagery or visualisation is used to achieve a specific therapeutic goal. Some methods of psychotherapy use symbolic visualisation to aid psychological integration and growth. Jung's (1963) active imagination and Leuner's (1969) guided affective imagery are two examples. During progressive relaxation exercises the person can be asked to identify tension-producing situations. She visualises one of these, then relaxes or eliminates the image, learning to reduce or eliminate the anxiety connected to a particular situation.

McCaffery (1979) reported on the use of guided imagery in the treatment of chronic pain. For these patients treated in a pain centre, the imagery was aimed at reducing the intensity of the pain, eliminating it altogether or producing temporary anaesthesia of a painful area. Gollop (1983) describes the technique and suitable visualisations with instructions for the teaching of such an intervention.

Implementation

The written care plan is a source of information for all the nurses who are to care for a particular person. The nurse planning the care involves the patient, explaining the care to be given and how it will help her. The literature discussed above suggests that allowing a person a measure of control helps to raise her self-esteem. Allowing the elderly person to control appropriate aspects of care can become an intervention to reduce chronic pain by raising self-esteem. The timing of certain aspects of care can be negotiated with the patient, helping her to realise that she is recognised as an individual person rather than one of a group of elderly patients in an institution. The communication of the person's preferences in food, drink, clothing or recreational activities by the written care plan helps each nurse giving care to see the patient as an individual person.

The care plan should be communicated to

the other professionals involved in the care of the patient and their advice sought about the interventions chosen to solve problems which involve their expertise. The physiotherapist and the nurse working together to fulfil the same goals will mobilise the elderly person more effectively. The speech therapist will have valuable suggestions for helping a patient to make her needs known more easily.

Evaluation

This is designed to measure the effectiveness of the care given. If the aims of care are stated using observable or measurable changes in the response of a person to pain, and the care given is designed to achieve the aims, then evaluation of the care involves assessing whether the aims are reached. The continued use of a pain chart will enable the nurse to document a change in the intensity of pain in different areas of the body and the frequency and dose of analgesics received. The patient's comments are recorded, as are the nursing interventions used. The nurse's comments should be relevant to the aims of care. Perhaps the older person is more alert and co-operative. Perhaps she is more active or seems happier and more outgoing.

The frequency of evaluation will depend in part on the type of intervention used and the length of time it takes to be effective. If oral analgesics are prescribed to be given on a 4–6 hourly, as necessary, basis, then the use of a pain chart at three hourly intervals will enable the nurse to establish how often the drug is needed. Once control is established, then the pain chart could be discontinued. Pain assessment should be continued for as long as the nursing interventions are carried out. If pain impairs mobility, then the continuing use of a mobility assessment tool could become part of the evaluation of pain relief. A deterioration in mobility or an increase in pain would then warrant reassessment of pain and the reintro-duction of a pain chart.

If progressive relaxation exercises are used, then the recording of pulse and respiration rates and blood pressure before and after the exercise will establish each person's response to it. A reduction in pulse rate and blood pressure can indicate relaxation and reduction of anxiety. An elderly person with cardio-vascular disease may respond to relaxation in an individual way and this response should be known by the nurse. If the blood pressure has dropped considerably the person should not attempt to get up too quickly, risking postural hypotension. The individual's comments on such an intervention are important, although physiological measurements are relevant. The person's view of how she feels and how effec-tive the intervention is being may give valuable insight into her willingness to continue. If a guided image is used, the person's response to the image may reveal anxiety aroused by part of it or her inability to visualise it fully. The image can be altered to suit the person's response and eliminate anxiety or enhance the visualisation.

Once the person has learned to use the technique effectively she can continue its use herself. Discussion with the old person will help the nurse to plan time when she can use the technique. By enabling the person to choose when she uses relaxation or an image, the nurse helps her to achieve some degree of control over her pain or discomfort, with a resulting rise in self-esteem and increased feelings of independence.

If several interventions are combined, then evaluation of the effectiveness of each one is important to determine its contribution to pain relief as a whole. The pain chart would be adapted to evaluate all interventions and so give a complete picture of the effectiveness of the whole regime. Both pain assessment and evaluation of interventions rely on the person's ability to communicate her experi-ence. Although measurable and observable responses are important, they give an incom-plete picture without the person's perceptions of her experience. The patient's satisfaction with pain relief is one of the most important indicators of the effectiveness of nursing care in this area.

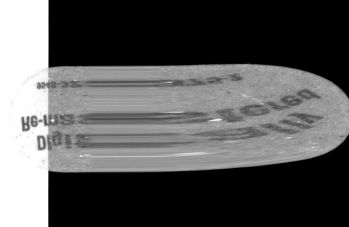

REFERENCES

Bourbonnais F 1981 Pain assessment: development of a tool for the nurse and the patient. Journal of Advanced Nursing 6: 227–282

Christoph P, Luborsky L, Kron R, Fishmal H 1978 Blood pressure, heart rate and respiratory responses to a single session of relaxation: a partial replication. Journal of Psychosomatic Research 22: 493–501

Cohen K P 1979 Hospice: prescription for terminal care. Aspen Systems Corps, Germantown, Maryland

Copp L A 1974 The spectrum of suffering. American Journal of Nursing 74: 491–495

Elton D, Stanley G V, Burrows G D 1978 self-esteem and chronic pain. Journal of Psychosomatic Research 22: 25–30

Gollop S M 1983 Pain and pain control. In: J Wilson Barnett (ed) Patient Teaching. Churchill Livingstone, Edinburgh

Hooker S 1978 Caring for elderly people. Routledge and Kegan Paul, London

Hunt J, Stollar J D, Littlejohns D W, Twycross R G, Vere D W 1977 Patients with protracted pain: a survey conducted at the London Hospital. Journal of Medical Ethics 3: 61–73

Jacobson E 1974 Progressive relaxation, 3rd edn. University of Chicago Press, Chicago

Jacox A 1979 Assessing pain. American Journal of Nursing 79: 895–900

Jung C G 1963 Memories, dreams, reflections. Vintage Books, New York

Leuner H 1969 Guided affective imagery. American Journal of Psychotherapy 23: 4–22

Lewis G 1978 The place of pain in human experience. Journal of Medical Ethics 4: 122–125

Longino C F and Kart C S 1982 Explicating activity theory: a formal replication. Journal of Gerontology 6: 713–722

McCaffery M 1972 Nursing management of the patient with pain. Lippincott, Philadelphia

McCaffery M 1979 Nursing management of the patient with pain, 2nd edn. Lippincott, Philadelphia

Merskey H, Spear F G 1967 Pain: psychological and psychiatric aspects. Baillière Tindall and Cassell, London

Pathy M S 1967 Clinical presentation of myocardial infarction in the elderly. British Heart Journal 29: 190–199

Pelletier K R 1977 Mind as healer; mind as slayer: a holistic approach to preventing stress disorders. Dell, New York

Raiman J 1981 Responding to pain. Nursing 31: 1362–1365

Reading A E, Reed C, Newton J R 1979 A card sort method for pain assessment in gynaecology: a multidimensional approach. Acta Obstetrics et Gynaecologica Scandinavica 58: 105–113

Schultz R 1982 Emotionality and aging: a theoretical and empirical analysis. Journal of Gerontology 37(1): 42–51

Skevington S M 1983 Chronic pain and depression: universal or personal helplessness? Pain 15: 309–317

Sternbach R A 1968 Pain: a psychophysiological analysis. Academic press, New York

Timiras P S, Vernadakis A 1972 Structural, biochemical and functional aging of the nervous system. In: Timiras P S (ed) Developmental physiology and aging. Macmillan, New York

von Knorring L, Perris C, Eisemann M, Eriksson U, Perris H 1983 Pain as a symptom in depressive disorders 1: Relationship to diagnostic subgroup and depressive symptomatology. Pain 15: 19–26

Weisenberger M 1977 Pain and pain control. Psychological Bulletin 84(5): 1008–1044

Welford A 1980 Sensory, perceptual and motor processes in older adults. In: Birren J E, Sloane R B (eds) Handbook of mental health and aging. Prentice Hall, Englewood Cliffs New Jersey

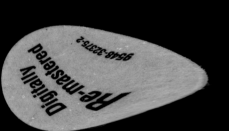

18

J. I. Brooking

Dementia and confusion in the elderly

INTRODUCTION

Distinctions between normal ageing, dementia and confusion

In old age many people suffer impairment of cognitive, emotional and social functioning. In mild form these are regarded as non-pathological age-related changes. There has been some debate about whether dementia could be distinguished from normal ageing. The current view according to Levy and Post (1982) is that dementia is quantitatively and probably qualitatively different from the normal ageing process.

In unfavourable circumstances, patients suffering from confusional states do not make a full recovery. Cognitive and personality defects may remain and stay static for many years. Such patients are not however dement*ing*, but have dement*ed*.

Nurses sometimes incorrectly use the terms dementia and confusion interchangeably. This difficulty arises because patients with dementia are invariably confused. It is hoped that this chapter will show that it is important to recognise the distinctions between the two conditions, as the care required for each may be very different.

Dementia can be defined as a steadily progressive and usually irreversible decline in previously normal mental function, which is associated with detectable brain pathology.

Confusion is an acute or subacute alteration in previously normal mental function, which is often temporary and reversible, associated with impaired brain function usually secondary to a pathological process outside the nervous system.

Classification of dementias

Dementias are termed senile or pre-senile, according to the age of onset—before or after 65 years. This chapter is mainly concerned with senile dementia. However, pre-senile dementia must be mentioned since these patients may come into the psychogeriatric services, as few provisions exist for them elsewhere. Others may appear in psychogeriatric wards some years after diagnosis. There has been uncertainty about appropriate terminology for two reasons. Firstly, scientific understanding of the nature of dementia has increased and some early diagnostic categories found to be inaccurate, e.g. evidence has accumulated that in the absence of infarcts, cerebral arteriosclerosis is unlikely to produce detectable dementia (Levy and Post 1982). Secondly, some believed that the term dementia carried a stigma. Many writers made cosmetic attempts to develop new names for the same disease, e.g. organic brain syndrome, brain failure and cerebral atrophy. These created endless misunderstandings.

The classification outlined below has the advantage of being simple, logical and based on research evidence.

Pre-senile dementias

Several rare diseases have been described as pre-senile dementias. These include Pick's disease, Huntington's chorea, Jakob Cruetzfeldt disease, normal pressure hydrocephalus and neurosyphilis (Miller 1977). Alzheimer's disease is more common and has a bimodal distribution with peaks at ages 40 to 54 and 70 to 84 (Katzman et al 1978). Thus early onset Alzheimer's disease accounts for many cases of pre-senile dementia.

Senile dementias

In the past, many subdivisions of senile dementia were described, but recent evidence shows these to have doubtful validity (Levy and Post 1982). A workshop in the United States (Katzman et al 1978) concluded that Alzheimer's disease accounts for over half of all cases. Less than a fifth of patients have what is now termed multi-infarct dementia. This is a more accurate term for what used to be called arteriosclerotic dementia.

Classification and mechanisms of confusion

Confusional states are classified according to whether or not the onset is acute and the condition of short duration, or subacute onset and longer duration. The condition may also be classified according to its underlying cause, which will be discussed later.

The mechanisms of confusion in the elderly are not fully understood. Grimley Evans (1982) hypothesised that they were more prone to delirium than the young because of increased neural 'noise' and an impaired blood–brain barrier. He suggested that when neural noise is further increased by random neurotransmitter activity, there is interference to perception, attention, memory, etc.

The pathology of dementia

Some or all of the following changes have been found in the brains of demented patients. The brain cells atrophy mainly in the cerebral cortex. The ventricles enlarge and the gyri are flattened with widening of the sulci. There may be a deficiency of acetylcholine in the cortical and subcortical areas. Microscopiscally, senile plaques, neurofibrillary tangles and granulovacuolar degeneration occur (Miller 1977).

The aetiology of dementia

Some possible risk factors identified by the American workshop (Katzman et al 1978) include a genetic link, increased brain aluminium concentration, latent viral infections, immunological factors and neuro-transmitters. There is thought to be no association with social class, previous intelligence or geographical distribution.

ASSESSMENT

Principles of assessment in psychogeriatric nursing

Initially, a normal comprehensive nursing assessment as used with all elderly patients should be carried out. However, some additional information is required for patients with psychiatric problems. This section will focus on these additional aspects.

Sources of information used to supplement the current nursing assessment

The psychogeriatrician's assessment will include a psychiatric history and mental status examination. Neurological examination and tests will be carried out as required, e.g. brain scans, lumbar puncture for cerebrospinal fluid (CSF), electro-encephalogram (EEG), etc.

Clinical psychologists use a range of psychometric and other types of tests to aid diagnosis and pinpoint functional deficits. These include tests of intelligence, various aspects of personality, memory, level of depression and dependency rating scales. Nurses must be willing to discuss the meaning of test results with psychologists.

Notes from other professionals' assessments may include assessments carried out by occupational therapists, social workers, physiotherapists, recreation officers, etc. They can provide valuable information and should be used to avoid time-wasting duplication of data gathering.

Nursing notes from previous hospital admissions and community care are useful to determine how the patient's condition has changed over time.

Developing an assessment schedule for psychogeriatric nursing

Various assessment schedules are available, mainly in American textbooks of psycho-geriatrics, e.g. Wolanin and Phillips (1981). Although comprehensive, these schedules tend to be complicated and time-consuming. In this country many hospitals have developed their own assessment schedules, designed specifically for the kinds of patient groups with whom they work, e.g. acute, rehabilitation or long stay. At local level it is helpful to develop methods of assessment which avoid excessive overlap with other professions. Nurses should assess all basic human needs (Henderson 1969) and associated activities of daily living, patterns of alcohol, drug and tobacco use, sexual functioning, sensoriperceptual capabilities, capacity for independent living and rehabilitation, suitability of environment in which care is taking place, mental status (discussed later), response of patient and family to the illness, and hospital care and treatment, the patient's life-history, socio-economic and cultural background, education and occupation and quality of relationships with family, friends and neighbours.

Mental status examination

A psychiatric history and assessment of current mental status would be carried out by an admitting psychiatrist or psychogeriatrician. However, many patients are treated by geriatricians or physicians whose primary focus may be physical and the psychiatric examination may be cursory. This information is thus given to enable nurses to decide what, if any, additional information they need to collect. The mental status examination describes in objective behavioural terms what the patient can and cannot do. It is usual to collect information using some or all of the following headings:
— General appearance and behaviour
— Speech—form and content
— Emotional state and mood
— Hallucinations and delusions
— Orientation
— Memory—recent and remote
— Comprehension
— Intelligence—reasoning, judgment, general

knowledge and ability to calculate
— Abstract thinking
— Level of insight.
For further information see a textbook of psychiatric nursing such as Wilson and Kneisl (1983).

Use of assessment scales

Psychogeriatric nursing is short of valid and reliable objective criterion measures to assess and evaluate nursing problems. There is an urgent need to develop instruments appropriate for use by nurses and sensitive to changes in patient status resulting from nursing interventions. There are, however, some fairly simple scales which can be used by nurses to provide objective assessment and which can be later used to evaluate changes. These include Goldfarb's (1960) simple 10-point scale of cognitive impairment, Beck's (1961) depression inventory, designed for completion by the patient, and Hamilton's (1960) depression scale, rated by the nurse or clinician on the basis of observations over a period.

General points about nursing assessment interviews

Privacy is vital to ensure confidentiality and reduce distractions. The interview should take place in a warm cheerful setting with the patient in a comfortable chair. The nurse should sit at the same level as the patient, ensuring that his or her face and lips are clearly visible. Extraneous noise should be reduced. The nurse should speak clearly, at moderate volume and avoiding jargon, slang and difficult words. She or he should create an unhurried, relaxed atmosphere, putting the patient at ease, and should be interested, empathic and encouraging. The interview should be kept fairly short to avoid fatigue. If necessary information could be collected over two or three meetings rather than tire the patient. The purpose of the interview should be made clear to the patient and potentially stressful questions kept to a minimum. The patient may find the interview therapeutic as she is reviewing and reminiscing. If using scales, the nurse should be aware that they can be tiring, stressful and tend to demoralise by emphasising weaknesses rather than strengths.

Assessing demented patients

Identification of patients' problems

Nursing assessment should focus on the following four areas of functioning within which demented patients experience problems.

Cognitive problems. Memory failure and global intellectual detioration are central. Some patients may confabulate, i.e. unintentionally fill in memory gaps with fabrications. Patients' experience disorientation of time, place, person and self. Disorientation means lack of awareness of one's position relative to the environment. There is an impairment of abstract reasoning and judgment.

Emotional problems. There is emotional blunting and lability, i.e. instability with rapid and inappropriate emotional changes. Some sufferers become depressed, suspicious and irritable. There may be exaggeration of the previous personality or the personality may alter markedly.

Social problems. There is narrowing of interests, loss of motivation, regression and desocialisation. In some cases, superficial social skills may be retained for a long time. Speech becomes anecdotal, repetitive and increasingly meaningless. Domestic skills decline.

Physical problems. There is general physical deterioration and eventually self-care capabilities are lost. Specific neurological features may occur.

Factors influencing the nature and severity of problems

Although the problems described above are all central to dementia, nurses will find that patients' problems vary in nature and severity. The following factors influence these variations and should be considered during the nursing assessment:

Stage of the dementia. Because dementia is progressive, nurses will meet patients at various stages of the disease. Initially, sufferers may exhibit only mild deterioration such as failure to cope with complex tasks or under pressure. The condition gradually deteriorates until eventually the patient is totally helpless and dependent.

Underlying pathology. The general features already described apply to most dementias, particularly Alzheimer's disease. However, each type of pre-senile and senile dementia has a different pathology and consequently slightly different clinical features. This is not important as a determinant of nursing care, but accurate diagnosis may be essential for other reasons. For example, Huntington's chorea is transmitted by a single dominant gene, thus genetic counselling of the offspring of sufferers is crucial.

Extent of compensation. Grimley Evans (1982) described how dementia may remain concealed within families for long periods. Families may engage in collusion, may accept deterioration as normal, may fail to notice because their interactions are always concrete and shallow, or fail to notice because the sufferer restricts her lifestyle so that deficiencies are concealed. This delicate balance can be disrupted by any alteration to the familiar environment, e.g. death of spouse, moving house or a family holiday. These events can lead to acute decompensation and the previously hidden dementia becomes obvious.

Self-fulfilling prophecy. Described by Merton (1957), this is a prophecy which is fulfilled solely because it was made. It may influence the behaviour or feelings of the person who made it, or the person about whom it was made. It was identified as relevant to dementia by MacDonald (1973) and Libow (1978). Nurses may increase dementia in several ways. They may expect 'senility' and treat patients as 'senile', which then fosters it. Secondly, patients may be nursed in an environment which is so unstimulating and lacking in orientation cues, that dementia is worsened. Thirdly, reversible confusional states may be assumed to reflect dementia and ignored, eventually resulting in permanent damage (LaPorte 1982).

Assessing confused patients

Identification of patients' problems

Nursing assessment should include the following four areas of functioning.

Cognitive problems. Patients are usually disorientated in time, place, person and self. They may experience perceptual problems, such as illusions i.e. misunderstanding of a real sensory stimulus, or visual hallucinations, i.e. a false perception occurring without any real sensory stimulus. Memory and learning will be affected and confabulation can occur. The patient cannot concentrate and is easily distracted. Thought processes are sluggish and confused. Information and events may be misunderstood.

Emotional problems. Patients may be anxious, apprehensive, fearful, agitated, perplexed and belligerent.

Social problems. Communication is inevitably disrupted by the cognitive deficits. Speech may become rambling, disorganised and verbose.

Physical problems. These are largely determined by the cause of the confusional state and some patients will be very ill. Confusion is often worse at night or in the dark and sleep may be disturbed. Some patients exhibit stereotyped and perseverating movements. Restlessness may be present.

Factors predisposing to confusion

Identification of the causes of a confusional state is an essential part of nursing assessment for three reasons. Firstly, to enable the nurse to understand and predict the pattern of problems experienced by a patient. Secondly, nurses can help to prevent confusion if they understand the predisposing conditions and try to reduce them at any early stage. Thirdly, the main principle of treatment and care is to search for relevant causes and remove or reduce them. The main causes are discussed under nine headings.

Pharmacological causes. Drug-induced confusion may be a side-effect or a withdrawal effect and even quite small dosages may induce toxicity in the elderly. Examples of drugs commonly associated with toxicity include levodopa, steroids, diuretics, anti-hypertensives, insulin and oral hypogly-caemics, digitalis, barbiturates, benzodiazepines and other psychotropic drugs. The high incidence of drug-induced confusion points to the need for regular drug review and close monitoring.

Nutritional deficiencies. This may be general malnutrition or specific vitamin deficiencies.

General medical conditions. These include cardiac, hepatic and renal diseases. Other conditions which may precipitate acute confusional states are alcoholism, anaemia, hypotension and hypothermia.

Infections. Any systemic infection with high fever involving dehydration and electrolyte imbalance may cause confusion. Most commonly, this includes pneumonia, septi-caemia and pyelitis.

Endocrine disorders. Any hormonal imbalance may be a causative factor. These include thyroid, pancreatic, pituitary or adrenal cortex disease.

Neurological conditions. These include trauma, neoplasms, anoxia, infections and haemorrhages involving the nervous system. Epilepsy, strokes and dementia also increase the risk of confusional states.

Surgical causes. Confusional states are sometimes precipitated by major surgery, especially to the heart, brain, eye and repro-ductive organs. Other causes include prolonged anaesthesia, shock, electrolyte imbalance, pain and anxiety.

Environmental causes. Patients may lack sensory supports such as spectacles and hearing aids to enable them to perceive their environment correctly. Hospital wards are often noisy and confusing, lacking familiar objects, clocks and calendars, etc. The general disturbance of the ward may cause sleep disruption and the normal cycle of light and dark may be interrupted, e.g. intensive care unit lights on all the time. Armstrong-Esther and Hawkins (1982) argued that admission to hospital could eliminate the social cues, which elderly people need to maintain synchron-isation of circadian rhythms. They argued that if desynchronisation occurred this could lead to confusion, sleep disturbances and incontinence.

Psychological causes. The importance of the self-fulfilling prophecy has already been mentioned. Once a patient has been labelled as confused, the ward staff often sustain the confusion by their behaviour (Chisholm et al 1982). Other important psychological factors include depersonalisation, loss of personal control over events and self, stress and anxiety and social isolation.

PLANNING AND IMPLEMENTATION OF CARE

Two types of goals need to be formulated for psychogeriatric patients: overall aims of care and specific problem-oriented goals. It is first necessary to consider the overall aim as this will largely determine goals for individual problems. The overall aims should include the appropriate level of independence likely to be achieved, the probability of full recovery and discharge home, or whether enhancing the quality of remaining life and ensuring a peaceful death are more appropriate. Nurses planning care should collaborate with the whole health care team, so that an overall policy for a particular patient can be agreed upon. Secondly, short- and long-term goals should be formulated for each specific patient problem.

The roles of nurse, doctor and other professional workers tend to be fairly blurred in psychogeriatric care. With the obvious exception of the medical treatments, the nurse could and should be the initiator of all the care and treatment activities which will be described. In practice, nurses too often concern them-selves only with routine physical care, and other treatments are initiated by occupational therapists, clinical psychologists, social workers, physiotherapists, doctors and volunteers. This need not be the case.

Care required for demented patients

Participation of the nurse in medical treatment

There are currently no effective medical treatments to reverse or slow down the degenerative process of dementia. Patients may be given tranquillisers, antidepressants or sedatives as symptomatic treatment. Cerebrovascular dilators such as cyclospasmol (cyclandelate) are occasionally used to increase cortical perfusion where cerebral arteriosclerosis exists. Ribonucleic acid (RNA), alleged to be a substrate of memory, has been used experimentally, but without convincing results. Hyperbaric oxygen treatment has also been tried experimentally, but reviewers conclude that there is little evidence of efficacy (Katzman et al 1978).

Psychological methods of treatment

Stimulation and activity. Studies reviewed by Holden and Woods (1982) suggest that the elderly are often deprived of sensory stimulation, which can increase confusion. Mental stimulation can have beneficial effects on cognitive function. Reviewing studies, Miller (1977) concluded that increased social stimulation of institutionalised demented patients would enhance the quality and quantity of their social interactions. But gains often disappear once the intervention is withdrawn. It is necessary to devise a permanently stimulating environment to maintain improvement. A range of interesting and engaging activities should be offered to patients, including discussions, music, films, games, outings, visitors, occasional parties, etc. Powell (1974) and Diesfeldt and Diesfeldt-Groenendijk (1977) found that structured physical exercise produced improvements in cognitive functioning. Physical activity offered to

demented patients should include walking, ball games, keep-fit exercises, skittles, dancing, etc.

Changes to the physical environment. This can be as simple as rearranging furniture so as to encourage social interaction. Peterson et al (1977) rearranged chairs in a psychogeriatric ward from straight lines round the walls to small groups. This led to an increase in social interaction among patients. Similarly, if patients eat at small rather than large tables they are more likely to talk to each other. Most people are not used to interacting in large groups. Furniture arrangements which bring together about four to six patients parallel family and work groups.

Environmental changes can be more drastic. Marston and Gupta (1977) suggested that large wards or old people's Homes should be divided into small living units of eight to 12 people. Holden and Woods (1982) reported that these arrangments seem to reduce confusion and incontinence and residents become more vocal and active. When making changes it is important to remember patients' needs for privacy and personal territory.

Increasing patient participation and choice. There have been several experiments with the institutionalised elderly in which patient participation, control and predictability were manipulated. Unfortunately the extent to which the subjects were demented is not indicated. Schultz (1976) in a well-controlled experiment found that predictable positive events had a powerful beneficial effect on indicators of physical and psychological status as well as level of activity. Langer and Rodin (1976) in a conceptually similar study gave an experimental group a communication emphasising their responsibility for themselves. They were given several choices and responsibility for looking after a plant. In comparison with a control group, the experimental group showed significant improvements in alertness, active participation, happiness, level of activity and general sense of well-being.

Both experiments included follow-up studies, but these produced equivocal findings. Rodin and Langer (1977) found that differences between the two groups were maintained and they concluded that decline of the aged can be slowed or reversed by inducing an increased sense of personal control. In his follow-up, Schultz (1980) found that the effects of the intervention had been temporary. This suggests that in order to maintain improvements, increased patient participation and choice need to be continued indefinitely.

Behavioural methods. These are based on the principles of operant conditioning developed by Skinner (1953) and later psychologists. The basic principle is that if a behaviour is rewarded or reinforced, this increases the likelihood of its being repeated. Conversely, if a behaviour is ignored or punished, the likelihood of repetition is decreased. Reinforcers take many forms, e.g. smile, praise, food, money or privileges. It does require that the subject is sufficiently cognitively intact to learn the association between her behaviour and the reward. Holden and Woods (1982) reviewed some evidence that demented patients could learn new things. Reward must be immediate. Delayed feedback or reward is not nearly so powerful in modifying behaviour.

Studies have been carried out with elderly patients demonstrating improvements in specific behaviours, such as eating, mobility, continence, participation in purposeful activities and social and verbal interaction. In a detailed review of studies, Holden and Woods (1982) concluded that behaviour modification is an extremely promising approach, but there is insufficient evidence of its effectiveness with demented patients.

General programmes for all patients on a ward have been tried. For example, Mishara and Kastenbaum (1973) evaluated a token-economy programme with elderly psychiatric patients. Patients were given tokens as rewards for specified behaviour, tokens which could be exchanged for privileges or cigarettes, wine, extra food, etc. The programme was successful in that patients became more independent in performing self-care tasks.

Reality orientation (RO) was originated in the United States by Folsom in about 1958 (Taulbee and Folsom 1966). The first published account of its use in Britain was by Brook et al (1975). It is one of the first therapeutic techniques of a psychological nature designed for use with demented patients. According to Murray et al (1980) RO is intended to maintain reality contact and to reverse or halt confusion, disorientation, social withdrawal and apathy. It enables the patient to relearn and then continually use a range of basic information relating to her orientation. RO consists of two main components—informal or 24 hour RO and formal or classroom RO.

Staff attitudes are an essential prerequisite and a consistent approach, geared to the patient's needs and personality, should be maintained by all staff. Staff should allow patients individuality, dignity, choice and independence. In informal RO orientation cues are provided in the environment, e.g. clocks, calendars, menus, name tags and names of rooms on doors. Staff present current information to the patient during every interaction. Realistic responses are rewarded with smiles and supportive statements.

During formal or classroom RO a small group of patients meet daily with a familiar staff member. This is to teach information related to orientation, establish group participation and develop interpersonal relationships. The content of the group work is adjusted to suit the level of cognitive functioning of the group.

Several reviews of evaluation studies have appeared recently, e.g. Burton (1982), Powell Proctor and Miller (1982), and Holden and Woods (1982). All have pointed out the difficulty of drawing conclusions about the effectiveness of RO because the evaluation studies tend not to be comparable and many are methodologically unsound. However, it is clear that RO brings about improvements in patients' orientation. Whether RO produces changes in other dimensions of behaviour is not certain. Powell Proctor and Miller (1982) concluded that RO needs to be continued indefinitely to maintain changes, and is good general background but no substitute for specific therapies geared to individual needs.

Several reviewers have examined the question of how the effects of RO are achieved. Possible mechanisms have been suggested: reactivation of neural pathways; increased stimulation; behavioural re-education; increased staff attention; patient participation; and overcoming depressive withdrawal.

Group work. Various approaches have been described as suitable for psycho-geriatric patients by Murray et al (1980). These include:
1. RO groups—already discussed.
2. Reminiscence and life review groups—to be discussed later.
3. Activity groups. These are notionally intended for the completion of a task such as making a collage. Other activities such as social participation, discussion of feelings and taking responsibility are equally important benefits.
4. Support groups. These are designed to help patients cope with the changes associated with old age. Topics are chosen by the group for discussion and might include loss, death, depression, isolation, etc. These discussions help the elderly realise the universality of their experiences and support one another.
5. Discharge groups. These are to help patients to plan for their discharge from hospital.
6. Remotivation groups. A topic of general interest is debated among the patients with a staff member as group leader. Such discussions are claimed to prevent disengagement, increase interest in reality and stimulate thinking. Gray and Stevenson (1980) included positive feedback for sensible utterances. They found that remotivation groups increased social interactions between group members.

Irrespective of the type of group, Murray et al (1980) suggest that the following general principles are helpful with psycho-geriatric patients. Groups should have clear goals, explicit rules about confidentiality, timing, membership, turn-taking, etc., a leader who provides structure, and a climate of acceptance and mutual appreciation.

Reminiscence and life-review. Butler (1963) first described the need to review one's life in old age, which may be responsible for the increased reminiscence of older people. He described life-review as a 'normal naturally occurring universal mental process characterised by looking back over life lived and recalling either pleasurable memories or unresolved conflicts which can be surveyed and integrated'. Ideally, life-review should result in new wisdom and insights, so that the old person can retire from life with an acceptable image and dignity.

Reminiscence in groups may be facilitated by a variety of items from the past, photographs and films. For example, Help the Aged Education Department (1981) produced the *Recall* package, which consists of tape/slide programmes about working-class life in London from the beginning of this century. These are designed to stimulate recollections and encourage communications between patients and carers. There is still much work to be done in evaluating the effects of reminiscence on the mentally infirm elderly.

The nurse's role is to encourage life-review and reminiscence by active listening, accepting, being interested, acknowledging achievements and providing constructive feedback. It should of course be remembered that recalling long-repressed emotions may be painful and that some patients may prefer to forget their past experiences, a preference which should be respected (Post 1982).

An overview of psychological methods of treatment. There is much overlap among the various treatments described and it is not intended that any one should be used in isolation from the rest. Most of the methods contain the following common elements, which are probably the most important to develop:
1. The patient's environment is enriched and compensates for gaps in functioning.
2. Meaningful activities and stimulation are provided.

3. Patients are encouraged to participate and make choices.
4. Social interaction and mutual help are encouraged.
5. Activities take place in small groups.
6. Appropriate behaviour is reinforced.
7. The ward staff are active and involved. The nurses' attitudes change from being custodial, emphasising physical tasks, to being rehabilitative, initiating care to meet all the patient's needs. These changes in nurses' behaviour and subsequently ward atmosphere, may be the most important factors in all the psychological treatments.

Meeting the basic human needs of demented patients

Nursing interventions which may be required for demented patients are discussed within the framework of Henderson's (1969) list of basic human needs. Those aspects of care which have already been discussed will not be mentioned here. It is important to remember that a patient's problems will vary according to the stage and severity of the disease, associated physical deficits and the pre-morbid abilities and personality. Therefore, care must be planned individually and the following notes used for general guidance only.

Nutrition. Ensure that the diet is adequate in quality and quantity, allowing the patient a choice of foods, which must be of manageable consistency. Modifications to china and cutlery may help the patient to feed him or herself. It is preferable to avoid bibs if possible as they look undignified. Encourage the patient to wear dentures and attend to oral hygiene. Check that she maintains a reasonable weight. Ensure adequate hydration with a wide selection of drinks chosen by the patient.

Elimination. Bladder retraining techniques should be tried for incontinence. Prevent constipation.

Movement and posture. Keep the patient ambulatory and encourage daily exercise, preferably out-of-doors. Provide shoes rather than ill-fitting slippers. Arrange regular chiropody. Provide clothes that encourage mobility. If bed- or chairbound, ensure good posture to allow chest expansion.

Cleanliness, skin care and grooming. Assess risk of pressure sores and take preventive measures. Help the patient to look attractive with regular hairdressing, removal of unwanted facial hair, and cosmetics if desired.

Dressing and undressing. If possible, allow patients to wear their own clothes. Provide dayclothes rather than nightwear during the day. If necessary modify clothes to make independent dressing and undressing easier. Ensure that clothes are attractive and well-matched. Encourage patients to choose what to wear themselves.

Body temperature. Be aware of the risk of hypothermia even for an ambulant patient. Keep the extremities warm but do not restrict mobility with unnecessary shawls and blankets over knees.

Sleep and rest. In many psychogeriatric wards, patients doze in chairs all day and are in bed at night for about 12 hours. Understandably, they become restless and are then given unnecessary sedation which increases confusion and creates daytime drowsiness. If patients are busy and active during the day and go to bed for about eight hours, night sedation is less likely to be needed. Many old people find an alcoholic drink is the best sedative. A short afternoon doze may be beneficial and restore energy for later activities.

Respiration. It is cruel to deny tobacco to demented patients if they enjoy it, but be aware of the serious fire risk and the effect on non-smokers, and observe unobtrusively.

Avoiding dangers in the environment. Ambulant demented patients are particularly prone to accidents as they may wander within the ward and away from the ward. Nurses are responsible for ensuring that the ward is a safe environment. Floors should be non-slip and there should be no frayed carpet edges. Dangerous items such as poisons and sharp knives should be locked away. Stairs and corridors should be well lit. Baths and lavatories should have handrails. Patients who tend to wander should be closely supervised and engaged in interesting activities.

The use of restraints. It is not uncommon for psychogeriatric patients to be restrained with the tacit approval of the institution, e.g. cot sides on beds, tables attached to tilting geriatric chairs, and sheets tying patients to beds or chairs. Miller (1975) reviewed the literature on the use of restraints and found a variety of adverse consequences: severe distress and regression; exacerbation of dementia; death wish; loss of ego strength; weight loss and incontinence. Miller cited several studies showing that the immobility resulting from the use of restraints produced muscle atrophy, osteoporosis, hypercalcaemia and other disorders. In addition to these medical and psychological reasons, there are also ethical objections to the use of restraints. They can rarely be justified.

Worship. Patients must be helped to continue practising their religion if they wish.

Communication. Help the patient to overcome sensory deficits by providing spectacles and hearing aids as necessary. Avoid excessive meaningless stimuli such as background noise from unwatched televisions. Make use of touch and remember the patient's needs for affection and friendship. Promote good communication between the patient and his or her family and friends.

Work and accomplishments. Maintain the patient's sense of worth, making use of his or her skills. If possible place the patient in a consultative role. Encourage creative expression, individuality, decision making and participation in care. Assistance with financial affairs and papers may be required.

Recreation. A wide range of recreational facilities should be available, e.g. games, cards, billiards, table tennis, books, newspapers, art, knitting and sewing materials, music and flower arranging.

Learning, discovery and curiosity. Demented patients need routine and order in their lives to increase predictability of events. Let the patient establish the daily routine, then maintain a structured and dependable programme.

Changes should be introduced slowly after careful preparation. Remember that if the patient is required to take part in activities and discussions which are too complex, frustration and disappointment may result.

Helping the families of demented patients

Hayter (1982) believed that the families had many unmet needs and she found little interest in this topic in the literature. She established family support groups which meet monthly. Families are encouraged to be involved in all stages of the nursing process. The groups allow an outlet for expression of grief or guilt. The groups tend to be very cohesive and mutually supportive. Working with demented patients' families, Hayter found a number of recurrent themes—topics about which families worried or about which they needed information. These included: need for information about the disease process—cause, course, prognosis and treatment; fear that they would develop the disease; need for information about their role and responsibility; guilt about having negative feelings towards the patient; worries about the patient's physical appearance; desire for contact with other sufferer's families; and desire to contribute to research and education about dementia.

Care required for confused patients

Prevention of confusion is of first importance. Given an understanding of the conditions prodromal to confusion, the nurse can attempt to reduce them. If a patient has developed a confusional state, then the main principle of treatment is to search for the cause and treat or reduce all precipitating factors.

Participation of the nurse in medical treatments

Hypnotics are rarely used as they cause dangerous sleepiness, make assessment difficult and increase confusion. Sometimes, however, the patient may be so agitated that sedation is essential. Post (1982) then recommends the use of promazine (Sparine), haloperidol or droperidol. Specific medical interventions will vary according to the cause of the condition.

Controlling the patient's environment

The environment should be kept constant to make it familiar and should be quiet and peaceful. These patients are best nursed in single rooms. The room should contain orientation cues such clocks, calendars, windows and familiar objects. Background noise from radios, conversations, etc. adds further to ambiguous and random stimuli, thus increasing confusion.

Dealing with psychological distress

Anxiety, hyperactivity, fear and screaming are not uncommon. A frightened patient should not be left alone. The nurse should be calm and supportive. If hallucinations and illusions occur, it is helpful to explain to the patient what is happening and reassure him or her. Realistic responses should be rewarded with simple operant conditioning techniques. The room should be well lit all the time to reduce confusion and fear.

Meeting the basic human needs of confused patients

The nursing interventions discussed here are required for most acutely confused patients, irrespective of the cause. However, other problems are likely to exist depending on the cause of the confusional state. The need for other nursing actions should be assessed individually.

Nutrition. Hydration is often a problem and patients must be offered drinks constantly. Many patients are anorexic and may need help and encouragement to eat a light but nutritious diet.

Elimination. Incontinence can be reduced if the patient is taken to the lavatory or commode every hour or two. Constipation is common.

Movement and posture. The patient may wander restlessly, but it is preferable not to restrict his or her movements too much.

Cleanliness, skin care and grooming. Patients can be helped to maintain their body image by wearing their own dayclothes or nightwear. Help may be required with grooming.

Dressing and undressing. The steps involved in dressing may be too complex for a confused patient, who will become frustrated at his or her own incompetence. Patients should be helped with dressing. Clothes which are comfortable and easy to wear, such as nightclothes, may be most appropriate.

Sleep and rest. Typically, confusion is worse at night and in the dark. The room should thus be well lit even at night. Other measures which will help to avoid the 'sundown syndrome' include: avoiding fatigue and pain; ensuring that bladder and bowels are emptied; giving clear explanations of all occurrences and keeping the environment constant.

Avoiding dangers in the environment. The safety of the patient is a major concern as he or she may be restless and wandering. These patients need careful constant observation within a safe and reasonably enclosed environment. Restraints should only be used as a last resort.

Communication. Ideally, the same nurses should care for the patient all the time. Any strangers should be introduced and the purpose of their visit explained. The patient should be informed of everything happening to and around him or her. Nurses should present a calm, concerned and understanding demeanour, speaking in a clear voice using simple statements. A quiet soothing voice helps to reduce agitation. Touch can be used to calm and reassure the patient. Occasional lucid intervals should be used to establish rapport. The patient should be encouraged to wear his or her spectacles and hearing aid to support sensory reception.

CONCLUSIONS

After reading this chapter we hope that nurses will appreciate the important differences between dementia and confusion and will be able to plan care accordingly. The reader should be able to carry out a comprehensive nursing assessment and understand the value of assessment in psychogeriatric nursing. We hope that the many methods of treatment and care discussed will encourage readers to realise that an optimistic approach to nursing demented and confused patients is entirely appropriate.

REFERENCES

Armstrong-Esther C A, Hawkins L H 1982 Day for night: circadian rhythms in the elderly. Nursing Times 78: 1263–1265

Beck A T, Ward C H, Mendelson M, Mock J, Erbaugh J 1961 An inventory for measuring depression. Archives of General Psychiatry 4: 561–571

Brook P, Degun G, Mather M 1975 Reality orientation, a therapy for psychogeriatric patients: a controlled study. British Journal of Psychiatry 127: 42–45

Burton M 1982 Reality orientation for the elderly: a critique. Journal of Advanced Nursing 7: 427–433

Butler R N 1963 The life review: an interpretation of reminiscence in the aged. Psychiatry 26: 65–76

Chisholm S E, Deniston O L, Igrisan R M, Barbus A J 1982 Prevalence of confusion in elderly hospitalised patients. Journal of Gerontological Nursing 8(2): 87–96

Diesfeldt H F A, Diesfeldt-Groenendijk H 1977 Improving cognitive performance in psychogeriatric patients: the influence of physical exercise. Age and Ageing 6: 58–64

Goldfarb A I 1960 Psychiatric disorders of the aged: symptomatology, diagnosis and treatment. Journal of the American Geriatrics Society 8: 698–707

Gray P, Stevenson J S 1980 Changes in verbal interaction among members of resocialisation groups. Journal of Gerontological Nursing 6: 89–60

Grimley Evans J 1982 The psychiatric aspects of physical disease. In: Levy R, Post F (eds) The psychiatry of late life. Blackwell, Oxford

Hamilton M 1960 A rating scale for depression. Journal of Neurology, Neurosurgery and Psychiatry 23: 56–62

Hayter J 1982 Helping families of patients with Alzheimer's disease. Journal of Gerontological Nursing 8: 81–86

Help the Aged Education Department 1981 Recall—a handbook. Help the Aged, London

Henderson V 1969 Basic principles of nursing care. International Council of Nurses, Geneva

Holden U P, Woods R T 1982 Reality orientation: psychological approaches to the confused elderly. Churchill Livingstone, Edinburgh

Katzman R, Terry R D, Bick K L (eds) 1978 Alzheimer's disease: senile dementia and related disorders. Raven Press, New York

Langer E J, Rodin J 1976 The effects of choice and enhanced personal responsibility for the aged: a field experiment in an institutional setting. Journal of Personality and Social Psychology 34: 191–198

La Porte H J 1982 Reversible causes of dementia: a nursing challenge. Journal of Gerontological Nursing 8: 213–216

Levy R, Post F 1982 The dementias of old age. In: Levy R, Post F (eds) The psychiatry of late life, Blackwell, Oxford

Libow L S 1978 Senile dementias and pseudo-dementias, clinical diagnosis. In: Eisdorfer C, Friedal R O (eds) Cognitive and emotional disturbance in the elderly. Year Book Medical Publishers, Chicago

Macdonald M L 1973 The forgotten Americans: a sociopsychological analysis of ageing and nursing homes. American Journal of Community Psychology 3: 272–292

Marston N, Gupta H 1977 Interesting the old. Community Care November 16: 26–28

Merton R K 1957 Social theory and social structure, revised edition. Free Press, Illinois

Miller E 1977 Abnormal ageing: the psychology of senile and presenile dementia. Wiley, Chichester

Miller M 1975 Iatrogenic and nursigenic effects of prolonged immobilisation of the ill aged. Journal of the American Geriatric Society 23: 360–369

Mishara B L, Kastenbaum R 1973 Self injurious behaviour and environmental change in the institutionalised elderly. International Journal of Aging and Human Development 4: 133–145

Murray R, Huelskoetter M M, O'Driscoll D The Nursing Nursing process in later maturity. Prentice Hall, New Jersey

Peterson R F, Knapp T J, Rosen J C, Pither B F 1977 The effects of furniture arrangement on the behaviour of geriatric patients. Behaviour Therapy 8: 464–467

Post F 1982 Functional disorders. In: Levy R, Post F (eds) The psychiatry of late life. Blackwell, Oxford

Powell R R 1974 Psychological effects of exercise therapy upon institutionalised geriatric mental patients. Gerontologist 14: 157–161

Powell Proctor L, Miller E 1982 Reality orientation: a critical appraisal. British Journal of Psychiatry 140: 457–463

Rodin J, Langer E J 1977 Long-term effects of a control-relevant intervention with the institutionalised aged. Journal of Personality and Social Psychology 35: 897–902

Schulz R 1976 Effects of control and predictability on the physical and psychological well-being of the institutionalised aged. Journal of Personality and Social Psychology 33: 563–573

Schulz R 1980 Aging and control. In: Garber J, Seligman M E P (eds) Human helplessness: theory and applications. Academic Press, New York

Skinner B F 1953 Science and human behaviour. Macmillan, New York

Taulbee L R, Folsom J C 1966 Reality orientation for geriatric patients. Hospital and Community Psychaitry 17: 133–135

Wilson H S, Kneisl C R 1983 Psychiatric Nursing, 2nd edn. Addison Wesley, San Francisco

Wolanin M D, Phillips L R F 1981 Confusion: prevention and care. Mosby, St Louis

19

J. I. Brooking

Depression and other emotional disorders in the elderly

DEPRESSION

According to Bergmann (1982) depression in the elderly is relatively common, but is often not recognised and even when recognised, often not treated. Two inaccurate assumptions are commonly held. Firstly, that depression is inevitable in old age and therefore not worth treating. Secondly, that depression is a prodromal phase of 'senility' and therefore not treatable.

Nurses will meet patients who have suffered from recurrent attacks of depression all their lives, and others who have developed a late-onset depression. The World Health Organis-ation Classification of Diseases describes a specific late-onset depression called invol-utional melancholia, with features of agitation, hypochondria and delusions of poverty. However, researchers such as Weissman (1979) and Weissman and Klerman (1977) found no evidence of this specific condition. Post (1982) suggested that depression in the elderly shows the influence of the ageing process, but is not essentially different from depression in other age groups. He considered that elderly depressives can appear anywhere in the classically defined spectrum from psychotic to neurotic manifestations with a large overlap in the middle. For a general discussion of depression see a textbook of psychiatric nursing, such as Murray and

255

Huelskoetter (1983), or a textbook of abnormal psychology, such as Davison and Neale (1978).

Factors causing depression in the elderly

There are many theories about the causes of depression, but the causes of depression in the elderly can be discussed under three main headings.

Social factors

Many stresses and losses occur in old age which may precipitate depression. Post (1972) reported the existence of precipitating events in more than 60% of the elderly depressives he studied. These social factors may include bereavement, retirement with its loss of status and income, reduced efficiency of the body and reduced mobility, awareness of one's own mortality and overt or covert messages from the rest of society about reduced worth.

Biological factors

Physical illness is known to be an important causative factor (Salzman and Shader 1979, Dovenmuehle and Verwoerdt 1963). A family history of depression is found in many patients. Other possible biological causes include changes in circadian rhythms, lower levels of biogenic amines and cerebral hypofunction.

Personality factors

Learned helplessness, associated with perceived loss of control was first identified as a major cause of depression by Seligman (1974) and shown relevant to the elderly by Schulz (1976). About half of elderly depressives have shown earlier neurotic tendencies with anxiety, depression or sexual maladjustment.

It is important for nurses to be aware of the causes of depression so that they are alert to the possible onset of depression. The two single most important antecedents are physical illness and bereavement, especially loss of spouse.

The relationship between depression and physical illness

Several possible relationships occur. Depression is a common reaction to serious illness or surgery, especially amputation, colostomy and chronic infections. Some physical illnesses, such as occult malignancies and giant-cell arteritis may present initially as depression (Grimley Evans 1982). 'Masked depression' (Pfeiffer 1977) may present as vague physical symptoms against a background of anorexia, weight loss, loss of energy, sleep disturbance and constipation. Elderly people with functional psychiatric disorders show higher morbidity and mortality rates than average for their age (Kay et al 1966).

The relationship between depression and dementia

The two commonly co-exist and according to Lader (1981) five forms of association can be found:
1. They can co-exist by chance.
2. The same brain pathology, e.g. multiple infarcts, can cause both.
3. Incipient dementia may make the patient become depressed as he or she realises that mental capacity is decaying.
4. Incipient dementia may lead to self-neglect and social isolation, resulting in situational depression.
5. Depression may lead to self-neglect with malnutrition and vitamin deficiencies, which in turn result in confusion and mental deterioration.

Whatever form the relationship takes, any associated intellectual impairment makes the assessment of depression more difficult, as symptoms may be masked.

Clinical features of depression

From the perspective of the medical model, depression can be viewed as a continuum with severely psychotic at one end and neurotic at the other. In a study of elderly depressives admitted to a psychiatric unit, Post (1972) found that approximately a third exhibited severe psychotic symptoms. These patients experienced bizarre, paranoid and ritualistic delusions. Some had auditory hallucinations. Many were physically retarded with sleeplessness, anorexia and weight loss. Hypochondria, bodily complaints, self-deprecation, guilt and ideas of poverty were common. Many communicated great sadness, fear, dread, agitation and despair. Another third of the patients exhibited more neurotic than psychotic symptoms. Generally they conveyed less overt sadness than is typical for younger patients and more anxiety. These patients preserved the capacity to see that their feelings were due to their emotional state. They had many physical complaints and sought constant reassurance about their health. They experienced feelings of worthlessness and self-reproach.

Nursing assessment

The general principles of assessing psychogeriatric patients have been discussed in Chapter 18. When assessing a depressed patient it is helpful to focus on commonly experienced problems outlined in the section above. Self-care capability should be considered and physical assessment should include level of activity, sleep pattern, appetite and bowel function. Physical complaints should be investigated. Psychological factors to be assessed include mood, self-esteem, level of anxiety, feelings of guilt and cognitive processes. The existence of psychotic symptoms such as hallucinations and delusions should be assessed and their content noted. It is important to examine the patient's social relationships with family and friends.

Participation of the nurse in medical treatments

Drug treatment

Tricyclic antidepressants are used most frequently. These include amitriptyline, imipramine and doxepin. The elderly tend to be more sensitive than younger adults to smaller dosages and may experience serious side-effects. Anticholinergic effects, i.e. signs of sympathetic overactivity, are common and include dry mouth, blurred vision, tremor and palpitations. Dangerous side-effects such as glaucoma, prostate damage and cardiotoxicity can occur. These drugs may take about two weeks to exert their antidepressant effect and they may also cause undesirable sleepiness. The tetracyclic antidepressants are newer drugs with fewer anticholinergic effects. They include mianserin hydrochloride. Monamine oxidase inhibitors (MAOIs), e.g. phenelzine and isocarboxozid, are now rarely used unless tricyclics are ineffective. They have very serious side-effects and special dietary restrictions are essential.

Nursing responsibilities include the following:
1. Administration—ordering, storing, checking, recording and administering the drugs using safe procedures.
2. Observation of the patient's responses to treatment. The effectiveness or ineffectiveness of the treatment should be reported back to the doctors to enable decisions to be made about continuing or changing the treatment.
3. Observation of unwanted side-effects. Nurses should familiarise themselves with all the possible side-effects of the drugs being taken by their patients.
4. Taking special precautions associated with particular drugs, e.g. dietary requirements for patients receiving MAOIs.
5. Patient and family education about the drug effects and side-effects, dosages, times of administration and the importance of compliance.
6. Ensuring drug compliance. This is a particular problem with patients receiving treatment at home.

Electroconvulsive therapy (ECT)

ECT is the administration of a controlled electrical current through the brain via electrodes placed on one or both sides of the forehead. The patient is anaesthetised and given a muscle relaxant beforehand. This is a complex and controversial procedure, which is claimed to be effective in the treatment of severe depression. The subject is comprehensively reviewed by Fraser (1982).

Old age is not a contraindication, although the risk of troublesome side-effects is somewhat increased. Reviewing the evidence on the use of ECT for the elderly Fraser (1982) concluded that the treatment is very effective against a wide range of depressive symptoms. It is particularly useful when drug treatment has failed, or with suicide risk or risk of serious self-neglect.

The nurse has a role in the physical and psychological preparation of the patient, communicating with the family, preparation of the ECT equipment, management of the convulsion, prevention of complications, and aftercare of the patient. For further information see the Royal College of Nursing's (1982) *Nursing Guidelines for Electro-Convulsive Therapy.*

Participation of the nurse in psychotherapy and counselling

There are various types of psychotherapy and counselling carried out with individuals or groups. All depend on the ability of the patient to discuss problems and achieve some insight into behaviour. It was traditional psychiatric wisdom that psychotherapy was useless with the elderly. Eisdorfer and Stotsky (1977) reported that this view is now changing and psychotherapy is being used with success. Studies reviewed by Post (1982) suggest that psychotherapeutic approaches with the depressed elderly should be directive and combined with somatic treatments.

The extent of nurses' involvement in formal therapy depends on their expertise in using these techniques. With appropriate training, nurses can function as psychotherapists and counsellors. Bereavement counselling may be particularly relevant as this is such a major cause of depression in old age. Group work was mentioned in chapter 18 and may be helpful. Discussion groups, support groups and activity groups could be led by nurses with relatively little extra training.

Nursing actions to help patients overcome depression

This is the central part of nurses' work with depressed patients, yet surprisingly there is little literature about what nurses can do to relieve depression. The nurses's attitude and manner can be therapeutic. (S)he should convey to the patient that (s)he accepts and appreciates him or her as valuable. The nurse should attempt to be calm, caring, supportive and empathic, communicating these qualities verbally and non-verbally.

The patient may be helped by information about the illness. It is important to convey that negative feelings are temporary and treatable. It is helpful to explain that physical symptoms may be a feature of the depression.

Patients should be encouraged to ventilate their feelings and negative emotions including sadness, anger and guilt. Conflicts and feelings of loss may be resolved by rational discussion with a sympathetic nurse. Thus patients can be helped to see that a happy future is possible.

The patient should also be encouraged to engage in a wide range of physical and mental activities. Positive responses and behaviour should be reinforced. At times of great adversity, many people turn to religion to seek meaning in their existence (Weber 1961). Attendance at church services and visits from a chaplain may be a great comfort to depressed patients.

Meeting the patient's physical needs

Elderly depressed patients, even if they have no associated physical illness, commonly experience many physical problems, each of which should be treated. Patients may need assistance and encouragement with basic hygiene and grooming. Loss of appetite, weight loss and constipation are common. Sleep disturbance may be associated with anxiety and inability to relax. Patients may become lethargic and unwilling to mobilise.

Helping the patient's family

Families may experience distress, anxiety and guilt about the patient's illness. Many relatives express a desire for increased participation in decision making about care and in giving care (Brooking 1982). This can be facilitated by encouraging and welcoming visitors and providing a pleasant and private place for visits. With the patient's permission, relatives should be given information about all aspects of care and treatment. One geriatric hospital established a 'relatives' corner' in each ward, where relatives could make tea, arrange flowers, wash clothes, help the patient with hygiene, grooming, hairdressing, etc. (Callaghan and Silver 1974). Success depended on the attitude and encouragement of ward staff. Relatives' groups, led by a staff member, can provide mutual support and discussion of problems common to all (Fuller 1979). It may also be possible to invite relatives to multidisciplinary meetings at which the patient's care is discussed (Leeming and Luke 1977).

SUICIDE

In western societies the incidence of suicide rises with increasing age, especially among men. About 25% to 30% of all suicides occur in the over 65 years age group, although they only represent about 10 to 15% of the population (Shulman 1978). In young people, there are at least half a dozen suicide attempts for every completed suicide. In elderly people attempted suicide (parasuicide) is very rare and usually represents genuine failure, rather than a bid for attention, which is common in the young. When an old person attempts suicide he or she usually fully intends to die. In a study in which men of all ages who had attempted suicide were followed up, Shulman (1978) reported that ultimately fatal acts occurred 20 times more frequently in old rather than young men.

Factors causing suicide

Suicide risk should be assessed in collaboration with the whole health care team, so as to determine the intensity of precautions required. Any threat of suicide must be taken seriously. A patient's predisposition to suicide should be considered under the following three headings:

Psychiatric predisposition

In young people suicide attempts are associated more frequently with personality disorders than with depression (Rees 1982). However, in the elderly, suicidal ideas and behaviour are almost always related to clinical depression (Gage 1971). A small percentage of elderly suicides are those of alcoholics, patients with organic brain disease and the terminally ill.

Social predisposition

An important characteristic of suicide is social isolation and lack of integration into the community. Typically there are few important ties, whether familial, religious, occupational, cultural or social. Sainsbury (1968) found that 39% of elderly suicides lived alone. Men are more likely to kill themselves than women.

Stressful events

Sainsbury (1968) found that 35% of elderly suicides suffered from a physical illness and 16% were recently bereaved. Any major crisis or interpersonal conflict can be seen as a risk factor.

Helping suicidal patients

Nurses' responsibilities to potentially suicidal patients include dealing with the factors precipitating suicide, developing a supportive relationship, close observation and providing a safe environment.

The care of depressed patients has been discussed earlier and is relevant here. Nurses can help to reduce social isolation by encouraging visits from family and friends, helping patients to make new friends, encouraging involvement in community activities, clubs, churches, etc. Bereavement counselling may be helpful.

The nurse should try to develop a supportive relationship with the patient and should find out what and whom still matters to the patient. The sources of distress should be identified and discussed openly. The nurse should assure the patient that he or she is not alone and that such feelings are not unusual. The nurse must be aware of her possible importance to the patient. If going off-duty this should be explained, and the patient introduced to the replacement nurse.

During the crisis period the nurse should take all precautions necessary to prevent suicide or self-mutilation. The first principle is constant unobtrusive observation by a designated nurse in a tactful way which will not be stressful or offensive to the patient. This is best achieved by sharing the patient's activities rather than scrutiny without participation. It is preferable to explain these basic precautions to the patient, using an honest but kindly attitude. Dangerous objects, such as razors, scissors, belts, drugs, matches, glass objects, should be removed. Windows should be locked or blocked. The patient should be supervised when bathing, using a razor or knife and when smoking.

Despite these precautions nurses should try to convey a feeling of empathic optimism that the patient will feel better. Staff should be aware of the dangers of the self-fulfilling prophecy if they feel hopeless about the patient.

OTHER EMOTIONAL DISORDERS

This section describes some of those psychiatric disorders (often termed 'functional' disorders) in which there is no currently demonstrable organic pathology. The aetiology of many so-called functional disorders is not yet fully understood, but may include organic factors such as biochemical abnormalities. Thus the distinction between organic and functional disorders is not clear cut, especially in geriatric psychiatry, where the effects of the ageing process and the deteriorating brain are relevant. It is traditional to subdivide functional disorders into neurotic and psychotic. Again there is no sharp demarcation between the two and it is preferable to view them as a continuum rather than a dichotomy. Personality disorders form a third category. For a more detailed discussion see Post (1982).

Psychoses

These are the major mental disorders where there is loss of contact with reality and lack of insight into the condition. In general psychiatry psychoses are broadly subdivided into schizophrenia including paranoid states, and affective psychoses, including mania and severe forms of depression.

Schizophrenia and paranoid states

There is a large population of schizophrenics who have been in psychiatric hospitals for decades and are now elderly. Although some classic symptoms, such as delusions and hallucinations may remain, their main problem is severe institutionalisation with flat affect, passivity and loss of capacity for autonomous action. Although the peak time for the onset of schizophrenia is young adulthood, there is a subsidiary peak in old age. Kay (1963) found that 4% of schizophrenia in men and 14% in women occurred after the age of 65 years.

Paranoia is the attribution to other people of motivations which do not exist (Pfeiffer 1977). In young people it is usually indicative of schizophrenia, but in the elderly it is very common and less serious. It is typically associated with solitary living, insecurity, anxiety and encounters with ageism. Reduced sensory input can lead to misinterpretation of the environment and suspicion. It should be remembered that old people can be persecuted, discriminated against and rejected by their families.

In mild forms of paranoid psychosis there is a transitory delusionary state, often precipitated by stress. In more severe forms this becomes paraphrenia, a form of schizophrenia, in which delusions and sometimes hallucinations occur. The delusions are always persecutory.

Psychotropic drugs have greatly improved what used to be a poor prognosis. Nursing interventions should be aimed at reducing stress, reducing any genuine persecution, helping the patient to explore reality, increasing self-esteem, maximising remaining cognitive capabilities, improving sensory input and developing a trusting relationship. It is pointless to contradict delusions, but nor should they be reinforced. It is best to admit puzzlement and gently suggest alternative explanations.

Affective psychoses

Depression, which may be neurotic or psychotic, has already been discussed. Mania, studied by Shulman and Post (1980) is much rarer than depression and typically occurs in women. Some cases are just mania, others are mixed manic-depressive. Shulman and Post argued that mania in old people rarely shows the classical 'flights of ideas'. A hostile, surly affect is more usual and depression is never very far away. The prognosis has been improved by drug treatment, such as lithium carbonate. Nursing interventions for manic patients should be aimed at ensuring that basic needs such as diet, elimination, hygiene and rest, are not neglected, providing a safe and calming environment and redirecting the patient's energies into purposeful activities.

Neuroses

These are the less severe disorders in which reality contact and insight into the condition are retained. Because elderly neurotic people are rarely referred to psychiatrists except after a suicide attempt, the study of neuroses in old age has been rather neglected (Kral 1982). Some people suffer from neuroses all their lives and little is known about the long-term course. According to Müller (1969) neuroses tend to become less disabling in later life. As the personality becomes less extroverted patterns of neurotic symptoms tend to shift from outward manifestations to more inwardly directed states. Post (1982) wrote that late-onset neurotics differ from lifelong neurotics in that they more often afflicted with real physical illness, have a higher mortality risk, are lonely and have low incomes.

Obsessive-compulsive neurosis is the only classical neurosis which appears for the first time in old age (Post 1982). Hypochondria is common, especially in women, due to increased concern with health and illness in old age. According to Vogel (1982) acute anxiety states are rare, but chronic anxious ruminations are common. Anxiety may arise from losses, changes and helplessness and is likely to exacerbate physical problems. Post (1982) suggested that complaints of physical disabilities should be investigated. Drugs should be used to treat neurotic symptoms, such as anxiety or depression. Distressing life circumstances should as far as possible be reduced. Individual and/or group psychotherapy may be helpful, unless denial is the patient's preferred coping strategy. It may be possible to work with relatives to improve family relationships.

Personality disorders

It is thought that 'deviant' personalities tend to become more normal with old age. Aggression reduces, but inadequacy worsens. Alcoholism is fairly common (Mishara and Kastenbaum 1980). Diogenes syndrome was described by Clark et al (1975). These eccentrics have a history of being independent, quarrelsome and secretive. They reject social contact and live in squalor, although they are not poor. They tend to have at least average intelligence and are often middle or upper class. On the other hand social isolation often occurs because of bereavement or rejection and can significantly reduce life satisfaction. That kind of isolation is remediable, whereas elderly eccentrics neither want nor need help.

CONCLUSIONS

This chapter has focused on the important problems of depression in elderly people. Nurses often feel incapable of helping these patients and consequently tend to ignore the problem. We hope that the nature and causes of depression in the elderly have been clarified and that we have given the reader some ideas that will facilitate effective treatment and care. Nurses without specialised psychiatric training often feel bewildered and helpless when they encounter suicidal patients. Our aim has been to make the problem more understandable and to indicate those approaches to care which will be most helpful. Other emotional psychiatric disorders that are seen in elderly patients have been briefly considered.

REFERENCES

Bergmann K 1982 Depression in the elderly. In: Isaacs B (ed) Recent advances in geriatric medicine 2. Churchill Livingstone, Edinburgh
Brooking J I 1982 Patient and family participation in nursing: a survey of opinions and current practices among patients, relatives and nurses. In: Hockey L, Keighly T C, Sisson A R (eds) Proceedings of the RCN Research Society 23rd Annual Conference, Royal College of Nursing, London
Callaghan J, Silver C R 1974 Relatives' corner. Nursing Mirror 138:76
Clark A N G, Mankikar G D, Gray I 1975 Diogenes syndrome. A clinical study of gross neglect in old age. Lancet 1: 366–373
Davison G C, Neale J M 1978 Abnormal psychology: an experimental clinical approach, 2nd ed. Wiley, New York
Dovenmuehle R H, Verwoerdt A 1963 Physical illness and depression symptomatology. Journal of Gerontology 18: 260–266
Eisdorfer C, Stotsky B A 1977 Intervention, treatment and rehabilitation of psychiatric disorders. In: Birren J E, Schaie K W (eds) Handbook of the psychology of ageing. Van Nostrand, New York

Fraser M 1982 ECT: a clinical guide. Wiley, Chichester
Fuller J, Ward E, Evans A, Massam K, Gardner A 1979 Dementia supportive groups for relatives. British Medical Journal 1: 1684–1685
Gage F 1971 Suicide in the aged. American Journal of Nursing 71: 2153–2155
Grimley Evans J 1982 The psychiatric aspects of physical disease. In: Levy R, Post F (ed) The psychiatry of late life. Blackwell, Oxford
Kay D W K 1963 Late paraphrenia and its bearing on the aetiology of schizophrenia. Acta Psychiatrica Scandinavica 39: 159–169
Kay D W K, Bergmann K, Foster E M, et al 1966 A four-year follow-up of a random sample of old people orginally seen in their own homes. A physical, social and psychiatric enquiry. Excerpta Medica International Congress Series No. 150, Proceedings of the Fourth World Congress of Psychiatry, p 1668–1670
Kral V A 1982 Neuroses of the aged: a neglected area. Clinical Gerontologist 1: 29–35
Lader M H 1981 Focus on depression. Bencard, Middlesex
Leeming J T, Luke A 1977 Multidisciplinary meetings with relatives of elderly hospital patients in continuing care wards. Age and Ageing 6: 1–5
Mishara B L, Kastenbaum R 1980 Alcohol and old age. Grune and Stratton, New York
Müller C 1969 Manuel de geronto-psychiatrie. Masson, Paris
Murray R B, Huelskoetter M M W 1983 Psychiatric/mental health nursing: giving emotional care. Prentice Hall, New Jersey
Pfeiffer E 1977 Psychopathology and social palthology. In: Birren J E, Schaie K W (eds) Handbook of the psychology of ageing. Van Nostrand, New York
Post F 1972 The management and nature of depressive illness in late life: a follow-through study. British Journal of Psychiatry 121: 393–404
Post F 1982 Functional disorders. In: Levy R, Post F (eds) The psychiatry of late life. Blackwell, Oxford
Rees L 1982 A short textbook of psychiatry, 3rd edn. Hodder and Stoughton, London
Royal College of Nursing (1982) Nursing guidelines for electro-convulsive therapy. Royal College of Nursing Society of Psychiatric Nursing, London
Sainsbury P 1968 Suicide and depression. In: Coppen A, Walk A (eds). British Journal of Psychiatry, Special Publication No.2
Salzman C, Shader R I 1979 Clinical evaluation of depression in the elderly. In: Raskin H, Jarvik L H (eds) Psychiatric symptoms and cognitive loss in the elderly. Wiley, New York
Schulz R 1976 Effects of control and predictability on the physical and psychological well-being of the institutionalised aged. Journal of Personality and Social Psychology 33: 563–573
Seligman M E P 1974 Depression and learned helplessness. In: Friedman R J, Katz M M (eds) The psychology of depression: contemporary theory and research. V H Winston, Washington
Shulman K 1978 Suicide and para-suicide in old age: a review. Age and Ageing 7: 201–209
Shulman K, Post F 1980 Bipolar affective disorder in old age. British Journal of Psychiatry 136: 26–32

Vogel C H 1982 Anxiety and depression among the elderly. Journal of Gerontological Nursing 8: 213–216

Weber M 1961 The social psychology of the world religions. In: Gerth H H, Mills C W (eds) From Max Weber: essays in sociology. Routledge and Kegan Paul, London

Weissman M M 1979 Environmental factors in affective disorders. Hospital Practice 14: 103–109

Weissman M M, Klerman G 1977 Sex differences and the epidemiology of depression. Archives of General Psychiatry 34: 98–110

J. A. David

20

Drugs and the elderly

As yet, no drug has been produced which can delay natural senescence. After all, age is not a disease even though many seek a 'cure'. With increasing age the likelihood that anyone will develop a chronic disabling condition increases; physiological ageing and the ravages of time make the body more susceptible to disease, accident or infection and reduce the ability to heal. Many of these conditions can be treated with drugs, allowing the elderly patient years of confortable, independent living, while others can be relieved without drugs if adjustments of life-style are made. For example, the introduction of bran to the diet can reduce the need for aperients as gut motility decreases.

Symptoms of age-related, diseases which in the past were suffered as 'part of life', are now treated and as a consequence the elderly expect more from doctors, nurses and the National Health Service (NHS), a situation which is both desirable and increasingly expensive. At the present time the elderly (over 65 years of age) make up approximately 15% of the population but consume 30% of the NHS drug budget. By 1991 the proportion of people over 65 years of age in our population is likely to be 37% (Office of Health Economics 1979). As a result, nurses can expect to care for more and more elderly patients as the years pass and more and more of them will be taking drugs. In spite of this, the understanding of how drugs act in the ageing body is not well understood. It is only comparatively recently that studies on drug handling have been attempted with the elderly and also an awareness of the problems which may be encountered by the patient in adhering to prescribed treatment. Although nurses are not responsible for diagnosis or the prescription of drugs, they are ideally placed where patients are concerned for observing the effects of drugs, administering the dose and monitoring progress. Their day-to-day contact allows them to assess the patient's ability to take their own drugs and to educate patients about drug effects.

THE USE OF DRUGS FOR TREATING ELDERLY PATIENTS

Drug treatment for elderly patients may be initiated for any reason, with the obvious exception of contraception. The conditions most commonly treated are those which are associated with ageing. Those not related to the patient's physiological degeneration must also be treated while taking into account other drugs used and the body's capability in dealing with drugs. Drugs prescribed fall into three main groups: therapeutic, replacement, symptomatic relief.

Therapeutic drugs

These are prescribed for specific curable conditions such as antimicrobials for infection, iron for anaemia and antidepressants. The course is usually short, but may need to be repeated if the problem recurs. Where the body fails to combat the condition (e.g. infection) the condition may become chronic with the continued use of antimicrobials together with anti-inflammatories.

Replacement drugs

These are chemicals, often endogenous substances, used to treat conditions where the chemical is reduced or absent because the body can no longer produce it. Many of these conditions, such as hypothroidism or diabetes,

occur often in elderly people and in such cases drugs can replace the lost chemical and allow the patient to lead a normal life. In Parkinsonism, drugs can rebalance the acetylcholine/dopamine levels in the brain allowing the patient relief from the symptoms. Drug replacement therapy does not, however, cure the condition and drugs will generally need to be continued for life.

Symptomatic relief

This can be given for many of the distressing symptoms which occur frequently with age, such as arthritis and rheumatism, cardiac failure, agitation and pain. Once initiated, treatment may need to continue for life and may, from time to time, require a change in dose. With long-term symptomatic relief there is always the problem of keeping a balance between desired comfort and the adverse effects of prolonged drug therapy.

PRESCRIBING PATTERNS

Initial diagnosis and treatment of elderly people is often made by the general practitioner. The presentation of disease symptoms in the older patient may be unusual or confused and current illness may be the culmination of a number of minor problems. Over the years the patient acquires more problems and consequently more drugs, which may themselves produce symptoms treated with more drugs.

It is not possible to determine from the overall figures the actual number of prescriptions made for the elderly, partly because 'free prescriptions' are issued to pensionable individuals (i.e. women at 60, men at 65 years) and partly because no age is included on the prescription for those over 12 years. A study made in a Southampton health centre showed that of the prescriptions written for patients over the age of 65, 25.6% were for cardio-vascular drugs, 16.5% for analgesics and central nervous system (CNS) drugs, 16.2% for psychotropic and 13.5% for metabolic drugs

(Freeman 1979). In a hospital in Dundee neuroleptics topped the list (33%), chloral derivatives accounted for 32% and benzodiazepines 16%; other drugs prescribed included diuretics 29% and laxatives 27% (Christopher et al 1979). The most commonly treated conditions of the elderly in both hospital and community care are therefore those of the cardiovascular and central nervous systems. The use of antimicrobial drugs is lower than in the community at large (16% of all NHS prescriptions): in hospital only 12% of drugs for the elderly and in the community 8.6% were for antimicrobials. These figures support the belief that cardiovascular symptoms are common in the elderly and that infection plays a prominent role in hospital admission. The frequency with which laxatives are prescribed in hospital is not, one hopes, a reflection upon the hospital diet. A more likely explanation is the imposed change of routine and the institutional take-over of the patient's self-medication responsibilities. Prescribing for the elderly is, therefore, costly. More then 60% of prescriptions are exempt from charges and many of these will be for the elderly. A large number of patients take more than one drug and some patients take as many as ten.

THE PROBLEMS ASSOCIATED WITH DRUG USE BY ELDERLY PEOPLE

The first problem related to drug use by the elderly is selecting the right drug since symptoms of disease are often different in old people compared with the young. Patients present with vague symptoms and unsuitable drugs may be used; patients treated for many years may develop new symptoms and these could require treatment with additional drugs. This can lead to interactions or even a situation where one drug is used to treat the side-effects of another. The addition of more drugs to the patient's programme leads to confusion, mistakes, wrong reporting by the patient and ultimately hospital admission. As

many as 15% of elderly patient admissions are for adverse drug reactions (Hurwitz 1969).

Case history

Mr M, aged 81 years, was admitted to hospital following a 'funny turn' which included inability to walk. A civil servant who retired at the age of 61 years with hypertension, he was prescribed at this time Decaserpyl plus a reserpine alkaloid by his general practitioner, who suggested also a change of lifestyle (early retirement). Over the follwing years the patient moved house and transferred to a new general practitioner, who continued his drug by repeat prescription, in spite of the advent of beta-blocking drugs, and without regular check up. When the patient was 75 years old his wife complained of his unsteadiness, fidgety movements and withdrawal. During a hospital consultation Parkinsonism was diagnosed and Sinemet (levodopa with carbidopa) was prescribed. Both drugs were then supplied on repeat prescription and no further consultation made until the present admission.

On Mr M's admission to hospital a cardiac monitor was set up and all drugs stopped. Blood pressure was only slightly raised and subsequently fell to within a normal range. No abnormality was detected and after 10 days the patient was discharged on a small dose of Sinemet to reduce slight rigidity. At an outpatient follow-up the drug was withdrawn and the patient remains well and drug free.

This problem was due to both side-effects and interactions; firstly, reserpine alkaloids (Decaserpyl-plus) deplete dopamine, the addition of the drug levodopa (Sinemet) rectified the condition—one drug nullifying the effect of the other. The patient's 'turn' was most probably due to postural hypotension, a known side-effect of levodopa, and an increasing sensitivity to the drug.

CHANGES IN DRUG RESPONSE WITH AGE

Many of the strange effects of drugs in elderly patients can be accounted for by the changes in drug handling which occur with increasing age. No two individuals are the same in their response to illness or drugs, and similarly they are not the same in the degree or sequence with which their organs age. The normal dose recommended and response expected of a given dose of drug is calculated using the dose response of normal healthy young men; from these recommendations the prescribing doctor must estimate doses for young, old and sick patients. This situation has been remedied for some drugs by comparative studies of young and elderly volunteers, but as yet there are many areas in which the appropriate dose for the elderly has to be determined by trial and error, based on the theoretical changes in drug handling which might be a consequence of ageing.

Changes in the ability to absorb drugs

Most drugs are administered orally. Before they can reach the site of action they must be absorbed into the body, enter the circulation and be transported to that site. Changes in the gastrointestinal tract associated with ageing could account for differences in the amount and timing of drug absorption.

Reduced gastric acid secretion as shown by a reduction in basal gastric acid and histamine-stimulated secretion occurs in the elderly. This could reduce the solubility of acidic drugs (aspirin) and could protect drugs (penicillins) destroyed by gastric acid.

Gut motility and the rate of gastric emptying are reduced. This increases the overall transit time of drugs to the site of absorption. A slower peak and prolonged overall absorption of the drug may result. In general this is of little consequence when drugs are given long term, but if a speedy high concentration is required (analgesia, antimicrobial chemotherapy) the expected effect may not be achieved. Delayed emptying of the stomach may also result in excessive irritation from known gastric irritants (non-steroid anti-inflammatories and levodopa) causing non-compliance by patients. Reduced gut transit time may result in an overall increase in drug absorption, and so lower doses of drug can be given.

Actively absorbed drugs such as the amines (methyldopa, levodopa) may have reduced absorption because of a decrease in absorbing cells resulting from the slower turnover of active cells with age. Most drugs are, however, unaffected since absorption is generally passive.

The destruction of drugs by gut metabolic enzymes is probably reduced as enzyme levels decrease, although where duodenal diverticula are present bacterial colonisation may result in bacterial enzyme destruction of some drugs and so account for unpredictable treatment failure.

The effects of ageing on drug absorption are therefore subtle, variable and unpredictable and can only be proved by the assay of plasma drug concentrations during the absorption period. Even then, more than one change may occur and one may counter the other, for example, a reduced ability to absorb may be unnoticed because decreased transit time allows a prolonged period for the slow absorption to take place.

The absorption of drugs from other sites

Changes in drug absorption from other sites may also be affected.

Injected drugs rely on subcutaneous or muscular circulation to carry the drug into the body circulation. Reduction in muscle tone and inactivity can mean that the injected drug remains in a tissue depot for longer than usual. Bruising may occur because of increased fragility of blood vessels, so that a careful rotation of sites is vital when repeated injections are necessary.

Locally administered drugs instilled into the eye, nose or ear and applied to the surface of the skin, mouth or vagina are generally not absorbed into the circulation, but produce an effect locally. With age, the elasticity, moisture and turnover of the body's surface cells is reduced and repeated applications may, therefore, result in irritation, soreness or local breakdown of the surface. A check of the surface condition should be made prior to each application, particularly in less visible places (ear, mouth) and any discharge (vagina) or soreness reported before another application is made.

Changes in drug distribution

The usefulness of any drug lies both in its specific action against the disease for which it is prescribed and in its ability to concentrate in the diseased organ. Alterations in the body's composition and physical activity which are the result of ageing can affect the distribution of drugs in the body.

The relative proportions of muscle and fat in the body change with increasing age. In young people, body fat represents 18% of tissue mass in men and 33% in women. By the age of 65 to 85 years these proportions are increased to 36% in men and 45% in women (Novak 1972). This increase in the proportion of fat to muscle means that there is a larger depot for fat-soluble drugs (barbiturates, anaesthetics, benzodiazepines) in elderly people. On administration the drug is rapidly taken up into the fatty tissue and subsequently released only slowly for metabolism and excretion. This accounts for some of the changes seen in elderly patients in their response to fat-soluble drugs including prolonged confusion after anaesthetics and reduced neuromuscular responsiveness after sedation (Cook et al 1983).

Body water reduces by as much as 15% between the ages of 20 and 80 years (Norris et al 1963). The reduction in fluid, with a parallel reduction in size, leads to the higher concentrations of some drugs recorded for elderly patients following a standard dose. This may result in unexpected signs of overdose following what is considered to be 'normal' dosage, particularly during long-term therapy.

Changes in plasma proteins occur in the elderly. Although the overall plasma protein concentration is not changed, a 19% reduction in albumin content has been recorded (Misra et al 1975). Albumin is the most plentiful protein in the plasma and acts as a vehicle for drug transport by binding drugs. Bound drugs are carried in the plasma and are not active or available for metabolism or excretion. A reduction in albumin may result in higher concentrations of unbound drug and increased drug action.

Changes in blood flow caused by reduced cardiac output have been reported in the elderly, reduction being about 30% between the ages of 30 and 65 years. The consequent reduction in blood flow to the organs is not uniform, flow to the liver and kidney being more reduced than that to the brain with little overall change to the circulation of the cardiac and skeletal muscle (Bender 1965). These changes are likely to reduce the speed of detoxification and excretion of drugs from the body.

Changes in metabolism

Drugs entering and circulating in the body are generally treated as foreign substances. They are actively destroyed and made harmless, a process which usually renders them more easily excreted. The most active site of drug metabolism is in the liver, where drugs absorbed from the gut are subject to breakdown and/or conjugation which renders them inactive. A considerable amount of any drug dose may be lost during this 'first pass' through the liver before entering the general circulation, and the dose is calculated accordingly. Theoretically, liver drug metabolism is reduced in the elderly by the combined factors of reduction in liver size (from 2.6% bodyweight in middle age to 1.6% at 90 years), reduction in blood flow, and in the capacity for enzyme production. Liver capacity is well in excess of requirements throughout life, and although studies have been made of the metabolism of some drugs in the elderly, little change in rate has been shown. With antipyrine, however, the drug usually used to test metabolic capacity, an increased half-life (the time taken for plasma concentration to reduce by 50%) and metabolic clearance has been demonstrated with age. It is therefore probable that the liver's capacity to metabolise drugs is impaired in elderly people, and that the normal response to repeated drug administration (i.e. an increase in the production of metabolising enzymes) is sluggish or delayed. In the same way the response of metabolising enzymes in the gut and other tissues will be lower. Diminished overall metabolism would lead to an increase in drug concentration and a great risk of toxicity.

Changes in excretion

Renal excretion is the principal route for the removal of excess toxins and waste from the body. Changes in the kidney's capacity as measured by renal function are, therefore, an important pointer to both the concentration and rate of excretion of drugs and metabolites in the elderly. Although serum creatinine levels remain constant in healthy individuals throughout life, the rate of creatinine excretion as calculated by the creatinine clearance rate decreases steadily thoughout life. For drugs which are excreted, unchanged, creatinine clearance can be a direct indicator of the rate of drug excretion. As we have seen, it is doubtful that the passive absorption of drugs is reduced in the elderly. Any increase in the plasma levels of drugs principally excreted in the urine is therefore likely to be due to reduced renal clearance. For drugs (e.g. digoxin) which have only small differences between the concentrations that are therapeutic and toxic, and are excreted unchanged in the urine, any build up of drug could be dangerous.

The elderly patient is therefore vulnerable to the risk of unintentional overdose effects. Patients on long-term therapy will, as they grow older, become more at risk so that dose adjustment will be necessary. Many elderly patients regulate their drug intake themselves according to side-effects or unintentionally by forgetting the odd dose. When admitted to hospital the full prescribed dose will be administered leading to the possibility of a toxic response.

Although the action, concentration and clearance of drugs metabolised before excretion will not be altered by reduced renal capacity, their metabolised products will be. As a consequence these metabolic products may accumulate in the body.

Other routes of excretion are possible. As with any other products of metabolism excretion via the bile, skin, lung or body fluids may occur with drugs. These routes are only of major importance in cases of renal damage. For elderly people, a general decline in the efficiency of these other routes makes the consequences of renal failure even more disastrous.

Changes in receptor sensitivity

The changes in the physiology of the gut, skin, circulation and liver account for the variations of drug concentration seen for elderly patients and hence unexpected symptoms of over- or under-dosage to a normal dose. For elderly patients a number of responses have been recorded which do not readily fit into the accepted categories of toxicity and which can only be explained as differences in sensitivity. For example, a single dose of a barbiturate can produce a whole range of responses, from restlessness to frank psychosis. Sensitivity may also be altered with diseases such as those of the vascular system where an increased sensitivity to warfarin can be expected. On the whole the unexpected symptoms of drug sensitivity are vague; rashes, dizziness, confusion and agitation are common symptoms which may often be passed off as signs of 'getting old'.

Adverse reactions

Adverse drug reactions are more common for the elderly than for younger individuals, firstly because more elderly people take drugs regularly. The elderly are also more likely to be taking a number of drugs, polypharmacy, which results from multiple symptoms. A number of the drugs prescribed are known to cause problems because of side-effects (anti-inflammatories) or because there is only a small difference between the toxic and therapeutic drug concentration (digoxin). Finally, the drug-taking habits of elderly patients may make them more vulnerable to adverse reactions. Where knowledge and understanding of the treatment is lacking and memory is needed to take the drugs effectively, mistakes are liable to occur.

Adverse reactions fall into three classes: dose related, hypersensitivity, idiosyncratic.

Dose-related reactions are apparent as overdose symptoms. These are either due to exceeding the dose or to changes in the individual's handling or sensitivity to the drug.

Hypersensitivity reactions are due to genetic or immunological abnormalities. Genetic differences may not be discovered even for elderly patients if the drug has not been taken before.

Idiosyncratic responses may also result from a combination of genetic, disease and age related causes. These reactions are bizarre, not being within the range of expected effects of the drug.

Drug-induced disease

Disease may result from either dose-related or hypersensitivity reactions and there are individual variations in the presentation of disease from the same drug. Drug-induced disease generally develops with prolonged use of the drug. The likelihood of gastric ulcer during anti-inflammatory use increases with age. Nutritional defects are more likely with the prolonged use of drugs which dull the appetite or reduce absorption (digitalis, anti-convulsants, amphetamines), create malabsorption (mineral oil, phenolphthalin, phenytoin), increase urinary loss of ions (diuretics, cortisone, alcohol) or act as vitamin K (warfarin), vitamin B6 (levodopa) or foliate (trimethoprim) antagonists.

The majority of deaths from adverse drug reactions are due to commonly used drugs such as digitalis, antimicrobials, insulin and diuretics, from overdosage or from predictable side-effects. The most common adverse reactions reported for elderly people are shown in Table 20.1.

COMPLIANCE WITH TREATMENT REGIMES

No drug can be effective unless it is taken. Non-compliance is therefore a major cause of treatment failure. True non-compliance (the complete refusal of treatment) is fortunately less common than repeated medication errors which can amount to treatment failure. In

Table 20.1 Problem drugs for the elderly

Drug group	Problems/symptoms
Cardiac glycosides	Overdosage easy—little difference between toxic and therapeutic dose. Overdose effects more common when combined with potassium depleting diuretics, hypercalcaemia and hypothyroidism. Adverse symptoms—nausea, vomiting, confusion, depression, gynaecomastia and acute abdominal syndrome. Any sort of arrythmia may occur
Diuretics	Thiazides—potassium deficiency, digoxin toxicity. Frusemide and ethacrynic acid—homeostatic upsets, transitory or permanent deafness, impaired glucose tolerance
Benzodiazepines	Reduced reaction time. Build-up of sedation with repeated dosage
Antidepressants	Tricyclics—accentuated side-effects, dry mouth, hypertension, drowsiness. Many interactions possible. MAOIs—potential hazard due to interactions with food and self-administered drugs
Anti-inflammatories	Age-related increase in incidence of gastric ulcer, bleeding and dyspepsia with both steroid and non-steroid drugs. Interactions with anticoagulants
Phenothiazines	Induce Parkinsonism, lethargy and hypotension. May cause cholestatic jaundice are reduce liver and thyroid function. Contribute to accidental hypothermia. Interacts with alcohol—effects enhanced
Oral anticoagulants	Increased anticoagulant response (warfarin), possibly due to reduced clotting factor production. Unpredicted haemorhagic complications. Possible interations, non-steroid anti-inflammatories, steroids, barbiturates, quinadine, thyroxine.

hospital it is the nurse's responsibility to ensure that drugs are administered correctly and that the patient actually receives the drug. Omissions do happen, the majority of which are due to the unavailability of either the patient or the drug (Bergman et al 1979). In addition administration may prove difficult because the patient fails to swallow the tablet. The patient should be offered a full glass of, preferably, water with tablets and possibly more liquid if there are a number of tablets. Rushing does not help, if the patient fails to swallow, remove the tablet with a spoon, offer a drink, and start again. A drink of water should also be offered following liquid drugs as these are often sticky and leave an unpleasant feeling in the mouth. Injections may be difficult or even ooze out of flabby skin, and bruising commonly occur with elderly patients. Such problems should be reported to the doctor so that, where possible, alternative routes of administration can be used either on a temporary or permanent basis.

Refusal of treatment

Some patients will openly refuse treatment and where the situation is known it can be easily dealt with. In most cases explanation of the reason for treatment and the benefits to be expected, or the suggestion that the patient tries the drug for a few days, will win confidence and get treatment started. If the patient dislikes the drug because of its taste or from, a change may be possible and should be made. Often the reason for refusal is this simple and seeing the patient's point of view makes all the difference. In other instances the refusal of drugs may be legitimate, for example when analgesics are given and there is no pain or when the patient knows of or is suffering side-effects.

The reason for refusal may, with elderly patients, appear to be for a relatively minor reason: suspicion, long-held belief or fears, the similarity of the drug name to others which are known to be dangerous. These problems are best dealt with by clear explanation at the initiation of drug therapy.

More difficult to deal with is the patient who conceals her non-compliance. Drugs may be hidden, spat out or hoarded; where failure of

treatment occurs, this possibility should be explored. Hoarded drugs are a potential danger, they may be found by other patients and used or distributed by the patient for others, without anyone being aware of the potential hazard.

Case history

Mrs N was originally prescribed nembutal as a sedative during a United States Air Force (USAF) alert in Norfolk—the noise of the planes kept her awake. The drug was added to those on her repeat prescription card by the general practitioner's secretary and on all subsequent occasions she was issued with a repeat prescription which included nembutal with her other drugs. When the USAF alert was over she only took the drug on 'bad nights' and accumulated quite a backlog of capsules. One day a friend complained of not sleeping well, so Mrs N kindly gave her a few capsules and then a bottle. Other customers followed and the prescription was subsequently accepted, so that she could supply her friends' needs. All these barbiturate-takers were elderly and fortunately well, and not taking much alcohol or drugs which might interact. Mrs N was amazed when she was told of the problems which could have developed and is now a reformed character.

Medication errors

Studies have shown that the main cause of non-compliance is lack of comprehension of the regime. This includes errors of omission, of addition and of mistiming of the treatment regime. In addition to the problem of a failing memory, poor vision, lack of manual dexterity and overall immobility contribute to non-compliance by elderly patients. Many complaints from elderly patients and their relatives, some of which are resolved only after hospital admission, are due to mistakes or misunderstanding of the treatment by patient and relatives.

Case history

Mr W, aged 70 years, came to the outpatients department with his wife who complained that he kept her awake all night and then went to sleep in the morning when she 'had all her work to do'. Mr W was being treated for cardiac failure and had been discharged from hospital three weeks before on a drug regime of digoxin, thiazide diuretic with potassium supplement, and nitrazepam. He had kept very well but admitted that he did have to get up several times at night to urinate. The pharmacist checked his tablets with him, except for the sleeping tablets which he kept by his bed. He explained that he hand 'little white ones' (heart tablest) twice a day and the 'white ones' (water tablets) in the morning together with the 'oblong ones' which 'were to put back what went out with the water'. Unfortunately all the containers were the same and the print rather small otherwise he might have noticed the he was in fact taking this sleeping tablets, white round tablets, in the morning instead of his 'water tablets' also white and round, which he had by his bed and took at night. The problem was solved by putting a different coloured label on the sleeping tablets and making sure that they and not the diuretic tablets were by his bed.

Muddling tablets is a common problem. Many patients keep all the day's drugs in one bottle and take them randomly. Some even keep their husband's or wife's tablets together with their own.

Measures to improve compliance

Acceptance

Making treatment acceptable to the patient is the first step to compliance. Many patients have fixed ideas about drugs or may expect strange things to happen to them, such as becoming impotent or 'queer in the head'. Such ideas are often based on old wives' tales or stories they have heard about completely different conditions. Even so, the worry is real and must be dealt with honestly, with the benefits and possible difficulties encountered by patients starting on the drug explained.

Helping patients to obtain drugs

Patients who leave hospital are supplied with drugs to take with them and subsequent prescriptions when required are generally obtained through the general practitioner. This should be explained to the patient and reassurance given that her doctor will know which drugs she is to take. The patient should be informed that the tablets she receives from the pharmacy may look different to those she receives from the general practitioner and that a repeat prescription should be ordered at least a week before supplies run out. In some cases it may be necessary for a relative or home help to collect repeat prescriptions. For

people of retirement age (60 years for women and 65 for men) prescriptions are free of charge if they fill in and sign the reverse of the prescription form and any patient receiving drugs after this age should be reminded of this.

Accurate administration

Memory aids

The routine for drug administration varies in different hospitals, but for patients starting a new drug it is the hospital routine which is taught. On discharge from hospital, this routine may need to be adapted to fit in with the patient's home life. Remembering when to take drugs is a difficult problem for elderly patients. The problem is increased in proportion to the number of drugs to be taken and the different regimes of administration. Where possible, patients should be taught to administer their drugs before discharge, an innovation which has proved a useful aid to compliance (Baxendale et al 1978). Simple measures such as linking drug-taking to events in the daily routine (getting up, washing, mealtimes) or marking a diary when the drug is taken may be all that is needed for some patients. Calender-packed drugs are also helpful in this respect. For patients with greater difficulties it may be necessary to make use of 'dose boxes' (Fig. 20.1). These are compartmented boxes, or collections of tablet containers, which are filled with a supply of drugs, generally weekly (Hatch and Tapley 1982). Each dose is placed in an individual compartment and the patient can check that the drug has been taken by seeing the compartment empty. This method requires the recruitment of a relative, neighbour or friend who can prime the box, but it means that the patient remains independent. The final resource for a patient who cannot remember drugs, is to employ another to administer them. This could be difficult, however, because elderly friends and relatives may also have memory problems.

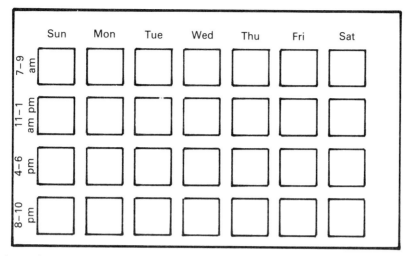

Fig. 20.1 Layout for multicompartment dose box. Design, printing, times and opening methods vary so that a suitable type can be chosen for the individual's needs.

Aids for physical disability

Many adults have difficulty in opening child-proof drug containers, and this problem increases with age. On request to the pharmacist drugs can be dispensed in conventional containers or in containers with winged lids (Fig. 20.2); these are very helpful for stiff hands. Small tablets may be difficult to handle and wide-necked bottles or tablet dispensers

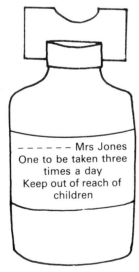

– – – – – Mrs Jones
One to be taken three
times a day
Keep out of reach of
children

Fig. 20.2 National Health Service container with 'winged' cap.

can help with this problem. Where these are used, they must be adequately labeled and help may be needed in filling them in. Calender packs may need to be snipped with scissors if the patient cannot tear the foil.

Poor sight should be compensated with large print or identifiable symbols for tablet container recognition. Braille labels are available, but not all blind people read Braille. Dose boxes are also useful as the patient can feel which compartments are empty. For liquid, a medicine measure cut down or painted clearly to the level of the exact dose, or a fixed volume syringe, may be useful.

All innovations should, however, be tried out with the patient to check that they work for her. As patients get older they may well require more help. For example, a nurse who can give an injection in a now inaccessible site would be welcomed by elderly diabetics. Reappraisal of the situation is important and should be remembered by nurses in outpatients and general practitioners' clinics, as well as by the visiting district nurse (see Chapter 26).

Complete compliance is only possible with obsessional patients. For most drugs the occasional omission has only a minor effect and may at times be useful in reducing side-effects, as with digoxin therapy. Additional doses can, however, be dangerous for the elderly (e.g. sedatives, digoxin, levodopa). The patient should be advised not to take an additional tablet just in case it may have been forgotten.

Case history

M J is a very fit, independent 78-year-old, successfully treated with Sinemet (levodopa and cabidopa) for Parkinsonism. One morning when he had an important meeting to attend at his local club and in his anxiety not to be late he suddenly wondered, 'Have I taken my morning dose of Sinemet?' Being very conscious of the benefits of the drug, he took another dose before he went out to be sure and drove to the club in his car. On arrival he felt dizzy and had to sit in the car again (postural hypotension), and on entering the club he rushed to the toilet and was sick (gastric irritation). The dizziness remained and a friend telephone his wife. She suggested phoning the doctor to which her husband responded by angrily knocking the telephone on the floor (aggression). All these manifestations, postural hypotension, gastric irritation and aggression, are symptoms of levodopa overdose. Mr J had, of course, taken his drug as normal with his breakfast.

SELF-MEDICATION

Self-medication, the prescribing of drugs for one's self has an important role in self-care and the maintenance of independence. Traditionally, the treatment of common ailments such as colds, coughs, headaches, constipation and symptoms such as aches and pains, together with first aid in the home, has rested on the individual or the family carer (mother). The purchase of medicines 'over the counter' (OTC) also rests with the individual or the one in charge of shopping. Choice of drugs may be traditional, influenced by advertising or by discussion with neighbours or friends. Occasionally, the advice of a nurse at the health clinic, the doctor, or the pharmacist may be sought, generally because the condition is one not encountered previously. The treatment of symptoms related to feeling 'unwell' is common. In 1972 a study made by Dunnel and Cartwright (1972) reported that nine out of every 10 people interviewed said

they had felt unwell in the previous two weeks, describing one or more symptoms. Drugs purchased OTC for self-treatment may be obtained from many outlets (slot machine, pharmacy, etc). The drugs taken most commonly, such as antipyretic analgesics (e.g. aspirin), are obtainable in many shops. The controls placed on them by the Medicines Act (1968) are related to the number and strength of tablet on sale through the different outlets. Large quantities of most OTC drugs are only allowed to be sold when a pharmacist is present. Many OTC drugs, including cold cures, contain a number of ingredients which may include aspirin, paracetamol, anti-histamines, stimulants and alcohol, all possible interactors with prescribed drugs.

The symptoms suffered by the elderly tend to be ascribed to 'old age', and these patients tend therefore to collect drugs in case they need them and to take drugs to maintain normality. This may delay their visit to the doctor or mask the symptoms of disease.

Problems associated with self-medication

Overdose may result from patients' 'doubling up' on drugs already issued on prescription, for example taking a 'cold cure' containing aspirin when prescribed soluble aspirin for rheumatic pain. This may result in frank overdose symptoms such as tinnitus or accentuated side-effects such as gastrointestinal bleeding.

Interactions with prescribed medicines may result if the patient is not advised of the possibility occurring, for example, between cold cures and monamine oxidase inhibitors (MAOIs) or between aspirin and coumarin anticoagulants. Patients tend not to consider that patent medicines are drugs, nor that they might cause problems in relation to prescribed drugs.

Masking symptoms as mentioned above can be a problem, the symptoms of illness of elderly patients often present in an unusual fashion. Pain which might be diagnostic of myocardial infarct in younger patients is often mild or absent in the elderly. Thus the taking (or giving) of an analgesic for mild chest pain or discomfort might rob the doctor of a useful diagnostic pointer.

Abuse of OTC drugs is common, particularly in relation to laxatives analgesics, and vitamins. In general, OTC drugs are only able to relieve symptoms; they are therefore of no use in prophylaxis. For example, the habitual taking of laxatives by elderly people who believe that only a daily motion is normal, can lead to dependence verging on addiction. The patient feels normal only if she has the laxative, and her bowel is incapable of evacuating without it. This may in time lead to fluid loss, malabsorption, irritation and a loss of normal function.

Non-drugs

Few people, other than pharmacologists, consider alcohol, tobacco, coffee, tea or herbs to be drugs. However, they all contain pharmacologically active ingredients with known action in the body. Many, such as alcohol, caffeine and nicotine, are known to have addictive properties as well as personal and social attributes. In moderation they may be useful and advantageous, but in excess can cause physical damage. Alcohol, for example, can be useful in the form of sherry as an appetite stimulant, whisky is a useful night sedative, and beer or stout provide useful energy and nutrients. Excessive use of alcohol is often a symptom of loneliness or depression and can lead to damage of the liver and brain.

In recent years herbalism has become more popular as an alternative to conventional medicine and is considered to be safer. The tests used on, and regulations such as quality control for, herbal remedies are less stringent than for drugs in spite of the fact that many contain pharmacologically active ingredients. For example herbs reputed to act on the heart or as diuretics (Adonis, False Hellebore, Yellow Foxglove) contain cardiac glycosides and will therefore potentiate the effect of prescribed drugs such as digoxin.

WHERE THE NURSE CAN HELP

When patients enter hospital they enter an institution which has organised routines, where many individuals from different disciplines with different levels of knowledge and at different stages in training, all have a role in the organisation of patient care. The routines of organisation are there to ensure that many activities are undertaken in an approved manner for many reasons such as efficiency, tradition and safety. The rules for drug ordering, care and issue are controlled for these reasons, but different activities are undertaken by different professionals. Prescription is generally the doctor's responsibility, issue the pharmacist's and administration the nurse's. At home the patient is responsible for administration and for the prescription and acquisition of non-prescription drugs. In taking over the role of drug administration the nurse imposes routines, generally based on tradition, which suit the hospital setting. For elderly patients who have been managing their drugs to home, these changes many be muddling and lead to non-compliance on discharge. Removing independence makes the patient incapable of self-care later and imposes physical changes which alter the drug response. Most of these problems can be avoided if the nurse appreciates the situation and the patient takes an active part in the drug routine.

On admission to hospital

The patient is usually asked to hand over the drugs taken at home when entering hospital. This action offers the nurse an ideal opportunity to obtain a drug history in which information on drugs currently taken, past problems with drugs and self-medication preferences can be acquired. Where possible, the hospital routine can be adapted to the patient's and changes in routine explained to the patient. Information on self-medication can be relayed to the doctor so that, where suitable, the patient's favourite laxative analgesic or indigestion mixture can be prescribed and be available when required. The drug history need not be collected all in one session, particularly if the patient is already exhausted with questioning. Some information may be more easily obtained from relations or friends.

Checklist for a drug history

1. *Prescribed drugs* from the general practitioner or hospital outpatients will already have been discussed with the medical staff. Information obtained by the nurse may, however, supplement and check this and some estimate of compliance gained. The list of drugs, numbers and times taken should be checked with the medical record. In the confusion of admission the patient may have forgotten one or told the doctor incorrectly that it was taken. These incidents occur particularly where there are many drugs or memory problems.

2. *The drug-taking routine* should be discussed, such as the times drugs are taken, their relationship to meals, sleep and other daily activities. Some patients will develop sleep problems if thyroxid or diuretic drugs are given too late in the day for them. A small alteration in nursing routine may prevent a sedative being given. A change in the routine of taking drugs either before or after meals will often alter the absorption pattern and response. Discussion of the routine will also give an estimate of compliance problems to be encountered on discharge.

3. *Self-prescribed drugs* are often forgotten but for many patients form a part of their everyday life. The discussion should include drugs routinely used, habits of use, any allergies, herbal treatment and dietary products such as bran, vitamins and slimming pills. The current fashion for dietary fads is often taken to extremes by people who do not fully understand what is intended, like the man who ate a pot of yoghurt after every meal because he was told it was good for slimming. The information given may provide clues to symp-

toms such as diarrhoea when laxatives are used daily, and may ensure that abnormal readings are not obtained in tests. Throat lozenges containing iodine can make the thyroid function test of a myxoedemic patient appear normal.

4. *Non-drug* stimulants (coffee, tea) or sedatives (alcohol) should also be discussed and their pattern of use established. Many people routinely use sherry to promote appetite (it activates gastric secretion) or whisky as a sedative, and there is generally no reason why this should not be continued for most people. Where bizarre treatments are established it may be necessary to wean the patient gradually from the drug, otherwise they could be physically upset and lose confidence in medical treatments. Such problems are best discussed with the doctor.

During the hospital stay

Through their role in drug administration nurses are in an ideal position to monitor the patient's drug progress, reporting responses and side-effects. They are also the people the patient asks about the drug, what it should do or how it works. Educating the patient about drugs is a very important task. The nurse should, however, be equipped to do so, checking in advance what response should be expected or the side-effects that are possible, so that the information is available when the patient asks questions. This education need not be restricted to current treatment but extended to cover first aid and self-medication. In the course of administration it is often possible to identify problems which may occur on discharge. The patient's physical ability to take drugs (vision, manual dexterity, swallowing) can be assessed and some idea of their ability to remember details obtained. Before discharge from hospital direct patient involvement in her own drug administration, under supervision, is desirable. Such steps have been used in some institutions (Hatch and Tapley 1982) but problems with rules and traditions are often encountered.

Throughout their hospital stay the nurse should be preparing for the patient's discharge, so that when the day comes the patient is not pushed (in a wheelchair) out of the door with a bagful of drugs and unprepared to take them.

On discharge from hospital

Going home might be as big a shock and change as hospital admission. The patient might be unsure about coping with meals at home, shopping, cleaning, is well as with drugs. If instructions and routines have been well established in hospital and are understood, the problems are reduced. Preparation should include liaison with the general practitioner, district nurse, pharmacist and relatives as the need arises. Instructions should be written clearly as well as given verbally. To ensure that they can be read and understood ask the patient to repeat the instructions. Advice on possible adverse effects and interactions with self-medication drugs should be included where they may occur.

Finally, for the patient going home discharge is often not the last contact with hospital. Nurses in the outpatients department can make use of their contact to help elderly patients with any problems which develop after discharge, to check and adapt their drug routine, or to help with compliance aids as they are required.

In many respects, the reaction of elderly patients to drugs and drug taking differs little from that of any other age group. The problems are, however, accentuated by the disease response, physical changes and expectations of the patient. In being aware of this the nurse can anticipate the problems and deal with them on an individual basis.

REFERENCES

Baxendale C, Gourlay M, Gibson I I J M 1978 A self-medication retraining programme. British Medical Journal 2: 1278–1279

Bender A D 1965 The effect of increasing age on the distribution of peripheral blood flow in man. Journal of the American Geriatric Society 13:192

Bergman U, Norlin A, Wiholm B E 1979 Inadequacies in hospital drug handling. Acta Medica Scandinavica 205: 79–84

Christopher L J, Ballinger B R, Shepherd A M M, Ramsay A, Crooks G 1979 A survey of hospital prescribing for the elderly. In: Crooks J, Stevenson I H (eds) Drugs and the elderly, Macmillan, London

Cook P J, Huggett A, Graham-Pole R, Savage I T 1983 Hypnotic accumulation and hangover in elderly inpatients: A controlled double-blind study of Temazepam and Nitrazepam. British Medical Journal 286: 100–102

Dunnel K, Cartwright A 1972 Medicine takers, prescribers and hoarders. Routledge and Kegan Paul, London

Freeman G K 1979 Drug prescribing patterns in the elderly: A general practice study. In: Crooks J, Stevenson I H Drugs and the elderly. Macmillan, London

Hatch A M, Tapley A 1982 A self-administration system for elderly patients at Higbury Hospital. Nursing Times 78(42): 1773–1774

Hodkinson H M 1980 Common symptoms of disease in the elderly, Blackwell, Oxford

Hurwitz N 1969 Predisposing factors in adverse reactions to drugs. British Medical Journal 1: 536–539

Misera D P, Loudon J M, Staddon G E 1975 Albumin metabolism in elderly patients. Journal of Gerontoloqy 30: 304–306

Novak L P 1972 Ageing, total body potassium, free fat mass and cell mass in males and females between 18 and 85 years. Journal of Gerontology 27: 438–443

Norris A H, Lundy T, Sheck N W 1963 Trends in selected indices of body composition in men between the ages of 30 and 80 years. Annals of the New York Academy of Science 110: 623–639

Office of Health Economics 1979 Compendium of health statistics. Office of Health Economics, London

FURTHER READING

Coleman V 1982 The good medicine guide. Thames and Hudson, London

David J A 1983 Drug round companion. Blackwell, Oxford

Heaney C R, Dow R J, MacConnachie A M, Crooks J 1982 Drugs in nursing practice. Churchill Livingstone, Edinburgh

Li Wan Po A 1982 Non-prescription drugs. Blackwell, Oxford

21

J. Hockley

Death and dying

> Nothing is more certain than death; nothing less certain than the time of its coming (Translation of the Latin inscription once present on official wills).

Discussion on the care of the elderly would be incomplete without some discussion on dying. Chalmers (1982) says that the best way to come to terms with old age is first to come to terms with death. This holds a great deal of truth, but as La Rochefoucauld (1613–80) wrote: 'Neither the sun nor death can be looked at with a steady eye.' Often there are no straightforward answers, only a willingness not to run away.

Each individual should take the opportunity to look at death, and, perhaps beyond, before it becomes a threat to his or her own life. A doctor or nurse who has not come to terms with the fact of his or her own death will find it difficult to support the dying (Twycross 1982). In the following few pages we hope that what is so often considered to be a taboo subject might be seen as a positive opportunity to care, so fulfilling the needs not only of elderly dying people but also of the relatives and carers.

Many patients have remarked, 'It is not death that I am afraid of but rather 'how' I am going to die that frightens me.' There is no doubt that this fear of the process of dying has not decreased over the years. Advance in medical science has enabled people to live longer, but many fear that it has been at the expense of dignity. However, with the advent of the hospice movement attitudes towards death and dying have started to change from that of a rather hopeless and depressing one into that of growth—growth not only for the patient, family and carers involved, but for society as a whole.

A century or so ago the greatest proportion of deaths occurred between the ages of 0 and 14 years. There has been an enormous change in this distribution over the past century, with 75% of deaths now occurring over the age of 65 years and as much as 50% of deaths taking place in those over the age of 75 (Office of Population Censuses and Surveys (OPCS) 1979). In dividing the elderly age group in two (those 65–74 years and those over 75 years of age) the percentage of male deaths in each category is much the same. However, when comparing female mortality in these two groups those dying at over 75 years of age are nearly three times as many as those dying in the 65–74 year age group (OPCS 1981).

CAUSES OF DEATH IN THE ELDERLY

In looking at the main causes of death in elderly people, heart disease accounts for just over a third of their deaths in England and Wales (OPCS 1981). Respiratory disease, cancer and cerebral vascular disease have consistently been the next most common causes of death. Up until recently deaths from cancer in the elderly were only significantly high in the 65–74 year age group, but statistics for 1981 show cancer deaths taking preference over cerebral vascular disease in being the third most common cause of death of people over 75 years of age. This may be because of the increased number of elderly people having more investigations to establish a diagnosis prior to death. All these diseases mentioned tend to cause a relatively *slow death* often being accompanied by a certain amount of physical and psychological distress. The gradual awareness of deterioration can appear a wearisome burden both for the patient and the carer.

Sudden death of the elderly is occasionally seen, and a recent national survey (Bowling and Cartwright 1983) showed that 4% of elderly deaths were sudden, without any warning of illness. For the partner who is left, this kind of death can be one of the most difficult to cope with as there is no warning or anticipation of loss. Other relatives, however, may say, 'It was a nice way to go . . . he [or she] did not suffer,' which the grieving spouse may not find particularly helpful.

Natural death of the elderly is rarely observed, partly because few of this age group die at home. Pneumonia, once known as 'the old man's friend' often continues being treated until it becomes a major decision whether to treat or not to treat. Cardiac resuscitation of old people may prevent natural death. A recent account of the attempted resuscitation of an 85-year-old man with a 10 year history of heart disease supports this. He had mentioned on several occasions that he did not wish to have his life prolonged, and the failed resuscitation only succeeded in producing unnecessary suffering for the patient, little comfort for the relatives and a feeling of failure on the part of the hospital staff. Bernard Levin (1980) reminds us of the macabre and repulsive scenes which accompanied the postponed deaths of General Franco of Spain and President Tito of Yugoslavia. Allowing life to move peacefully towards its close is much more preferable for dying people than endeavouring to keep them alive at all costs.

In many primitive societies where one might expect to see the acceptance of natural death, one sees a different concept—that of the acceleration of death. Hinton (1967) describes how nomadic tribes would leave the frail old person behind at the camp site to die, while the rest of the tribe moved on. In other societies it was traditional for the aged to request to be buried alive once they thought they were dying.

Suicidal deaths occur especially amongst the elderly bereaved. They may feel that, now their lifelong partner has gone, there is no incentive to go on living.

Mr Day was a 75-year-old man who was admitted having attempted suicide by taking an overdose of sleeping tablets. His wife had died six months previously and although he went to luncheon clubs and got invited out by his attentive daughter at the weekend, he could not cope with the fact of being in the house alone.

The adjustment many bereaved elderly have to make especially after a long happy marriage is often an uphill struggle, even with willing family and friends to help. (Suicide is discussed in more detail in Chapter 19.) If an actual suicide is not attempted one commonly hears of a widow or widower dying of a 'broken heart'.

WHERE PEOPLE DIE

In 1973 Cartwright et al estimated that about 60% of deaths occurred in hospital or similar institutions; 10 years later it is estimated at nearer 70%. In America, as many as four out of five elderly people spend their last days in a hospital, nursing home or other type of institution (Lerner 1970). However, Bowling and Cartwright (1983) found that if a patient was aged 80 or over at the time of death these were the ones least likely to die in hospital.

General hospital

The 'acute' setting of the general hospital, although having all the facilities, in many ways is not the most ideal place for dying elderly people. The rigid routine and pressing physical needs of other patients easily takes time away from the psychosocial and spiritual care of the dying. The opportunity to just 'be' with dying people is given lower priority than all the things to 'do' for those patients getting better. Bowling and Cartwright (1983) found that patients dying in hospitals were more likely to die alone and even when the spouse had stayed overnight at the hospital they were often absent at the time of death. Nurses, medical students and doctors often lack the teaching and experience to initiate the different care the dying require, and so dying patients may feel isolated.

Hospice

A hospice incorporates a homely atmosphere with medical and nursing expertise. Since hospices are small (the largest in England having only 62 beds) patients are able to receive individualised physical, psychosocial and spiritual care. Within these units tests and observations are kept to a minimum so that the patient is not unnecessarily disturbed. The grieving family will be cared for for as long as is necessary even after the death of the patient. Hospices are ideal for caring for dying patients and their families because nurses and doctors are trained and motivated to do this work. Unfortunately, except in a few cases, beds are provided only for those dying from cancer.

Home for incurables

These long-stay units provide excellent care for patients dying from non-malignant disease. There is the time to build relationships between staff and patient in a homely atmosphere. Both this kind of Home and the hospice rely heavily on voluntary help and well-motivated personnel for practical and financial support.

Continuing care unit/geriatric ward

These units are perhaps the most used to caring for dying elderly people outside the hospice setting. People working in these units are often highly motivated but they can become frustrated because low staffing levels prevent them from giving adequate care. Many of the patients are in this setting because they have no one to care for them at home, and consequently few visitors are available to help with needs such as feeding and sitting with these patients. The great demand on the physical needs in these units again often detracts from the needs of the dying. However, because patients dying on these wards may have been nursed in the unit many months and sometimes years, a close relationship has often been established between patient and nurse and between patient and doctor, which helps in understanding the patient's specific needs.

The standard of care varies greatly from unit to unit, but unfortunately public and professional opinion is, often mistakenly, rather gloomy. There is still a stigma attached to being a patient in a geriatric ward.

Nursing home

These Homes vary in the quality of care they give to dying elderly residents. They rely on the community service of general practitioners and district nurses and although often providing a more homely setting than hospital, they might not be able to provide the expertise required to nurse the dying. The current pilot scheme in England of National Health Service nursing Homes may provide the necessary expertise. These are discussed briefly later in the chapter.

At home

For old people, dying at home is often preferred. They will suffer tremendous hardships to be able to stay in the familiarity and comfort of their own home where they can feel in control of what happens to them. However, few relatives can stand the pressure of giving 24-hour care over a long period of time without considerable back-up, medical care and support.

With the gradual emergence of domiciliary terminal care support teams attached to both hospitals and hospices, keeping the dying patient at home has been made a possibility in some areas. This would appear to be the ideal sort of care, but unfortunately this limited service is generally confined to those dying of cancer.

MANAGING THE PROBLEMS OF THE DYING ELDERLY PERSON

Hinton (1967) states that most people will have a terminal period lasting a few days or weeks—not usually exceeding three months. The art of caring for the dying refers mainly to this period of terminal illness and, irrespective of the length of the terminal phase of an illness, control of the problems that may arise is essential in order to achieve a good quality of life. Unfortunately, the terminal phase for the old person dying from a non-malignant disease is not always easy to define.

In Cartwright et al's (1973) study, relatives or friends of the deceased reported several symptoms which either they or the patient had found distressing: pain (66%), sleeplessness (49%), loss of appetite (48%), dyspnoea (45%). As was said earlier, it is often 'how' someone is going to die that frightens them more than the actual concept of death.

Pain

Most people fear pain more than anything (Saunders and Baines 1983), and many patients associate this fear with dying. It is important to remember that what presents as physical pain in the dying might be due to psychological, social or spiritual factors. 'Total' pain (Saunders 1978) is a phrase used in a deliberate attempt to encourage people to look at various factors of a dying patient's distress. Twycross (1978) states that pain is often not just a physical sensation but an emotional reaction to it. People's pain thresholds vary considerably but can be lowered and raised by certain factors (see Table 21.1).

Table 21.1 Factors modifying pain threshold. From Twycross 1978

Threshold lowered ↓	Threshold raised ↑
Anger	Diversion
Anxiety	Sympathy
Depression/sadness	Elevation of mood
Discomfort	Relief of symptoms
Fatigue	Rest
Fear	Understanding
Insomnia	Sleep
Introversion	Drugs
Mental isolation	Analgesics
Past experience	Anxiolytics
	Antidepressants

There has been a considerable improvement in the control of pain over the past 10–15 years through the work of hospices and the wider use of opiates, nerve blocks and electrical stimulators, but Parkes and Parkes (1984) showed that pain was still a problem at home causing a 'very great anxiety' for spouses.

To believe the patient when he says he has pain is essential, but must not stop there. The nurse's duty is not just to report pain but to know its site or sites, duration and description, whether it is most likely the result of the illness or of other factors such as infection, position or constipation, and how long after analgesia it recurs. Both body and pain charts can be helpful in recording and assessing pain on certain patients and allow for a better continuity of care. The assessment of pain has been described in detail in Chapter 17.

For the dying patient adequate relief of 'useless' or 'chronic' pain is paramount—without it, patients will often die sooner. Analgesics must be given regularly in a therapeutic dose before the pain returns. Charles-Edwards (1983) explains in detail the various analgesics available. The use of opiate medication (morphine and diamorphine) for the dying will almost always relieve any discomfort or suffering. The right dose of elixir for each patient (beginning with 2.5 mg) must be given every four hours for the proper control of pain. The 'Brompton cocktail' (a mixture of diamorphine, chlorpromazine and cocaine in an alcoholic base) was for many years the drug of choice, and still is used by some doctors. However, more recently it has been found that just diamorphine or morphine made up in chloroform water gives adequate pain relief without making the patient too sleepy.

An anti-emetic is also given with the opiate but prescribed separately to prevent any nausea. It can be discontinued after 2–3 days if nausea is not a problem. If and when a patient is unable to take oral medication, then suitable alternative measures must be taken, such as giving the analgesia sublingually, by suppository or by subcutaneous injection. Four-hourly subcutaneous injections can be substituted by a battery-operated 'syringe driver' which administers a steady dose of medication, usually diamorphine, over a 24-hour period.

Anorexia and mouth care

Cartwright et al (1973) and Ward (1974) found that 76% and 61% respectively of their terminally ill patients complained of anorexia—second only to pain. Although a lot of people when they are very ill do not feel like eating, factors which reduce the appetite must be detected.

Dirty mouths, sore gums, constipation, nausea and badly presented food are all factors contributing to anorexia. Alcohol before or with a small, nicely presented meal with the willing offer of assistance can be a great help. Prednisolone 5 mg three times daily or dexamethasone 2 mg daily are both used to stimulate the appetite of the terminally ill. However, these drugs can cause fungal infection in the mouth, and so strict and regular mouth care is most important.

Cleaning the teeth with toothpaste and brush is the most effective way of keeping the mouth clean, together with a reasonable fluid intake. Alternatively, a gloved hand and swabs can be used. Once the mouth has become dirty, corsodyl mouth-wash (and if infected, nystatin suspension) is effective. Betadine 'gargle' 1:3 parts of water can be used as another antifungal agent. A solution of lime cordial on swabs is refreshing for the weak and dying patient whose sucking/swallowing reflex is often present right up until near the end. Small pieces of crushed ice placed in a piece of gauze can also be given to the patient to suck on or even be placed between the gums and the cheek. In this way the ice slowly dissolves without the danger of the patient choking. Relatives will often feel more relaxed and 'useful' if they are shown how to assist with this care.

Breathlessness and cough

Breathlessness can be one of the most distressing symptoms for the patient and carer (whether relative or nurse). It is most often present in patients dying from chronic bronchitis, fibrosing alveolitis, heart failure and carcinoma of the lung. Breathlessness produces a vicious circle of anxiety, fear, tension and increased breathlessness. All possible factors causing the breathlessness must be considered and treated appropriately. When these measures are ineffective, small doses of oral morphine or diamorphine with or without a phenothiazine given four hourly (or just at night for some people) can reduce anxiety without reducing the rate of respirations. The use of oxygen via a humidifier and Ventimask can be continued if this is what the patient is accustomed to, but often acts as a barrier to conversation with relatives and staff.

A tiresome cough can be extremely irritating and exhausting for the terminally ill patient. Benylin expectorant is often quite adequate but, if the sputum is thick and tenacious, bromhexine (bisolvon) tablets or elixir is more effective in making the sputum less thick. Linctus methadone 5–10 ml is especially useful at night. In the last stages, if excessive secretions have accumulated ('death rattle') in the lungs, then hyoscine 0.4–0.6 mg given subcutaneously with an opiate can be helpful in drying up secretions.

Nausea and vomiting

Nausea and vomiting can be two of the most demoralising of all symptoms, and adequate control is essential. Hinton (1963) found that these two symptoms as well as breathlessness were the three most difficult to relieve and were particularly common for patients dying from heart and renal failure. Distinguishing between the causes of nausea or vomiting before prescribing the most appropriate antiemetic is the first important step in finding a solution to the problem. Often the cause is one or more of the following:

(a) the use of certain drugs prone to produce nausea, e.g. opiates, gastric irritants;
(b) obstruction of the alimentary tract due either to disease or constipation;
(c) raised intracranial pressure;
(d) metabolic disturbances (e.g. uraemia, hypercalcaemia).

Insomnia

Insomnia in the terminally ill is a lot more common than is generally believed. Unfortunately, this problem is often accepted by both patient and nurse as part of being in hospital and is not taken seriously. A good night's sleep is very important if the terminally ill patient is going to be able to cope with the next day. Cartwright et al (1973) showed that sleeplessness in the dying patient is most common for patients suffering from a malignant or respiratory disease. If symptoms such as pain, breathlessness, anxiety, depression or urinary frequency can be relieved, insomnia should improve. However, if not, medication such as Welldorm, temazepam, or heminevrin should be given. The mistake is often made of omitting night sedation when a patient is receiving opiate medication. This is not a sedative.

Pressure sores

Immobility, incontinence and malnutrition are some of the factors contributing to pressure sores in the elderly dying person. Once these patients get pressure sores it is extremely unlikely that they will heal, and so prevention is paramount. Unfortunately, pressure sores often appear to be accepted as a necessary evil in terminal care. With more people dying in hospital, pressure sores will increase (Barton and Barton 1981). Norton et al (1975) found that 54% of elderly dying patients had pressure sores, 24% developing them while in hospital. In a more recent but smaller study (Hockley 1983), where the average age of the elderly dying patient was 71 years, 61% of the patients had one or more pressure sores, 38% developing them after admission to hospital.

Nurses often appear to be more alert to the risk of sores developing in patients dying from malignant disease rather than other diseases. We hope this will change now that the approach to nursing is more 'problem oriented' than 'disease oriented'. Good observation and nursing care with the help of 'ripple' mattresses, soft sheepskins, Spenco Silicore mattresses should prevent sores from developing. Time taken to explain the necessity of relieving pressure to both patient and relative is time well spent.

Constipation and incontinence

Constipation and urinary incontinence are the two problems likely to make the dying patient feel most undignified. The constipating effect of opiates, weakness, and lack of fluid intake are a few of the factors making the regular prescription of aperients important.

Bulk aperients such as lactulose (Duphalac) syrup and dioctyl sodium sulphosuccinate (Medo or Forte) are very useful for softening the stool. Stimulant aperients to increase peristalsis such as bisacodyl (Dulcolax) tablets or sennoside B (Senokot) tablets can be used. More often than not, however, for the terminally ill patient a combination of a bulk softener and bowel stimulant is preferable, Dorbanex or Dorbanex Forte being the most commonly used.

When the elderly dying patient has had good bladder control, incontinence is often only a problem in the last few hours of life. Continued incontinence is an additional factor in the breakdown of pressure areas, and catheterisation should be considered if incontinence persists over a period of 24–36 hours. However, catheterisation should not be performed as a matter of routine and patients should be given a clear understanding of what is going to be done whether they are able to respond or not.

Confusion and terminal restlessness

Confusion in the dying can be a difficult problem to cope with, especially if the patient is restless at the same time. It can cause a lot of distress to both family and staff. Pain, dyspnoea, a full bladder or rectum may be contributing factors exacerbating confusion, and appropriate treatment of these should be carried out first. For the patient suffering from senile dementia a move to unfamiliar surroundings is bound to increase the confusion, and isolation may easily make the situation worse.

The use of sedatives and tranquillisers must be selective but the following may be helpful:
— haloperidol (Serenace) 5–10 mg daily in divided doses.
— thioridazine (Melleril) 25 mg three times daily.
— chlorpromazine (Largactil) 25–50 mg three times daily.

If muscle twitching is present during the last day or so, diazepam (Valium) 5–10 mg intramuscularly or by suppository is effective.

When a crisis occurs, such as an acute exacerbation of breathlessness, haematemesis or haemoptysis, an injection of diamorphine 2.5 mg and hyoscine 0.4 mg with or without chlorpromazine can be effective. This, together with a nurse to sit and hold the patient's hand, will almost always calm the situation.

Emotional reactions to dying

In describing people's emotional reactions to dying, Kubler-Ross (1973) mentions five stages: denial (disbelief), anger, bargaining, depression and acceptance. These are not necessarily everyone's experience but some of these descriptive stages may be present and patients should be allowed to express them and to work through all their feelings.

Hinton (1963) found that depression and anxiety increased for the dying patient with the length of illness and the degree of distressing symptoms. However, intense anxiety is often only really seen when patients are dying with breathing difficulties or where they have continued to deny the imminence of their death. It is very difficult to measure anxiety although Carr (1982) states that moderate anxiety is experienced by between one quarter and one half of patients, but is less often seen in patients over 60 years of age. Fear of the unknown, the unexplained, being a burden, becoming helpless can often 'paralyse' the dying into an inability to communicate. If these fears can be identified and discussed it will help decrease anxiety and reassure the patient of the love and care surrounding them.

Hope is a very important ingredient to life and should not be excluded from the care of the dying. To be 'written off' by the doctor with the statement 'There is nothing more we can do for you' is extremely devastating. This need never be said—one can always care. Hope for each day or a realistic event should be encouraged, but there is no place for false hope.

Dying does not usually call for specialised skills in counselling—just a willingness to try to understand and stay near. However, when the question 'Am I going to die, nurse?' is suddenly and unexpectedly thrust upon us it is too easy for the denial 'No, of course not' to be the immediate response. It is important to remember that often a patient does not want an immediate answer and this in itself can be a worthwhile pause. To take time to decide what to say is most valuable and can be found by returning the patient's question with a further question.

The relatives and carers

Relatives of dying patients are now more often recognised as part of the emotional network from which the patient has come, and they often need as much help to adjust to the situation as the patient does. In trying to help them they must be allowed to express the confusion, fear, anger and grief they feel. The loss of a family member can be the single most feared event in the life of an individual (Kalish 1977). Whatever age one is, this has to be true; but for the elderly spouse there is the heartbreak, loss and loneliness after many years of marriage. To try and encourage the building of links with close friends or family at this time, before the death, can prevent the relative from isolating her or himself and so help in the bereavement process to follow.

Richmond and Waisman (1955) emphasised that the family's involvement in the physical care of the dying person is extremely important—allowing the family to feel they have been able to 'do' something. They should not be made to feel guilty if they cannot help, or do not want to help, in these tasks. Hampe (1975) has identified eight needs of the spouse of a dying patient: visiting at any time; helping with physical care; prompt and competent attention to physical and emotional needs of the patient; awareness of diagnosis and daily progress by the nursing staff; awareness of impending death; expressing anxieties regarding the care given; comfort and support; friendliness by the health professionals to the spouse.

Some relatives feel it is best that the truth be kept from the dying patient. This, unfortunately, causes a conspiracy of silence to be built up, isolating the patient from those around. Relatives often make excuses to go to the toilet in order to see the doctor, and soon further 'lies' have to be told to keep up the façade. Families should be warned beforehand how easy it is to lie to the patient about her condition but how difficult it is to handle the problems and tensions that this creates.

Inevitably there comes the time when the dying are too weak to 'entertain' their visitors and many relatives feel awkward and helpless. At this point encouraging both relatives and staff to sit by the bed and 'just be there' is often helpful. To the weak and dying patient, the comfort of knowing someone is there is all she needs—knowing that she is not alone. This can, however, be very exhausting for relatives and they may well need to be told to go for a break or go home for a meal with the reassurance that someone will keep a close watch on the patient's condition. One of the dangers of open visiting can be that relatives get overtired, especially if a patient is dying over a number of weeks. In these circumstances, following the idea of many hospices, to make sure the relative has a complete 'day off' is very important.

The anticipation of loss of the loved one should not be discouraged in the case of a terminal illness. Parkes (1972) states that as much as 50% of the grieving should be done beforehand if the person is to cope with the bereavement process. Where anticipatory grief has not been allowed to take place, as with sudden loss, it can cause serious physical or mental breakdown of the bereaved person afterwards. The following case illustrates this point. An elderly widow was admitted with an acute attack of asthma, never having had asthma before. She happened to be admitted to the care of the same doctors who had looked after her husband the previous year. Through tears she related how she had been told by the doctors that her husband had chronic bronchitis and when asked if she wanted to nurse him at home, she agreed. After a rapid deterioration he died four days after discharge and on his death certificate the wife noticed the cause of death to be carcinoma of the bronchus. She had not suspected that her husband was going to die and was utterly distraught—'If I had known I would of done so much more for him, and now he is dead.' With a lot of belated support this lady was slowly able to recover. In being able to give the elderly dying and their relatives the care and respect they deserve enables society once again to recognise a depth of human compassion and understanding.

The following extract describes beautifully how many of us feel when faced with bereaved relatives but it is our duty in caring to reach out to them.

> I did not know what to say to him, I felt awkward and blundering. I did not know how I could reach him, where I could overtake him and go hand in hand with him once more. It is such a secret place the land of tears. (Antoine de Saint-Exupery 1945.)

THE HOSPICE MOVEMENT—COULD ALL ELDERLY PEOPLE BENEFIT?

> To do all we can to help you, not only to die peacefully, but also to live until you die (Cicely Saunders 1978).

The growth of what has become known as the 'hospice movement' now has its influence reaching far and wide across the world. The United Kingdom alone has 70 hospices each varying in size from 8–62 bedded units. The advent of the hospice movement has revealed an attitude of care that is relevant not only to the cancer sufferer but to all who are dying, the elderly included. Evidence of the gratitude shown by our needy society must be seen in the amount of financial support and voluntary help people have given to this movement.

The word 'hospice' was first used in the Middle Ages to describe a 'resting place' or inn, where travelling pilgrims throughout Europe could stay, find food and spiritual comfort to equip them for their journey ahead. This same idea of a resting place for weary travellers, but those weary from life's journey, has been adopted by the hospice movement to describe their philosophy of care. The emphasis is still that of a resting place and not a terminus, as death is not seen as the end, but a passing on.

Within a hospice, basic nursing care is the same as that in hospital but the working environment and philosophy differ greatly. All members of a hospice ward team are motivated to the individualised care of each patient, who in turn receives continual assessment of his or her physical and psychosocial needs as well as sensitive spiritual care. Honesty and openess allow patients to feel secure in the answers to their questions and time is given to talk things through. Families are considered an important part of the patient's emotional well-being and every effort made to meet all the different needs from the youngest grandchild facing his or her first loss, to the wife, mother, sister or husband of the person dying.

Some hospice units have a few beds for those dying from other diseases, such as motor neurone disease. Others provide a 'holiday relief' service that enables relatives caring full-time for someone to go away for a two week break.

To accommodate within hospices all those dying would not be appropriate and certainly was never the idea behind setting them up. If this occurred, death still would run the danger of being hidden away—not in a side-room, as happens now, but in a hospice. Instead, hospices should be seen as a tool for the education of doctors, nurses and the general public in the art of caring for the dying. Cartwright et al (1973) in their nationwide study on 'Life before death' recognised this and recommended that there should be a wide dissemination of these principles into the acute and geriatric hospitals. In this way they felt all terminally ill patients, whether old or young, dying from an acute or chronic illness, could benefit from the hospice expertise. To a small degree this has started to emerge with the setting up of symptom control support teams and palliative care units in a few district and specialist hospitals. Unfortunately, the emphasis is often concentrated on patients with malignant disease.

The recent development in this country of state nursing Homes similar to those in Denmark (Dopson 1983) could provide places where the quality of life for elderly dying people is best achieved. These three experimental NHS units, accommodating around 20–30 people, plan individualised care for each resident. The Department of Health and Social Security (1983) states that an important requirement of the new nursing Homes is to meet the emotional, psychological and spiritual needs of residents. Although these Homes are not specifically intended to provide terminal care, it is recognised that patients may require support and treatment relating to terminal illness and such care will be provided in the Home. This is a further way in which the elderly may benefit from the dissemination of hospice care principles.

EUTHANASIA AND THE ELDERLY

Over the last 20 years euthanasia, the literal meaning of the word being 'an easy death' (Gr. *eu*, Well, *thanatos*, death), has become one of the moral issues of our day. People have had the power to induce death for many hundreds of years but euthanasia is probably at present more widely discussed, (a) because of the greater ability man now has to prolong life owing to medical advances, and (b) the

increasingly secular approach society has towards life. All of us would want an easy death in the sense of its being free from pain and other distressing symptoms, but this is not what is currently being meant by the word 'euthanasia'. It has now become to mean 'the deliberate termination of the life of a person who is suffering from a distressing irremediable disease.' (British Medical Association 1973).

Euthanasia first became a social issue with the formation of the Voluntary Euthanasia Society (or EXIT, as we now know it) in 1935. Since then, pressure has been put on Parliament to try and legalise the action of bringing about death when certain criteria are met. Four Bills have been introduced and debated since 1935 but all have been rejected. In 1969 the Representative Body of the British Medical Association passed a resolution that the medical profession had a duty to preserve life and to relieve pain, and they condemned euthanasia.

Carr (1982) states that public support for euthanasia is probably based upon the expectation that death will be unduly lengthy and prolonged because of current medical knowledge and techniques. It is true that for some elderly people dying now produces fears of dependence and pain, as well as physical and psychological indignities. However 'requests' for an 'easy way out' are heard most often from relatives and friends of these patients, rather than elderly people themselves. It would appear that one's hold on life is often as strong at 70 or 80 years as it is at 30 or 40 years.

The legalising of euthanasia poses a very real threat to the elderly especially the invalid, the demented and the chronic sick. Providing for the sick elderly is not cheap in both economic and social values; and it will not get any cheaper with nearly half the elderly population of England and Wales now living longer than 75 years. But the question must be, 'What is life about—wealth or people?'. The incurable and elderly exist as real people and should be seen as the opportunity for our society to express compassion, patience and understanding. What is needed is not a change in the law but a change in people's attitudes towards the dying. If society holds strong ageist attitudes towards the elderly, the atrocities of Germany in 1939 could be repeated. Then, state institutions were required to report on patients who had been ill for five years or more, or who were unable to work. From brief information such as name, race, marital status, next of kin, who visited them and who bore the financial burden, decisions were made on their extermination (Shaeffer and Koop 1980).

Reliance on their families or on the state for help can become an enormous burden for old people. This burden can easily pressurise them into thinking that 'they are a nuisance' or that 'they would be better off dead'. With the legalisation of euthanasia this pressure could be even greater, and could run the risk of making elderly people feel obliged to decide when to die. Every tablet or injection prescribed or given would be a threat to the original trust between patients and their carers if doctors and nurses had the right to 'kill'.

Euthanasia, in its current meaning, is also inconsistent with the biblical view that human life should be cherished. In saying this, one is not advocating life being preserved at all costs; this would be as unacceptable as euthanasia. Each person, old or young, should be seen as a unique individual, and loved right up until the end of his or her life.

Over the last 10 years it has become increasingly popular in the United States to sign a 'living will'. Although the legal status of such a document is unclear, its purpose is to record the person's own preference for medical treatment in the event of his or her having a critical illness or injury. This seems to be a reasonably safe compromise which Britain could also adopt. There will always be the distinction between tender, loving and appropriate care for the elderly and that of deliberate killing. The former kind of care has been exemplified in the work of the hospice movement.

Postcript

This poem was written by an old lady of 90 years shortly before her death.

Thoughts at ninety

If I could choose the method of my death
Would it be sinking into soundless sleep?
The wild confusion of a storm-swept sea?
Or the sharp mercy of the headsman's sword?

There is no dread in these, no trembling fear
When swept in silent speed to the unknown.

Or with a smile, as did my little son—
Eyes closed as if in sleep, but his small hands
Curling around my hand until he felt
The golden circle of my wedding ring
And stroked that finger as he always had
From smallest babyhood. He found the ring,
Smiled a contented smile . . . and went to heaven.

Or as my mother, opening suddenly
Eyes that lit up to see a happy vision
And cried a loving greeting with their names
Of those of us who had gone before.
Any of these so varied deaths I'd die
But with the wistful hope that I might be
Not quite alone to face what waits for me.

Adelaide de Cabsonne.   September 1983.
(Published with the author's permission.)

REFERENCES

Barton A, Barton M 1981 The management and prevention of pressure sores. Faber, London
Bowling A, Cartwright A 1983 Life after a death—a study of the elderly widowed. Tavistock Publications, London
British Medical Association 1973 The problem of euthanasia. In: Trowell H (ed) The unfinished debate on euthanasia. SCM Press, London
Carr A T 1982 Dying and bereavement. In: Hall J (ed) Psychology for nurses and health visitors. Macmillan, London

Cartwright A, Hockey L, Anderson J L 1973 Life before death. Routledge and Kegan Paul, London

Chalmers G L 1982 Caring for the elderly sick. Pitman, London

Charles-Edwards A 1983 The nursing care of the dying patient. Beaconsfield Publications, London

de Saint-Exupery A 1945 The Little Prince. Heinemann, London

Department of Health and Social Security 1983 The experimental NHS nursing homes for elderly people—an outline. DHSS, London

Dopson L 1983 Having your own front door. Nursing Times 79 (October 19): 10–12

Hampe S O 1975 Needs of the grieving spouse in a hospital setting. Nursing Research 24(2): 113–119

Hinton J M 1963 The physical and mental distress of the dying. Quarterly Journal of Medicine 32: 1–21

Hinton J 1967 Dying. Penguin, London

Hockley J 1983 An investigation to identify symptoms of distress in the terminally ill patient and family in the general medical ward. Unpublished report. St Bartholomew's Hospital, London

Kalish R A 1977 Dying and preparing for death: a view of families. In: Feifel H (ed) New meanings of death. McGraw-Hill, New York

Kubler-Ross E 1973 On death and dying. Tavistock Publications, London

Lerner M 1970 Why and where people die. In: Brimm, Freeman, Levine and Scotch (eds). Dying patient. Russell Sage Foundation, New York

Levin B 1980 Generalissimos die in bed. The Times April 29: 24–27

Norton D, McLaren R, Exton-Smith A N 1975 A study of factors concerned in the production of pressure sores and their prevention. In: An investigation of geriatric nursing problems in hospital. Churchill Livingstone, Edinburgh

Office of Population Censuses and Surveys 1979 Trends in mortality. HMSO, London

Office of Population Censuses and Surveys 1981 Mortality statistics. HMSO, London

Parkes C M 1972 Bereavement studies of grief in adult life. Penguin, London

Parkes C M, Parkes J L N 1984 Hospice versus hospital care: re-evaluation of ten years of prognosis in terminal care. Post-Graduate Medical Journal 60 (February): 120–124

Richmond J B, Waisman H A 1955 Psychological aspects of management of children with malignant disease. American Journal of Diseases of Childhood 89 (January): 42–47

Saunders C 1978 The management of terminal disease. Arnold, London

Saunders C, Baines M 1983 Living with dying. Oxford University Press, Oxford

Shaeffer F, Koop C E 1980 Whatever happened to the human race? Marshall, Morgan and Scott, London

Twycross R G 1978 Relief of pain. In: Saunders C (ed) The management of terminal disease. Arnold, London

Twycross R G 1982 Euthanasia—a physician's viewpoint. Journal of Medical Ethics 8: 86–95

Ward A 1974 Telling the patient. Journal of the Royal College of General Practitioners 24: 465–468

PART THREE

The organisation of care for elderly people

22

H. K. Evers

Care of the elderly sick in the UK

In this chapter some of the topics which seem important in understanding contemporary trends in the organisation of care for sick old people are discussed. In the first part of the chapter we outline some of the characteristics of our elderly population and the implications regarding need for and availability of care. Most old people live in private households, and the bulk of the care they need comes not from services but from families and other lay people.

Today's array of services and the division of labour among them is complex and not always logical. This reflects the process of historical development. In the second part of the chapter, we note briefly some of the landmarks in historical development of services for the elderly, together with the implications of government policies for old people and their carers, both lay and professional. The needs of old people seldom fit neatly with the organisational divisions among services.

Although most dependent elderly people are looked after at home by lay carers, the development of geriatric medicine as a specialty has had a profound influence on health care for the elderly. In the third part of the chapter, we give a short summary of its history in the United Kingdom and outline the major ways in which it is organised. As the dominant health care profession, medicine and its organisation is the prime influence in setting the parameters for the work of other health professionals, and we go on, in the fourth part of the chapter, to review what we know of the practice and organisation of geriatric nursing. We explore some tentative ideas about its relationship with geriatric medicine; and offer some thoughts about approaches to what seem to be perennial problems in care provision.

DEMOGRAPHIC TRENDS AND SOCIAL CIRCUMSTANCES

Size of elderly population

In 1981, there were 8.3 million people aged 65 years and over living in Britain (Central Statistical office 1983), constituting around 15% of the total population. The proportion of the population who are more than 65 years old has risen dramatically during this century. In England and Wales, less than 5% of the population was aged over 65 years in 1901. Of these, a quarter were more than 75 years old. In 1982, almost half the numerically much larger elderly population were 75 or older (Department of Health and Social Security (DHSS) 1983). By the end of the century, the proportion of the population aged 65 years or more will not increase dramatically, but within the elderly population, there will be a slight decline in the proportion of 'young' elderly, and an increase in the proportion of 'old' elderly people. These changes in population reflect in part the fact that fewer people die during earlier stages of the life-cycle. This has resulted primarily from environmental improvements: better housing, sanitation, clean water, adequate diet and general improvements in the standard of living.

Women and men

What do we know about these growing numbers of elderly people? Women tend to live longer than men do, thus they outnumber men by 2:1 in the 75 years and over age group. Women also tend to marry men who are older than themselves. For both reasons widowhood among women is very common: in 1980, 49% of women aged 75 or over were widows and 38% were still married, whereas only 17% of men in

the same age group were widowed, and 75% were still married. Given these facts, it is no surprise to find that 45% of women, but 17% of men, lived alone in 1980 (Office of Population Censuses and Surveys (OPCS) 1982).

Housing and income

What of the circumstances in which elderly people live? Tinker (1981) reviews a range of evidence which shows that standard of housing and access to household amenities tends to be worse, on average, in households containing an elderly person. Old people are among the poorest members of society (Townsend 1979). Although financial circumstances in late life bear a relationship to financial circumstances at earlier phases in the life-cycle—the retired professional person will be relatively well off compared with the retired manual worker—income is drastically reduced for almost all after retirement. For a majority of old people, the state old age pension is their main source of income (Abrams 1980; DHSS 1981a). Women are usually worse off than men of comparable social status and age: they have had fewer opportunities to acquire occupational pension rights or to accumulate savings from paid work. Widows living alone are a particularly disadvantaged group: nearly half of those elderly women who live alone are receiving supplementary benefit (Abrams 1980). Extreme old age is the life stage featuring the greatest material poverty, just at a time when extra expenses may accrue if life is to continue to be possible; e.g. better heating, transport and special diet.

Dependency

A survey by Hunt (1978) and a special section of the General Household Survey for 1980 (OPCS 1982) provide data on health problems reported by old people, mobility and capacity for self-care. The incidence of problems in all these areas rises with increasing age, and there are various sex differences worth noting. In all age groups, old women are more likely to report a long-standing illness which limits their activities and more likely to report mobility problems (Hunt 1978, OPCS 1982).

Most elderly people—about 95%—live at home. Some of those living at home are heavily dependent on others for many kinds of essential help. What does the demographic picture mean in human terms, and who helps those elderly people who become sick or disabled?

Care of dependent or sick elderly people

A majority of old men have wives to look after them if they become sick. But their wives, although on average a little younger, are likely, as they age, to have their own health problems, which may limit their activities. In contrast, a minority of women have husbands to take on the care-work should they become unable to do this for themselves. Female spouses are thus a major source of help, after which children—primarily daughters or daughters-in-law—make an essential contribution (Equal Opportunities Commission 1982; Nissel and Bonnerjea 1982, Rossiter and Wicks 1982). To a lesser extent help is provided by neighbours and friends, which is probably very important for those living alone and who have no children, i.e. about 30% of today's old people (Abrams 1980).

What role, then, do formal services play? Government policy (examples are DHSS 1976, 1981b) has for some time indicated that home-based rather than institutional-based care provision is to be preferred on humanitarian grounds, and because it may be cheaper; though this last assumption is now widely challenged. Policy also explicitly states that services are intended only to supplement what the major care givers, the women of the family, provide by way of support (DHSS 1981a). Data on patterns of service provision are scant and suffer from limitations. They tell us nothing about the circumstances of those who receive no services, yet we cannot assume these non-recipients need no help.

Elderly people are major users of the health and social services. But the available evidence on community services suggests that 'unmet needs' are commonplace (e.g. Chapman 1979)

and that allocation of services depends not just on need but also on availability and mix of services in a given geographical area (Levin et al 1983), local professional policies—implicit as well as explicit—and gender-based assumptions. An example of the last was Hunt's (1978) finding that men were more likely than women of comparable age and disability to receive a home help just because they are old and living alone: women are assumed to be able to cope with far more on the domestic front than are men.

Since most old people live in private households, health care is in the main provided by the primary care team. People over 65 years old account for about a fifth of all general practitioner (family doctor) consultations (Age Concern 1977). Rossiter and Wicks (1982) state that people of 65 years and over accounted for nearly half all home nursing cases in 1980 in Great Britain, and about 13% of the caseload of health visitors.

With increasing age, the probability of contact with the hospital services also increases. As with primary health services, the elderly are also major users of hospital services. Around 50% of all hospital beds (excluding maternity and geriatric departments) are occupied by people who are 65 years of age or older.

Some implications

The decreasing proportion of 'young elderly' in relation to 'old elderly' means that fewer relatively fit people in the 65–74 age group will be available to look after increasing numbers of frail and much older kin: parents, spouses or siblings. Where carers come from a pre-retirement generation, not only are demands and obligations to look after an older family member more likely to arise, but also the women carers must cope with other pressures. These include the needs of their own families, and the need and often the desire to work outside the home. The increasingly common incidence of divorce, followed perhaps by remarriage, may have profound effects on family structure which will affect availability of younger-generation carers for sick elderly people.

At the same time, government policy endorses community-based care without obvious diversion of resources into state community services. In effect, this places greater demands on family carers. The current picture, in a period of economic austerity, holds little promise for any of the interested parties: old people, family carers or formal service providers.

DIVISION OF LABOUR IN CARE PROVISION FOR ELDERLY PEOPLE

Although lay people provide the bulk of care received by dependent or sick old people, a formidable array of professional and non-professional paid and voluntary workers is also involved, not to mention complex arrangements for a range of cash benefits: from attendance allowances to special needs payments. The paid workers include members of the primary health care team—doctors, nurses, remedial therapists and health visitors—and hospital staff, home helps, social workers, providers of the meals-on-wheels service, day centre and day hospital staff, staff of residential Homes and ambulance drivers, to mention only some. While this proliferation of types of worker and the services they supply may have obvious advantages for their clientèle, our present systems of service delivery feature many anomalies and confusions. It is not unusual to find elderly people or their carers bemused by the distinction between the roles of social worker and health visitor, or health visitor and district nurse, for instance. There seems little inherent logic in the fact that a person who comes to require institutional care on a semipermanent basis, pays nothing for this if it is provided in a hospital, yet faces a weekly charge for local authority residential care. And this despite repeated evidence that long-term hospital beds and residential places do not cater for discrete populations (Wade et al 1983).

Services for the elderly have evolved in a piecemeal fashion. Some understanding of the pattern of care services we have today can be gained through a brief look at how they have developed.

HISTORICAL DEVELOPMENT OF SERVICES FOR THE ELDERLY

Many writers have traced the historical development of government policies and of services vis-à-vis elderly people. Macintyre (1977) and Tinker (1981) are two recent and excellent examples, and Brocklehurst (1975) provides an overview of the development of geriatric services.* In this chapter, we have space only for a very brief summary of these complex developments.

Legacy of the Poor Law

At the turn of the century, the main provision for elderly people in Britain derived from the Elizabethan and the New Poor Law of 1834. Outdoor relief was provided to the destitute and infirm, from Poor Rates collected from all occupants of property in a parish. The workhouse became the repository of the destitute and infirm, and in 1834 the principle of 'less eligibility' was enshrined as a deterrent. Provisions in the workhouse were to be less attractive than the lowest level of subsistence 'enjoyed' by anyone outside, although it was suggested that the elderly of 'good report' might deserve some special arrangements. Workhouse infirmaries provided accommodation for the aged and chronic sick.

The beginnings of change

The Old Age Pension Act of 1908, which gave people over 70 years a small weekly—but at first means tested—pension, was an important landmark. It began to establish provision for elderly people outside the framework of the Poor Laws. As to institutional provision, in

* Since going to press, an important book has been published which has analysed the development of welfare services for the elderly, including reference to health care services (Mears and Smith 1985).

1929 the Local Government Act made the local authorities responsible for the work of the former Poor Law guardians, including the administration of Poor Law institutions. These now became known as public assistance institutions. The stigma of Poor Law relief of destitution was probably significantly diminished as a result of this new arrangement. Amulree (1951) considers, however, that this Act had an unexpectedly negative consequence for the elderly sick. Under a permissive clause, local authorities could choose to transfer infirmaries attached to public assistance institutions to the health authorities, the idea being to improve standards. This happened: but as standards improved, these infirmaries became highly selective of the patients they admitted, and many elderly people could no longer gain access. The statutory right of admission had been lost with the transfer of control of infirmaries to the health authorities.

Health and social services

The National Health Service Act of 1946 and the National Assistance Act of 1948 were both important in setting the stage for the development of today's pattern of health and social service provision for elderly people. The 1946 Act brought the former public assistance infirmaries, the municipal hospitals, the voluntary hospitals and community-based health services together into the National Health Service. It also empowered local authorities to employ home helps and to make provision for the care and aftercare of the sick. The 1948 Act enabled local authorities to concern themselves with the welfare of those who were deaf, dumb, blind or otherwise substantially handicapped. Under Part III of this Act, local authorities were required to make accommodation available for all who needed care and attention because of age, infirmity or other circumstances. Many large former workhouses were used to this end and are now referred to as 'Part III' accommodation. Section 31 of the 1948 Act empowered local authorities to make a financial contribution in support of the work

of voluntary organisations, for example voluntary homes and meals services.

In 1971, the Local Authority Social Services Act (1970) was implemented. This aimed to provide for a co-ordinated approach to the family by bringing together in social services departments, the former children's and welfare departments. Some writers (e.g. Harris 1979) imply that the generic approach to social work has served to reinforce the pre-eminence of work concerning children—deriving from numerous statutory imperatives—to the detriment of professional social work with elderly people.*

Government policies on the elderly

Macintyre (1977) shows how policy concerns about the elderly as a 'social problem' between 1834 and 1976 oscillated between organisational considerations such as the 'burden' on society of the cost of supporting a dependent sector of the population, and humanitarian concerns about responding to the health or welfare problems occasioning hardship to old people. The tensions between organisational and humanitarian perspectives are evident today, for example in policy statements about community care (DHSS 1976, 1978, 1981a, b). The official line is that service provision for old people should be grounded in the assumption that being looked after at home is best, both because old people prefer this and because it is cheaper. If it is in fact cheaper, this may be because types and levels of service provision are inadequate (Opit 1977). This is now implicitly recognised in the present government's policy line for the 1980s: that family care of old people, supported by community services, is the 'best' model for service development on both organisational and humanitarian grounds. The tension between these two perspectives has been 'resolved' by firmly locating responsibility with the family, thus, among

* Others (e.g. Court 1976) have suggested that preventive health services for children have suffered through increasing involvement of health visitors with elderly people.

other things, rendering the human plight of some sick old people less publicly visible.

Some practical implications of service organisation and government policy

In the post-war period, both the health and personal social services have, chameleon-like, undergone various changes in their respective organisations. Yet the needs of their elderly clientèle cannot be so neatly divided between health and social services—not to mention housing or financial considerations, which have not been discussed here. Furthermore, needs do not remain static: classification and response is not a once-for-all activity. Thus, in order to carry out their work with dependent or sick elderly people, collaboration among families, health and social services professionals is essential. The historical development of separate health and social service organisations—whose territorial boundaries often do not coincide—in some respects militates against easy co-ordination. The mix of institutional and community bases of provision in both services compounds the difficulties. Undoubtedly, there are many examples of effective co-ordination in service delivery, but one may speculate that these eventuate despite rather than because of service organisational features, and are mediated through the efforts of individual workers and managers to establish mutually harmonious and complementary inter-relationships.

Voluntary and private sector provision must be mentioned in this context. Voluntary and charitable organisations have a long history of providing community and institutional services for the elderly; and old people with the financial means to do so have always had the option in practice of buying the support they deem themselves to need, whether at home or in an institution, provided they can find this. In the early 1980s, a reading of the professional journals suggests that the private sector is growing in its importance in provision of residential and nursing Home care for dependent elderly people. McCoy, for example, documents this. He also suggests that private

and voluntary facilities may be catering for different categories of resident from those to be found in state-run facilities (McCoy 1983).

Concern about monitoring standards and controlling developments in the private sector is expressed by some writers, for example Johnson (1983), and 1983 saw the passing of new legislation governing standards for the mandatory inspection and registration of residential Homes (Health and Social Security and Social Security Adjudications Act).

Today's professional carers for elderly people work within a complex pattern of service organisation. The territorial and functional boundaries of its components have assumed their present limits after years of development and change, shaped significantly by Acts of Parliament. These boundaries do not necessarily coincide neatly with the presenting problems of real old people and their lay carers.

ORGANISATION OF GERIATRIC MEDICINE AND NURSING

We have emphasised that care of sick and dependent old people is provided by many different workers, paid and unpaid, and that this work is mainly done outside the hospital. Why, then, is it necessary to pay specific attention to the hospital-based specialty of geriatric medicine, and to geriatric nursing? There are four main reasons.

1. The organisation of professional hospital-centred delivery of care for elderly people has received, perhaps, a disproportionate amount of professional and research attention as compared with health care provided in other settings. There are good reasons for this: the prestige of hospital-based medicine; the 'visibility' of the hospital; the managerial challenges and economic costs of today's hospital care. Rightly or wrongly, hospital-centred care of the elderly occupies considerable attention. Thus we need to analyse its implications for nursing and for patients.

2. The geriatric department is important for its contribution to raising expectations and

status of health care of the elderly as a legitimate and valuable occupation, whether it is done in primary care, geriatric departments, other hospital departments or settings outside the hospital.

3. Most health professionals receive much of their education and training in the hospital, and, increasingly, the geriatric department features—if fleetingly for some—on the agenda. As such, it has a vital role to play in educating those who will meet elderly people in their professional practice, in whatever setting it may be carried out.

4. Solution of problems in geriatric nursing care, as we hope to show below, are more likely to be found if nurses have a clear understanding of how medical philosophy, priorities and organisation of practice affects their own position and that of their patients.

Geriatric medicine: The specialty*

Geriatric medicine as a specialty is generally deemed to have begun with the work of Marjory Warren at the West Middlesex Hospital in 1935. The patients of a former Poor Law infirmary became her responsibility, and she carried out assessments of the patients contingent upon which treatment and rehabilitation was started. The effects of this were soon apparent: it became possible to discharge some patients and to challenge the prevailing practice of nursing a majority of elderly and chronic sick patients in bed. The concentration of elderly chronic sick patients in London's peripheral hospitals during the war provided opportunities for development of practice. The setting up of the National

Health Service, more than 10 years after Warren's pioneering work, added impetus to the beginnings of geriatric medicine. When the NHS brought the voluntary and the municipal hospitals together, the largely custodial role of the latter in the care of the elderly and chronic sick was increasingly questioned.

Also there were fears that the acute beds of the former voluntary hospitals could be overwhelmed by elderly people who previously would have had the right of access only to the municipal hospitals. For example, Thomson et al (1951) wrote: 'When the National Health Service Act became operative . . . it seemed certain that many of the aged sick, no longer able to obtain admission to overcrowded infirmaries under statutory orders, would either remain at home or find their way into the wards of acute general hospitals and choke their beds with cases it was impossible to move. In either event grave hardship and public scandal would result' (p 1).

Dr Trevor Howell, who established one of the early geriatric units in London, and the first geriatric research unit, was instrumental in establishing the Medical Society for the care of the Elderly in 1947, to become the British Geriatrics Society (BGS) in 1959. The first appointments of physicians in geriatric medicine were made from the 1940s onwards, since when the specialty has continued to grow. In 1982 there were more than 470 consultants in England and Wales and the first university chair in geriatric medicine was established in 1965, and by 1983 there were 14 chairs in Great Britain.

Despite its rapid growth, the specialty faces continuing dilemmas over its relationship with other medical specialties which are involved in care of the elderly sick, and a range of organisational solutions is to be found in practice. These can best be discussed in the context of a description of trends in the organisation of the hospital geriatric service.

In the early days, as a legacy from the former workhouse infirmaries, geriatric departments tended to have the image of custodians for long-stay patients who had proved irremediable in other departments of the hospital. Thus almost all admissions came

---

* There is no definitive history, to date, of the development of geriatric medicine in the UK. A number of geriatricians have written about aspects of the specialty's history; and others provide a resumé as a preface to considering contemporary themes. I have drawn on various sources of this kind in my account of the specialty's development; including Amulree, 1951; Brocklehurst, 1975; Macintyre, 1977; Ferguson Anderson, 1981; and Clark, 1983.

Another important book, located after this chapter was written, has compared the development of geriatric medicine in the UK with its non-development in the USA, and provides some fresh insights (Carboni 1982).

from other wards or hospitals, and the geriatric wards were very often housed in under-resourced buildings remote from the general hospital. It was quickly realised that if geriatric medicine was to establish itself on a par with other medical specialties, and to provide a service for a defined elderly population, it had to do more than serve as custodian for the failures of other branches of medicine. Two things had to be done: geriatricians needed to establish that they had a unique contribution to offer to the care of the elderly sick; and they had to change the practice and organisation of their departments, and their relationship with other hospital departments and the community.

The claim to a unique contribution in care of the elderly sick seemed to derive primarily from two arguments. First, that the presentation of illness in old age is often distinctive as compared with illness in younger adults. Not only may the clinical picture present differently, but very often multiple conditions are found, which may also be directly related to social and environmental factors. Geriatricians have special knowledge and skills in understanding the presentation, and thus the management, of illness in old age.

The second argument is that geriatricians have special expertise in rehabilitation, and experience in organising hospital care so as to meet patients' rehabilitative needs. Thus many of the patients whom the acute wards find hard to discharge and who come to be seen as 'bed blockers' would perhaps never have found themselves in this predicament, it is argued, had they been admitted directly to the geriatric department and received the benefits of its expertise and special organisation from the outset. On the acute ward, mobilising the patient with a fractured femur or stroke illness when the patient is elderly may receive low priority, and the chance of rehabilitation may be completely lost if the management of the early days of the illness does not pay close attention to mobilisation.

A vital change in the organisation of practice is the acceptance of direct admissions to the geriatric department. Achieving direct rather than second-hand admissions both enables geriatricians to demonstrate their special skills, and requires a different kind of departmental organisation from that which featured in the largely custodial long-stay, back wards. Various ways of receiving direct admissions are possible, for example adopting a policy of taking all hospital emergency admissions of medical patients of a particular age; or taking age-defined emergencies of particular diagnostic categories. Direct acceptance of all, or of defined types of, emergency patients above a certain age referred by general practitioners is another strategy, as well as accepting general practitioner requests for home assessments. As a result of this at least some elderly patients may be admitted directly to the geriatric department. Taking direct admissions means that the variety of patients' services will need to increase: besides those needing long-term hospital care, there will be increasing numbers of acutely ill patients for whom active treatment, perhaps followed by a period of rehabilitation, will be needed prior to discharge. Assessment of patients becomes very important, including seeking out factors which the patient may erroneously attribute to 'old age', and positive rather than residual criteria for admission must be identified. Emphasising treatment in the geriatric department also requires a reorientation of work priorities among existing staff—nurses and doctors—and greater involvement with other professionals having a therapeutic role to play, e.g. physiotherapists, occupational therapists and social workers. A wider repertoire of skills will be needed by all these staff when they are dealing not just with long-term care, but also with acutely ill patients and rehabilitation. Thus the nature and quality of their training, experience and calibre become crucial.

Successful discharge of an elderly patient who has responded to treatment and rehabilitation requires different strategies, very often, from discharge of 'cured' patients in younger age groups. Remember that the elderly patient may have some limitations of day-to-day activities even when deemed 'cured'; that she is very likely to live alone or with an elderly spouse and in less than ideal housing circumstances. So it is an advantage if staff of the geriatric department know something of the social and environmental circumstances of the elderly patient at home, such that steps can be taken to compensate for inherent problems through initiating provision of aids, adaptations or services. Health education in its broadest sense, including practical ways of making self-care or care of an elderly spouse, easier, is also essential to achieving a successful discharge.

'Community orientation' of the medical specialty has for many years been seen by geriatricians as a basic requirement for providing a good service to a defined elderly population. Home assessments originally offered a way of screening patients referred for admission and reducing waiting lists by suggesting alternatives to hospitalisation. When a patient is admitted to hospital, first-hand knowledge of their home environment and social and family circumstances may help in planning the treatment strategy and in organising a well-supported discharge when the patient recovers. Home assessments also enable geriatricians constantly to review their admissions policies in relation to the range of presenting needs among the elderly population, as well as maintaining working relationships with primary health workers, and other agencies involved in providing care for elderly sick people. The development of day hospitals, the increasing importance of out-patient clinics run by geriatricians and the provision of beds for short-term admissions to relieve caring relatives are other features of the specialty's community orientation.

In establishing its unique contribution and evolving new approaches to organising its practice, geriatric medicine has come to set great store by multidisciplinary teamwork. The needs of elderly patients are so varied, and health factors so often inextricably linked with environmental and social factors, that a range of professional skills must be brought to bear in assessment, treatment and rehabilitation and planning a patient's discharge.

Ferguson Anderson (1981) summarises the features which differentiate geriatric medicine from general medicine as follows:

1. The practice of health education for the elderly.
2. The use of the members of the health care team . . . to seek out unreported illness.
3. The knowledge of the home conditions of the individual patient before admission; of the atypical presentation of disease in older people, often accompanied by multiple pathology; of the frequent combination of physical and mental illness in the elderly, and of problems with medication.
4. The need for comprehensive patient management and for continuity of care.
(Ferguson Anderson 1981, p 122.)

Much of this could, incidentally, be applied to other branches of medicine not organised around specific disease processes, for instance general practice, or paediatrics, which, like geriatrics, is concerned with an age-defined rather than disease- or organ-defined patient category. Isaacs (1981) reflects that geriatric medicine has been mainly concerned with problems of organising practice in order to provide a quality service to the elderly population. For the future, Isaacs sees increasing emphasis on exploiting the opportunities for the scientific study of human ageing which the specialty of geriatric medicine affords.

Geriatric medicine: contemporary organisation

Like other mainstream medical specialties, geriatric medicine is now firmly committed to active treatment and patient turnover, and it is around this general aim that most geriatric departments are organised. Providing long-term care, which was the most common base from which the early geriatric departments developed, now fits uneasily into a cure-oriented service.

There seems to be an unresolved tension here. The existence of large numbers of chronically sick elderly hospital patients, on whom medicine had 'given up', provided the early impetus to the development of the specialty. And today, the British Geriatrics Society (1983) notes, 'The largest number of patients under the geriatrician's care at any one time are those in need of continuing nursing care which cannot be given at home . . . the continuing care wards are very much part of the "shop window" of the specialty. . . . The medical attention given to such patients is relatively small but the way in which it is given is absolutely vital' (p 3–4). Yet, at the same time, geriatric departments are striving to establish themselves by the same criterion of 'success' commonly applied to other medical specialties: high rates of patient turnover. The issue of long-term care is one about which many geriatricians are both profoundly concerned and profoundly uncomfortable. The Hull geriatrician Peter Horrocks (1982) is committed to the organisation of geriatric medicine as an age-related specialty. In explaining why, he provides an excellent review of the three major approaches to organisation, which are a 'residual', an integrated and an age-related service.

A 'residual' service

Horrocks' view is that the quality of service for the elderly population would remain poor if geriatrics were only a rehabilitation and long-term care specialty taking its admissions largely from other hospital departments. This is probably uncontroversial. That policy serves to deny the special contribution of geriatric medicine in care of the elderly sick; to reinforce the second-class status of geriatric medicine, which would in turn ensure that the specialty's claim on scarce resources and on staff would always be secondary, and that training and recruitment in the specialty— lacking any coverage of acute illness, and suffering inadequate resources—would always be a problem.

An integrated service

A model which has been adopted by various departments, and which was favoured by a working party of the Royal College of Physicians (1977), features integration between geriatric and general medicine. This might take the form of appointing general physicians with an interest in geriatric medicine, who would divide their attention between general and geriatric beds; or, Horrocks describes, a geriatric physician working alongside general physicians, all of whom would admit patients to the same wards. There might be back-up wards, under the sole control of geriatricians, for slow-stream rehabilitation and long-term care.

An integrated service—a model put into practice in some areas—is said to have the advantages that the special skills of the geriatrician would be available to sick old people; that the access of sick old people to diagnostic and treatment facilities would be secured; that recruitment and training in the specialty would be assured since it would be a part of mainstream medicine; and that the status and resource control of geriatric medicine vis-à-vis other specialties would be improved. But Horrocks has reservations about integration. He questions whether the physician with an interest in geriatric medicine, or even the full-time geriatrician within an integrated service, would in practice be able to accord sufficient priority to work other than with acute patients; and suggests that there are practical difficulties in providing the appropriate equipment and environment for sick old people in a general medical ward. Horrocks cites other medical writers who are worried that the geriatrician's patient in the general ward may be resented and accorded low priority.

The integration model has much to commend it as a strategy for securing higher levels of recruitment into geriatric medicine. Indeed this consideration was a major influence on the deliberations of the Royal College of Physicians' working party, at a time when numerous articles and letters in professional journals were both bemoaning the persistent shortage of geriatricians relative to funded consultant posts, and discussing with alarm the possible effects on medical care generally of the rising numbers of elderly people, in particular the very old.

An age-related service

In this third type of service, which Horrocks reviews, the geriatrician offers comprehensive care—acute, rehabilitation, long-term care, community involvement and continuing responsibility when needed for patients known to the department—for all patients with non-surgical conditions above a particular age, commonly, 75 years old and over. Organisationally, this requires that emergency cases are admitted at the discretion of the patient's general practitioner or via the casualty department, along with patients who have been assessed at home by the geriatrician. A department set up along these lines would feature relatively high turnover rates (Horrocks provides some data on the age-related service he manages) and would deal with a wide variety of medical conditions. As such, the department would offer valuable experience, and would be in a good position to attract doctors and other staff of the necessary calibre to work in this broad-based and challenging arena. For patients, continuity of care by specialists in geriatric medicine has obvious advantages. It improves their chances of recovering their former well-being. The need for long-term care is said to be minimised where appropriate diagnostic, treatment and rehabilitation skills, along with advance planning of appropriately supported discharge, are brought to bear from the very moment of first presentation of the sick old person at the hospital. Thus the turnover rate can be maintained, and beds be kept available to meet the needs as they arise from the geriatric department's catchment area. Horrocks notes his experience that actual numbers of beds are less important than the quality and range of services associated with available beds. That is, a good proportion of the patients need to have full access to all the facilities of the district general hospital.

In comparing the resources and performance of several geriatric services, run along differing lines, Grimley Evans (1983) endorses this point. He also observes that various modes of service organisation can achieve the desired objective of ensuring access of elderly patients both to the facilities of the district general hospital and to appropriate—i.e. geriatric—expertise (Grimley Evans 1981).

Horrocks quotes data from a 1980 survey carried out by the British Geriatrics Society of 49 geriatric departments. This showed that consultants having dual responsibilities for general and geriatric medicine were very much in a minority. Twenty-nine of the 49 departments took emergency admissions, and 20 of these only admitted patients above a certain age. When asked about 'ideal' policies, four out of five respondents favoured age-related admissions, the majority opting for a rule-of-thumb age limit somewhere above the minimum pensionable age.

Isaacs (1981) remarks that the age-related model can be criticised 'on grounds of illogicality, segregation, ageism, duplication—but it succeeds' (p 228). He also notes that most departments of geriatric medicine embody some characteristics of an age-related service. Grimley Evans (1983) uses data on the operation of his 'integrated' service compared with data from three other services including Horrocks' service in Hull, to argue that an 'integrated service' is the most viable option where access to district general hospital beds for elderly patients is very restricted.

A 'best buy'?

Having set out the basic elements of three general approaches to organising geriatric departments, it is not our intention to attempt to identify a consumer's 'best buy'. Expediency and professional interests may have a great influence on chosen strategies of organisation, and we have already mentioned that the stark realities of unfilled consultant posts in geriatric medicine may have influenced the Royal College of Physicians' hearty endorsement of an integration model.

An age-related model, if it succeeds in achieving a healthy turnover level and minimising its devotion of resources to long-term care, has clear advantages in raising the prestige of geriatric medicine as a specialty on a par with mainstream acute hospital specialties. This may in turn have real advantages for patients: the prestigious geriatric department is likely to be able to muster stronger claims to resources and staff than its less prestigious counterpart, and to gain support from other specialties, if it is seen to be taking care of its share of the older age groups, from among whom the 'bed blockers' of the acute wards would otherwise emerge.

Local contingencies may reinforce or preclude particular possibilities; valuable accounts of the practicalities of developing effective psychogeriatric and geriatric services in two different locales are provided by Jolley et al (1982) and Harrison (1984).

Geriatric nursing

Having discussed the medical context, we now turn to the implications for geriatric nursing. The discussion is divided into four sections: origins; research-based analyses of practice and problems; relationship with geriatric medicine; towards organisational solutions?

Origins

Baker (1978) draws out the parallels between the development of geriatric medicine and geriatric nursing. She refers to White's (1978) study of the development of nursing, and argues that the voluntary hospital nurses shared the prestige accorded to the medical élite who serviced the voluntary hospitals and developed their mainly curative work with acutely ill patients. The Poor Law nurses of the workhouse infirmaries, which became the municipal hospitals, worked with chronic sick, bedridden patients who embodied all the stigma of the workhouse, providing routine bedside care. This was in stark contrast to the nursing work of the voluntary hospitals, and it was this low status group, the Poor Law nurses, who became the first geriatric nurses.

Research-based analysis of practice and problems

The British literature on geriatric nursing does not seem to have begun to emerge until well after the founding fathers had become established in medicine. The work of Doreen Norton and her colleagues (1962) is perhaps the pioneering research-based text in the field. Their *Investigation of geriatric nursing problems in hospital* reported detailed studies of patients and of nursing work, aimed towards practical ends of improving patient care and easing the workload of nurses. Specific areas included individual patient care studies; assessment of patients; furniture and equipment; design of suitable clothing; and, perhaps best-known, a study of the identification of patients liable to develop pressure sores, and nursing care strategies for their prevention and treatment.

Two of the most important British studies which illuminate the nature of geriatric nursing are those of Baker (1978) and Wells (1980). Wells' research began in 1972, before Baker's, and her aim was to describe current nursing practice in order to develop a potential model for geriatric nursing. She felt that the specialty lacked a distinctive body of nursing knowledge and skill. Her three starting assumptions were: that nurses' behaviour was influenced first by their physical work environment; second, by their attitude towards geriatric ward patients; and third, by their knowledge of the causes and treatment of patients' needs. The findings of Wells' research were on the whole depressing. She concluded that the environment posed many problems and, on top of that, most nurses lacked the understanding and knowledge necessary to cope with the nursing care problems of their patients, never mind to promote change. This was true of both trained and untrained staff. But trained staff had positive attitudes towards old people, and saw the answer to all their problems as resting in the provision of more staff. Wells shows that life is not so simple: she found that nursing problems often featured lack of awareness about current practices; unclear aims; lack of planning; and lack of communication and co-ordination of routine and innovative work practices. Commonly, there was no monitoring of work progress either. In observing how geriatric nurses spent their time, Wells found:

> The nursing work on the geriatric wards was not focused on the patients' needs but on ward routines which might or might not be appropriate for each patient. The work routines were based on minimal, universal needs such as meals, commoding/changing wet pads, "getting up", and "going to bed". Work was not organised in the sense that it was assigned in any manner. Routines were determined by the time of day, and the work progressed in bursts of frantic activity by nurses working in pairs or a group of three to complete the routine from one end of the ward to another.
>
> Further, not only was work not assigned or even focused on individual patients but there was no nursing record of individual patient preferences and such information was not regularly transmitted verbally in nurse communication. Moreover, individual patient preference or even necessary variation in care appeared to be obstructive to the work goal, which was completion of the routine. Thus, the problem of nursing work in geriatric wards was not so much shortage of staff as the fact that such work was neither sensibly organised nor provided the likelihood of helpful care for patients.
>
> Patients' physical care problems were not the central issue. Nursing staff were not concerned about any specific patient problem; their prime concern was the completion of ward routines.
> (Wells 1980, p 127–128)

Baker (1978) was interested in the relationship between nurses' perceptions of their work and their actual work behaviour. In a participant observation study, she found that patients in geriatric wards were on the whole perceived as enjoying less than adult status, and that the prevailing style of nursing was what she called 'routine geriatric'—the application of broad-based routines to whole groups of patients, irrespective of considerations of individual need or preference. She accounts for this in terms of medical priorities and expectations, first of all. Little medical attention is accorded to those patients deemed unlikely to make a speedy recovery to

a point at which they can be discharged. The low status accorded to patients who do not fit this category is mirrored in nurses' perceptions of such patients, on the whole. This arises through the traditional primacy of the doctor's role and the pervasiveness of the idea of and desirability of cure and discharge—a widespread emphasis in most departments of geriatric medicine. The 'routine geriatric' style of nursing is reinforced by various organisational factors. Wards which attract low levels of medical attention tend to have poorer levels of staff and other resources; administrative priorities of nursing managers and some doctors—tidy wards, a quiet life, for example—are best met by following the 'routine geriatric' style. A patient-centred style might mean, for example, that beds remained unmade for long periods while patients' needs were attended to; or that doctors might have to wait for the completion of essential personal care of patients by nurses before beginning a ward round.

There were some exceptions to the 'routine geriatric' style, for which it was only possible to speculate as to the explanation. Overall, Baker's findings, suggesting as they do a lack of humanitarian concern for patients in the delivery of care, lead her to consider some radical changes. She calls for a complete reorientation of the nursing profession such that nursing care is provided to individual patients *as* individuals: remember that Baker's research pre-dates the nursing process 'revolution' in the United Kingdom. She also states that raising the status of geriatric nursing is a prerequisite to improving things: the caring along with the curing role of nursing care deserves and indeed demands proper recognition. Baker is an advocate of organising long-stay institutional care outside the hospital system, under the clinical management of the nursing profession.

By the 1980s, we have seen the emergence of optimistic literature from geriatricians concerning the successes of their departments judged by medical criteria—e.g. increased turnover. It is often implicated that a better service for a larger slice of the elderly population of a catchment area results (Harrison 1984).

What evidence do we have from other sources that things are in fact better from the nursing and the patients' angle? There are some instances where improved practices have been described—e.g. Cullen (1983), Storrs (1982), and Stevens (1983), and by finalists in the West Midlands Institute of Geriatric Medicine and Gerontology's Ward of the Year Competition (1982). But one suspects that, from research done in the late 1970s and early 1980s the problems described by Wells and Baker remain part of the scene in many geriatric departments.

Godlove et al (1981) found that apathy and inactivity were major features in long-term care wards. In my own research, I found that, in eight unremarkable geriatric wards in different hospitals, housing predominantly long-stay patients, a 'warehousing' approach to geriatric care, similar to that described by Miller and Gwynne (1972) in residential homes for the physically handicapped, predominated. There was some evidence of personalised care in five of the eight wards (Evers 1981, 1984) But there remained considerable evidence of inhumane treatment of patients, and patterns of care in many respects failed to match the various professional and policy statements about appropriate standards of care, e.g. the joint statement by the British Geriatrics Society and the Royal College of Nursing (1975). Wards providing some personalised care were distinguished from those which did not in the stance adopted by the consultants towards the work of slow-stream rehabilitation and long-term care. They expressed the belief that such work was valuable and important, no less so than cure-work. In different ways, they provided positive support in practice of the nurses' primacy in this area of patient care. In the other wards, the consultants saw care-work as necessary but less attractive and interesting than cure-work. They had in effect handed the responsibility to the nursing staff and withdrawn from the arena. Not surprisingly, these nursing staff felt discour-

aged and disaffected in their work because patients were implicitly labelled by the doctor as 'second class', or 'less eligible'.

The medical argument that a modern, high turnover geriatric department is offering a quality service to the elderly population of the catchment area rests not only on what happens to its patients for whom rapid cure and discharge is the aim, but also—less explicitly—on the presumption of quality non-medical care for its 'backstage' patients (those for 'slow-stream' rehabilitation and possibly eventual discharge; patients needing long-term care; and some dying patients). They occupy the majority of geriatric beds, so what goes on in these beds is crucially important. Writing about their services, many geria-tricians devote little explicit attention to the organisation of care for patients other than 'fast stream' treatment and rehabilitation patients. Could this be because they believe that if their practice and organisation succeeds in relation to discharging patients, then appropriate practice and organisation of care for the other patient categories will automatically follow?

From my own research findings—in line with common sense—it seems that the opposite may be true, unless active measures are taken to identify and institute positive care strategies for *all* categories of patient. That is, where high turnover is a chief criterion of success, work with patients who do not fit this category is in danger of becoming devalued medically and therefore in nursing and remedial therapy terms too. In some of the wards I studied there was a mixture of patient types. There were three common trends in the provision of care, which sometimes occasioned much suffering—albeit unintentionally—to patients. First, efforts were sometimes made to define patients as candidates for rapid cure and discharge and treat them accordingly, when from the patient's perspective this was not necessarily appropriate. Second, there was often an avoidance of explicitly defining care goals for manifestly 'non-cure' patients, who then suffered from aimless residual care. A third trend was to reject or ignore patients who did not fit a ward's preferred repertoire of care and treatment strategies and its established routines; or even—more rarely—to eject them, by redefining them as psychiatric cases for example (Evers 1984). Multidisciplinary teamwork, commonly assumed to be beneficial for patients, seemed not to be successfully applied in practice to any patients other than those for whom rapid cure and discharge was the agreed goal (Evers 1982). Fairhurst's work (1977) also suggests that teamwork fails to fulfil its promise for patients, but serves instead as a medium for professionals to try to resolve conflicts over status and resources.

Nursing and social research, then, continues to paint a picture of geriatric care and attendant quality of life for patients which is not altogether cheerful. What, if any, are the implications of research evidence for the nature of care provision within the differing medical strategies for organising geriatric departments?

Relationship of geriatric nursing and geriatric medicine

For the future, the main viable alternatives seem to be age-related and integrated types of service; thus just these two will be considered. We do not know of any research analysis of the relationship between overall medical policy and organisation of geriatric departments and the nature and organisation of non-medical care. But on the basis of the studies discussed above, some tentative speculations can be made. Perhaps these might form the basis for a future research study. In both the age-related and integrated geriatric department, acute-type nursing care aimed towards cure or amelioration and rapid discharge, is likely to be done satisfactorily if we assume minimal levels of competence and resources. This is what all nurses learn to do during their training, and is directly and obviously linked with the miracles of modern medicine. In our 'ageist' society, however, people who have chosen to work with the elderly in a geriatric department may not have to confront the

same dilemmas regarding priorities which could arise for those working with acutely ill patients of all ages. Where pressure of work is extreme, elderly acutely ill patients may be accorded less priority than younger ones in an integrated service.

The research studies described above show that work with types of patients who command little medical attention and regard tends to feature depersonalisation, routinisation and unintended suffering for at least some patients. Thus, so long as patient care is carried out within a medicalised arena, the age-related type of service, whose staff have largely chosen to work there, is perhaps best placed to confront these perennial problems.

Towards organisational solutions?

Organizational strategies for continuing to improve the status and quality of work with sick elderly people are needed. The medical emphasis on turnover serves a vital purpose in this regard, and has succeeded in mobilising improved resources to offer a service to larger numbers of elderly people. However, there may be room for improvement in the extent to which the needs and problems of patients who cannot be rapidly 'turned over' are met. A case can be made for removing what is primarily care-work outside the medicalised arena of the hospital. A nursing-based care facility could, in the British context, enhance the status of nursing care-work, and at the same time create the conditions in which the practice of nursing *care* could be expected to flourish. The feasibility of this is currently being researched by Bond and his associates for the DHSS (Bond 1984). This approach perhaps offers fresh promise; it certainly embodies familiar problems. Such an arrangement could serve simply to aggravate existing fragmentation of care of the elderly sick. It could also create a new kind of institutional ghetto for nurses and patients. To avoid this, access to material and professional resources would need to be assured, and 'openness' of organisational boundaries actively maintained.

But, so long as care of the elderly sick

continues along established lines in this country, it is vital for the medical profession to articulate and practise explicit and positive strategies in relation to *all* categories of elderly patient. The medical strategy, rightly or wrongly, sets many of the parameters within which patient care work done by others is practised.

Education and training are important in spreading the word throughout the caring professions that care-work as well as cure-work is important and valuable, even when performed with the very old. As Norton (1965) pointed out, geriatric nursing well done epitomises good nursing care. Yet care-work is often described as 'basic', and by implication seen as boring, low status and less important. I sometimes heard, during my research, newly qualified nurses remarking sadly that geriatric nursing was 'a waste of all that training'. On the educational front there are promising developments. Geriatric experience is now compulsory for all nursing pupils and students—and the quality of that experience is, we hope, improving along with developments in nursing practice and education more generally, as well as in geriatric care and its organisation. In 1974 the Joint Board for Clinical Nursing Studies established curricula for two post-basic training courses in geriatric nursing, which should be contributing to elevation of both status and practice of the specialty.

A more obviously patient-centred and flexible service should in our view incorporate ways of bridging the Great Divide between the hospital and the rest of the world. We have already noted that hospital-centred care commands a disproportionate level of attention. Although geriatricians see themselves as fostering a community orientation and indeed may spend much of their time working outside the hospital, geriatric nurses commonly have no community involvement. First-hand knowledge of the patient and his or her home, family and social environment might result in numerous benefits for patients and nurses; most obviously, the enhanced opportunity for planning, together with the patient, a person-alised care regime. Conversely, community-based health professionals might usefully cross the boundary into the hospital more often than is currently the case. The importance of a 'community orientation' cannot be overstressed, given that that is where 95% of the elderly population live—and cope and are likely to continue to do so.

Conclusion

In the 1980s services for care of the elderly sick in the United Kingdom are, like other health care services, feeling the effects of austere economic policies. Even greater responsibility for care will, as a result, be vested in families and other lay carers, given the facts of demography.

Innovative responses to the needs of elderly sick people and their lay carers are called for on the part of service providers. Despite problems of the cost, and of putting new ideas into practice, our formal and voluntary services have a strong tradition of developing innovative responses to unmet needs, and we hope this tradition will continue (Isaacs and Evers 1984).

Health care professionals who work with elderly people can do a great deal, individually and collectively, to capitalise on the strengths and combat the problems of our current patterns of service provision. Nurses, being the largest group, perhaps have the greatest responsibility here. We have suggested that the conventional relationship with geriatricians might be challenged and revised in the interests of improved long-term care. Further, there is a strong argument for an extension of nurse-controlled patient-centred care environments—with some caveats. Fostering interchangeability of hospital and community staff is urgently needed, and nurses are well placed to take a major initiative here. Breaking down some of the barriers between hospital-centred and other bases of care provision would facilitate continuity of care in the endeavour to understand and respond to the needs of old people and their lay carers in their own social environment. The hospital is a small but disproportionately visible part of the care network. The family and other lay carers contribute the greatest part, and are the least visible. The nursing profession does much, but could do more, in support of the latter.

REFERENCES

Abrams M 1980 Beyond three score and ten: A second report on a survey of the elderly. Age Concern, Mitcham

Age Concern 1977 Profiles of the elderly 4: Their health and the health services. Age Concern, Mitcham

Amulree 1951 Adding life to years. National Council of Social Service, London

Baker D 1978 Attitudes of nurses to the care of the elderly. Unpublished Ph.D thesis, University of Manchester

British Geriatrics Society 1983 Geriatric medicine: a career guide. Geriatric Medicine 13 (Mimeo): 3–4

British Geriatrics Society and Royal College of Nursing 1975 Improving geriatric care in hospital. Rcn, London

Bond J 1984 Evaluation of long-stay accommodation for elderly people. In: Bromley D (ed) Gerontology: social and behavioural perspectives. Croom Helm, London

Brocklehurst J (ed) 1975 Geriatric care in advanced societies. MTP, Lancaster

Carboni D 1982 Geriatric medicine in the United States and Great Britain. Greenwood Press, London

Central Statistical Office 1983 Social Trends 14 for 1984. HMSO, London

Chapman P 1979 Unmet need and the delivery of care. Occasional papers on social administration No. 61, Bedford Square Press, London

Clark A 1983 The historical perspective: development of geriatrics in the United Kingdom. In: Graham J, Hodkinson M (eds) Effective geriatric medicine. Department of Health and Social Security, London

Court S 1976 Fit for the future. Report of the Committee on Child Health Services. HMSO, London

Cullen M 1983 Nursing care. In: Denham M (ed) Care of the long-stay elderly patient. Croom Helm, London

Department of Health and Social Security 1976 Priorities for health and social services in England and Wales. HMSO, London

Department of Health and Social Security 1978 A happier old age. HMSO, London

Department of Health and Social Security 1981a Growing older. HMSO, London

Department of Health and Social Security 1981b Care in the community. HMSO, London

Department of Health and Social Security 1983 On the state of the public health for the year 1982. HMSO, London

Equal Opportunities Commission 1982 Caring for the elderly and handicapped: community care policies and women's lives. EOC, Manchester

Evers H 1981 The creation of patient careers in geriatric wards: aspects of policy and practice. Social Science and Medicine 15A: 581–588

Evers H 1982 Professional practice and patient care: multi-disciplinary teamwork in geriatric wards. Ageing and Society 2: 57–75

Evers H 1984 Patients' experiences and the social relations of patient care in geriatric wards. Unpublished Ph.D thesis, University of Warwick

Fairhurst E 1977 Teamwork as panacea: some underlying assumptions. Unpublished paper read at Annual Conference of the Medical Sociology Group of the British Sociological Association, University of Warwick

Ferguson Anderson W 1981 The evolution of services in the United Kingdom. In: Kinnaird J, Brotherston J, Williamson J (eds) The provision of care for the elderly. Churchill Livingstone, Edinburgh

Godlove C, Richard L, Rodwell G 1981 Time for action. Joint Unit for Social Services Research, University of Sheffield

Grimley Evans J 1981 Institutional care. In: Arie T (ed) Health care of the elderly. Croom Helm, London

Grimley Evans J 1983 The appraisal of hospital geriatric services. Community Medicine 5: 242–50

Harrison J 1984 Making a geriatric department effective. In: Isaacs B, Evers H (eds) Innovations in the care of the elderly. Croom Helm, London

Harris J 1979 More than going grey: a preliminary examination of gerontological theory and social work practice with old people. Unpublished MA thesis, University of Warwick

Horrocks P 1982 The case for geriatric medicine as an age-related specialty. In: Isaacs B (ed) Recent advances in geriatric medicine. Churchill Livingstone, Edinburgh

Hunt A 1978 The elderly at home. HMSO, London

Isaacs B 1981 Is geriatrics a specialty? In: Arie T (ed) Health care of the elderly. Croom Helm, London

Isaacs B, Evers H (eds) 1984 Innovations in the care of the elderly. Croom Helm, London

Johnson M 1983 A sharper eye on private homes. Health and Social Services Journal August 4: 930–32

Jolley A, Smith P, Billington L, Ainsworth D, Ring D 1982 Developing a psychogeriatric service. In: Coakley D (ed) Establishing a geriatric service. Croom Helm, London

Levin E, Sinclair I, Gorbach P 1983 The supporters of confused elderly persons at home. Extract from the main report. National Institute for Social Work Research Unit, London

McCoy P 1983 Private lives. Community Care September 22: 18–19

Macintyre S 1977 Old age as a social problem. In: Dingwall R, Heath C, Reid M, Stacey M (eds) Health care and health knowledge. Croom Helm, London

Mears R, Smith R 1985 The development of welfare services for elderly people. Croom Helm, London

Miller E, Gwynne G 1972 A life apart. Tavistock, London

Nissel M, Bonnerjea L 1982 Family care of the handicapped elderly: who pays? Policy Studies Institute, London

Norton D 1965 Nursing in geriatrics. Gerontologia Clinica 7: 51–60

Norton D, McLaren R, Exton-Smith A N 1962 An investigation of geriatric nursing problems in hospital. Reprinted 1975, Churchill Livingstone, Edinburgh

Office of Population Censuses and Surveys 1982 General household survey for 1980. HMSO, London

Opit L 1977 Domiciliary care for the elderly sick—
economy or neglect? British Medical Journal 1: 30–33

Royal College of Physicians 1977 Report of the Working
Party on Medical Care of the Elderly. The Lancet
1: 1092–1095

Rossiter C, Wicks M 1982 Crisis or challenge? Family
care, elderly people and social policy. Study
Commission on the Family, London

Stevens P 1983 It's not the tidiest ward in the hospital.
British Journal of Geriatric Nursing 3: 6–8

Storrs A 1982 What is care? British Journal of Geriatric
Nursing 1: 12–14

Thomson A P, Lowe C R, McKeown T 1951 The care of
the ageing and chronic sick. E and S Livingstone,
Edinburgh

Tinker A 1981 The elderly in modern society. Longman,
Harlow

Townsend P 1979 Poverty in the United Kingdom.
Penguin, Harmondsworth

Wade B, Sawyer L, Bell J 1983 Dependency with dignity.
Occasional papers on social administration No. 68
Bedford Square Press, London

Wells T 1980 Problems in geriatric nursing care.
Churchill Livingstone, Edinburgh

White R 1978 Social change and the development of the
nursing profession: a study of the Poor Law Nursing
Service 1848–1948. Kimpton, London

23

B. E. Wade

Choice and flexibility in long-term care settings

INTRODUCTION

Over the past 10 years there has been a great deal of research on old people, both in the United Kingdom and in other western nations. This upsurge of activity reflects a recognition of the problems posed by the demographic changes already described (see Chapter 22), but it also reflects an expectation that research, by creating new knowledge, can help in the solution of problems (Illsley 1983). This chapter will draw on some of this research, especially where it is relevant to the long-term care of the elderly in institutional settings.

Approximately 5% of the elderly are currently receiving long-term care in institutions. The majority of these patients are catered for in hospital geriatric units and residential Homes run by local authorities (Part III Homes) but a considerable proportion is sponsored by some local authorities in private or voluntary residential Homes. Private nursing Homes, catering mainly, or exclusively, for the elderly tend to be concentrated in certain geographical areas in the southern countries of England.

The wide range of care provision might lead one to suppose that there is a degree of choice available to that minority of elderly people who require long-term care. Indeed we are told that 'maintaining choice and flexibility in care provision should be a guiding principle underpinning all policy decisions'

311

(Fennell et al 1983, p 28). However, choice and flexibility do not just depend on the provision of a range of services. The levels of provision, the pressure exerted on that provision and the degree of collaboration and co-operation between professionals, as for example between health and social services, are also important. Choice and flexibility will be possible only if we have a fully functioning co-ordinated care system with ease of transfer between the different parts.

In 1978 Plank criticised the care system, commenting that 'the major forms of service provision are developing, like Topsy, in an uncoordinated and isolated manner without benefit of a considered framework of policy and professional practice' (p 17). The evidence to support these allegations is not hard to find. Elderly people waiting to transfer to other accommodation are seen as 'blocking' beds; admissions to care are mainly crisis-based; there is a high degree of overlap in self-care ability between the elderly in hospital, residential Homes and sheltered housing; there is unmet need in the community and there is evidence of considerable strain upon relatives who undertake the caring role (Wade et al 1983).

The overall picture of care provision given at the beginning of this chapter conceals wide variations in both level and type of provision between different authorities. For example, the number of geriatric beds per 1000 population aged 65 years and over in England varies from 6.2 in the South West Thames region to 9.7 in the Yorkshire region. Similarly, the number of residents catered for or sponsored by local authorities varies enormously from one local authority to another. It is this variation in levels of provision that has enabled researchers to gauge the extent to which pressure in one part of the care system may be associated with demand in another part of the system. For example, a low level of provision in local authority residential Homes (Part III accommodation) is associated with greater sponsorship of the elderly in private and voluntary Homes (Gorbach and Sinclair

1982). Overall, approximately 11% of the elderly supported by local authorities are sponsored in private and voluntary residential Homes. Similarly, a high turnover of patients occupying geriatric beds and lower levels of geriatric bed provision are associated with a higher average age of old people in Part III Homes and with increased caseloads for home helps. However, it is suggested that this inter-relationship does not necessarily mean that services have been planned in this way but that the relationship derives from transmission of pressure from one part of the system to another (Gorbach and Sinclair 1982).

The discussion document 'A Happier Old Age' (Department of Health and Social Security 1978) noted the large number of hospital beds occupied by the elderly. It was suggested that nursing Homes could cater for physically dependent elderly people who do not require hospital-based resources, and a research project was funded by the DHSS to provide information about the potential clientèle (Wade et al 1983). This research showed that one quarter of the elderly on community nurse lists and almost one quarter of elderly residents in part III Homes had high or very high nursing care requirements and were directly comparable with the majority of elderly patients receiving long-term care in hospital. On the other hand, 11% of long-stay patients in hospital geriatric wards had minimal nursing care requirements. In view of these findings it is not surprising that care staff considered that the needs of almost one quarter of residents in Part III accommodation could be more appropriately catered for in a different environment. Similarly, ward sisters considered that approximately 40% of the long-term care patients could be more appropriately catered for elsewhere, the largest number of single suggestions being for Part III Homes.

Interviews with care staff in this study illustrated the difficulties involved in transferring elderly people from one care setting to another. These interviews also illustrated the lack of collaboration between health and social services. For example, some of the consultants suggested that the problem of highly dependent residents in Part III Homes arose because problems which were initially treatable were left until people deteriorated and became more dependent: 'It may be too late to get them fit by the time I am presented with them, they should be referred much sooner.' On the other hand, officers in charge of Part III Homes often complained that they could not gain access to hospital beds: 'If it is somebody that we feel needs geriatric care then we contact the general practitioner, the general practitioner contacts the geriatrician and nine times out of ten they're turned down.' The interviews held with the relatives of people being cared for in Part III Homes reinforce this view. It was exceptional for the elderly to have been given a choice of Home. Some people had to wait a very long time before being discharged from hospital to Part III accommodation, and requests for elderly people to be placed in a Home nearer to their relatives were often refused, due either to lack of vacancies or local authority boundaries: 'I'd love to be able to get him nearer but he's not a resident.'

This brief resumé of research clearly illustrates a care system which is under pressure and strongly suggests that the interrelationship between the different parts of the system is due to this pressure, rather than to planned co-ordination. The evidence also suggests that it can be very difficult to transfer elderly people from one care setting to another. The general picture is one of inflexibility and, as far as placement is concerned, it would seem that there is little choice for the consumer.

Yet, the notion of choice can be considered at a different level—that of service delivery. At this level choice is dependent upon organisational factors and is open to manipulation by the people concerned. To what extent do nurses or other care staff safeguard or restrict the control that elderly people have over their own lives?

Interviews with care staff and with the rela-tives of elderly people being cared for in hospital geriatric units, Part III Homes and private nursing Homes shed some light on this issue. These will be examined in the next section.

THE ORGANISATION OF CARE

Conceptual analysis of the interviews with care staff has been reported elsewhere (Wade 1983). Briefly, four models of care were described. These were derived from the identification of two continua relating to the organisation of care. The first of these ranged from an emphasis on the socio-emotional well-being of the elderly to an emphasis on routine and task completion. The second ranged from an open organisation, in which efforts were made to increase the involvement of the elderly with the wider community, to a closed organisation wherein contacts with the wider community were restricted.

The supportive model

This model is characterised by consultation and involvement of elderly people in the care regime. They are recognised as adults and efforts are made to maximise their physical and mental independence. For example:

> Maybe a patient has one bad arm, but she can use the other, why take that away from her too? (Ward Sister)

There is thorough involvement of visitors including relatives, volunteers and children, and a breaking down of barriers between the institution and the wider community:

> All my nurses come back, they bring their children, they come home from school and wait here for Mum. They go and see all the patients, sometimes bring a few flowers, a few sweets, sometimes patients give them sweets. The patients know all the nurses' children, but it's home you see (Matron, Private Home).

The elderly are encouraged to participate in activities which they see as relevant. For example, one residential Home organised escorts so that the old people could take advantage of late-night shopping facilities.

Suggestions for activities/outings are made by the elderly people themselves, possibly through patient/resident committees.

The protective model

This model of care is characterised by some degree of choice and consultation, but there is an undue emphasis on safety. Staff decide which activities are suitable for elderly people, thus denying them their adult status. For example:

> No, I wouldn't let them [go into the garden unaccompanied] because they are responsible to the hospital (Ward Sister).
>
> No, I wouldn't risk kettles or anything (Matron, Private Home).

There is little or no attempt to involve visitors in the care regime:

> You know they're very pleased that they don't have to do it [give help in caring] (Warden, Part III Home).

Under this model of care, contact with the wider community is restricted. For example, children may be seen as a source of infection. Diversional activities are provided by staff.

The controlled model

Under the controlled model of care the elderly person is subordinate to the care regime. For example:

> Most of them want to go fairly early [to bed], because we are dragging them out early (Ward Sister).

Choice is circumscribed by staff:

> Yes, we have got a choice of menu, but we choose for them (Ward Sister).

Staff arrange all activities and outings. Although there is open visiting, attitudes towards visitors are related to their possible contribution to routine:

> They give them tea or feed them for us (Ward Sister).

The restrained model

The restrained model of care operates purely for the convenience of care staff:

> Well, of course, you have to appreciate that you have to fit into a certain routine (Ward Sister).

The elderly are deprived of choice, there is restricted visiting and little therapeutic input. They are 'batch processed'.

THE VIEWS OF RELATIVES

The above analysis was based on interviews with professionals; those who organise and deliver care. Although examples of the supportive model of care were seen in all the different settings, interviews with the relatives of 21 heavily dependent hospital patients, 26 heavily dependent elderly people living in Part III Homes, and 26 heavily dependent elderly people in private nursing Homes provided a different perspective. These interviews, which often revealed great perception of the problems inherent in long-term care, will now be considered separately for each care setting.

Hospital long-term care

When asked directly about the care given to elderly people, responses from relatives ranged from 'The staff are very kind' to 'The staff are marvellous'. Direct questions gave rise to little criticism and this was limited to comments on cleanliness or the quality of the food. On the other hand, responses to more detailed questions about the care regime were much more discerning.

More than one third of the people interviewed described their elderly relatives as 'withdrawn'. Some attributed this withdrawal to the lack of opportunity to participate in meaningful activities.

> She loves the outside, but she never goes out. I can't see why they couldn't push her out in her wheelchair down to the garden.
>
> She hasn't been outside for the last three or four years.

Their brains need stimulating.

She sits and looks out of the window and there's a row of old Victorian terraced houses and she said the other day, 'I sit and look at those houses, I wonder who the people are.' She peoples the houses in her imagination and that passes the day until she falls asleep.

I've never seen her close her eyes and all she can do is just sit and look around. I notice when I'm there she'll watch the nurses, probably she's sitting there and she says in her mind, 'Look at that silly old so and so.'

Approximately one third of patients in hospital long-term care wards had been assessed by staff as having difficulty in hearing or being completely deaf, with a similar proportion as having difficulty in seeing or being completely blind. A further third had speech difficulties. Relatives were sensitive to the problems posed by these sensory impairments:

She's left a lot on her own because she's deaf.

She always has a laugh with me and jokes. They can't communicate with her. I notice when the others are doing therapy she's not.

She can't see but she needs to be talked to and she likes to talk. Sometimes they're forgotten you know, those that can't see.

If she'd had her ears done and a hearing aid then they could have done her glasses. Consequently she's living in a world of her own and she just dwells back on the past.

The problems of withdrawal and the lack of meaningful activities were seen by some people as contributing to the further deterioration of their relatives:

She gradually deteriorated. I'm convinced that if these hospitals had more physiotherapists we wouldn't have so many disabled people.

She deteriorated mentally after going into hospital.

I don't think she knows where she is, which is maybe a good thing.

While they are in their own homes and they are busying about and they have things that interest them they remain mentally and physically active much longer. Once they go into an institution everything is more or less done for them and they sit about and start to deteriorate.

The question of salience was also brought up by this relative:

Once when we saw her she was sewing bits of leather together. But there is no purpose, is there? It isn't the same as if you had to make yourself a cup of tea. There must be some purpose, I think that is terribly important.

The contrast between the rehabilitation ward and the long-term care ward was noted by one distressed relative who was herself disabled:

The atmosphere there was so different, everyone was alive and visitors were coming. In this ward people sit like zombies. In the first ward she was being nursed, in this ward she is only cared for.

Some of the problems perceived by relatives of the elderly were attributed to shortage of staff:

There is not the necessary staff to take them [to the toilet] and they eventually have to do it where they sit, and I think that really takes away all their self-respect.

It has already been shown that some people saw the mental withdrawal of their elderly relatives as the only means of coping with an environment which was devoid of stimulation. Occasionally, this was taken a step further when staff were seen as contributing to the regression of their elderly patients.

They say you go back to your childhood, don't they? But I think it doesn't help a lot to be called by your first name; it's going back to your childhood for them. They stop being Mrs So and So, they're called like children again.

The sister used to speak to her very sharp when she fell down; she said she'd been a naughty girl.

Approximately one third of the people interviewed stated that the clothes that they had taken in for their relatives had been lost or 'swapped'.

We take her nightdresses and jumpers and that sort of thing and we've never seen them. I suppose somebody else has got them on.

In view of the above comments it should not be surprising that more than one half of the people interviewed said that their elderly relatives were unhappy.

She says, 'I'm fed up I think I'll run away.'

I don't see how anybody could be happy there because they just sit all day. It's a long time just to sit.

He cries because he's parted from his wife. It's sad for both of them.

It breaks their hearts, I think they get worse.

Part III Homes

When asked directly about the care given to the elderly the responses of these relatives were similar to those received from the relatives of elderly people in hospital. There was little criticism. However, more detailed questioning led to some revealing comments:

She has special permission to stay in her room after lunch and for the rest of the day except for meals.

They put him in a high chair with a tray across it and the trouble is that he can't get out and he gets frustrated.

She keeps talking about her freedom.

One third of those interviewed described their elderly relatives as bored or withdrawn:

She goes to bed at about half past five because she's so bored.

They have a service for them on Sundays and, apart from that, there isn't much else.

I realise they do the best they can but I feel they're all like zombies. They're in the same room, the same chair, they never move. He doesn't speak to a soul.

If they could be given something to do. They could be taken out for a day or a few hours, or if someone came there and, well—tried to talk to her. Life is so boring, isn't it when you just sit there, you know, the whole day, every day? They just get up to have their meals and they sit down again. I have seen them get up and walk around and immediately they said to them, 'Now sit down on that chair.' Well they're not really doing any harm, just walking around in the corridors are they?

The lack of meaningful activities was also pointed out, together with the loss of role:

They wouldn't let her do any work. She thought that she should have hoovered up the carpets and washed the dishes and they wouldn't let her do it.

She used to like to have a little walk in the gardens but there is nobody to take her out.

If they could be given something to do, they could be taken out for a day or a few hours.

When she comes here at weekends she sings and she wipes up. They said to me, 'Well she doesn't do anything here,' but they don't ask her to do anything.

There's an old guy there who can play the piano. Now wouldn't it be a great idea to give him a piano and he can sit there and tinkle away and people can sing. That's all part and parcel of a bit of therapy. It's no good sticking the telly on in a corner.

Make them do something, it doesn't matter how small it is, but make them do something.

The lack of activities was also seen by some of these relatives as contributing to the further deterioration of the elderly:

I think it's very nice but there's nothing for them to do. I think my mother's deteriorated, they sit there like zombies. You know, the old people just sitting there—they must deteriorate much quicker. The television is always on, nobody watches it.

More than one quarter of people being cared for in Part III Homes were rated as having difficulties in hearing or being completely deaf, one fifth were rated as having difficulty in seeing or were blind, and a little less than one fifth of all residents were dysphasic. The additional problems posed by these sensory deficits were also pointed out by relatives:

She's hard of hearing and of course people can't talk to her. We know how to handle her because she could read our lips you see.

She can't communicate because of deafness and she's a bit blurred in her vision.

The blindness is the greatest single handicap. Whatever she would do she wouldn't be happy.

She's very deaf and she moans at the Home about shouting at her, but it's the walking problem and eyes are the main problem.

Relatives were asked whether the elderly person had taken personal possessions into the Home.

They can't take furniture of their own, there isn't enough room. They didn't want her to wear any jewellery, watch or anything; it's a temptation to others to lift things.

The problem of pilfering was one which was commented on several times.

She went in there with quite a few bits and pieces of her own and they went missing. She lost a lot of things—cherished possessions.

Clothing, too, was often lost, this was mentioned by one third of those interviewed:

They lose her clothes and they're marked with great big letters and they still get lost. She's a size 44 and they sent her home in a size 36 slip. The other Friday I got really upset because they sent her home in a man's vest.

Less than one third of the people interviewed thought that their elderly relative was happy in the Home and approximately the same number were unsure.

She doesn't complain.

I don't know if she's happy but she doesn't laugh or sing so much.

I think she's happy—every time I go she says, 'When am I going to come out of here?' But basically she's quite happy.

However, more than one third were said to be unhappy:

She's very miserable actually. She says quite openly, 'Please God, take me.'

Absolutely broken-hearted. He's never been away from his sister.

He definitely isn't happy. They try their utmost, but I think it's too impersonal. I think they need a room of their own where they can go on their own and keep their own little things.

Private nursing Homes

The relatives of those being cared for in private nursing Homes were asked about their choice of Home—what did they look for in a Home? One relative who had visited 15 private nursing Homes gave the reasons for her choice:

I chose this one because they don't expect the patient to conform to the Home, they conform the Home to the patient. They don't pressurise her, they let her do exactly what she likes in her own way. She has eccentricities—at 91 we are all going to have them—and they just accept her.

Other relatives stated their priorities:

It's very well run, as the matrons says, 'This is their home. You can come and go and there are no rules.'

I think every person has the right to privacy and an individual room where he can have his own bits and pieces around him.

Yet, despite the greater degree of choice, some people still complained that their relatives had become withdrawn:

It's painful to go—there's no conversation.

I wish it had a sitting room. I wish it had a proper lift.

I think if you mix with people it keeps you more alert, there's incentive. They are all in their own rooms, they never see each other.

She likes to sit in the sitting room. She likes a bit of life. She's not like the others, she likes to get out. The others don't seem to want to go out.

Sitting rooms were, however, the subject of some criticism.

They sort of all sit round the outside of the room which does seem to me to be a bit austere. If they could divide it up . . .

Yet the privacy afforded by a private room was also valued.

My mother would hate a place where she had to go and talk to people, where they all had to go for meals or something.

One relative took a more positive view of withdrawal:

She's now living in the past and very much happier for it, too, I think.

These relatives also referred to the lack of activities for the elderly.

There is nothing for her to do all day.

That's what is so awful about old people's Homes. I've been in three or four and you see these old people just sitting, not doing anything. Oh, it fills me with despair just to see it.

The importance of keeping elderly people purposefully occupied was readily perceived. For example, one old lady spent a great deal of time knitting blanket squares:

We can hardly keep her going in wool but her hands have unscrambled as a result.

The problem of sensory deprivation was also noted:

Her sight is very poor. She cannot read. She can barely see the television. She cannot walk. So her world is very limited and she is very bored.

The problems of secondary deterioration were also mentioned:

My mother has gone downhill mentally since she's been there because she hasn't had to think for herself very much.

He doesn't get enough exercise. He is losing the use of his limbs.

> I just wish they hadn't allowed Mother to vegetate.

> She feels she should be dressed and undressed and of course the reason why they don't do it—if they dress and undress her she'll not do anything. It's terribly important.

One third of those interviewed thought that the elderly were unhappy in these private Homes. For example:

> It's a very caring place and she has got her bits and pieces round her but, I mean, it isn't your home and the company is not exactly exhilarating.

> Sometimes she says, 'I wish I was back home,' or, 'I wish I was dead.'

LOSS

These two sets of interviews give us quite different perspectives on the care of the elderly. Interviews with the professionals, which enabled the different models of care to be identified, show quite clearly that, under a supportive care regime, choice can be given to the elderly. Equally clearly, supportive care can be given in any setting, but its success depends on the attitudes of care staff.

The interviews with relatives illustrate their concern and, on occasions, their all too apparent despair. Loss of choice was highlighted in interviews with care staff: 'We think it is better to more or less think for them.' However, loss of choice was seen by relatives as one component of loss on a much greater scale. Such loss included:

Loss of clothes—'They sent her home in a man's vest.'

Loss of possessions—'She went in there with quite a few bits and pieces of her own and they went missing.'

Loss of privacy—'It wouldn't take a minute to cover him up.'

Loss of dignity—'They eventually have to do it where they sit and I think that really takes away all their self-respect.'

Loss of adult status—'She said she'd been a naughty girl.'

Loss of role—'They were sewing bits of leather together, but there is no purpose.'

Loss of freedom—'They put him in a high chair with a tray across it and the trouble is that he can't get out and he gets frustrated.'

Loss of identity—'They sit there like zombies.'

The loss of independence incurred by elderly people who enter a long-term care facility is often superimposed on the loss which precedes admission. Such loss may include the death of a spouse, friends or relatives, sensory loss and the decline of physical health. Admission in itself can also mean being parted from loved ones: 'He cries because he's parted from his wife, It's sad for both of them.'

Coping and confusion

Bonar and Maclean (1983) argue that the many crises and losses which occur in old age may contribute to a breakdown. They suggest that psychological defences such as regression and withdrawal may be construed as symptoms of 'senility', whereas if these symptoms were recognised as evidence of coping behaviour, steps could be taken to alleviate the underlying distress. Slater and Lipman (1977) make a similar point: 'Staff in homes for old people can readily assume that the expression of confused behaviour by a resident is pathological in origin rather than as signalling efforts to comprehend and/or cope with the experiences of ageing in an institution' (p 523).

One study revealed that 71% of staff working in residential Homes particularly liked working with the 'confused' whereas the lucid and physically able residents were seen by many to be difficult and demanding and provided little in the way of job satisfaction (Evans et al 1981). This same study revealed that a number of residents thought that they were in school.

There is a certain circularity in the designation of patients as 'confused' on the basis of childlike behaviour if, at the same time staff refer to and admonish patients as children, thus reinforcing the behaviour on which they base their 'diagnosis'. The interviews with relatives described above illustrate this very point: 'They say you go back to your childhood, don't they? But I think it doesn't help a lot to be called by your first name; it's going back to your childhood for them.'

Wolanin and Phillips (1981) also suggest that confused behaviours may be positively reinforced and that attempts at control and autonomy may be negatively reinforced. They argue that a patient's credibility is first questioned by staff and later by the patient herself. They suggest that patients are reinforced for withdrawing behaviour. For example, when a patient does not respond, staff give extra attention to draw the patient out. Similarly, patients who indulge in bizarre behaviour are likely to receive extra attention from staff. 'The end result is positive reinforcement for behaviours that are both aberrant and withdrawn.' (p. 21)

Sensory impairment

In a recent article on stress and coping, Clarke (1984) suggests that one of the most disagreeable situations known to man is the absence, or a low level, of stimulation. For many elderly people the lack of stimulation in an institutional environment is made worse by sensory impairment and this too was readily perceived by many relatives, some of whom saw withdrawal as one means of coping with an unstimulating environment: 'She peoples the houses in her imagination and that passes the day until she falls asleep.'

Wolanin and Phillips (1981) discuss this problem in great detail, citing the experiments of Bexton et al (1954) and others which have shown that sensory deprivation, sensory overload or sensory distortion in an isolating situation can give rise to profound behavioural changes in normal, healthy, young people. It would seem that there is an optimal range, level and variety of stimulation to maintain awareness.

Depression and loneliness

The work of Herbst and Humphrey (1980) has demonstrated a strong relationship between deafness and depression, and Clarke (1984) suggests that hospital patients who have little control over the environment may be particularly prone to feelings of depression and helplessness. The interviews described above would lead us to believe that considerable proportions of the more heavily dependent elderly in all three settings were either unhappy or depressed. This impression is borne out by interviews with the old people themselves; less than half of those in hospital or residential Homes who were able to respond to questioning said that they were happy in their current situation (Wade et al 1983). For example: 'There is no freedom. I get depressed a lot, I've not been out for a year' (Hospital Patient).

The comment which follows was made by an elderly man for whom admission to hospital had meant parting from his wife: 'I'm fed up with sitting in this chair day after day. I've been sitting in this blooming chair since last September. I never go anywhere, sit here all day long. Nobody to talk to. I wish I could go home.' This patient was completely blind and extremely deaf. He was rated 'confused' by the ward sister.

A small pilot study of patient satisfaction reported by Morle (1984) suggests that loneliness may be experienced by the majority of patients, even in a modern geriatric assessment unit. Wolanin and Phillips (1981) argue that the problems of loneliness and lack of meaning are further compounded in long-term care settings where oneday may be very like another. Of those who were able to respond, almost one third of old people in residential Homes and long-term care wards said that they were often lonely (Wade et al 1983).

Freedom and purpose

The importance of providing meaningful

activity was something which was expressed by many relatives who clearly perceived that inactivity led to apathy, secondary deterioration and, finally, loss of identity.

Diversional activities may be provided by staff but to provide *for* meaningful activity implies making provision for greater participation in the life of the ward or home. In her book *Rights and Risk* Alison Norman (1980) cites a DHSS study of 124 local authority, private and voluntary Homes in the London area. This survey showed that there were very few Homes in which residents were consulted about the way life was organised. In most of these Homes residents were not encouraged to help with chores or to do things for themselves. Similarly, Brooking (1982) conducted a survey of the practices and opinions of staff, patients and their relatives in 16 wards in two hospitals. Findings indicated only very limited involvement of patients and relatives in the planning and implementation of care.

The regimentation of institutional living can weaken an old person's awareness of self (British Geriatrics Society & Royal College of Nursing 1975). If we accept, as Alison Norman suggests, that elderly people should enjoy the liberty granted to other adult citizens—that is, to order their activities, finances and personal affairs—then restrictions should be limited to those which are necessary to provide the level of care they need and to protect the quality of life of others.

This chapter began by focusing on choice and flexibility both with regard to the range and level of provision and at the point of service delivery. Those involved in caring for the elderly have a dual responsibility, as policy makers on the one hand and as carers on the other. 'What I can't get across to people—it seems to me that they all talk about the old and the young as though they're separate, they're not, they're us. They're us in another 20 years. So what would you like done to you?' (Relative).

REFERENCES

Bexton W H, Heron W, Scott R H 1954 Effect of decreased variation in the sensory environment. Canadian Journal of Psychology 8: 70–76

Bonar R, MacLean M J 1983 Senility symptoms as a psychological defense. Paper presented at Systed 1983 Conference, Montreal, 15 July

British Geriatrics Society and Royal College of Nursing 1975 Improving geriatric care in hospital. Report of Joint Working Party of the British Geriatrics Society and the Royal College of Nursing, London

Brooking J I 1982 Patient and family participation in nursing: a survey of opinions and current practices among patients, relatives and nurses. In: Proceedings of the RCN Research Society XIII Annual Conference, University of Durham, p 97–120

Clarke M 1984 Stress and coping: constructs for nursing. Journal of Advanced Nursing 9(1): 3–13

Department of Health and Social Security 1978 A Happier old age. HMSO, London

Evans G, Hughes B, Wilkin D, Jolley D 1981 The management of mental and physical impairment in non-specialist residential homes for the elderly. Research Report No. 4, Department of Psychiatry and Community Medicine, Manchester University

Fennell G, Phillipson C, Wenger C 1983 The process of ageing: social aspects. In: Elderly people in the community: their services needs. HMSO, London

Gorbach P, Sinclair I 1982 Pressure on health and social services for the elderly. Working Paper, May

Herbst K G, Humphrey C 1980 Hearing impairment and mental state in the elderly living at home. British Medical Journal 28: 903–905

Illsley R 1983 The contribution of research of the development of practice and policy. In: Elderly people in the community: their service needs. HMSO, London

Morle K M F 1984 Patient satisfaction: care of the elderly. Journal of Advanced Nursing 9(1): 71–76

Norman A J 1980 Rights and risk. National Council for the Care of Old People (now Centre for Policy on Ageing), London

Plank D 1978 Old People's homes are not the last refuge. Community Care 202: 16–18

Slater R, Lipman A 1977 Staff assessments of confusion and the situation of confused residents in homes for old people. Gerontologist 17(6): 523–530

Wade B E 1983 Different models of care for the elderly. Nursing Times 79:12 Occasional Papers 33–36

Wade B E, Sawyer L, Bell J 1983 Dependency with dignity. Occasional Papers on Social Administration No. 68. Bedford Square Press, London

Wolanin M O, Phillips L R F 1981 Confusion, prevention and care. Mosby, St Louis

24

J. I. Brooking

Services for the elderly mentally infirm

THE DEVELOPMENT OF PSYCHOGERIATRIC MEDICINE AND NURSING AS SPECIALTIES

Specialised psychiatric services for the elderly began during the 1960s (e.g. Macmillan 1960, Robinson 1962) and since then has come increasing recognition and acceptance of the need for special services in each locality. The Royal College of Psychiatrists established a specialist section for the psychiatry of old age, which has been important in the development of ideas, and has generated a series of policy statements and guidelines for practice (Royal College of Psychiatrists 1973). A Working party of the Department of Health and Social Security (DHSS) also endorsed the trend towards special psychiatric services for the aged (DHSS 1981).

Factors which have contributed to the development of psychogeriatric services were described by Arie and Jolley (1982) as the increase in the number of elderly people, especially the very old; developments in psychiatry leading to more effective treatments for the elderly; and acceptance that health services should be planned for defined populations. The purposes of psychogeriatric services were described by Arie and Jolley (1982) as maintaining mental health; preserving independence; and providing permanent or intermittent institutional care when necessary.

After years of neglect, psychogeriatric medicine is becoming a recognised specialty. Both psychiatrists and geriatricians have chosen to specialise in this subject. By the end of 1980, 120 consultant psychiatrists described psychogeriatrics as their main activity, which was 10% of all consultant psychiatrists in the National Health Service (Wattis et al 1981). There should be at least one psychogeriatrician in each health district whose role should include the organisation of facilities and staff in the district, representing the specialty in planning committees etc., clinical practice, education and research (Arie and Jolley 1982).

The care of the elderly mentally infirm has traditionally been regarded as an unattractive and low-prestige area of nursing. There is however, evidence that attitudes are beginning to change. For example, in a small Scottish survey, Jones and Galliard (1983) found very positive attitudes among nurses to geriatric-psychiatric nursing.

General and psychiatric nursing students gain experience in the care of the elderly during training, although general nursing students may not work with psychogeriatric patients. As these patients may be cared for in general or psychiatric settings, their carers may be either general or psychiatric nurses. It is possible that a combination of both kinds of nursing experience provides the best preparation for work in this specialised area.

There are now many nationally recognised post-basic clinical courses for qualified nurses to update knowledge and acquire specialist skills. Courses relevant to psychogeriatric nursing include Nursing Elderly People, Community Psychiatric Nursing and Advanced Psychiatric Nursing. There are no clinical courses currently available which are specific to psychogeriatric nursing. The setting up of such a course would provide a major landmark in establishing the care of the elderly mentally infirm as a recognised branch of nursing.

Scope of the problem

Psychiatric disorders in the elderly are very common. Estimates of the prevalence of dementia vary, but different researchers suggest that between 5% and 15% of those over 65 years and between 20% and 30% of those over 80 years suffer from senile dementia. In Newcastle Kay et al (1964) found dementia to be the main determinant of the need for institutional care. Bergmann (1971) found that 10% to 20% of old people suffer from neurotic disorders. Psychiatric disorders seem to be more prevalent among old people in institutions than at home (Kay et al, 1962). Bergmann and Eastham (1974) found that about half the patients over 65 years of age in general hospitals suffered from some kind of psychiatric illness. Symptomatic confusional states are common in acute medical and surgical wards (Millar 1981), but dementias and affective disorders are common in geriatric wards and among residents in old people's homes.

CATEGORIES OF PSYCHOGERIATRIC PATIENTS AND FACILITIES REQUIRED

A DHSS document published in 1972 classified mentally ill old people into four groups, and defined the relative responsibilities of geriatric, psychiatric and medical units and social services departments in caring for this population. The four categories were as follows:

1. Patients who entered psychiatric hospitals before modern treatment was available, have grown old and are likely to live out their lives in hospitals. They comprise about 20% of the current psychiatric hospital population (Macdonald 1982). The fate of their successors, the middle-aged chronic schizophrenics, is uncertain, but it is likely that many will remain in psychiatric hospitals. These groups of patients are the responsibility of psychiatrists within the general psychiatric services.

2. The elderly with 'functional' mental illnesses who contribute more than half the referrals to most psychiatric services. They are also likely to remain within the spectrum of general psychiatry.

3. Patients with a mild degree of senile

dementia but no physical disease who can usually be managed in their own home. Their social circumstances may require residential or day care under the social services department.

4. Severely demented ambulant patients who could be cared for in psychogeriatric day hospitals or admitted to psychiatric care. Demented patients with an associated physical illness are mainly the responsibility of the geriatric medical services, whether as in-patients or day patients.

Services for patients living at home

Government policy in Britain emphasises the importance of treatment and care in the community rather than in hospital (DHSS 1972, 1978). Hemsi (1982) described reasons for the community emphasis in psychogeriatric medicine. The disorders are such that no hospital investigations may be required and little is gained by admission. Old people are members of social networks which should be maintained. Institutional resources are scarce and expensive and there are well-recognised disadvantages of hospital care. Therefore, Hemsi (1982) argued that it is better to support the patient (and his or her carers) in the community. In trying to achieve the goal of community care, obstacles arise because of the administrative separation of the health services, provided by central government, and the social services, provided by local authorities.

It is usual in psychogeriatric practice for initial assessment to take place in the patient's home (Arie and Jolley 1982). This is because functioning at home gives an accurate picture of the patient's capacities, whereas moving the patient can increase confusion. Hemsi (1982) argued that hospital assessment is only appropriate when special investigations are necessary.

Many mentally infirm old people receive no help at all, but others are cared for by relatives. According to Pasker et al (1976) families carry a formidable burden, yet rarely receive adequate support from the domiciliary services. Services which should be available include home helps, meals-on-wheels, laundry services, telephones, emergency call systems, etc. Bergmann et al (1978) argued that if resources are limited, more domiciliary services should be directed to people living with their families than to those living alone. This is because the former can often remain at home given adequate support, whereas many of the latter will inevitably require eventual admission.

In Britain general practitioners (family doctors) deal with most of the problems of the elderly mentally infirm, without referring them to consultants. However, a study by Williamson et al (1964) found that general practitioners were unaware of many of the psychiatric disorders suffered by their elderly patients. It also appeared that patients do not always receive adequate long-term medical supervision. A review by the Royal College of Psychiatrists (1981) suggested that these problems are due to the organisation of general practice as a patient-initiated service and to the doctors' lack of knowledge about psychiatric illness.

Community psychiatric nurses are playing an increasing role in the care of mentally abnormal old people (Ainsworth and Jolley 1978) and many specialist posts have been created within general community psychiatric nursing teams. District nurses, health visitors and social workers are also likely to be involved in home care.

Day care facilities

Day care is a natural link between institutional and home care, and may provide enough support for patients who would otherwise be unable to remain at home. Patients can benefit from social interaction, nursing care, medical treatment and stimulating activities. Day facilities are entirely dependent on the availability of transport. Discharge from day care is most often by death or admission to another form of care (Greene and Timbury 1979). Psychogeriatric day care may be an extension of the hospital service, or it may consist of local authority day centres, social clubs or luncheon clubs. It is often possible to arrange short-term admissions to enable overburdened relatives to take a holiday.

Residential care

Part III of the National Assistance Act of 1948 gives local authorities responsibility for providing old people's Homes and other sheltered accommodation. Britain has no significant nursing Home sector to fill the gap between old people's Homes and hospitals. Indeed, nurses have very limited involvement in this type of care. In a comparison of New York and London, Gurland et al (1979) found that both cities provide residential care for about 4% of their elderly population. In New York about two thirds were in nurse-run nursing Homes, whereas in London about two thirds were in local authority Homes staffed by wardens and domestic helpers.

Residential Homes have a proportion of mentally infirm residents and this is likely to increase (Wilkin et al 1978). The question of whether mentally alert and mentally infirm residents should live in integrated Homes or whether they should be segregated has been debated. Those in favour of integrated Homes argue that confused people are less likely to be subjected to 'infantilising processes' in mixed Homes (Meacher 1972) and that rational residents assist and encourage confused residents. Arguments in favour of segregated Homes are that a safer environment can be created in which wandering can be contained without resort to restraint (Bergmann 1973). Staff in integrated Homes are unlikely to have been adequately trained in the specialised management of old people with psychiatric disorders. A compromise may be integration but with some separate facilities, so that the needs of each group can be met.

Hospital care

Elderly mentally infirm patients may be found in geriatric hospitals, psychiatric hospitals, general hospitals and in specialised assessment units.

Psychogeriatric assessment units

Studies in the 1960s, e.g. Kidd (1962), concluded that extensive misplacement of patients between geriatric and psychiatric hospitals led to poor treatment, prolonged stay and unnecessary mortality. Concern about misplacement led to an official policy of developing psychogeriatric short-stay assessment units, jointly directed by psychiatrists and geriatricians (DHSS 1970). Arie (1981) argued that they should be located in general hospitals because diagnosis, especially of acute confusional states, requires painstaking investigation. Some assessment units have worked well, but many have had difficulty functioning effectively, because of the lack of places to which patients could be transferred following assessment.

Psychiatric hospitals

In Britain, psychiatric in-patient services have been moving from large psychiatric hospitals to psychiatric units in general hospitals. This has resulted in a two-tier system with the general hospital units tending to take young acute patients, leaving the large psychiatric hospitals increasingly occupied by long-stay patients and the elderly. This has had serious consequences for staff morale and quality of care. Many psychiatric hospitals are geographically remote from their catchment areas, thus weakening social ties and reducing the likelihood of the patients returning to the community.

Fifty per cent of all mental illness beds are occupied by patients aged over 65 years and they account for 20% to 40% of psychiatric admissions (DHSS 1976). Describing the distribution of elderly patients in a typical large psychiatric hospital, Macdonald (1982) found 8% suffering from acute 'functional' illness, 30% severely demented, and 20% had 'graduated' from the long-stay wards and were mainly chronic psychotics. There was also another large group of middle-aged institutionalised schizophrenics who were likely to grow old in hospital.

General and geriatric hospitals

Elderly mentally infirm patients may be found in geriatric, medical, surgical and orthopaedic wards. They are also in geriatric hospitals. If patients are suffering from physical illness or disability, the medical geriatric services should provide care and should be able to cope with associated mental disturbance. It is understandable that geriatric services are often reluctant to take ambulant demented patients, as their wandering takes up much nursing time and they may disturb mentally alert patients.

CHARACTERISTICS OF HIGH QUALITY IN-PATIENT FACILITIES

It can be argued that elderly patients with 'functional' disorders should be placed alongside younger patients with similar disorders. However, there are also advantages in an age-related service, and it should be possible to care for patients with organic and functional disorders together, especially as there are often blurred boundaries between the two groups.

It may be preferable for assessment, acute and long-term treatment to take place in the same unit. This facilitates continuity of care as patients are cared for by the same staff throughout their stay in hospital. It also eliminates the stigma and problems of low status associated with long-stay wards and is likely to result in a more vigorous unit with enthusiastic staff.

The unit should be small and should accommodate men and women. It should be close to the catchment area to encourage visiting and family participation. Ideally, patients should have their own bedrooms or cubicles to allow privacy and personal space. Patients should be encouraged to have personal belongings in their bedrooms. There should be a sitting room and ideally a separate room for noisy activities such as television.

It should be possible to deal with uncomplicated physical illness and disability within a psychogeriatric unit, rather than having to transfer patients to geriatric medical wards. The unit should be able to offer vigorous, individually planned, psychiatric and physical treatments as discussed in chapters 18 and 19. But there should also be recognition when active treatment and rehabilitation are no longer appropriate. The unit should be able to provide skilled terminal care.

Nursing the elderly mentally infirm is different from both geriatric and psychiatric nursing. It requires particular motivation and specialised education. There are currently few educational opportunities, either at pre- or post-registration level and an in-service educational programme is essential to a successful unit. The presence of students can be helpful in developing new ideas and maintaining enthusiasm.

Working with demented and depressed patients is emotionally draining. Staff can easily feel inadequate and discouraged when patients fail to improve. Support is essential if high calibre nurses and doctors are to be attracted into this area and stay. Clear communication among staff at all levels is a first essential. Frequent patient review by the multidisciplinary team and nursing care planning meetings facilitate this. All staff must be fully informaed about the goals for their patients. Support groups can help staff to become aware of their own reactions and to ventilate their worries and frustrations, but they only work if the ward atmosphere encourages mutual respect and acceptance.

LEGAL ASPECTS OF PSYCHOGERIATRIC CARE

Compulsory admission

The decision to admit a person compulsorily to a psychiatric hospital under Part II of the Mental Health Act 1983 rests on two judgments: firstly, that the person is suffering from a mental disorder; and, secondly, that the person is a danger to him or herself or to others. Separate sections provide for admission for assessment and for treatment. Hemsi (1982) considered that compulsory detention under the Mental Health Act is rarely justified in psychogeriatric medicine. He points out that basic care rather than treatment is required for dementia, and so the Act is irrelevant. A possible exception identified by Hemsi (1982) is the patient with an insight-impairing functional psychosis who may respond to physical treatment but refuses it, and can be detained in the interests of his or her own health and safety.

Section 47 of the National Assistance Act 1948 as amended in 1951 applies to the elderly who are living in unsanitary conditions and who are not able to give themselves, nor receive from others, proper care and attention. The Act enables such a person, under clearly defined procedures, to be taken to a hospital for three weeks. Muir Gray (1980) found that about 200 people a year were removed from their homes to hospitals or old people's Homes each year under the provisions of Section 47.

Finance and property of patients

If patients are lucid, financial decisions are entirely their own. If they are physically incapable or choose not to manage their own affairs, they can transfer that function by giving another person the 'power of attorney'. This can be revoked at any time and it lapses in law if the patient ceases to be lucid.

The Court of Protection exists to protect and control the administration of the property of persons who become physically or mentally incapable of doing so themselves. The Court derives its statutory authority from Part VII of the Mental Health Act 1983. It is part of the Supreme Court and is staffed by judges nominated by the Lord Chancellor. A medical recommendation is required to place a patient under the jurisdiction of the court and enquiries may be made by officers of the court. The court can appoint a receiver, often a family member, to administer the property under its direction. In 1983 about 23 000 people were under the jurisdiction of the Court of Protection (Bluglass 1983). Many are elderly people.

PREVENTION OF PSYCHIATRIC DISORDERS AND PROMOTION OF MENTAL WELL-BEING

Pfeiffer (1977) viewed psychopathology in the elderly as a failure to adapt to this stage of life, and he identified three main adaptive tasks of old age:

1. Adaptation to losses such as spouse, work and social roles, income and mobility. The task is replacement and learning to cope with loss.
2. Life review. The task is to mark out an identity which integrates the diverse elements of life and allows a positive view of one's life work.
3. The task of remaining active to retain physical, emotional, social and intellectual function.

Nurses have a role in helping elderly people to carry out these adaptive tasks and to reduce the likelihood of illness.

Ferguson Anderson (1978) considered that the two main causes of emotional disturbance in the elderly are physical disease and an adverse environment, including loneliness. Both have implications for nursing. Nurses can help to prevent physical disease by health education, patient teaching and health visiting. In order to improve the living environment of elderly people, nurses may need to broaden their perspectives beyond the individual to whole families and communities. Changing negative social attitudes towards the elderly and campaigning on their behalf are legitimate nursing activities.

In addition to the ideas outlined, it is also beneficial to enhance family relationships; to change attitudes towards retirement and educate people to use their extra leisure time productively; to change the negative attitudes of care-givers, and to facilitate elderly people's participation in former interests and activities.

CONCLUSIONS

This chapter has considered the development of the specialty of psychogeriatric medicine and nursing and the scope of the problem. The types of patients and facilities required have been categorised. The current provisions for the elderly mentally infirm have been described and briefly discussed. These include community and day care, residential care and hospital care in assessment units, psychiatric and general hospitals. The characteristics of high quality hospital care for these patients were considered. Some legal aspects of psychogeriatric practice, including compulsory admission and patients' property, were outlined. The chapter closed with a consideration of the prevention of psychiatric disorders in the elderly.

REFERENCES

Ainsworth D, Jolley D 1978 The community nurse in a developing psychogeriatric service. Nursing Times 74: 873–874

Arie T 1981 Consideration for the future of psychogeriatric services In: Kinnaird J, Brotherston J, Williamson J (eds) The provision of care for the elderly. Churchill Livingstone, Edinburgh

Arie T, Jolley D 1982 Making services work: organisation and style of psychogeriatric services In: Levy R, Post F (eds) The psychiatry of late life. Blackwell, Oxford

Bergmann K 1971 The neuroses of old age In: Kay D W K, Walk A (eds) Recent advances in psychogeriatrics. British Journal of Psychiatry, Special publication, no. 6

Bergmann K 1973 Letter. New Society 22:531

Bergmann K, Eastham E J 1974 Psychogeriatric ascertainment and assessment for treatment in an acute medical ward setting. Age and Ageing 3: 174–188

Bergmann K, Foster E M, Justice A W et al. 1978 Management of the demented elderly patient in the community. British Journal of Psychiatry 132 441–447

Bluglass R 1983 A guide to the Mental Health Act 1983. Churchill Livingstone, Edinburgh

Department of Health and Social Security 1970 Psychogeriatric assessment units. Circular H M (70) 11, DHSS, London

Department of Health and Social Security 1972 Services for mental illness related to old age Circular H M (72) 71. DHSS, London

Department of Health and Social security 1976 Health and social services statistics for England 1975. HMSO, London

Department of Health and Social Security 1978 A happier old age: a discussion document on the elderly in our society. HMSO, London

Department of Health and Social Security 1981 Growing older. HMSO, London

Ferguson Anderson W 1978 Preventive medicine in old age In: Brocklehurst J C (ed) Textbook of geriatric medicine and gerontology, 2nd edn. Churchill Livingstone, Edinburgh

Gurland B et al 1979 A cross-cultural comparison of the institutionalised elderly in the cities of New York and London. Psychological Medicine 9: 781–788

Greene J G, Timburgy G C 1979 A geriatric psychiatry day hospital service. Age and Ageing 8: 49–53

Hemsi L 1982 Psychogeriatric care in the community In: Levy R, Post F (eds) The psychiatry of late life. Blackwell, Oxford

Jones R G, Galliard P G 1983 Exploratry study to evaluate staff attitudes towards geriatric psychiatry. Journal of Advanced Nursing 8: 47–57

Kay D W K, Beamish P, Roth M 1962 Some social and medical characteristics of elderly people under state care. Sociological Review Monograph No. 5, Keele

Kay D W K, Beamish P, Roth M 1964 Old age mental disorders in Newcastle upon Tyne. Part 1: A study of prevalence. Part 2: A study of possible social and medical causes. British Journal of Psychiatry 110: 146–158, 668–682

Kidd C D 1962 Misplacement of the elderly in hospital. British Medical Journal 2: 1491–1493

Levy R, Post F (eds) 1982 The psychiatry of late life. Blackwell, Oxford

Macdonald C 1982 A psychogeriatric rehabilitation programme In: McCreadie R G (ed) Rehabilitation in psychiatric practice. Pitman, London

Macmillan D 1960 Preventive geriatrics. Lancet 2: 1439–1440

Meacher M 1972 Taken for a ride. Longman, London

Millar H R 1981 Psychiatric morbidity in elderly surgical patients. British Journal of Psychiatry 138: 17–20

Muir Gray J A 1980 Section 47. Age and Ageing 9: 205–209

Pasker P, Thomas J P R, Ashley J S A 1976 The elderly mentally ill—whose responsibility? British Medical Journal 2: 164–166

Pfeiffer E 1977 Psychopathology and social pathology In: Birren J E, Schaie K W (eds) Handbook of the psychology of ageing. Van Nostrand, New York

Robinson R A 1962 The practice of a psychiatric geriatric unit. Gerontologia Clinica 1: 1–19

Royal College of Psychiatrists 1973 Joint Report of the British Geriatric Society and the Royal College of Psychiatrists on matters relating to the care of psychogeriatric patients. News and notes. August. Royal College of Psychiatrists, London

Wattis J, Wattis L, Arie T 1981 Psychogeriatrics: a national survey of new branch of psychiatry. British Medical Journal 282: 1529–1533

Williamson J, Stokoe I H, Gray S et al 1964 Old people at home: their unreported needs. Lancet: 1117–1120

Wilkin D, Mashiah T, Jolley D 1978 Changes in behavioural characteristics of local authority homes and long-stay hospital wards, 1976–77. British Medical Journal 2: 1274–1276

P. Fielding

25

Nursing old people in hospital

The idea that nursing old people in hospital is a specialised activity has been growing since the 1930s, when Marjorie Warren established the first department of geriatric medicine. But it is not a nursing speciality which any nurse can afford to ignore—the ailing aged over 65 years are not only to be found in geriatric beds but are major users of all other hospital beds with the obvious exceptions of paediatrics and maternity. In 1973, the elderly occupied 49% of general medical beds, 38% of orthopaedic beds and 47% of psychiatric beds (Owen 1976). This means that the National Health Service resources are directed towards the elderly more than towards any other age group. In 1978, the average per capita cost of care and treatment of people over the age of 75 years was seven times greater than that of a person of working age (Department of Health & Social Security (DHSS) 1978). It is therefore apparent that nurses working in hospital settings, particularly on medical, orthopaedic and psychiatric wards, should have a working knowledge of the special needs of the elderly and should demonstrate a willingness to cater for those needs.

PATTERNS OF CARE

Many of the issues which confront the geriatric ward nurse stem from the historical development of geriatric medicine which has emphasised early diagnosis, and the assessment and treatment of reversible conditions in the fashion of acute medicine. This is reflected in the report of the Royal College of Physicians' Working Party on Medical Care of the Elderly (1977), which in turn reflects the attempt to rationalise priorities in health and personal social services in a consultative document (DHSS 1976). This document stated that a primary objective must be to enable the elderly to remain in the community for as long as possible. To this end, emphasis should be placed on the development of domiciliary services and the provision of adequate facilities in general hospitals with easy access to diagnostic, therapeutic and rehabilitation resources. The aim is that eventually 50% of geriatric beds would be located in general hospitals. However, because of local hospital and community resources, geographical consideration and the influence of the interest of a particular physician, geriatric hospital services throughout the United Kingdom take many different forms (see Chapter 22 for further discussion on the historical development of services for the elderly).

Admissions policy

Central to this diversity is the admissions policy of the geriatric unit. On the one hand, the unit may accept any new medical patient over a certain age and provide an extensive range of diagnostic and therapeutic resources. On the other hand, the unit may accept referrals from other specialties once the acute phase of an illness has passed and rehabilitation or social problems hinder resettlement in the community. Often linked to the admissions policy or consequent upon local hospital resources is the placement of geriatric beds. These may be 'scattered' throughout the general hospital, a policy which has serious implications for the provision of appropriate resources and a therapeutic environment. However, even if beds are provided in a single unit there are two main patterns of organisation which have differing strengths and weaknesses.

Multipurpose wards

Firstly, multipurpose wards cater for patients who may require short-term diagnostic and therapeutic facilities, rehabilitation and continuing or extended care services, or a mixture of these (Bagnell et al 1977). Amongst the benefits claimed for this type of service are: higher staff and patient morale; continuity of care; and the need for relatively few long-stay beds. However, Pathy (1982) points out that to provide extended care in a district general hospital is unduly expensive and suggests that the use of smaller local hospitals would be better for this purpose and may also maintain patients near to relatives and friends. Pathy also indicates that, in multipurpose wards, relatives are often reluctant to agree to discharge when it is apparent that other patients receive extended care.

The effects of multipurpose wards on nursing and on patient outcomes are unresearched. One might suppose that some of the problems identified in long-stay care such as depersonalisation and institutionalisation would be ameliorated if long-stay patients shared facilities with the more acutely ill elderly, but such evidence as exists suggests that 'long-stay' patients on general medical wards fare badly when in competition with patients in more urgent need of attention (Fielding 1982).

Single-purpose wards

Secondly, a unit may be divided into wards with separate facilities for assessment, rehabilitation or continuing care. This functional separation allows resources to be applied discriminately where they are most needed and permits an appropriate 'homely' environment to be provided for those patients needing extended care. Pathy (1982) argues that, with efficient organisation, this system of functional separation is compatible with a high turnover and a minimal number of long-stay beds provided that the active treatment beds are sited in the general hospital.

In addition to such 'straightforward' geriatric

beds, some hospitals have established units for particular areas of need, e.g. joint orthopaedic-geriatric units (Devas and Irvine 1963, 1969) and stroke units (Garraway et al 1980).

BASIC REQUIREMENTS

Wherever geriatric beds are sited, there are certain basic requirements in terms of space and facilities which must be considered. The nurse involved in commissioning a new unit must be aware of these, but the nurse working in a well-established environment can often recommend improvements in existing facilities at little cost, providing she has a good grasp of the issues involved.

Bed areas

The DHSS has outlined minimum standard requirements with regard to bed areas for geriatric wards (DHSS 1972). These prescribe a minimum of 60 square feet per person. This should be the floor space available when suitable arrangements have been made for privacy, e.g. bed curtaining or cubicles. Once the minimum standard for space has been met, there are a variety of bed arrangements which can be used, e.g. long and open 'nightingale' wards, four to six beds grouped in bays, or individual rooms. Proponents of the traditional nightingale ward maintain that patients prefer them because nurses are always in view and there is plenty of activity to watch. Opponents of this style of ward cite the lack of privacy such an arrangement affords. These two issues, the need for social stimulation and the need for privacy are the prime factors to be considered when planning bed areas.

Privacy is a basic human need and the difficulties associated with its provision in institutions are well documented. Townsend (1962) writes: 'In the institution, people live communally with a minimum of privacy, and yet their relationships with each other are slender. Many subsist in a kind of defensive shell or isolation' (p 379).

Being admitted to hospital is, for most people, a stressful event. The lack of privacy which follows hospitalisation often compounds such stress. Davies and Peters (1983) have shown that nurses are somewhat insensitive to stressful items such as noise, privacy and toileting procedures, so it is important that the structured environment affords the maximum amount of privacy for the patient.

Tate (1980) suggests that the functions of privacy are fourfold. Firstly, personal autonomy—the ability of the individual to exercise control over her life. In a hospital ward this would include her ability to have privacy when she wished. In an acute assessment ward this provision may not be possible at all times because of the competing need for surveillance and monitoring of health by staff, but in less acute settings, professional workers of all kinds should recognise the need for the elderly person to exercise control in her dealings with others. Secondly, privacy affords the opportunity for emotional release. The demands on an elderly person who is also a patient, in terms of pleasantness, compliance and availability, are considerable. Periods of 'time-off' are an important feature in any role and are essential in order to alleviate concomitant tensions. Thirdly, privacy affords the opportunity for self-evaluation. This is particularly important for elderly people whose hospitalisation may mark a significant life crisis and herald a major change in lifestyle. Tate (1980) suggests that everyone needs time for reflection, creative imagination and integration of life experiences and that most institutions for the elderly are not conducive to such activity. Fourthly, privacy provides a base from which the individual can have limited and protected communication. One can share confidences with chosen and trusted individuals and, with the knowledge that privacy is available, one can seek social contact with others. This latter function of privacy has implications for nurses and other health workers who need to give information to, or obtain information from, elderly patients. Personal matters which may be causing great distress may not be dealt with adequately or satisfactorily for either party if the only privacy provided is a thin curtain.

Delong (1970) has shown that single rooms served to decrease aggression amongst the institutionalised elderly and suggests that this is because there is less need to establish personal territory in public spaces such as corridors and lounges. Furthermore, Lawton (1970) found that younger psychiatric patients in single rooms engaged in more social interactions than patients in multiple occupancy rooms.

From the evidence available, it would seem that single rooms in long-stay facilities have much to commend them and may indeed be valuable in the more acute areas if the need for surveillance can be met.

Day space

Again, the DHSS has specified minimum standards for geriatric wards (DHSS 1972). These state that at least 10 square feet per person should be provided. This specification is usually interpreted to mean a dayroom for the recreational use of patients. However, in some units space is at a premium and dayrooms may double as rest-rooms for staff, interviewing rooms, case conference rooms and physiotherapy or occupational therapy rooms. Multiple use of dayroom facilities often means that the furniture is less homely and the room less comfortable than is desirable. Ideally, no such duplication of use would occur and patients would be free to use the dayroom for a variety of activities at any time.

It is generally considered appropriate that dayrooms in geriatric units should be carpeted. Recent advances in the design of floor coverings and in the management of incontinence have rendered the arguments against carpeting dayrooms null and void. Indeed, there is much to be said for carpeting fostering a positive expectation of continence in patients. A carpeted area is also valuable for the patient who is learning to walk with a frame or for the wheelchair user as many difficulties associated with floor coverings often come to light only when the patient is at home. Useful information on floor coverings and other items of design can be found in Goldsmith (1976).

Décor in the dayroom is a matter of personal taste but wallpaper rather than painted walls may be appropriate for the elderly; several blending colours may be easier to maintain than one rigid colour scheme when new items of furniture are added; pictures will help to lessen the institutional impact, and lighting should provide both general and local illumination. Even in acute units it is appropriate to provide television and radio in the dayroom for selective use whilst in rehabilitation or extended care facilities one might expect record and cassette players or perhaps a piano. Thought should also be given to the provision of facilities for patients and relatives to make drinks or snacks as appropriate. This may be provided in the dayroom area or in a separate kitchen.

The arrangement of furniture in dayrooms is a vexed issue. Most nurses are familiar with the chairs-against-the-wall arrangement which does not appear to facilitate social interaction between patients. However, attempts to manipulate seating arrangements have shown that patients feel more secure and comfortable with their backs against either a wall or other physical barrier (Sommer and Ross 1958). In a large dayroom the need for a secure vantage point and for close face-to-face interaction can be provided by the careful use of room dividers. Whatever the seating arrangement, however, staff should always try to respect the individual's claim on a particular chair or a particular space.

Dining areas

The importance of mealtimes in the day of any patient of any age cannot be overemphasised. In the case of hospitalised elderly people, the dining experience can influence recovery and rehabilitation to a great extent and can affect the maintenance of dignity and independence. For most adults, social life is linked to a great extent to the pleasures of eating and drinking. Social and psychological significance is attached to eating at certain times and for certain purposes. Beck (1981) points out that meal-times still assume importance even in institutions, as shown by the fact that in some long-stay units residents will resort to queuing for an hour or more waiting for the dining room to open.

It is essential, therefore, that mealtimes are not merely a physiological event of food supplying nutrition but that they are a social and satisfying experience. Indeed, it could be argued that if they are not the latter, then there may be a failure to meet nutritional needs. Beck (1981) cites the increased dependency of the elderly patient, staff attitudes and sensory loss as vital factors to consider. The elderly may be confronted by strange food at unusual times. Clarke and Wakefield (1975) showed that nutritional scores were lowered when elderly nursing Home residents changed the nutritional habits of a lifetime. Whenever possible, mealtimes should provide continuity with the patient's pre-morbid state. Disabilities and sensory losses should be properly assessed by an occupational therapist who will recommend appropriate aids. Staff attitudes are crucial in promoting and maintaining independence in eating. The change to plated meals service in many hospitals has taken the provision of food away from nursing staff and encouraged the easy serving of food on trays to individual patients. This should not be allowed to detract from the social experience of mealtimes. Even with a plated meals service it is still possible to provide dining areas where patients can dine in groups of four to six to encourage socialising. Dining tables attractively laid with tablecloth, cutlery, crockery and condiments suitable for the meal will create an environment where independence becomes a real possibility. Nursing staff should be encouraged to circulate at mealtimes not only to assess nutritional intake but to facilitate conversation which will in turn increase interest in eating (Clancy 1975).

Toilet facilities

Continence promotion is an essential part of the work of any geriatric ward and the location of lavatories is crucial. It is generally acknowledged that lavatories should be within 40 feet of bed and day areas. Greater distances will inevitably lead to a high level of incontinence in a disabled population. The amount of space required within the lavatory is debatable. In a rehabilitation unit, too much space may give an unrealistic picture of the patient's level of independence, if her home circumstances are cramped and less than perfect. But in an assessment or long-stay unit it will be essential to have sufficient space to enable a patient to be assisted by one person or to use a wheel-chair. A patient with a walking frame needs up to 30 square feet in order to turn around. Ideally, all wards should have a variety of facilities and standard aids such as grab-rails should be provided. These and raised toilet seats can easily be supplied when the patient returns home. Bailey (1982) suggests that lavatory paper should be provided on a roll and in sheets to facilitate independence for hemiplegic patients.

It should be remembered that outward-opening doors leave more room on the inside and increase the likelihood of doors being closed for privacy.

A range of washing facilities is also desirable. For those patients who will be returning to their own homes, bathrooms with standard aids such as bath seats should be provided. For the more disabled person, hoists or cabinet baths may be necessary, but many elderly people can use showers successfully if seating is provided. Mirrors over wash-basins are essential in order to encourage patients to take pride in their appearance, and some should be fitted at the right height for wheel-chair-bound patients. Where wash-basins are located in a communal area, nurses should remember that their elderly clients are probably quite unused to sharing such facilities. It is only in recent years that shops and swimming baths have provided communal fitting and changing rooms. The nurse should endeavour to provide privacy for the often laborious and painstaking procedures of washing and dressing.

Lighting

Good lighting is greatly enhanced by natural sunlight and if the building is well positioned, then this can be used to good effect. Low level windows will enable patients to look outside even when seated. Blinds or curtains can be used to protect from direct sunlight and to darken the ward at night. If the ward is not naturally well lit, fluorescent lighting may be necessary, provided it is shaded to eliminate glare. In dayrooms, local lighting can be used for specific areas. Bailey (1982) suggests that lighting at floor level can be particularly useful at night—patients who are getting out of bed can see where they are going but the light does not shine in the eyes of those who are in bed.

Furniture

Beds

It is desirable that a good range is available to take account of the varied needs of patients. However, in most UK units it is the 'King's Fund' general purpose bedstead which is supplied and the need for diversity is often overlooked. There are certain general points, however, which should be borne in mind when considering any bed (Andrews and Atkinson 1982).

(a) Every bed should be adjustable in height. This enables the patient to transfer from bed to chair or commode with the minimum of difficulty.
(b) There should be a safe, simple and effective braking system.
(c) All beds should have the possibility of having safety sides attached to them which can be stored when not in use.
(d) All beds should be designed to accommodate poles for intravenous infusions, overhead handles and a few should have facilities for traction in combined orthopaedic/geriatric wards. More specialised beds should be available if they are needed, e.g. turning and tilting beds, flotation beds, low air loss beds and some of the many others now marketed.

Chairs

A wide range of chairs is essential. Nurses should resist uniformity for the sake of appearances in favour of being able to provide a specific chair for a particular patient's need. This will mean chairs with a range of seat heights and angles. General points to be considered are:

(a) A stable base is essential to avoid over-balancing for patients who may be able to push themselves up with only one arm.
(b) Handgrips should be positioned so that patients can use them when attempting to stand.
(c) There should be no crossbar at the front which would prevent correct positioning of feet under the chair for standing.
(d) Padded armrests and wings may be comfortable but wings can discourage social interaction if the chair is badly positioned.

The maintenance of chairs, as of all equipment, is extremely important. Vinyl seat covers, which are favoured because of their easy-to-clean feature, can become very hard and brittle with repeated washing. Splits may occur, particularly if the underlying foam collapses. This is not an uncommon sight and it is a potential fire hazard. Wells (1980) in a study of 749 chairs in one geriatric unit found that approximately one third were unsuitable for use because of very low seat heights, low backs, instability and grossly uncomfortable seats. A further 8% were severely damaged and had extensive seat welling and tears in the upholstery. In total, 48% of the chairs in the unit needed immediate replacement.

Lockers

All patients should be provided with a locker which has hanging space as well as drawer space for clothes. Doors and drawers should be easily opened with large handles to accommodate arthritic hands. It should be possible to use the locker on either side of the bed either for patient preference or for some therapeutic purpose such as encouraging a stroke patient to pay attention to her affected side. A mirror should be provided on the outside of the locker and the whole thing should be easily movable on castors.

Over-bed tables

These should be easily adjustable and easily movable and be suitable for use from chairs also.

Equipment

There are three areas of work in which the nurse caring for elderly people in hospital should be an expert and which require the use of special equipment. These are pressure sore prevention, the management of incontinence, and the lifting and handling of patients.

Pressure sore prevention

The major factors implicated in the development of pressure sores are direct pressure, shearing force and friction (see Chapter 14). It is, of course, essential that a detailed assessment of each patient's propensity to pressure sore development is carried out on admission and thereafter at regular intervals. Treatment should be directed at alleviation of pressure, shearing force and friction and there are several mechanical devices which the nurse may wish to use. Torrance (1983) describes these devices under three headings.

1. Devices which minimise pressure by increasing and varying the area which supports the body: These include alternating pressure mattresses and support systems which mould to the shape of the body such as foam, sawdust or sand—this concept has lately been modernised in the Clinitron bed using tiny particles of glass agitated by air currents which can be stabilised for easy transfer of the patient. Also in this group are the Mediscus low air loss bed and the water-bed. Major disadvantages of both these items are their expense and their size and weight. The low air loss bed has a sizeable pump system and control panel which must be accommo-

dated in addition to the bed itself. The deep tank water-beds which are more effective in relieving pressure than the shallow tank beds are necessarily heavy (approximately 660 kg) and may be too heavy for some old hospital floors.

2. Devices which aid turning and movement: This group ranges from such simple items as overhead handles which help the patient to change her own position, to sophisticated beds which the nurse can use to turn the patient or which turn automatically. The Egerton turning and tilting bed and the Stryker Circolectric bed are motorised whilst the Mecanaid Mecabed is an example of a manually operated turning bed. A major consideration of all patient support systems should be the effectiveness with which they relieve pressure and the effect on the patient in terms of mobility. If the patient has a pressure sore or is 'at risk', the use of a particular piece of equipment may relieve the pressure effectively at the cost of reducing mobility. A compromise must be sought and the relative advantages and disadvantages weighed carefully.

3. Devices which will support and protect specific areas. Perhaps the most commonly used of these are the sheepskins which are said to reduce friction and absorb moisture. They are particularly useful as a preventive measure against the development of heel sores in conjunction with the use of a bed cradle to take the weight of bedclothes off the feet. The development of heel sores is particularly catastrophic for the rehabilitation patient and is not related to a low score on the Norton pressure sore risk scale (Norton 1975). The use of preventive measures for all elderly patients is therefore justified, and the nurse may want to consider the use of sheepskin boots, sorbo boots, or leg troughs such as the Dermalex Pediprop which suspends the heel above the mattress. Gel pads and pressure relieving cushions also fall into this third group. Air-rings should not be used because of the danger to the blood supply of the sacrum and they are often overinflated. Sorbo rings are a more satisfactory substitute. A detailed analysis of the many different types of wheelchair cushions available can be found in Jay (1983). Further discussion on prevention of pressure sores is in Chapter 14.

Management of incontinence

Again, detailed assessment of incontinence is essential but in the control and management of incontinence there is a bewildering profusion of aids available. A directory of aids has been produced by the Association of Continence Advisors (1983), who suggest that five points should be considered when choosing an aid:

1. The amount and occasion of leakage
2. Whether used during the day, night or both
3. Whether the patient is up and dressed or in bed
4. The degree of mobility and dexterity
5. The extent of the patient's dependence on others.

This directory includes information on catheters, clothing, drainage bags, pads and urinals and is a valuable resource. See chapter 12 for a detailed discussion of incontinence.

Lifting and handling patients

There are many occasions when the nurse, quite appropriately, lifts or handles the patient without any recourse to special equipment. She or he should, therefore, be familiar with the various techniques recognised for safe handling and lifting. Some of these are discussed in Chapter 8. Where special equipment is necessary, there are many aids available which cater for patients with varying degrees of independence. Lloyd et al (1981) group these under three headings.

1. Aids for the independent patient with a residual disability. Included here are sliding boards which enable a patient to transfer from bed to chair; overhead handles or trapeze lifts which may be attached to the ceiling above the toilet for example to facilitate transfers; and bath seats which encourage independence in getting into and out of the bath.

2. Aids for the dependent patient who can

offer some assistance. In this group are turntables for transfers through 90° for patients who can take some weight through their legs; transit seats or slings which enable the nurse to move a patient from one sitting area to another without having to grasp painful joints. A makeshift sling of this kind can be made by rolling up a drawsheet to either side of the patient, then turning the four corners into 'handles' for the lifters.

3. Aids for the dependent patient for whom hoists may be necessary. Hoists may, of course, be used to facilitate bathing in less dependent patients. They may be fixed to the floor, to the ceiling, or they may be mobile. Hoists are described in more detail by Tarling (1980) and it is essential that the nurse knows how to use them to their best advantage. Information on their use can always be obtained from the Disabled Living Foundation.

ASSESSING THE ELDERLY PERSON IN HOSPITAL

Thus far the importance of adequate assessment of the patient has been stressed several times particularly with regard to the prevention of pressure sores and the promotion of continence. Consideration should also be given to a general assessment of the patient's level of independence. This is particularly important if the nurse is to have any indication of the type of nursing intervention needed and is also important in terms of evaluating the effect of interventions on the patient's progress.

Function versus pathology

During the past 20 years or so, there has been a shift of emphasis away from the 'pathology' of the patient, to a functional assessment of the patient's ability to carry out the 'activities of daily living'. Hall (1976) illustrates this well by pointing out that many disabilities commonly seen in a population, such as anaemia, cardiac failure, urinary symptoms, deafness and defective vision, could possibly co-exist in a single individual and yet that person may lead a quite satisfying life with no functional problems in terms of her activities of daily living. It is important, therefore, that assessment of the elderly person in hospital should focus not simply on a medical diagnosis but on functional disability. For the nurse, the latter is paramount.

Advantages of functional assessment

The advantages of functional assessment are at least threefold.

1. It can be used and understood by all members of the multidisciplinary team and provides a tool whereby patient and carers can converse in the same language about common goals. The patient's problem, in this functional sense, will not be her rheumatoid arthritis but will be her inability to perform the fine finger movements necessary for dressing herself.
2. It can be used to assess the degree of independence before, during and after treatment and if used in conjunction with some visual display, such as a wall chart, gives essential feedback to the patient so that she can monitor her own progress.
3. It provides a means of identifying specific functional deficiencies when the total score is broken down into individual items. Crucial items can also be weighted numerically in order to reflect their importance for certain levels of independence.

A fourth possible use may be in order to predict recovery of rehabilitation patients. Work by Stewart (1980) suggests that functional scoring can be used in order to select those patients who will benefit most from rehabilitation and the present author is currently looking at this possibility.

Perhaps the best-known functional assessment tool is the Barthel index (Mahoney and Barthel 1965) but there are several which the nurse might consider for a variety of purposes—the Kenny rehabilitation index (Schoening et al 1965), the nursing depen-

Table 25.1 An activities of daily living (ADL) score (*based on Stewart 1980*)

Function	Level of independence	Score
Bowel	Faecal incontinence (complete loss of bowel control and/or occasional soiling)	0
	Complete control	15
Bladder/catheter	Urinary incontinence	0
	Dry by day or catheter dry	10
	Complete control and/or manages own catheter	15
Walking	Requires at least two nurses	0
	Walks with one person or an aid	5
	Complete independence safely	10
Dressing/undressing	Requires complete help	0
	Requires limited help, e.g. fastenings	5
	Dresses independently	10
On/off toilet	Requires help at some stage	0
	Independent safely	10
Feeding	Requires feeding	0
	Independent but may need help with food preparation	10
Wheelchair (only for those unable to walk)	Unable to control safely	0
	Complete control	15
Stairs	Unable or unsafe	0
	Able to climb five stairs safely	5

dency index (Walton et al 1978) and the ADL score used by Stewart (1980). See Table 25.1.

Reliability and validity

There are certain issues of reliability and validity, however, which need to be addressed when using a functional assessment. Firstly, do two observers testing the same patient arrive at the same result? Before any index is used, the inter-rater reliability should be established. Secondly, do the tests in hospital correlate sufficiently well with the tasks facing the patient in her own home? If they do not, then the test's usefulness for information relevant to discharge will be limited. A third question has to do with the likelihood that the patient will perform at home to a similar standard as when in hospital. Many more factors may be involved here including responses to a different environment or a deterioration in physical or mental status. Assessment in the home will usually be standard practice before discharge from hospital.

DISCHARGE/TRANSFER FROM HOSPITAL

It should be emphasised that planning for discharge should begin early in hospital treatment. The nurse is in a good position when establishing goals with the patient to find out her wishes vis-à-vis returning to the community, and (s)he must try to judge, along with other members of the team, whether or not the patient is realistic in her plans for the future. Many people will be involved in returning the patient to her own home or to some other residential accommodation but it is vital that all arrangements are co-ordinated, that one person has an overall view and the nurse may be the best person to fulfil that role, because of her extended contact with the patient.

Standard checklist

In planning for discharge, it may be useful to follow a standard checklist. McFarlane and Castledine (1982) discuss the use of standard care plans and point out that it goes against the philosophy of individualised care planning. However, they also argue that it helps to establish safe and helpful routines of nursing care. The value of a standard discharge checklist is that it provides a visible record of arrangements made or to be made and reduces the risk of patients being sent home from hospital with inadequate preparation. It can be particularly useful for those wards who are not used to making the complicated

arrangements for discharge which are normally associated with geriatric ward patients.

Any checklist should include the following items with room for indicating special arrangements, names of contact persons and the signature of the nurse responsible:

1. The patient's family/friends to be informed.
2. The home is to be prepared, i.e. clean and warm, food and drink available.
3. Access to the home to be confirmed, i.e. key available or someone already present.
4. Transport to be arranged.
5. All clothes and property to be given back to patient.
6. Occupational therapy assessment carried out in hospital.
7. Occupational therapy assessment carried out at home or in simulated environment.
8. All aids or home adaptions to be provided or completed.
9. All medicines or dressings to be provided.
10. The patient or carer to be instructed (with some check for understanding) in:
    (a) the taking of medicine;
    (b) treatment;
    (c) exercises;
    (d) prosthesis/appliance functioning.
11. Community services to be arranged:
    (a) home help
    (b) meals-on-wheels
    (c) community nurse
    (d) other.
12. Follow-up appointment to be made with or without transport.
13. General practitioner to be informed of discharge.

This checklist is not exhaustive and the nurse will need to liaise closely with social workers, health visitors and various other professionals, depending on local arrangements and the level of service provision available. It is also useful if the patient is provided with the name address and telephone number of someone to contact should services not begin as arranged. Service provision may also be precarious at weekends and on public holidays and the nurse needs to bear this in mind when arranging the patient's transfer to community care.

CONCLUSION

Ethos of the geriatric unit

The overall ethos of the geriatric unit should not be ignored. For many elderly people whose hold on independent living is tenuous a sudden crisis resulting in hospitalisation can be a major life event of enormous proportions. In the acute phase of their illness they should receive all the necessary diagnostic and therapeutic treatments which are available for younger patients. However, the elderly patient's resistance to the negative effects of institutionalisation should not be overestimated and the nurse is in a key position to protect the patient. Depersonalisation can occur in several ways. The mode of addressing patients for example, can reveal something of the nurse's attitude towards them and can also convey something of their perceived social worth. Consider the relative merits and demerits of 'Hello, Granny' and 'Hello, Miss Frankland'. The use of first names by nurses and patients should be a matter of individual negotiation.

Depersonalisation can also occur by material means. One often sees in institutional environments, a misuse of articles for other than their original purpose, e.g. saucers used as ashtrays or cups used as sugar basins. This can convey the message to the patients that they are not worth the provision of the proper item. Routinisation also encourages depersonalisation. Whilst in any institution certain routines are essential, such as the provision of meals at specific times, other routines, e.g. bathing, getting up, going to bed, going to the toilet, are often instituted for staff convenience rather than for patients' benefit.

The wearing of hospital garments is another means whereby the person is stripped of personal identity. Unless the patient is acutely ill and confined to bed, there is no justification for wearing nightclothes during the day.

Indeed, valuable dressing skills may be lost by such a practice.

However, if elderly patients are to wear their own clothes, then some suitable means of laundering will have to be provided for those patients without relatives, and a personal clothing service would need to be installed for a long-stay unit.

The absence of personal possessions may also have a deterious effect on the elderly patient. Holzapfel (1982) suggests that being able to surround oneself with familiar items such as pets, albums, heirlooms, not only provides a sense of continuity with the past in a new environment, but also serves as a means whereby one can review one's life constructively. In an acute hospital setting, it may not be possible to accommodate large items of furniture but patients could be encouraged to keep photographs and small keepsakes by their beds. In a continuing care establishment every effort should be made to provide as homely an atmosphere as possible.

REFERENCES

Andrews J, Atkinson L 1982 Ward furniture equipment and patient clothing. In: Coakley D (ed) Establishing a geriatric service. Croom Helm, London
Association of Continence Advisors 1983 Directory of aids. ACA, London
Bagnell W E, Datta S R, Knox J, Horrocks P 1977 Geriatric medicine in Hull: a comprehensive service. British Medical Journal 3:102
Bailey R 1982 The hospital unit. In: Coakley D (ed) Establishing a geriatric service. Croom Helm, London
Beck C 1981 Dining experiences of the institutionalised aged. Journal of Gerontological Nursing 7: 104–113
Clancy K 1975 Preliminary observations of media use and food habits of the elderly. Gerontologist 13: 329–532
Clarke M, Wakefield L M 1975 Food choices of institutionalised vs. independent living elderly. Journal of American Dietetic Association 66: 600–604
Davies A D M, Peters M 1983 Stresses of hospitalisation in the elderly: Nurses' and patients' perceptions. Journal of Advanced Nursing 8: 99–105
Delong A J 1970 The micro-spatial structures of the older person: Some implications of planning the social and spatial environment. In: Pastalan L A, Carson D H (eds) Spatial Behaviour of Older People. University of Michigan, Ann Arbor
Devas M B, Irvine R E 1963 The geriatric orthopaedic unit. Journal of Bone and Joint Surgery 418:630

Devas M B, Irvine R E 1969 The geriatric orthopaedic unit. British Journal of Geriatric Medicine 6:19

Department of Health and Social Security 1972 Minimum standards in geriatric hospitals. DHSS, London

Department of Health and Social Security 1976 Priorities for health and personal social services in England. HMSO, London

Department of Health and Social Security 1978 A happier old age. HMSO, London

Fielding P 1982 An examination of student nurses' attitudes toward old people in hospital. Unpublished Ph.D. Thesis, University of Southampton

Garraway W M, Akhtar A J, Prescott R J, Hockey L 1980 Management of acute stroke in the elderly: Follow-up of a controlled trial. British Medical Journal 281:827

Goldsmith S 1976 Designing for the disabled. Royal Institute of British Architects, London

Hall M R P 1976 The assessment of disability in the geriatric patient. Rheumatology and Rehabilitation 15: 59–63

Holzapfel S K 1982 The importance of personal possessions in the lives of institutionalised elderly. Journal of Gerontological Nursing 8: 156–158

Jay P 1983 Choosing the best wheelchair cushion. Royal Association for Disability and Rehabilitation, London

Lawton M P 1970 Ecology and ageing. In: Pastalan L A, Carson D H (eds) Spatial behaviour of older people. University of Michigan, Ann Arbor

Lloyd P, Osborne C, Tarling C, Troup D 1981 The handling of patients: A guide for nurse managers. Back Pain Association and the Royal College of Nursing, London

Mahoney F I, Barthel D W 1965 Functional evaluation of the Barthel index. Maryland State Medical Journal 14: 61–65

McFarlane J, Castledine G 1982 A guide to the practice of using the nursing process. Mosby, London

Norton D 1975 Research and the problem of pressure sores. Nursing Mirror 143: 1965–67

Owen D 1976 In sickness and in health. Quartet Books, London

Pathy J 1982 Operational policies. In: Coakley D (ed) Establishing a geriatric service. Croom Helm, London

Royal College of Physicians 1977 Report of the working party on medical care of the elderly. RCP, London

Schoening H A, Anderegg L, Beighstrom D, Fonda M, Steinke N, Ulrich P 1965 Numerical scoring of self-care status of patients. Archives of Physical Medicine and Rehabilitation 46: 689–697

Sommer R, Ross H 1958 Social interaction on a geriatric ward. International Journal of Social Psychiatry 4: 128–133

Stewart C P U 1980 A prediction score for geriatric rehabilitation prospects. Rheumatology and Rehabilitation 19: 239–245

Tarling C 1980 Hoists and their use. Heinemann, London

Tate J W 1980 The need for personal space in institutions for the elderly. Journal of Gerontological Nursing 6: 439–449

Torrance C 1983 Pressure sores: aetiology, treatment and prevention. Croom Helm, London

Townsend P 1962 The purpose of institutions. In: Tibbets C, Donahue W (eds) Social and psychological aspects of ageing. Columbia University Press, New York, p 379

Walton M, Hockey L, Garraway W M 1978 How independent are stroke patients? Nursing Mirror 147: 56–58

Wells T J 1980 Problems in geriatric nursing care. Churchill Livingstone, Edinburgh

26

F. M. Ross

Nursing old people in the community

Nursing old people at home is complex, challenging and rewarding. The patient is seen as part of a family, in her own home with memories, rights and dignity; community nursing functions in this context. Nursing care is patient-oriented and family-centred and aims to support old people to live independently.

PRIMARY HEALTH CARE

Primary care in the United Kingdom is the first level of health care provided outside institutions. It is characterised by patient initiated consultations for health or social problems or a case-finding approach. This patient encounter with a health professional triggers a sequence of events that results in the patient becoming part of the health care system.

Access to primary care has particular significance for the old and disabled. A survey carried out for the Royal Commission on the Health Service found that because of frailty and poor transport many old people found difficulty in obtaining a consultation (Royal Commission on Health Service 1979).

There are different forms of primary health care delivery, and these will be discussed in terms of the organisation of district nursing.

Geographical organisation

This describes a system whereby a district

nurse is responsible for a defined geographical area. Her patients may be registered with more than one general practitioner. This has the advantage that the district nurse becomes knowledgeable about the neighbourbood, is known to local people and is therefore accessible for unplanned encounters. However, because the district nurse has a functional relationship with several general practitioners there are frequently problems of communication and continuity of care, particularly with the complex social and medical needs of old people.

Attachment

A district nurse may be 'attached' to one, or a group of general practitioners. She is responsible for the nursing care needs of all patients registered with these general practitioners. Doctors and nurses are formally based in the same location, health centre or general practice surgery. In reality there are several interpretations of this system. Some attached nurses pay only fleeting daily visits to the practice, others may genuinely use it as a working base. This is not always related to the availability of premises. Other professionals such as social workers involved in the care and welfare of the same patients are based elsewhere in offices with poor access to health records and few opportunities for the exchange of information. Although attachment provides a structure for improved communication it does not necessarily imply effective teamwork; success probably depends on attitudes and facilities available for the key workers.

The primary health care team

The primary care team has been defined as 'an interdependent group of general medical practitioners, secretaries, receptionists, health visitors, district nurses and midwives who share a common purpose and responsibility, each member clearly understanding his or her own function and those of other members, so that they can all pool skills and knowledge to provide an effective primary care service' (Standing Medical Advisory Committee 1981, p 2).

Fundamental to the concept of teamwork is the division of labour, co-ordination and task sharing, each member making a different contribution, but of equal value towards the common goal of patient care. A multidisciplinary approach is essential for the care of elderly people because of their complex social, psychological and physical health care needs.

Primary care teams work either in health centres or a general practice setting with facilities for professional activities, office space and clerical support.

Health centres

Health centres are units where family doctor services, child health and health education services are carried out. Accessible to the community, they provide a non-institutional setting for the integration of specialist skills. The special needs of old people may be catered for by chiropody, audiology, dentistry, optical, medical and nursing services. In addition, the health centre may serve as a setting for welfare advice or an outlet for publicity such as the Age Concern prevention of hypothermia campaign.

Health centres have several advantages. First, they provide a base for different professionals which facilitates interdisciplinary communication and the exchange of information. Second, they enable experiments such as a shared, centralised patient record system to be accessible to all members of the team. Evidence submitted to the Royal Commission on the Health Service recommended that, for teams to be co-ordinated and effective, professionals must share a core of knowledge and have access to the same reliable clinical information (Batchelor and McFarlane 1980). This kind of experiment clearly has important implications for the delivery of informed care to the elderly. Finally, health centres may be the focus of primary care developments such as computerisation of records, or multidisciplinary screening of the elderly using an age–sex register.

It is DHSS (Department of Health and Social Security) policy supported by the Royal Commission on the Health Service (1979) that teams should be the natural providers of primary care for the elderly with general practitioners and community nurses forming the core. A working party set up to review the primary care team recommended that it should be strengthened using three main approaches:

1. multidisciplinary education for trainee nurses and doctors in community care;
2. promotion of effective interprofessional communication;
3. multidisciplinary planning of health centre premises to encourage and maximise communication (Standing Medical Advisory Committee 1981).

THE ROLE OF THE DISTRICT NURSE

The district nursing sister is employed by the health district to give skilled nursing care to all persons living in the community including the home, health centre and residential accommodation. She (or he) is the leader of a nursing team which includes registered nurses, enrolled nurses and nursing auxiliaries to whom she delegates work as appropriate. She is accountable for the work delegated in addition to her own. District nurse training has been mandatory since 1981. It is a nine month course organised at institutes of higher education and includes three months supervised practice.

Functions of the district nurse

1. Identification of physical, emotional and social needs of patients in their own homes.
2. Planning and provision of appropriate programmes of nursing care particularly for the following groups: the chronic sick,

disabled, frail elderly, terminally ill and post-operative patients.
3. Mobilising community resources both professional and voluntary.
4. Identification of the special needs of the carer and family.
5. Ensuring continuity of care between home and hospital in both directions.
6. Promotion of health education and self care with individuals and groups.
7. Rehabilitation.
8. Counselling.

Other activities may include nursing care in the health centre and participation in multidisciplinary screening.

The district nurse spends 75% of her time with old people, the majority of whom are female (Dunnell and Dobbs 1982). The following discussion will use a nursing process framework to focus on the key issues of the district nurse's role, referred to above, that are particularly relevant to the care of the elderly.

Assessment

The aim of the assessment is to obtain sufficient information to identify problems. It includes information gathered during the patient interview, observation of the patient, family and environment, and information from the medical records, referral agency and other health workers.

Some assessment tools for the community have been developed, but not evaluated (O'Hare 1980, Robertson 1981). Basically, there are three approaches to assessment:

1. The body systems approach is based on the medical model and organises information in terms of diseases and clinical problems.
2. The top-to-toe approach uses a graphic representation of a person, for example the 'Gingerbread man', as a visual reminder of the assessment process (O'Hare 1980). Although useful as an aide-mémoire the mechanical nature of this approach implies a compartmentalised and dogged comprehensiveness with a physical focus that fails to explore some of the complex social

and personal issues of community care.

3. A needs model such as Maslow's (1970) is based on a hierarchy of needs embracing physiological, safety, love and belonging, self-esteem and self-actualisation. The central and important idea here is that these needs are interdependent and interrelated. The assessment concentrates on the connections between the individual, family and society. Although no formal assessment tool has been developed for the community using this model it would seem an appropriate framework for the district nurse to adopt, combined with a memory aid.

It is the conceptualisation of assessment in terms of nursing rather than medical problems that is important. Instead of a series of predetermined questions, the district nurse's approach should be the exploration of needs and feelings which are common to everyone, but may have assumed troublesome significance for the patient.

The first visit is of enormous importance in establishing a relationship with the patient and determining a baseline of information which can be built on over a period of nursing intervention. Handling information in an accepting, non-judgmental way is essential. The ability to do this in some circumstances is a challenge to and a measure of the district nurse's professional skills. The nurse is a guest in the patient's home, with no right of entry. The patient therefore has ultimate authority and can play a major part in negotiation for change.

Important information is obtained on the doorstep at the first visit. The appearance, access to the property and state of the garden give useful clues. The response when the doorbell rings, whether there is the noise of boisterous children, a dog barking or a long silence followed by the shuffle of bedroom slippers. This, combined with observation of the person's expression of anxiety, relief, fatigue or despair contribute to the nurse's assessment.

There may only be a single problem contained in the referral, but others may emerge during the interview and through discussion with neighbours, family, etc. A referral for the assessment of a patient with a leg ulcer may reveal an isolated old man, cut off from his remaining family, with grossly oedematous legs, sleeping in an armchair because the bed evokes the pain of his wife's terminal illness.

Care planning

Information obtained during the assessment is used to define the patient's problems. Both patient and carer should be involved in setting realistic goals in priority order preferably using their own words. The reason for this is twofold. It involves the patient directly in goal setting and self-care and, secondly, as the care plan is left in the home and is accessible it may avoid anxiety and misunderstanding if the language is that of the patient rather than the jargon of the nurse.

Identifying to what extent the problem is that of the patient and not the nurse is central, for example: persuading the old man to sleep in his bed, to allow passive drainage of the leg and therefore promote healing of the ulcer is pointless if the real problem is unresolved grief for his wife. This raises several key issues. The patient must determine the pace of the nursing intervention. There would be no value in setting up a comprehensive rehabilitation programme that failed to include counselling if the patient is unprepared to cope with change. Secondly, there may be a conflict between the patient's and the nurse's values and priorities, for instance an old lady may be preoccupied with unbearable loneliness and not a weekly bath. Finally, there may be a conflict of the nurse's aims with the resources, services and staff available. For example, the nurse may agree that the problem with the chairfast patient is stress incontinence, that the long-term aim should be the promotion of continence with the short-term goal to strengthen the muscles of the pelvic floor by exercise and regular toileting. However, staff shortages may make this kind of labour-intensive rehabilitation programme difficult to implement.

Implementation

The implementation of the care plan combines clinical skills with those of health education and counselling. This approach will be illustrated by the nursing management of venous leg ulcers. It is said that 0.5% of the population have leg ulcers (Seville and Martin 1981). It is commonly a problem of the elderly and is on the increase. The district nurse spends 27% of her time looking after patients with leg ulcers over the age of 65 years (DHSS 1982). It is important that nursing care embraces the psychological and educational needs of the patient and avoids focusing entirely on the ulcer. Many patients have strongly held beliefs about their ulcers based on folklore that the ulcer was the outlet for bad humours from the body (London 1981). Because of the chronic, intractable nature of many ulcers patients may be anxious, protective and even obsessive about their treatment. In order to treat the underlying condition the nurse must adopt a strategy to teach the importance of good nutrition, losing weight, exercise and rest with leg elevation. Furthermore, it has been found that the majority of ulcers are a recurrence, and so the nurse has an important role in prevention and in teaching maintenance care, such as the use of support stockings.

The home circumstances may pose constraints and limitations on the implementation of nursing care. If the only table is littered with papers and cigarettes then it may be better to use a chair or the end of the bed to do the dressing. The kingsize double bed which the 74-year-old overweight amputee shares with her husband may make nursing very difficult. The patient, with justification, may resist advice for a hospital bed because of the symbolic importance it has for their relationship.

Adaptation and improvisation in the home depends on the patient's condition, the environment and the available equipment. It may mean that in the final stage of a terminal disease a decision not to carry out an insensitive and probably unnecessary dressing using a meticulous aseptic technique would be wise because it would cause anxiety to the patient and additional stress for the family. Improvisation and the imaginative use of available equipment and resources are important, for example using a metal coathanger to make a catheter stand.

Suggesting or making too many changes at once, particularly in a new, complex and personal situation, may be stressful for the patient. It may also be interpreted as interference or a painful reminder of the loss of independence and deterioration in health, or it may threaten the balance of a relationship where the carer's role is sustained by looking after a dependent member of the family.

Evaluation

Assessing the effectiveness of nursing care for the elderly is central and should be done regularly. Evaluation completes the cycle making the process continuous. Sometimes changes take place almost inconspicuously either in the patient, carer, or care given. Care must therefore be adjusted gradually to meet changing needs.

The community nursing record is a legal statement of care given in the home. Conventionally, records are kept in the home as well as the health centre or nurse's working base with the inevitable problems of duplication. Problem-oriented recording is developing alongside the nursing process. These allow the clear definition of nursing goals and interventions and facilitates audit and the evaluation of care.

Future developmental strategies in the community should recognise the importance of the record as a vehicle for multidisciplinary communication not only between members of the primary care team, but also between primary and secondary care.

1. A shared professional record kept in the home at the point of delivery of care would

promote co-ordination and prevent frag-mentation of professional resources es-pecially for the housebound elderly.

2. Communication between hospital and community through the transfer of nursing care plans in both directions would posi-tively enhance the exchange of information.

Prevention and health education

Prevention has been classified by Caplan (1961) as primary, secondary and tertiary. District nurses are involved to a varying degree in all three. The following discussion will focus on the district nurse's role in prevention of ill health in the elderly.

Primary prevention entails intervention to prevent the incidence of disease, for example, by immunisation. An old person with an abra-sion following a fall may alert the district nurse at an encounter either in the home or health centre to organise tetanus toxoid through the general practitioner.

Secondary prevention involves the early detection of illness using tested screening techniques, for instance measuring blood pressure or testing the urine for glucose. This may take place routinely at a first visit or if a clinical problem is suspected. District nurses increasingly participate in multidisciplinary screening programmes. In addition to under-taking some technical procedures such as venepuncture for haemoglobin levels, sight testing and electrocardiographs, they may be involved in promoting health advice on diet, exercise and leisure activities.

Tertiary prevention is defined as the measures taken to alleviate an existing condition, prevent complications and modu-late the effects of illness. The district nurse uses this preventive approach in many ways:

1. Implementing a rehabilitation programme for the aftercare of a stroke patient at home, helping with adjustment to disability and preventing complications.
2. Teaching patient safety such as measures to prevent accidents and falls caused by unsuitable footwear, torn floor coverings and unlit passages.
3. Teaching old people about environmental problems that may cause ill health such as the risks of hypothermia, the problems of muscle wastage caused by immobility, apathy and withdrawal and constipation owing to a low roughage diet and insufficient exercise.
4. Teaching relatives how to prevent pressure sores, and demonstrating the principles of safe lifting to ensure comfort to the carer and prevent damage to the patient's deli-cate skin tissues. Preparing relatives to come to terms with imminent death in order to avoid abnormal grieving behaviour.

Health education may take place in the home at an individual level with the patient or carer, or in a group in a health centre, community centre or day centre. The district nurse is in a unique position to promote health education as an accepted visitor in the home. She may become a well-known and trusted figure over time and therefore will be in the position to influence and change existing behaviour. Group work may take several forms and is usually a response to a community health need or a personal interest in a particular area such as an obesity group, exercise sessions for maintaining mobility of the well elderly or a leg ulcer group associated with a clinic.

It is clear from the above that the district nurse has a crucial role to play in prevention and health education. This is in line with government policy that district nurses as well as health visitors should be committed to advising about prevention and health mainten-ance (DHSS 1977). However, the evidence is that only 17% of the district nurse's time is spent on 'advice, counselling, reassurance and health education' (Dunnell and Dobbs 1982). It is even more disturbing that 41% of a national sample of district nurses in the same survey reported that there were no areas of counselling and health education that they would like to spend more time on. There are many possible explanations for this: management's short-sighted view that the district nurse's role stops at treatment and that prevention is a luxury, shortcomings in previous training programmes, workload constraints and district nurses' own uncertainty about their role and position in the primary care team.

Having said this, there are many innovative experimental programmes where district nurses are using a preventive approach in patient care. Changing attitudes, an improved curriculum in district nurse training and developing opportunities within the primary care team will provide the foundation for future initiatives.

Counselling

Counselling is a purposeful relationship in which one person helps another to explore her feelings, thoughts and behaviour to reach a clearer self-understanding and to use her strengths so that she copes more effectively with her life by making appropriate decisions. Counselling is non-judgmental and non-directive and presupposes the nurse has some insight into her own feelings. District nurses are in an excellent position to develop a counselling role, because of their continuous, regular, often long-term contact with patients in their own homes. The process of giving practical, personal help often elicits trust.

There are many different circumstances when counselling is appropriate:

1. The nurse's interest and sensitive directed concern for the old person may help to promote change and allow discovery of new methods of coping.
2. Insight into the feelings of an old person may be explored by looking at the barriers to communication and defensiveness about illness and disability.
3. The traumatic life event of rehousing can be very stressful for old people. There may be intense ambivalence such as the longing to move out of the damp, cold flat with the peeling wallpaper and the conflicting

sadness at leaving the familiar and the known.
4. The relatives' involvement in care should be continuously valued, supported and regenerated. Attentive listening may help carers come to terms with role changes and the effects of illness in the family and share some of the burden of the caring task.

Decision making and the district nurse

District nursing involves making complex decisions. The isolation of district nursing practice increases the responsibility for making decision alone with few opportunities for sharing with peers. Several studies have reported that district nurses have difficulty with decisions especially those affecting the elderly. McIntosh (1979) found that decisions were frequently ritualised, task oriented and unsystematic.

Kratz (1978) looked at nursing care given to patients recovering from a stroke at home. She developed a continuum of care theory that identified appropriate valued and focused care for the acutely ill and inappropriate and diffuse care for those patients who were getting better, but still suffered from a residual disability. The conclusion reached from this study was that district nurses have difficulty defining goals for the long-term and chronic sick and fail to value their care as highly as for the acutely ill. It was confirmed by White (1979) that district nurses found it easier to discharge patients following a clearly defined programme of treatment such as post-operative dressings than the elderly chronic sick requiring 'supervisory' visits.

These findings highlight a real dilemma faced by district nurses today. On the one hand, a goal of community care is to promote self-care. However, to an elderly person independence may mean loneliness and isolation (Gray and McKenzie 1980). How much anxiety is generated when finally the venous ulcer has healed? The nurse may feel a sense of achievement but the old lady may only feel the loss.

District nurses are often criticised on the grounds that their long-term nursing intervention fosters patient dependency. The real problem is more complex. The district nurse may fill the gap between the termination of professional care and the absence of community support because the alternative is making a complete statement of withdrawal.

Drugs and old people in the community

The district nurse gives parenteral, rectal, and oral medication to elderly people and drugs by inhalation. She has a responsibility for monitoring compliance or adherence and observation for adverse reactions and ensuring safe storage. The reader is referred to Chapter 20 for a detailed discussion of drugs and the elderly. In this section, the problems experienced by patients at home, which are encountered by the district nurse, are highlighted.

Drugs are the property of the patient for whom they are prescribed. The administration of drugs in the community therefore involves adapting principles of safe practice to the particular needs of the patient at home. The rules governing controlled drugs may seem more relaxed in the home, but the nurse must be vigilant to make sure that written prescriptions are available, meticulous records are kept, storage is safe and the patient's or family's permission is obtained for disposal of the drugs when no longer required.

The district nurse should be aware of the factors associated with poor compliance such as multiple pathology, polypharmacy, complex drug regimes and isolation from medical advice (Parish et al 1983). It has been found also that complex drug regimes cause considerable anxiety to the elderly patient (MacDonald et al 1977) and reduce comprehension and compliance (Parkin et al 1976).

One of the most serious problems in the community is the breakdown of communication which often occurs at the interface between primary and secondary care. The separate systems of hospital and community often lead to failure or delay in the communication of a patient's drug information in both directions (Bliss 1981). For example, the patient often does not understand that the list of drugs given on discharge have replaced the old ones she was taking before admission.

There are several strategies that the district nurse can follow to help the patient understand and follow drug regimes. First, the problem-oriented approach of the nursing process enables individual assessment and encourages active participation and understanding of drug regimes. In practical terms drug regimes can be tailored to the patient's own routine and requirements. Second, the district nurse has an important role in prevention. Because of her continuous regular contact with elderly people she is in an excellent position to notice early signs of adverse reactions, and to anticipate and prevent drug misuse. This is a sensitive area because some old people may feel checked up on, or criticised, if too intrusively supervised. Therefore, it is important to adopt tactful, imaginative, innovative strategies with the aim of preventing hazards and at the same time protecting the patient's independence. These measures may include ensuring that labels are clearly typed in large print including name, strength of drug, date of dispensing and expiry (Kiernan and Isaacs 1981). Directions for use should be simple, but specific, using words patients understand. Old people find child-resistant containers notoriously difficult to open and often transfer tablets to alternative bottles with inappropriate labels, which is an obvious potential source of error.

Simple systems to aid memory can be devised, for example counting tablets into an egg-box to be taken at specified times of the day, or devising charts with instructions on time and dosage. Written instructions for drug use have been found to be an inexpensive and effective method of improving compliance amongst hypertensive patients (Laher et al 1981), and particularly effective when used in conjunction with counselling (Macdonald

1977). Kiernan and Isaacs (1981) found a lack of co-ordination in the management of patients' medicines leading to inappropriate drug use.

Clearly, a multidisciplinary approach is important in the prevention of medication error, particularly for the high-risk dependent housebound elderly. This has implications for the development of a personal health record including current medication, kept in the home at the point of delivery of care, and accessible to all health workers.

Community nursing aids and equipment

Nursing aids are obtained through the health district, voluntary organisations or on prescription. The health district supplies a range of nursing aids to assist nursing care at home. Most departments stock standard items such as aids for the promotion of continence—commodes, male urinals, incontinent pants and pads, aids for the prevention of pressure sores—ripple mattresses, air-rings, sheepskins and mobility aids, etc.

In the absence of an appropriate aid the district nurse often needs to be imaginative and adaptive, for instance using a cardboard box as a bed cradle. Realistic and careful planning is important. Often the solution is a compromise between the ideal piece of equipment and that preferred by the patient. Some old people find it hard to accept the use of aids which may be a reminder of their deteriorating health, loss of independence and represent a threat to an accustomed way of life. For example, the 90-year-old lady living alone in a neglected basement flat with restricted mobility, spending all sleeping and waking hours in her armchair, refused to contemplate reorganisation of her room to accommodate the single bed because of the disruption it would cause to the work on her autobiography. The personal space of this lady was intensely private, and no reassurance would change her mind. In this situation the nurse must recognise that her patient's priorities are different from her own and that the nursing environment is far from ideal.

There are common problems with the supplies system of many health districts. Nurses often have a limited choice of aids available, although appropriate goods are on the market. There is often a delay in obtaining equipment, because of a long waiting list, stock shortfall or slow delivery system, and frequently communication failure exacerbates these problems.

The day hospital

Day hospitals provide a bridge between hospital and the community. They are often located within the geriatric department of a general hospital. The aim is to provide a therapeutic environment during office hours, with multidisciplinary specialities including occupational therapy, physiotherapy, speech therapy and chiropody. The reasons for referral to a day hospital include continuity of care on discharge, rehabilitation, treatment to maintain the progress of an intensive hospital programme, medical and nursing procedures that cannot be carried out at home, and social care.

Day hospitals have been criticised for low patient turnover, and an emphasis on social care other than rehabilitation.

The community hospital

The concept of the community or general practice hospital is an exciting new development in primary care. Staffed by, for example, members of the primary care team the aim of the community hospital is to provide a service for rehabilitation, respite care, terminal care, and for patients with acute medical problems not requiring intensive treatment.

A study that set out to evaluate a 24-bed general practice hospital in Bayswater, London, found that carers valued the service and felt confident in the continuity of care given by known medical and nursing staff. Clearly, the community hospital as an extension of the primary care team has a valuable part to play in planned admissions and phased care for old people (McKay et al 1983).

Aftercare for the elderly

There is considerable evidence to suggest that the co-ordination of aftercare is unsatisfactory (Skeet 1974, Roberts 1974, Turton & Wilson-Barnett 1981). Skeet's study (1974) identified the discharge of old people as a matter of particular professional concern. The Continuing Care Project set up in 1977 was a result of her work. The aims of this organisation are to improve arrangements made for the support and care of elderly discharged patients in the community. In addition it sets out to promote experimental schemes and interdisciplinary education.

There are three major problems in the provision of follow-up care: communication between hospital and community, absence of discharge planning by hospital staff and family expectations.

1. Communication. The exchange of information between hospital and community in both directions has been found to be unsatisfactory. There is often a delay of up to three weeks before the general practitioner is notified of a patient's discharge (Continuing Care Project 1979). Parnell (1982) found that in 93% of cases the district nurse received information, but in only 48% of these was it 'reasonable' enough to plan appropriate care. There are three methods of communication that take place: direct contact between professionals, which in practice happens rarely; referral forms, which vary in quality; liaison nursing staff who function as co-ordinators. Communication from the community to hospital has also found to be lacking (Continuing Care Project 1979). Forty six per cent of hospital nurses 'rarely' or 'never' receive information (Parnell 1982). This communication failure in both directions has implications for the elderly. Reliable information should be transferred with the patient in order to prevent this major change being traumatic and unsettling. Future developments of the nursing process could adopt a problem oriented care plan to promote the exchange of information.

2. Discharge planning. The urgent need of a hospital bed often results in a precipitate and ill-conceived decision to discharge a patient. Lack of time to co-ordinate services, an unprepared home and uninformed relatives means confusion and insecurity for the old person.

3. Family expectations. Relatives are the main carers for recently discharged dependent patients (Roberts 1974, Age Concern 1980). Poor communication between the services places additional strain on the family. Whereas the old person may minimise her health and social problems, because of an overriding desire to return home, families may have different expectations. They may undervalue their own role, feel guilt for previous failure which led to hospital admission or they may resent renewing the inevitable exhausting and continuous caring tasks.

Where an old person lives alone many relatives find it hard to accept the element of risk. This raises the question of how much support to give. Too much can lead to over dependence and too little may expose undesirable risk. Coping with the anxiety of risk is as hard for relatives as it is for involved professionals.

Alternative strategies for aftercare

A number of studies have identified the need for a follow-up home visit to consolidate advice and give reassurance during a period of adaptation (Roberts 1974, Skeet 1974). There is a difference of opinion on who should give this follow-up care. Some advocate the health visitor, because of her preventive function. The opposing argument is that because the district nurse mainly looks after old people then she is the member of the primary care team to combine her skills of caring with those of prevention and health education to provide continuity of care. In some areas there are liaison nurses, either health visitors or district nurses whose function it is to co-ordinate services. There has been little evaluation of these posts, and although individuals have made important contributions, the job by definition is unsatisfactory, because it entails conveying messages between two organisations demonstrating communication failure.

Planned early discharge is the practice of discharging selected surgical patients to the follow-up care of community nurses and family doctors after a minimum stay in hospital. Candidates may in the past have been excluded because of age, but this is likely to change, because of pressure on beds. Various experiments of this type have been reported. Hockey and Buttimore (1970) demonstrated that 600 bed days could be saved in a 23-week period. Although this project evaluated the effectiveness of a specially appointed district nurse, other studies have successfully involved existing community nursing services for follow-up care (Ruckley et al 1980, Plant and Brendan Devlin 1978).

PERSONAL SOCIAL SERVICES

The local authority personal social services are responsible for important supportive care of old people in the community including services in the home, day centres and residential accommodation. The elderly and particularly the very elderly represent one of the largest care groups for social services. A study by the National Institute of Social Work found that over 20% of referrals to the social work department were from the 75+ years age group (Phillipson 1982).

Social service provision includes:

1. Social workers employed by and based in the social work department of the local authority. Occasionally, they may work in a health centre, which clearly facilitates communication with the primary care team.
2. Domiciliary occupational therapists based in social work departments. They assess old people's needs for aids to daily living. The Chronically Sick and Disabled Person's Act, 1970 obliges local authorities to make necessary adaptations to the home such as ramps, handrails, hoists, stair lifts, etc. Other services provided under this Act include help in obtaining radios and tele-

visions, the allocation of telephones and enabling elderly people to have holidays.
3. Social services are also responsible for specialists such as social workers for the blind, laundry for the incontinent, and welfare benefit advice.
4. Respite care is organised by social services to give relatives a rest from the continuous and exhausting demands of caring. This may entail organising a bed in residential accommodation or perhaps arranging board with the growing number of families willing to look after an elderly person for payment.

Services in the home

Home help

The home help service is a vital part of helping old people to maintain their independence at home, but only 9% are recipients (Phillipson, 1982). Home helps provide regular help with domestic and household tasks including shopping, collecting prescriptions, cleaning and the preparation of meals. There have been some recent developments in the service, for example, the 'early discharge team', or 'flying squad'. The aim is to provide short-term intensive personal care following discharge of an old person from hospital. The frequency of visits are reduced as the client adjusts to home life. Joint funded programmes are being set up for home aides. The aim is to train a carer to provide domestic help as well as assisting with personal care.

It is important that there is a good working relationship between the home help and the primary care team in particular the district nurse. In some areas regular liaison meetings are organised and in others informal meetings at health centres exchange information and provide mutual support for stressful and demanding care giving.

Meals-on-wheels

This is a domiciliary service to provide a subsidised, hot two-course dinner for frail elderly or disabled people. More than 50% of the 26 million meals in 1978/79 were provided by the local authority, and the remainder by the Women's Royal Voluntary Service (WRVS) (DHSS 1981). The availability of the service is variable. In some areas the elderly are restricted to weekly visits, and in others clients may receive meals on seven days a week according to need. Most receive three meals or less a week, although this may be an overestimate, because of current cuts in spending. Special diabetic or low roughage diets can be arranged on request. The meals service also fulfils a surveillance function. If an old person fails to answer the door or suddenly deteriorates, then the appropriate agency can be informed.

Social day care

Day care is provided by the local authority or a voluntary organisation. Day centres offer a hot lunch, entertainment diversionary activities, adult education, bathing, chiropody service and facilities for self-help or health education groups.

The majority of elderly people do not go to any social centres (Abrams 1978, Hunt 1978). One of the reasons for low uptake may be the problem of access and transport. It is for the housebound, isolated old person that day centre provision is important and it is for precisely this group that places are restricted, because of the shortage and unpredictability of transport. Many old people are frustrated by long circuitous journeys, the uncertainty of picking up times and uncomfortable seating. This illustrates the frequent absence of collaboration between services when planning new programmes. The social work response to the elderly has been criticised as failing to develop progressive and imaginative programmes (DHSS 1978, Phillipson 1982). Old people's problems are commonly given a low priority and frequently allocated to untrained workers.

HOUSING

The majority of elderly people live at home, often in inappropriate accommodation (DHSS

1978). There is a strong, but complex, relationship between health and housing. The Black Report identified a link between tenants in the private and public rented sector and a high mortality rate (Townsend and Davidson 1982). The district nurse may often care for old people in substandard accommodation. In certain circumstances she may take the role of patient's advocate working with environmental health officers or housing welfare officers to instigate repairs or facilitate rehousing.

Sheltered housing

Sheltered housing or Assisted Independent Living Accommodation has been developed in Britain over the last 20 years by local authorities and housing associations and now houses about 6% of the elderly population in England and Wales, although provision is patchy (Tinker 1982). Sheltered housing consists of grouped accommodation (flats or bungalows) with some communal facilities, an alarm system and a warden on site. The resident warden provides a regular and continuous 'friendly neighbour' support, making daily visits, providing emergency domiciliary care and liaising with other community workers and members of the primary care team (Heumann 1981). Sheltered accommodation provides a vital part of assisted housing stock for the old. Proposals from the present government to offer sheltered housing for sale means that the available stock will be seriously reduced.

There are some schemes to support old people to stay in their own homes. Examples of these include joint approaches between housing and social services to promote the Crossroads scheme whereby a paid worker helps old people with personal care and household tasks, the short- and long-term boarding of the elderly, the caring repair service and grants for home improvements for the elderly owner-occupier.

One of the main conclusions arising from research on sheltered housing and old peoples' Homes is that for some people they are there for want of an adequate alternative.

Concern for the frail, confused elderly and absence of funds for new capital expenditure must prompt new multidisciplinary housing strategies.

SOCIAL SECURITY BENEFITS

The evidence suggests that the old in Britain are poor. Two million old people live at or below the poverty line (Phillipson 1982). There is an expectation that impoverishment is an inevitable part of ageing amongst the working class. It is important that the district nurse is aware of the benefits her patients are entitled to and if necessary assists them in the complicated process of claiming, or refers them to appropriate advice centres such as the Citizens' Advice Bureaux, social services or local neighbourhood advice centres.

The system of state financial support for old people is complex and the following section will outline the four main groups of benefit available. The government department responsible for administering social security benefits is the Departement of Health and Social Security. The benefit level is adjusted annually, and current information and further details can be obtained from the DHSS Information Service, Leaflets Unit, Block 4, Government Buildings, Honeypot Lane, Stanmore, Middlesex HA7 1AY, or the Child Poverty Action Group, 1 Macklin Street, London WC2B 5NH.

National insurance benefit

This is based on insurance contributions. The retirement pension is payable to men at 65 years and women at 60 years. There are two rates, the basic and additional pensions, the latter being related to earnings and contributions. There is an age addition of 25p per week for those over 80 years.

Non-contributory benefit

Attendance allowance is tax free and is not means tested. It is payable at two rates. The higher rate for a dependant requiring continual supervision both day and night or a lower rate for a person requiring frequent attention by day. This allowance is not payable for the first six months, but before qualifying it is possible to claim for the attendance needs payment.

Invalid care allowance is payable to non-married women of working age unable to enter employment because of responsibilities to care regularly and substantially at least 35 hours a week for a dependant. This discriminates against married women who do not qualify for benefit even though they, too, must forego paid employment and career opportunities.

Supplementary benefit

Pensioners form the bulk of the claimants for supplementary benefit in spite of the rise in the unemployed. Although many old people are eligible, figures for the take up of supplementary benefit in 1979 show that £145 million was unclaimed, (Hansard 1983).

There are many discretionary benefits that fall into this category:

1. Supplementary pension
2. Heating allowances payable on grounds of chronic ill health or inadequately heated accommodation
3. Laundry allowance payable to the incontinent
4. Bath allowance—an extra 25p payable to anyone needing more than one bath a week, usually granted to the incontinent
5. Diet allowance for diabetics and people with ulcerative colitis
6. Single payments for draught proofing, repair of heating appliances. Grants to purchase essential items of furniture, extra bedding and clothing.

Other benefits

These include rent and rate rebate for those on supplmentary pension or those who have had adaptations to property under the 1970 Chronic Sick and Disabled Persons' Act.

Included are exemptions from National Health Service charges for drug prescriptions, spectacles and dental treatment. Carers of the elderly may be eligible for tax allowances, e.g. dependent relative's allowance, daughter's service allowance.

THE ROLE OF THE VOLUNTARY SECTOR

The activity of the voluntary sector in the United Kingdom is dynamic and changing according to local need and individual initiatives. It includes the work of the formally constituted voluntary organisations, neighbourhood care groups, mutual support groups and informal carers.

Voluntary organisations

These provide support for old people in the community and include groups such as Age Concern, Red Cross and WRVS (Women's Royal Voluntary Service). They offer services such as transport, help with gardening, shopping, visiting the isolated elderly, offering respite for carers, bereavement counselling, aids for nursing old people at home, supplementary linen and hypothermia packs.

Neighbourhood care groups

These are organised attempts to mobilise local resources to increase the amount and range of help and care they give to one another, such as offering support to someone during an acute phase of illness or skill swapping, for instance exchanging plumbing expertise for knitting a pullover.

Mutual aid groups

These offer mutual support and a focus for social contact for people with similar problems or a common concern such as stroke clubs, carers' organisations and pensioners' self-help groups. There is often an intrinsic element of pressure group activity, which has meant that many professionals regard their existence with suspicion.

In recent years there has been a growth in radical mutual aid groups such as pensioners' action groups. Often with a strong community identity they fight local campaigns to improve services for old people, such as providing evidence on the association between number of falls by the elderly with disrepair of pavements.

Informal carers

Informal carers give the majority of care to the old at home (Hunt 1978). Carer is an inexact term, because it is used in a wide range of circumstances. It can be defined broadly as those caring for dependants on an unpaid basis in either the carer's or dependant's home. In the majority of cases the carer is a family member, either the frail, elderly spouse or closest female relative. Occasionally, the responsibility for care is taken by a close friend or neighbour. The figures for numbers of dependent elderly with carers are scanty. However, it has been demonstrated that carers are predominantly women. A survey carried out by the Equal Opportunities Commission (1982) found that three times as many women as men were looking after elderly or handicapped relatives. It has been estimated that the numbers of female carers aged 45–60 years will decline from 1980 onwards (Royal Commission on the National Health Service 1979), and this will have clear implications for family care.

Nissel and Bonnerjea (1982) carried out a survey to look in depth at the effect of caring for a handicapped elderly relative in 22 families. The burden of care was carried by the woman. It was found that the continuous emotional demands, fatigue and resulting heightened tension in the family were more difficult to cope with than the physical tasks of caring.

Family breakdown is a common cause of hospital admission. In a recent study that looked at the effect of admission of old people on their carers, it was found that in the majority of cases the carer was the prime mover in the decision for hospitalisation. Sanford (1975) found that sleep disturbance and faecal incontinence were two common reasons poorly tolerated by relatives and were causal factors for precipitating admission.

Nissel and Bonnerjea (1982) found that not only were carers commonly unsupported by their family except in a crisis, but also help from the services was patchy and often scarce. Patients with similar disabilities received a disparate level of care—some above the average and some below. It is not surprising that, since the carer's greatest need was for emotional support, the help most appreciated from district nurses was of the 'listening kind'. It is sad, therefore, that in this study the help most frequently given was with physical tasks or specific disease oriented advice. There is no doubt that caring for a sick, disabled elderly relative at home is exhausting, stressful and often frustrating, producing many conflicts such as the sadness of witnessing the slow deterioration and illness of a close relative, the unfamiliar nature of a changing relationship, and the powerful, often opposing feelings of love, commitment and resentment.

The evidence shows clearly that district nurses' supportive visiting should be given higher priority to prevent in particular the breakdown of the caring situation, undue stress and non-accidental injury to old people. The conclusions of the study on community care (DHSS 1981) were that the resources of voluntary networks are not limitless and that the statutory services should devise strategies for collaboration and support. Knowledge of the existence and role of informal self-help organisations is important for the district nurse, whether facilitating hairdressing for the housebound old lady or motivating someone recovering from a stroke to visit a patient during an acute phase of the same illness. Furthermore, acknowledging political and social responsibilities at a local level is a measure of effective professional practice, e.g. involvement in community activities and membership of local committees.

THE IMPLICATIONS FOR DISTRICT NURSING OF COMMUNITY POLICIES FOR OLD PEOPLE

Policy documents during the 1970s emphasised the need to shift from institutional to community care and identified the frail elderly as a priority group. At the same time recommendations were made for an extended role for community nurses involved in the care of old people and a corresponding growth rate of 6% in the numbers of district nurses and health visitors (DHSS 1976, 1977). The preventive function of the district nurse was clearly identified (DHSS 1976) and it was suggested that whereas health visitors should spend proportionately less time with the elderly, district nurses should spend proportionately more (DHSS 1978). This was backed up by the recommendation of the Royal Commission that nurses take more responsibility for the surveillance of vulnerable groups and that an extended role should entail making first contact decisions, prescribing nursing care programmes and mobilising other services (e.g. community physiotherapy), as long as this was not at the expense of the nurse's caring role (Royal Commission on the National Health Service 1979).

The findings from a survey of all chief nursing officers and regional nursing officers in England showed that one of the fastest developing areas in the community nursing service are schemes involving district nursing and the elderly, and a large number of priority areas for future research identified the elderly and district nursing (Baker and Bevan 1983).

Clearly, there is role interchangeability and overlap between the health visitor and district nurse. However, given that the majority of the district nurse's time is spent with the elderly (Dunnell and Dobbs 1982) and with the higher expectations from the mandatory nine-month professional course it seems a sensible use of resources that she should fully exploit her skills in clinical practice, health education, prevention and counselling to become the key worker for old people in the primary care team.

CURRENT DEVELOPMENTS IN DISTRICT NURSING PRACTICE FOR THE ELDERLY

Specialisation

The district nurse is usually described as a generalist. In recent years there has been an adaptation of her role in specialist areas which includes work in stroke rehabilitation, coronary, terminal, stoma and diabetic care, promotion of continence, hospital/community liaison, care of children and patients with venous leg ulcers.

The argument put forward in favour of specialisation is that it provides greater nursing expertise and support to patients and other practitioners. There are also misgivings and anxieties that specialisation not only devalues the role of the district nurse but also fragments care.

Hospital-at-home scheme

This experimental scheme which started in Peterborough, England, using the district nursing service aims to provide intensive nursing care for patients during an acute phase of illness at home (Peterborough Health Authority, undated). Evaluation of the project shows that the average age was 71 years, 33% were aged 80 years and over and 31% lived alone. The specific events that precipitated referral to the scheme included 14% who rejected hospital admission and 25% of families no longer able to cope. It is interesting that in 4% of cases district nurses identified the inseparability of the patient and spouse as a clear personal problem affecting treatment choices. The advantages of the scheme were that it allowed families to stay together and avoided expensive social service support for the frail or disabled partner left behind at home. Families, patients and nurses were positive about the programme. Relatives were able to take a more active role in care

and the district nurse found the work gave her more job satisfaction.

Out-of-hours nursing care

An out-of-hours service is defined as functioning between 5 p.m. and 8 a.m. There are two sorts of provision, the evening service which covers the 'twilight hours' between 5 p.m. and 9.30/10 p.m. and the night service which provides cover throughout the rest of the night.

The evening service provides mostly long-term nursing care for the elderly, disabled and chronic sick. Patients are often highly dependent, living alone or with frail relatives. Nursing care may be the administration of drugs by injection such as insulin, antibiotics or opiates, help with activities in preparation for bed such as washing, toileting, pressure area care or contributing to a rehabilitation programme such as the promotion of continence. Occasionally, help is needed during a crisis, for instance helping relatives to nurse a patient through the early stages of a stroke. For many, the evening nurse is often the last visitor of the day before the long and probably lonely night.

The night service covers 8 p.m. to 8 a.m. It overlaps with the evening service, and the functions are twofold. First, crisis or short-term care. This may take place during an episode of acute illness or an acute phase of a terminal disease. Referrals may be made to unblock a catheter, give an enema or sort out a patient who has been discharged from hospital with a leaking wound and no dressing supplies. The second type of care is long term and may involve providing a night sitter to give exhausted relatives a good night's sleep.

Unfortunately, provision of out-of-hours service is patchy. Some districts are carrying out experimental programmes. Where schemes have been implemented and monitored they have been found to be valued highly by patients and their relatives (Martin and Ishino 1981).

Joint funded schemes

These schemes include:

1. Combined programmes with social services for district nurses to work in day centres and residential accommodation to provide health advice to residents and staff.
2. Intensive domiciliary care for the sick elderly through the home aid programme.
3. Liaison between housing departments and health districts to promote closer working relationships between district nurses and wardens of sheltered housing.
4. Alignment with social work teams of geriatric visitors who are trained district nurses.
5. Utilisation of day care facilities to provide night nursing care for the elderly.

In summary, there are several key issues central to the provision of community nursing services for the elderly. Research should be carried out into the nursing needs of old people. Future developments of housing schemes, social service provision and primary care programmes should recognise the professional implications for other relevant departments and adopt joint planning strategies. The primary care team should be aware of the implications of cuts in spending on social and health services in a system already constrained by regulations in health care (Townsend and Davidson 1982). In particular the district nurse, practising at the sharp end of policy implementation, should recognise her professional responsibilities to oppose social and economic policies that militate against the well-being of the community (Journal of District Nursing 1984).

Finally, the district nurse's work with the elderly raises many questions such as her own attitude to ageing, dependency, uncertainty and the stress of coping with the complex problems culminating from many years of neglect. Sharing, listening and finding support from her peer group, opportunities for professional development and close working relationships with other members of the primary care team are central strategies for the delivery of effective community nursing care to old people.

REFERENCES

Abrams M 1978 Beyond three score and ten. Age Concern, London
Age Concern 1980 Discharge from hospital—the social worker's view. Age Concern, London
Anonymous 1984 Editorial Journal of District Nursing 2(7): 3
Baker G, Bevan J 1983 Developments in community nursing within primary health care teams. Health Services Research Unit 46 Part III. University of Kent, Canterbury
Batchelor I, McFarlane J 1980 Multidisciplinary clinical teams. Project paper. King's Fund, London
Bliss M R 1981 Prescribing for the elderly, including problems of instructions, supervision and liaison between hospital and general practice. British Medical Journal 283: 203–206
Caplan G 1961 An approach to community mental health. Tavistock, London
Continuing Care Project 1979 Organising aftercare. National Corporation for the Care of Old People, London
Department of Health and Social Security 1976 Priorities for health and personal social services in England. A consultative document. HMSO, London
Department of Health and Social Security 1977 Prevention and health—everybody's business. HMSO, London
Department of Health and Social Security 1978 A happier old age. HMSO, London
Department of Health and Social Security 1981 Report of a study on community care. HMSO, London
Dunnell K, Dobbs J 1982 Nurses working in the community. Office of Population Censuses and Surveys, London
Equal Opportunities Commission 1982 Caring for the elderly and handicapped. EOC, Manchester
Gray J M, McKenzie H 1980 Take care of your elderly relative. Allen and Unwin, London
Hansard Parliamentary Debates, House of Commons 1983 Written answers. Nov. 30 Col. 542
Heumann L F 1981 The function of different sheltered housing categories for the semi-independent elderly. Social Policy and Administration 15(2): 164–180
Hockey L, Buttimore A 1970 Cooperation in patient care. Queen's Institute of District Nursing, London
Hunt A 1978 The elderly at home. HMSO, London
Kiernan P J, Isaacs J B 1981 Use of drugs by the elderly. Journal of the Royal Society of Medicine 74: 196–200
Kratz C 1978 Care of the long term sick in the community. Churchill Livingstone, Edinburgh
Laher M, O'Malley K, O'Brien E, O'Hanrahan M, O'Boyle C 1981 Educational value of printed information for patients with hypertension. British Medical Journal 282: 1360–1361
Loudon I S L 1981 Leg ulcers in the eighteenth and early nineteenth centuries. Journal of the Royal College of General Practitioners 21: 263–269

Maslow A U 1970 Motivation and personality, 2nd edn. Harper and Row, New York

MacDonald E T, MacDonald J B, Phoenix M 1977 Improving drug compliance after hospital discharge. British Medical Journal 2: 618–621

Martin M H, Ishino M 1981 Domiciliary night nursing service, luxury or necessity? British Medical Journal 282: 883–885

McKay B, North N, Murray Sykes K 1983 The effect on carers of hospital admission of the elderly. Nursing Times 79(48): 42–43

McIntosh J B 1979 Decision making on the distirct. Occasional paper. Nursing Times 75(29): 77–80

O'Hare E 1980 The gingerbread man. Nursing Times 76(8): 318–320

Nissel M, Bonnerjea L 1982 Family care of the handicapped elderly. Policy Studies Institute, London

Parkin D M, Henny C R, Quirk J, Crooks J 1976 Deviation from prescribed drug treatment after discharge from hospital. British Medical Journal 18: 686–688

Parish P, Doggett M A, Colleypriest P 1983 The elderly and their use of medicines. King's Fund, London

Parnell J 1982 Continuity and communication. Occasional paper. Nursing Times 78(9): 33–40

Peterborough Health Authority Undated Hospital at home, Peterborough. The pilot scheme, April 1978–March 1981. Peterborough Health Authority

Plant J A, Brendan Devlin H 1978 Planned early discharge of surgical patients. Occasional paper. Nursing Times 74(7): 25–28

Phillipson C 1982 Capitalism and the construction of old age. Macmillan, London

Roberts I 1974 Discharged from hospital. Royal College of Nursing Series 2, no. 6, Royal College of Nursing, London

Robertson R 1981 The nursing process in community nursing. Nursing Times 77(30): 1299–1304

Royal Commission on the Health Service 1979 Report, Cmnd 7615. HMSO, London

Ruckley C V, Garraway W M, Cuthbertson C, Fenwick N, Prescott R J 1980 The community nurse and day surgery. Nursing Times 76(6): 255–256

Sanford R A 1975 Tolerance of debility in elderly dependants by supporters at home: its significance for hospital practice. British Medical Journal 3: 471–473

Seville R H, Martin E 1981 Leg ulcers. Nursing Times 77(29): 1249–1251

Skeet M 1974 Home from hospital. Macmillan, London

Standing Medical Advisory Committee and the Standing Nursing and Midwifery Advisory Committee 1981 Report of a joint working group on the primary health care team. (The Harding Report.) Department of Health and Social Services, London

Tinker A 1983 Housing elderly people: some theories of current research. Public Health 97: 290–295

Townsend P, Davidson N 1982 Inequalities in health. Penguin, Harmondsworth, Middlesex

Turton P, Wilson-Barnett J 1981 Two aspects of nursing care. In: Simpson J E, Levitt R (eds) Going home. Churchill Livingstone, Edinburgh ch 22, p 265–280

White C 1979 A study of some of the factors influencing the district nurse's decision to discharge patients from her care. Unpublished MSc thesis. University of Manchester

27

A. E. While

Health visiting and the elderly

Health is a matter of prime importance to the elderly because it is in staying reasonably well that enables them to remain independent. In order to enable the elderly to remain healthy, attention should be given to prevention of ill health, detection of deviation from the healthy state and rehabilitation. It is this positive approach upon which the health visitor's contribution is based. Indeed, the idea of health visitors working with the elderly is not new. In 1976, it was suggested that health visitors should increase their involvement with this age group (Department of Health and Social Security (DHSS) 1976a).

HEALTH VISITORS AND THE ELDERLY

The health of the elderly is one of the major concerns of the National Health Service since large financial resources must be devoted to their care. The present economic climate has raised issues of efficiency and effectiveness in the health service and cost effectiveness has become a major concern. In 1976, the DHSS (1976b) suggested that early detection of disability among the elderly would be of great benefit. Detection of early signs of illness is achieved by a variety of methods, including prophylactic visiting and screening clinics. This is important because not all old people readily report their medical problems, seemingly because they do not know that many symptoms constitute ill health rather than the assumed natural process of ageing (Williams et al 1972, Currie et al 1974, Brocklehurst 1975, Hay 1976, Williams 1979, Barber and Wallis 1982). Such failure to acknowledge ill health can lead not only to serious illnesses being unnoticed in their early stages, but also to failure to treat minor conditions which later have a cumulative effect.

The health visitor is unique in the field of health care in that she (or he) determines her own clientele by selection from the population. She is able to make contact with people on her own initiative without waiting for a specific request for help, although she has no statutory right of entry into people's homes. In practice, it seems that health visitors have drawn their clientele from families with young children (Clark 1973, 1978) whom they have a statutory responsibility to visit. This apparent concern for the welfare of young children and their families may be a reflection of the early history of the health visiting service (MacQueen 1962). The health visitor's ability to determine her clientele according to need and her professional responsibility should enable her to exercise her function in the prevention of ill health, surveillance and rehabilitation to the full among the elderly population.

As long ago as 1955, Anderson suggested extending the role of the health visitor to include promotion and health maintenance of the elderly. Anderson identified the health visitor's role in terms of offering support during family crises and potentially improving the elderly person's morale. This is an interesting perspective in view of recent research (Hodkinson 1975) which suggests that a successful outcome owes more to mental factors such as personal motivation than to the degree or nature of the physical disability. Health visitors can, therefore, make a significant contribution to the rehabilitation of elderly people after episodes of ill health, assisting them in the achievement of the optimum level of independence.

A number of studies have been undertaken in which the health visitor's contribution to the care of the elderly has been analysed in terms of surveillance and community support.

This work is reviewed later in this chapter. The appointment of specialist health visitors has not been adopted widely, preference being given to health visitor assistants, sometimes known as geriatric visitors, who are registered nurses working under the supervision of health visitors. Curnow et al (1975) found that, in a pilot scheme in Reading, England, specially appointed health visitors visiting only those aged 65 or over did not find their work sufficiently satisfying nor was such work considered good for their career prospects. It seems that most geriatric health visiting is undertaken by health visitor assistants where such appointments exist (Office of Population Censuses and Surveys 1982).

Dingwall (1977) considers that health visitors have a role as the principal case finding agency of the welfare state. The health visitor is qualified for this in view of her training in health and social work skills and her knowledge of the individuals and services in her area. She is therefore able to refer clients appropriately or apply for aids on their behalf. This is an important point since it identifies the health visitor as a facilitator in the community and perhaps also as a 'stop gap' in a large bureaucratic health care system. Indeed, primary health care provisions in the inner cities undoubtedly require a health worker with a flexible role. Possible role overlap between health visitors and district nurses has been of concern in some quarters, but the demands of the acutely sick or those requiring fundamental physical care must and will always take precedence in the district nurse's caseload. Health visitors have no such conflict since they make no curative or physical contribution to care, which leaves all their time for case finding, health teaching and surveillance.

From the evidence currently available there is much variation in the number of elderly people receiving visits from a health visitor (Fig. 27.1). Luker (1979) suggests that this variation is due to a number of factors: age structure of the population in an area; health visitor organisation, that is, attachment to general practice (family doctor practice) or geographical location; local health district

Area	%	Source	
Brighton (Pilot GP attachment)	36.2	Gilmore	(1970)
Brighton (all HVs)	24.6	Gilmore	(1970)
Berkshire	18.0	Clark	(1973)
London	2.1	Marris	(1971)
Scotland	19.5	SHHD	(1975)

Fig. 27.1 Number (%) of health visitor visits to people over 65 years as a proportion of the total number of visits made by health visitors. *Source: Luker 1979. Reproduced by permission of Newbourne Publications.*

policy and the personal preference of the health visitor. In 1977, 15% of clients handled by health visitors were elderly compared with 10% in 1971, thus in 1977 about half a million old people were in touch with a health visitor (Tinker 1981), a figure representing only 6% of those over 65 years of age. The Royal Commission on the National Health Service (1979) thought there was considerable scope for expanding the role and responsibilities of health visitors and district nurses. 'We consider that there are increasingly important roles for community nurses, not just in the treatment room, but in health surveillance for vulnerable groups and in screening procedures, health education and preventive programmes, and as a point of first contact, particularly for the young and elderly' (p 79).

SURVEILLANCE AND PROMOTION OF HEALTH

A number of studies have been carried out in which the health visitor was involved in screening for problems among elderly patients. Barber and Wallis (1976) describe a system in which the health visitor made assessments of elderly patients (65 years and over) who were already in contact with a general practioner or health visitor. Apparently no extra staff were required to carry out the comprehensive assessments, but the newly identified problems generated more work for the primary health care team. Interestingly, the health visitors felt that their visits based upon the assessment schedule were more useful than their previous visits had been. Barber and Wallis (1978) discuss the benefits to the elderly of a

surveillance programme based upon a comprehensive assessment using their schedule. The schedule requests demographic data about the elderly person, together with details of her acceptance of the interview. The second section includes questions on such topics as mobility, vision and hearing, which are all socially as well as physically important. Another section of the schedule notes the domiciliary services and support currently being provided. The final section includes questions of a specifically medical nature. Barber and Wallis conclude that such a continuing programme of geriatric assessment is valuable. The greatest improvements for clients were found in such areas as clothing, bedding, heating, dentition, diet, vision and hearing, and the least improvement in level of dependency, home hazards and problems with a caring relative.

Subsequently Barber et al (1980) developed and tested a postal questionnaire (Fig. 27.2) as a screening procedure in a comprehensive geriatric assessment programme for all elderly people over 70 years of age. The authors conclude that the questionnaire was acceptable to the elderly and that it safely identified all those who could benefit from further assessment by a health visitor. This successfully reduced the enormous workload that would be generated in routine assessment visiting of all elderly people.

Where no screening procedures exist, it seems that the subsequent implementation of screening substantially increases the workload

---

Do you live on your own?
Are you without a relative you could call on for help?
Are there any days when you are unable to have a hot meal?
Are you confined do your home through illhealth?
Is there anything about your health causing you concern or difficulty?
Do you have difficulty with vision?
Do you have difficulty with hearing?
Have you been in hospital during the past year?

Fig. 27.2 Questions in the screening letter of a geriatric assessment programme for the elderly. *Source: Barber, Wallis and McKeating 1980. Reproduced by permission of the Journal of the Royal College of General Practitioners.*

for all health workers during the 'intervention' phase. However, after this phase the general practitioner's workload decreases considerably, whereas although the district nurse's and health visitor's workload with the elderly decreases it is still higher than before the 'intervention' (Barber and Wallis 1982). Once a surveillance scheme is established, Barber and Wallis (1982) have estimated that the time required to continue a full screening and assessment programme for those aged 75 years and over is 11 hours per week throughout the year. Jones (1976) attempted to extend Tudor Hart's Inverse Care Law to geriatric screening. This states that the quantity of unmet need discovered at geriatric screening reflects the lack of care that elderly people usually receive from their general practitioner. Thus Barber and Wallis's estimate may need to be considered with caution.

Munday's research (1979) revealed that between 9% and 21% of those aged 75 years or over registered at four general practices in Devon were not seen by either a doctor or a health visitor during the course of a year. This research developed and tested an Elderly At Risk record card (Fig. 27.3) to facilitate the care offered to the elderly in the community. The record card is similar to Williams' (1974) schedule and was considered not only a useful assessment tool but also a means of co-ordinating the support available to the elderly.

Luker (1981) attempted to evaluate the effect of 'focused health visitor intervention' on a group of elderly women. Using two groups of elderly people in a 'cross-over' study (that is, both groups alternately acted as the 'experimental' and 'control' groups), it was found that health problems did improve with 'intervention' although there was no clear improvement in 'life satisfaction'. Ninety-five per cent of her sample (*n*=100) reported that they had enjoyed the health visitor visits. Luker attributes this to the benefits accruing from 'therapeutic anticipation' before the next expected visit, and to the well-being generated through another person taking an interest in their welfare, described by Luker as 'worthy of interest syndrome'. Sixty-two per cent of the sample reported that they had been helped by the visits if only through the social contact, while others felt that they had been helped directly with health-related matters such as the maintenance of a reducing diet or identifying possible household hazards. The overseeing or surveillance function of the health visitor was also acknowledged with 92% of the sample agreeing that it was a good idea for health visitors to visit elderly people. Luker's study also demonstrated the long-term effect of health visitor intervention with the benefits of 'intervention' continuing to accrue at the follow-up after six months.

ALTERNATIVE MEANS OF HEALTH VISITING FOR THE ELDERLY

An alternative approach to the care of the elderly is the establishment of screening clinics, clubs and self-help groups under the auspices of health visitors. One scheme set up clinics to which those over 50 years of age were invited for some screening and health advice (Figgins 1979). This scheme was not within a general practice context but in an area noted for the large number of single-handed general practitioners in a large city.

Few health visitors have written or conducted research into their work with elderly people so that the literature pertinent to health visiting and the well elderly tends to focus on the health visitor as the doctor's assistant in screening programmes rather than on independent health visitor surveillance (Luker 1980). This scarcity of studies extends to the contribution of health visitors to independent health visitor screening clinics, clubs and self-help groups although this work exists throughout the United Kingdom. Some health visitor have established teaching programmes within the context of luncheon clubs and warden-assisted housing schemes or fostered contact groups within their own locality.

Health visitor skills have been used in several experimental schemes to give special attention to the needs of the elderly. A health visitor was seconded to a social services

Front

NAME

ADDRESS

Date of Birth

Social Worker

G.P.

Special Disability

Telephone

H.V.

Address 2

Address 3 (or next of kin)

ASSESSMENT/SERVICES: Requested (R) Provided (√)

YEAR & AGE	ASSESSMENT DATE	CATE-GORY OF RISK	OTHER RISK FACTORS	G.P.	Health visitor	District Nurse	Chiropody	Day Care	Social Worker or O.T.	Home Help	Meals on Wheels	Warden Scheme	Resi-dential Home	OTHER	MARITAL STATE (M.S.W. D. Sep.)	HOUSING

ELDERLY AT RISK REGISTER

Rear

CATEGORY OF RISK

Codes for use overleaf

Minimal or No Risk (0) (√)	Some Risk (1) (√)	Severe Risk (2) (√)
Adequate mobility	Mobility restricted/Housebound	Movement restricted to 1 or 2 rooms
Can shop, clean & cook unaided	Unable to shop	Unable to cook
Cheerful mental state	Mental deterioration present (a) Mood (b) Memory	Severe mental deterioration (a) Self with danger to (b) Others
No incapacitating illness	Risk of physical illness	Debilitating illness

OTHER RISK FACTORS

X – Social isolation
Y – Financial need
Z – Family under strain
ZZ – Family cannot cope

V – Inadequate housing
W – Inadequate heating

HOUSING

A – Lives with spouse
B – Lives alone
C – With friends/relatives

H – Own Home
J – Rented Accommodation
K – Sheltered Accommodation
L – Lodgings

DATE	NOTES

Fig. 27.3 'Elderly at Risk' record card—modified version. *Source: Munday 1979. Reproduced by permission of the King's Fund Centre.*

department under a joint finance scheme with responsibilities for preventive care, health education and liaison (between health and social services staff). She also had a particular responsibility to foster the welfare of the elderly and handicapped in that district (Day and Magridge 1981). This scheme is currently under evaluation but it demonstrates that the particular training and skills of health visitors can be utilised in the community and not just within the primary health care team. Indeed, health visitors may have a role in community action to improve the care of local elderly residents.

In a pilot scheme in Manchester funded by inner-city money, a geriatric team is led by a health visitor who acts as the liaison between hospitals, community health services and social services (Halladay 1981). Geriatric liaison health visitors increasingly are being appointed throughout the country in an attempt to ensure continuity of care of patients on discharge from hospital. Thursfield (1979) reports on such a scheme which aims to give support to elderly patients and assess their progress while also avoiding the duplication of visits by care workers. Griffiths and Eastwood (1974) describe the work of a psychogeriatric liaison health visitor.

GROWING OLD IN INNER CITIES

Enough is known about the decay, poverty and socially unstable nature of our inner cities for the conclusion to be reached that such environments can exert strong negative influences upon many of the people who live there. Elderly people are a vulnerable group who feel particularly threatened by their apparent demise in our youth-oriented society.

Housing is often substandard and some areas are poorly maintained or polluted and are clearly a hazard to health. The deprived inner city frequently lacks the kind of social institutions in which the elderly, black or white, can participate and, in view of the indisputable evidence of higher crime rates (Smith 1981) many perceive the environment

as physically threatening. The environment is further disadvantaged by its often poor aesthetic appearance—uncollected litter, pavements covered with broken glass, graffiti-covered walls and deserted buildings. Despite this catalogue of negative features, residents in inner city areas frequently display tolerance. Lawton (1980) points out that it is possible to ignore disturbing or irritating elements of the environment. Indeed, one must be wary of imposing outsiders' judgments of what it is like to live in inner city neighbourhoods upon individuals who have spent much of their life in them. Sometimes it is possible to overstate the degree of change to which the physical appearance of inner-city areas has been subjected. For example, rebuilding does not necessarily mean a new layout of the facilities because in many instances the shops are rebuilt on their original sites. Thus the basic geography of the shops and other facilities continue to be familiar.

It is generally accepted that the inner-city environment is less healthy than others. However, Lawton (1980) cites American data to show that elderly people living inner-city areas are significantly more mobile and less hampered by chronic illness than those living in rural areas. There is also the positive advantage of the relative ease of access to health service facilities in densely populated areas. In general, however, the disadvantages for inner-city elderly in comparison with suburban elderly are great and extend into their health as well as other areas of daily life.

AGEING EXPERIENCE OF ETHNIC MINORITIES

Blakemore (1983) studied the difference experiences of the elderly white compared with the elderly black population in inner Birmingham. He found that two fifths of the total population of elderly people in this area live alone. The elderly whites tend to be objectively better off with regard to personal circumstances than the elderly blacks while at the same time they express a greater sense of deprivation.

Blakemore suggests that most elderly blacks have a fatalistic, accepting attitude towards their environment, although he points out that West Indian old age is not without its problems. There is a higher incidence amongst West Indians of poverty and ill health coupled with the need to cope with the potentially lonely role of being an ageing immigrant. However, he suggests that immigrants are able to divert their angry or resentful feelings about the environment towards an acceptance of the situation viewing their initial migration as the cause of these unsatisfactory conditions. He found that poverty, isolation and the sense of not being welcome in British society was frequently interpreted by elderly blacks as evidence of personal failings, bad luck or God's will. The act of migrating set in motion a chain of events leading to either personal success or failure. Blakemore suggests that higher general practitioner consultation rates not only reflect the elderly blacks' morbidity but also their level of personal anxiety and insecurity, with the general practitioners acting as agents of reassurance and sympathy. It seems that growing old is accepted with resignation or fatalism by elderly blacks and, contrary to expectation, it also seems that the presence of more blacks in a neighbourhood does little to enhance the elderly blacks' sense of identity, security or engagement.

Blakemore found that elderly whites in inner Birmingham were disturbed by their environment. It seems that it did little to support their morale or sense of identity, rather it became a permanent reminder of their marginal role as strangers in their own land. The elderly whites expressed the feeling of loss of a valued community and frequently displayed their anxiety by focusing their concern on the 'strange ways' of black people and their neighbours. Blakemore suggests that elderly whites are much more critical than elderly blacks of their environment and their experience of deprivation is much keener.

In summary, it seems that both groups suffer a loss of the anticipated pattern of ageing, the whites having built up their model in middle age before the ethnic composition of the inner city had changed, while the blacks had memories of the pattern of ageing as it used to be in the West Indies. Quite different solutions are needed to resolve the isolation, loneliness and anxiety of inner city elderly people according to their ethnic background and their wishes. The health visitor should be aware of the differences that exist among inner-city elderly in their different cultural backgrounds and seek appropriate ways of ameliorating the personal experiences of this vulnerable group. For example, the establishment of contact groups may be helpful.

VIOLENCE AGAINST THE ELDERLY

Violence outside the home

Prominent press coverage of violence against the elderly may lead one to suppose that they are under continuous threat from the mugger and vandal. However, there seems to be a discrepancy between fears of such crimes and the risk of it (Mawby 1983). The 1975 Sheffield victim survey (Bottoms et al 1981) found that old people were statistically less likely to have been victims of crimes than younger respondents, and this finding was supported in a London victim survey (Sparks et al 1977). Thus contrary to popular opinion the elderly are relatively safe from crime.

The research indicates, however, that elderly men are more at risk than elderly women, and those living in 'problem' areas are not more at risk than those living in any working-class area. It seems also that those previously employed in unskilled work are less likely to be victims. The research indicates that household size is unimportant while those with few local friends are at more risk. Although criminal assault is a very traumatic experience and should attract intensive care for the old person wherever it occurs, the research findings do not support the impression that the elderly are a particularly vulnerable group in comparison to others.

Mawby suggests that violence against the elderly is relatively low because they venture out of doors less frequently than younger people and so expose themselves less to the possibility of attack. Indeed, where crime is rationally planned it would seem that the elderly offer little reward since old age is associated with poverty (Townsend 1979). However, the fact remains that much crime is unplanned. Mawby also points out that certain locations are especially vulnerable to crime, such as public houses, city centres and near-empty streets. These are places not often frequented by elderly people since they are more likely to be at home. It is also worth nothing that crimes against property are more likely if the property is empty so that those remaining at home are doubly protected. Unfortunately, if policies are pursued which encourage more participation by the elderly in activities outside the home, the risk of crime against them may be expected to rise. The Sparks et al (1977) survey clearly demonstrates a relationship between age, crime and activities.

A health visitor can assist in the prevention of crime against elderly people. She can influence the various vulnerability factors by mounting crime prevention campaigns, encouraging neighbour support and minimising the isolation of the elderly. She may affect the 'visible target attractiveness' by encouraging old people to refrain from displaying obvious signs of possessions which may attract offenders. She can inform the elderly of dangerous locations, and she can sponsor the rehousing of those who feel trapped or endangered by their environment, especially those who have been victimised. She can also contribute to the care of victims and perhaps help in setting up schemes similar to Victims-Aid to which the police are asked to refer elderly victims of crime so that they may be counselled or referred to others.

Violence inside the home

It is difficult enough to find valid statistics of violence against the elderly outside the home. It is even more difficult to assess the extent to which 'granny-battering' inside the home occurs. As with crime against elderly people

outside the home, abuse in the domestic setting is a popular subject for the press. However, as Cloke (1983) points out there is no unanimous view among researchers as to what constitutes 'old age abuse'. A working definition has been provided by Cloke: 'The systematic and continuous abuse of an elderly person *by the carer*, often, although not always, a relative, on whom the elderly person is dependent for care' (para 2.2, emphasis added).

Eastman argues that abuse includes physical assault, threats of physical assault, neglect, exploitation and abandonment, sexual abuse and psychological abuse (Eastman and Sutton 1982, Eastman 1982, 1983). Eastman contends that this is not an exhaustive list but a useful framework in which to view granny-battering, with abuse by people other than caring relatives constituting something quite different.

Eastman and Sutton (1982) estimate that 500 000 elderly people in the United Kingdom are at risk from old age abuse. This is based upon their report that 42% of those over 65 years of age in the United Kingdom are supported by care-giving relatives. They use American research which suggests that 10% of such people are at risk from abuse. However, the application of American research findings to a different society is dubious. America does not have a comprehensive welfare system for the elderly, which forces most elderly people to be wholly dependent upon their younger relatives. The suggestion that 42% of those over 65 years are supported by care-giving relatives is not supported by the Office of Population, Censuses and Survey study (1978) which found only 12% of elderly people living with their children. In summary, although it has been established that old age abuse occurs in the United Kingdom there is insufficient research evidence to indicate its prevalence.

Similarly, knowledge about the predisposing variables of old age abuse is scanty. The only data for analysis have been gleaned from the limited number of reported incidents where adequately detailed case history information is seldom available. A number of factors individually or jointly may contribute to old age abuse: lack of support to carers, low income, poor and overcrowded housing, poor family relationships and poor communication within the family, carer also looking after another person such as a spouse or child, history of violence in the family, emotional stress, psychological defects in the carer, an alcoholic carer, changes in the carer's lifestyle, and a lack of understanding by the carer of the ageing process and the capabilities of elderly people (Cloke 1983). The lack of research findings in this field means that health visitors must be mindful of the possibility of abuse in all settings and should be particularly supportive to caring relatives. Warr (1980) gives a moving account of her personal experience as a carer of an elderly relative clearly outlining some of the problems involved. Adequate support to carers seems to be all too readily overlooked. Cartwright et al (1973) revealed that relatives often struggle on with inadequate help from professionals and community services, and in some instances there was no co-ordination of services to support families.

THE VALUE OF HEALTH VISITING FOR THE ELDERLY—CONCLUSION

Clearly, health visitors have a role to play in the care of the elderly. In the future they should perhaps become the principal case finding agency at work in the community, exercising their training and skills to the full so that every elderly person may be aware of their entitlements to welfare as well as knowing the facilities and services to which they could have access in their locality. The use of age–sex registers in general practices is one means of locating elderly people, which is an extremely difficult task if no such register exists. Alternatively, active case searching by health visitors may prove more rewarding, making use of registers concerning those in receipt of meals-on-wheels or the home help service, or attendance registers at luncheon clubs or the fostering of self-help groups.

Health visitors have a major role to play in the maintenance of well-being among the elderly. Uninvited visits allow the health visitor to carry out regular surveillance, anticipating future needs while educating old people about diet, hypothermia, financial entitlements and so on. There is an enormous contribution health visitors can make to health teaching among the elderly, and I have reviewed some of the work in this field (While 1983).

The counselling skills of health visitors are particularly important with regard to the care of the bereaved. The elderly are more likely than any other age group to lose the companionship of someone close to them, and the loss of a partner or friend may cause grief, shock, anger and bitterness. In 1977 13% of men and 40% of women between 65 and 75 years were widowed or divorced. For those over the age of 75, the proportion is higher, being 34% for men and 67% for women (Tinker 1981). The importance of understanding mourning and the need for skilled professional help is underlined by Parkes (1975) and Pincus (1976). Williams (1974) suggests that there is a need for a higher priority to be accorded this work and that perhaps health visitors should allocate more of their time to this type of work.

The application of the nursing process to health visiting may become a helpful innovation in the care of the elderly and overcome Luker's (1983) criticism that health visitors do not focus their interaction with the elderly clients. Rogers (1982) describes the successful introduction of the 'health visiting process' and the development of a new record card in a health district in southern England. The use of such an approach offers a systematic method of record keeping in which client needs and problems and health visiting plans can easily be identified. It also enables health visitors to audit the effectiveness of their care and intervention. This is important because the needs and problems of an elderly person constantly change, and so the health visitor must continually assess whether her actions are effective. If they are not, she must make alternative plans, and these in turn must be evaluated. As Hedley et al (1982) point out, in a situation of limited working time and unlimited health needs there is much to be gained from using an improved method of record keeping. They suggest that the use of the health visiting process records has promoted logical thought which enables them to formulate the needs of their clients. They also suggest that it has helped their assessment of priorities and their planning on a daily and weekly basis. Furthermore, they argue that the use of the health visiting process has improved their practice with the formulation of short and long-term plans for clients helping to focus the health visitor intervention and including an evaluation of the effectiveness of the advice or subsequent action.

The health visitor is an ideal link between the individual in need and available help. The adoption of focused health visitor intervention should offer much for the future welfare of elderly people. The use of one of the described assessment tools together with the health visiting process may provide a helpful starting point for improved health visitor care of the elderly.

Taylor and Ford (1983) suggest a hierarchy of 'at risk' elderly which provides health visitors with a potential priority scale from which to organize their work. They suggest, contrary to popular opinion, that the isolated, childless and never married are the least disadvantaged elderly, whereas the recently widowed, those living alone, the poor and social class V form an intermediate group. The most 'at risk' elderly are those who have recently moved, those recently discharged from hospital, the divorced or separated and the very old.

The functions of the health visitor as outlined by the Council for the Education and Training of Health Visitors (CETHV) (1976) are as applicable for the elderly as for any other age group:

(a) prevention of mental, physical and emotional ill health or alleviation of its consequences;

(b) early detection of ill health and the surveillance of high risk groups;

(c) recognition and identification of need, and

mobilisation of resources where necessary;

(d) provision of care; this will include support during periods of stress, and advice and guidance in case of illness.

Health visitors should use their skills to assist in the care of elderly people so that the wish of most to remain in their own homes may be a reality. This should enable old people to enjoy the maximum quality of life.

REFERENCES

Anderson W F 1955 A consultative health centre for old people. Lancet 1: 239–240

Barber J H, Wallis J B 1976 Assessment of the elderly in general practice. Journal of Royal College of General Practitioners 26: 106–114

Barber J H, Wallis J B 1978 The benefits to an elderly population of continuing geriatric assessment. Journal of Royal College of General Practitioners 28: 428–433

Barber J H, Wallis J B, McKeating I 1980 A postal screening questionnaire in preventive geriatric care. Journal of Royal College of General Practitioners 30: 39–51

Barber J H, Wallis J B 1982 The effect of a system of geriatric screening and assessment on general practice workload. Health Bulletin 40(3): 125–132

Blakemore K 1983 Ageing in the inner city—a comparison of old blacks and whites. In: Jerrome D (ed) Ageing in modern society. Croom Helm, London

Bottoms A E, Mawby R I, Xanthos P D 1981 Sheffield study on urban social structure and crime, Part 3. Unpublished Report to the Home Office

Brocklehurst J C 1975 Geriatric care in advanced societies. Blackburn Times Press, Blackburn

Cartwright A, Hockey L, Anderson J 1973 Life before death. Routledge and Kegan Paul, London

Clark M J 1973 A family visitor. Royal College of Nursing, London

Clark M J 1978 What do health visitors do? Royal College of Nursing, London

Cloke C 1983 Old age abuse in the domestic setting—a review. Age Concern, London

Council for the Education and Training of Health Visitors 1976 The health visitor: function and implications for training. CETHV, London

Curnow R N, Macfarlane S B J, Gatherer A, Lindars M E 1975 Visiting the elderly. Health and Social Service Journal 15: 79–80

Currie G, MacNeill R M, Walker J G, Bernie E, Mindie E W 1974 Medical and social screening of patients aged 70 to 72 by an urban general practice health team. British Medical Journal 2: 108–111

Day L, Magridge J 1981 Health visitor who stayed. Health and Social Services Journal 91: 1114–1115

Department of Health and Social Security 1976a Priorities for health and social services in England. HMSO, London

Department of Health and Social Security 1976b Prevention and health: everybody's business. A reassessment of public and personal health, HMSO, London

Dingwall R 1977 What future for health visiting? Evidence to the Royal Commission on the National Health Service. Nursing Times 73: 77–79

Eastman M 1982 Granny battering: A hidden problem. Community Care 27: May 12–13

Eastman M, Sutton M 1982 Granny battering. Geriatric Medicine 12(11): 11–15

Eastman M 1983 Who'd bash their granny? She(Feb): 72–73

Figgins P 1979 Screen now benefit later. Nursing Mirror 149(9): 24–25

Griffiths A, Eastwood H 1974 Psychogeriatric liaison health visitor. Nursing Times 70: 152–153

Halladay H 1981 A geriatric team within the health visiting service. Nursing Times 77: 1039–1040

Hay E H 1976 A geriatric survey in general practice. Practitioner 206: 443–447

Hedley C, Grieve L, Hood J, Leyshon Y 1982 Health visiting and the nursing process. III: Using the need/problem orientated method of record keeping. Health Visitor 55: 211–215

Hodkinson H M 1975 An outline of geriatrics. Academic Press, London and New York

Jones R V H 1976 Recognition of geriatric problems in general practice. Update 13:643

Lawton M P 1980 Environment and ageing. Brooks/Cole, New York

Luker K A 1979 Health visiting and the elderly. Midwife, Health Visitor and Community Nurse 15: 457–459

Luker K A 1980 Screening of the well elderly in general practice. Midwife, Health Visitor and Community Nurse 16: 222–229

Luker K A 1981 Elderly women's opinions about the benefits of health visitor visits. Occasional Paper. Nursing Times 77(9): 33–35

Luker K A 1983 An evaluation of health visitors' visits to elderly women. In Wilson-Barnet J (ed) Nursing Research—Ten Studies in Patient Care. Wiley, Chichester

Mawby R I 1983 Crime and elderly: experience and perceptions. In: Jerome D (ed) Ageing in modern society. Croom Helm, London

MacQueen 1 1962 From carbolic powder to social counsel: centenary address to Battersea College of Technology. Nursing Times 58: 886–888

Munday M 1979 Care of the elderly in Devon. King's Fund Centre, London

Office of Population Censuses and Surveys 1978 The elderly at home. Audrey Hunt. HMSO, London

Office of Population Censuses, and Surveys 1982 Nurses working in the community. Dunnell K, Dobbs J, HMSO, London

Parkes C M 1975 Bereavement: studies of grief in adult life. Pelican, London

Pincus L 1976 Death and the family. Faber and Faber, London

Rogers J M 1982 Health visiting and the nursing process. I: Introducing the health visiting process. Health Visitor 55: 204–208

Royal Commission on the National Health Service 1979 Report. (The Merrison Committee) Cmnd. 7615. HMSO, London

Smith S J 1981 Negative interaction: crime in the inner city. In: Jackson P, Smith S J (eds) Social interaction and ethnic segregation. Academic Press, New York

Sparks R, Genn H, Dodd D 1977 Survey victims. Wiley, Chichester

Taylor R C, Ford E G 1983 The elderly at risk: a critical examination of commonly identified risk groups. Journal of the Royal College of General Practitioners 33: 699–705

Thursfield P J 1979 The hospital that doesn't say goodbye. Nursing Mirror 150(6): 50–52

Tinker A 1981 The elderly in modern society. Longman, London

Townsend P 1979 Poverty in United Kingdom. Penguin, Harmondsworth

Warr J 1980 Caring for an elderly relative: a personal experience. Health Visitor 53: 525–529

While A E 1983 Teaching those in need in the community. In: Wilson-Barnett J (ed) Patient teaching. Churchill Livingstone, Edinburgh

Williams E I 1974 A follow-up of geriatric patients' socio-medical assessment. Journal of the Royal College of General Practitioners 24: 341–346

Williams E I, Bennett F M, Nixon J V, Nicholson M R, Garbert J 1972 Sociomedical study of patients over 75 in general practice. British Medical Journal 12: 445–448

Williams I 1979 The care of the elderly in the community. Croom Helm, London

Williams J 1974 Death and bereavement. Age Concern, London

PART | FOUR

Care of elderly people: conclusions

28

The elderly person: the challenge of an aged society

In this chapter an attempt is made to draw together the earlier discussions concerning the impact of the ageing population in western societies in general, but particularly in Britain. We have highlighted some of the experiences that women, men and people from ethnic minorities have in being old, victims of discriminatory attitudes and dependent on inadequate services. Finally, and more positively, we have discussed some aspects of successful ageing, and what nurses can do to help old people stay healthy.

THE IMPACT OF AN AGEING POPULATION

The demographic trend in all western industrialised countries is much the same. As discussed by Malcolm Johnson (Chapter 1) and Helen Evers (Chapter 22), the proportion of very old people in Britain is rising. In actual numbers there are 8.3 million (17%) old people in Britain and although the total number is not expected to increase very much, by the year 2000 the rise in the over 75 age group will be substantial, and this will be accompanied by a proportional reduction in the fitter 'young elderly', aged 65–74 years (Shegog 1981, Acheson 1982).

The position in the United States is similar, although the proportion of old people relative to the total population is smaller than in Britain. The 1980 census showed a 27% growth in the 65+ age group since 1970, that is from

20 million to 25.5 million people. This represents just over 11% of the total American population, and by the year 2000 it is forecast that this proportion will increase to 13% (Ernst and Glazer-Waldman 1983).

Given the association of disability and dependency with increasing age, the consequences of this rise in the very old and most frail are regarded as grave. At least half the expected additional over 85 year olds will need help with bathing, one fifth of those living at home are likely to be housebound, and many will be incontinent (Acheson 1982). Coupled with other social patterns such as the increasing mobility of younger families, smaller families, more married women doing paid work, and more marital breakdown leading to double the number of old people who live alone and who have no children, the present level of caring services will be stretched to breaking point and beyond.

Although it is important to keep a sense of proportion in that a substantial number of old people have no incapacitating disabilities, nonetheless, the size of the 'crisis' or 'challenge' and the impact on the health services should be assessed. The commonest health and disability problems experienced by very old people are immobility, instability, incontinence, mental impairment, disturbances of hearing and vision, foot troubles and toxic drug effects (Isaacs 1981, Rossiter and Wicks 1982). Reduced mobility leads to a vicious cycle of decreasing social contact, isolation, and inability to keep warm and to prepare food. Mentally frail, demented and depressed elderly people experience greater physical decline and are particularly at risk from malnutrition, burns, falls and other diseases (Rossiter and Wicks 1982).

Even with ill health and disability, old people are the survivors; they have survived in spite of exposure to disease, poor nutrition, defective immunity, and multiple drug taking, which leaves them unfit but does not kill them. The multiple diseases of very old age converge on the four Giants of Geriatrics (Isaacs 1981)—immobility, instability, mental impairment and incontinence. As Isaacs makes

clear, these Giants, although not exclusive to the elderly, have four common properties which cause great difficulties for old people: they have multiple causes, they destroy independence, there is no simple treatment, and they need human helpers. They are not inevitable consequences of old age but do require the skills of the specialist. 'Too often they evoke a cry for removal and storage rather than for investigation and treatment' (Isaacs 1981, p 145).

Population statistics do not emphasise the practical consequences for society of an ageing population. Grimley Evans (in Hodgson 1984) maintains that the British government has based its future policies for health and social services on two fallacies. First, the phenomenon of 'rectangularisation', described by Malcolm Johnson in Chapter 1, in which the death rate curve is shifted towards a maximum lifespan. This shift is evident in most industrial countries, and the fallacy is that the government assumes that the shift will also occur in the need for care. This is to say, if life expectancy increases by 10 years, nursing, medical and social services care will be needed 10 years later than at present. There is no evidence for this.

The second fallacy highlighted by Grimley Evans is the assumption that any increase in the care burden can be borne primarily by the community rather than the state. Yet all the evidence indicates that an ageing population generates increased health care needs in general, and there is a huge proportionate increase of old people with conditions requiring skilled nursing care. Grimley Evans predicts that by the twenty-first century, in order merely to maintain present standards, home visits by general practitioners must increase by 9%, district nurse and health visitor visits by 14%, home help by 18%, meals-on-wheels by 23%, and chiropody by 9%. Expert and dedicated 24-hour nursing supervision is needed for demented old people. There is no evidence that dementia itself shortens life, but there is plenty of evidence that lack of care does.

The social context of ageing and retirement

reflects negative attitudes. As discussed elsewhere (Chapters 1 and 7) society is still in the early stages of understanding and interpreting old age. It views the 'age explosion' with alarm and regards the elderly as a 'social problem', creating an intolerable economic and social burden. Old age is still seen as a period of 'social redundancy' with an emphasis on the non-productiveness of the elderly. This stereotype of inevitable physical and mental decline and of the elderly as consumers of excessive amounts of health and social services, even if true of large numbers of old people today, is not an inevitable consequence of survival into very old age. The backgrounds, social and financial status, and environmental and health factors of today's elderly are unique and different from those of the next generation of old people.

Financially, many elderly people are living on or near the officially defined 'poverty' line. As Amanda Stokes-Roberts points out in Chapter 7, the state pension is the sole source of income for many old people. They are dependent on additional supplementary benefits, although by no means all who are eligible claim these benefits. This point is made by Fiona Ross in Chapter 26, who describes the social security benefits available in England for old people. Most of their income is spent on necessities like food, fuel and housing, and it is the working-class single women and widows, who have no access to occupational pensions, who are most likely to be below the poverty line. It is women who bear most of the poverty in this country.

WOMEN IN RETIREMENT AND OLD AGE

In many ways ageing is a woman's issue. Of those over 75 years, there are two women to every man and many live alone, a large proportion of these having done so for a long time (Phillipson 1982; and see Chapter 22 of this volume). They are, therefore, very used to being alone and, one would think, are particularly prone to feelings of isolation, loneliness, depression and alienation. Many are on the poverty line and so cannot afford the communication commodities (car, telephone, etc.) which would enable them to be with others more often and be less likely to suffer these negative psychological experiences.

It is not really known what this isolation and the health problems and disabilities experienced mean for older women. We know something about the famous exceptions to the old age stereotype (Pablo Picasso, Sybil Thorndyke, Bertrand Russell, Marlene Dietrich, etc.), and about life in institutions for the elderly, but we know very little about what the isolated elderly woman living alone does with her time, although Evers (1983) has been investigating this recently. Evers found the commonest response to a question about what they had been doing the day before was 'nothing much' or 'nothing at all'. However, on further questioning, these women had in fact been doing many things, like personal and household tasks, leisure activites and meeting people. Evers speculates on why such activities were not mentioned, and she offers three explanations of the 'doing nothing much' syndrome. It may reflect a relative reduction in the number and importance of activities with age, or a gloomy out-look on life, or a devaluation of 'women's work' which is not considered worth mentioning. Evers found that the women interviewed could be classified crudely as either 'passive responders' (PR), who seemed to have little control over their lives or 'active initiators' (AI), who were very much in control and had purpose in life. Ill health and dependency were not apparently characteristics exclusive to either group but were represented in both, nor were the groups different according to class, education level, affluence, or contact with surviving children.

Evers has made the link between AI women and 'engagement' and PR women and 'disengagement'. She suggests that AI women had pursued activities in their lives in addition to the traditional work of women as carers, whereas PR had filled most of their lives with caring activities. The categories are unlikely to be as simple as suggested here, but if confirmed, the implications of Evers' hypothesis are important for health care workers. They should understand the psychological characteristics of women in their care, otherwise AI women may resent a loss of control over their lives, and PR women may be unable to respond to enforced independence. Nurses are the workers in the best position to identify such characteristics and to ensure that they and others meet the individual needs of each old woman in their care.

Because they are the survivors, old women are much more likely than old men to spend their final years in an institution. The generally low standards in institutions may be partly a result of there being more women residents. It may reflect external, societal beliefs about the status and rights of elderly women in particular and of women in general (Phillipson 1982).

The effectiveness of future problem solving and social policy on care of the elderly will depend on whether past and present ageing patterns and needs of women are incorporated into professional and popular perceptions, or are ignored as they are today. Social, professional and legislative systems do not recognise women's needs as a priority or as different from men's (Roebuck 1983). As Roebuck observes, writers on the elderly, be they philosophers, literary writers, gerontologists from classical Greeks to the present, from Aristotle to Shakespeare, write about old age in male terms. Jacques' speech in 'As You Like It' views ageing in terms of the seven ages of man. Writers and politicians continue in this vein even though numerous censuses have confirmed the numerical dominance of old women. They assume that all elderly people either possess male characteristics or are homogenously sexless.

Elderly women are victims of two stereotypes, sex and age. Even though, as discussed in other chapters in this book (e.g. Chapters 2 and 16), the 'sick and helpless old person' does not apply to most old women or men, the stereotype remains powerful and little is expected of them as a result. They are thought too feeble to have demands made on them.

This leads to the self-fulfilling prophecy of asocial functioning, incompetence and dependency (Roebuck 1983). Old people themselves hold these stereotypes and the effect may be disastrous for them because they think they are decrepit burdens to families and to society. They may hate themselves and their contemporaries, and believe that late life can offer nothing useful or interesting.

Roebuck maintains that women are labelled as old sooner than men are, that is, at the menopause. This is the time when women are 'cast off' as old because they can no longer bear children and fulfil the reason for their existence as defined by male-oriented society. In contrast, men at this age may be at the height of their careers. The view that women are old, sick and useless from the menopause to death is not an uncommon one, and this period may be nearly half their lifetime. Negative stereotypes are physically, psychologically and socially damaging to the victims and are extremely difficult to erase because they are rooted in society's deep past. The old people suffer despair and impotence, and the rest of the population either ignore the reality or reinforce the negative stereotype. It is not by chance that the negative descriptors which are applied to old age are similar to those often used to describe women, such as lack of vigour or initiative or dynamism, inferior mental capacity, low social status, weak and economically dependent.

Many writers (e.g. Roebuck 1983) support the view that women have coped better than men with old age. They may have a more diverse social world with friendships outside the family, are more accustomed to widowhood and the need to build new lives without a spouse, and are less used to being looked after. Women are said to be more likely to make and retain strong friendships and so female patterns of life and response to major change are generally more successful than male. Women are, they think, successful survivors and their greater life expectation, which is continuing to increase relative to men's, bears witness to this.

Phillipson (1982) disputes this view and suggests that women have a more difficult time coping with retirement and old age than is suggested. He bases his argument on three factors. First, the position of women in women's studies. Even though women outnumber men after retirement from work most of the research focuses on the experiences and problems of men in retirement. It is a cause for concern that the feminist literature also puts very little emphasis on older women, who when joining women's groups feel resented as outsiders (Lewis and Butler 1980, Macdonald and Rich 1984). This may, however, disappear as the women's movement grows and its present members become old. In America elderly women are gaining in political strength, and they have time to be actively involved in consciousness-raising, as Maggie Kuhn has shown with her Gray Panther movement (Kuhn 1980). Such pressure groups have not yet become visible in Britain. Malcolm Johnson (Chapter 1) discusses the development of corporate consciousness and action by older people.

Phillipson's second factor relates to women as workers. As unpaid workers, retirement is seen to be less of a crisis compared with that for men because they continue to keep active with household chores. On the contrary, Phillipson argues that women's domestic and work responsibilities may create considerable stress in middle and old age. The identity of women only as mothers is outdated because many of those who have children spend a fairly small proportion of their lives caring for them full-time. Even so, the mothering role remains and is extended into women's work, as volunteer carer, nurse, home help, etc., all of which roles concern the sick and elderly. Even though women may try to escape from the caring role when they no longer have dependent children, society limits the work opportunities available and expects them to take on the more nurturing roles. Social policies are, in today's climate of economic restraint, increasing the pressure on women to accept such roles, especially in the care of elderly relatives, and it is well known that

women take on the major burden of caring for old people (see Chapters 22 and 26 of this book). Thus, just when a woman feels free to pursue studies or a career, she finds she is tied to yet more dependants, a pressure which is much greater for her than for men. Then, when her parents die, she is faced with caring for an ailing husband.

There has been a large increase since the Second World War in women over the age of 45 years doing paid work, many women coping with the dual role of worker and mother/homemaker. The jobs they do are usually poorly paid, unskilled, and auxiliary work which may not carry an occupational pension. Furthermore, social attitudes still regard paid work for women as secondary to their primary homemaker role, and this is reflected in low levels of pay. The Conservative government in the United Kingdom today emphasises that the woman's place is at home, she should not take jobs away from men, and should care for young and elderly dependants. In other words, she should provide extra domestic labour to compensate for the public services which are cut.

The third factor outlined by Phillipson refers to the implications for later life of female labour under capitalism. Women can experience discrimination at premature retirement when their own careers are sacrificed to care for parents or husband on his retirement. The transition from work to retirement may be extremely stressful for women, especially financially if there is no occupational pension. The full-time homemaker may find that her workload and financial burden have increased with husband at home all day. Women workers are often more resistant than men to retirement because many have already experienced the isolation of working at home all day with young children, although in some cases, especially the better off, retirement may provide long sought opportunities for growth and recreation for both women and men.

The twentieth century has been a period of very rapid modernisation in the western world and women's adaptability to change has been more marked than men's. Women have had to learn to make the most out of scarce or dwindling resources because they tend to bear the major burden of poverty in a period of decline.

> Within "the aged" those most likely to teach us not only how to make the most out of the least but also how to cope successfully with major personal and social changes are women. The future promises to hold challenges very different from the past, but to be no less a time of massive change than the rest of the modern era has been. Perhaps the greatest difference is that the most logical revolutionary leader for the future is that hitherto most unlikely candidate—grandma (Roebuck 1983, p 264).

MEN IN RETIREMENT AND OLD AGE

This section is much shorter than the previous one on women in retirement and old age. This deliberate bias occurs not because we have less to say about men, but because so much less has been written about elderly women who are clearly more at risk as a group, as evidenced by the demographic data.

In Chapter 2 of this volume, Sally Robbins observes that the attainment of 'retirement age' is a life event which, for both sexes, is accompanied by many stresses, whatever the quality of the change.

Phillipson (1982) has described three main variations in the transition from work to retirement for men. The 'stable withdrawer' prepares for a change in lifestyle and may feel that he has achieved all he can in his work role. The 'unstable withdrawer' may experience retirement as a result of redundancy and perhaps ill health, accompanied by feeling rejected and discarded, and dwindling resources. The 'abrupt withdrawer' may experience anxiety before retirement which interferes with his successful preparation for it. Evidence shows that most men do not prepare for retirement but just let things happen. This clean break from work to non-work is a crisis for most people; it may bring loneliness, and requires adjustment as with any loss. Coupled with a drop in income and perhaps poor health, the main problem may be bewilderment at how to cope with such change, rather than boredom. Social class is important, with middle-class men in professional jobs more likely than working-class men in unskilled jobs to take social roles after retirement. The former may have more skills that can be used in retirement than manual workers.

Even though many men enjoy the sense of freedom and escape from the clock, retirement is not generally seen as a period for growth and self-development. The idea of an active, purposeful retirement is being encouraged, but as Phillipson argues, it is difficult to see how it can be reconciled with declining income and living standards. On the one hand the government promotes retirement as being healthy for the individual (more leisure) and for the state (new job opportunities), yet on the other hand the resources provided are small. Retired people are bound to feel marginal citizens. This low status may not be felt early in retirement but comes later when finances and health decline and contemporaries die.

Phillipson highlights the conflict inherent between work and leisure in a capitalist and bureaucratic society. The opportunities for development of human potential become more and more limited, especially for office and factory workers, yet the expansion of educational, cultural and other activities to fill our leisure time encourages us to realise this potential. Phillipson suggests that improvements would occur if the worker could enter and re-enter the workforce at different times in his career, and spend time on paid educational leave and sabbaticals so that work and education were more closely linked. This would also suit women who need time out from paid work for child-rearing. Also, if workers had more control over the nature and pace of their work, older workers would not become obsolete so quickly and could continue on a part-time basis. Such flexible links between work, education and leisure would make retirement easier, but existing structures are currently too rigid for this to occur on any scale.

OLD PEOPLE FROM ETHNIC MINORITIES

Confining the term 'ethnic' to people from erstwhile colonies outside Britain, India, Pakistan, the West Indies, Africa, etc. is inaccurate. These people are no more 'ethnic' than older British groups which consist of English, Scots, Welsh and Irish, all with different customs and lifestyles. There is evidence that people from the newer 'ethnic minorities' are retaining their distinctive lifestyles, demanding recognition and respect along with those of the multi-ethnic British. But as long as 'being British' is equated with being white, Christian and of indigenous ancestry, the ethnic minorities will continue to be regarded as alien (Ballard 1983).

The black and Asian elderly in Britain are heterogenous, with different languages and religions. A Punjabi Indian following the Sikh religion may be no more familiar with the lifestyle and language of a Muslim Pakistani or a Hindu Gujarati Indian than with a white British Christian or a Rastafarian West Indian.

Most elderly black and Asian people living in Britain have needs and problems similar to the indigenous poor. They tend to live in inner-city areas and are relatively deprived of financial security, health and social services, adequate housing, education and enhanced chances in life. Traditionally, as Amanda Stokes-Roberts observes in Chapter 7, these old people would have been the respected heads of their households, but they find this difficult to achieve in Britain. They experience discrimination because of their colour, language and culture, they tend to be lonely and isolated, and their dietary needs are not often met by the health and social services (Barker 1984). Barker sees little evidence of 'active racism' by the services, but plenty of what he calls 'passive racism and cultural arrogance' and considerable insensitivity towards these vulnerable people. This is because those providing services are ignorant about immigrants' home countries, their reasons for migration, the cultural norms of the different groups, and their experiences and perceptions of living in Britain. Barker emphasises that care providers, policy makers and service planners must learn about these people, why they come to Britain, what makes them stay, and their disillusionment about British life and the welfare services. Alison While, in Chapter 27, describes the different expectations and experiences of elderly black and white people living in inner city areas.

There are some 50 000 elderly people of New Commonwealth and Pakistani origin and 32 000 of these live in London (Davies 1982). It is not unusual for local authorities to assume that they are cared for by their families who also take care of their special needs. But in 1982, 500 Afro-Caribbean and Asian elderly people attended conferences in London to voice their concern about their needs and the lack of services. They lack knowledge of the services available, 88% of Asian elderly people cannot speak English, they live in overcrowded housing, they experience financial hardship (only 46% of the Asian elderly receive pensions compared with 83% of Afro-Caribbeans and 94% of British), and they suffer a high degree of ill health (Davies 1982). Asians find the diet served in hospitals, old peoples' Homes and meals-on-wheels unacceptable, although Birmingham now provides Asian meals-on-wheels and employs Asian home helps.

Although, on the whole, little effort has been made by either statutory or voluntary agencies, Davies describes a number of new initiatives. The West Indian community in Birmingham, with AFFOR (All Faiths for One Race), are setting up sheltered housing schemes for the elderly from ethnic minorities, and their leaders are arguing for separate services (housing, day centres, old people's Homes) for their old people, as exist for elderly Jews and Poles. In London, the Brent and Lambeth boroughs do have separate day centres and Task Force, the London organisation which works with pensioners, is becoming increasingly involved with black pensioners' groups. The Pepper Pot lunch club in London's North Kensington, set up in

1981 by the Citizens' Advice Bureaux, offers Caribbean food once a week cooked by a West Indian worker, and it provides companionship as well as food. Projects like these are valuable but insufficient. The statutory and voluntary organisations have been painfully slow in meeting the needs of these old people. Nurses, too, should inform themselves of these needs, and the Royal College of Nursing has recognised the problem. Its education centre in Birmingham has organised a week's course on the 'nursing needs of ethnic minorities' (Nursing Standard, July 12, 1984), although how much material relates to old people is not clear.

'NEW AGEISM' AND 'GERIATRICS'

We have seen how old people may be discriminated against on grounds of their age, sex and race, but the elderly frail and dependent are subject to even more discrimination. 'New Ageism' is a term introduced in the late 1970s (Borkman 1982). It indicates an implicit ageist attitude amongst some gerontologists, geriatricians and other health professionals who care for old people. They pay lip service to the heterogeneity and diversity of old people, but in practice, see them as unhealthy, incapable, unalert, helpless and dependent on services. 'New Ageism' is a more subtle and damaging form of discrimination than ageism because it is held by professionals actually engaged in the care of old people, who ought to embody and promote anti-ageist attitudes and education.

Alison Norman (1984) reminds us of Humpty Dumpty who said that when he used a word it meant what he chose it to mean. This has been the case with 'geriatrics'. It was coined by Nascher in 1909, 'geras' meaning old age and 'iatrikos' meaning relating to the physician, the antithesis of paediatrics. Geriatrics gained acceptance as a new medical specialty but it became corrupted to 'geriatric' meaning an old person, often a confused old person. We never call a child a 'paediatric'. Misuse of language is a serious issue because it creates stereotypes of identity and behaviour which have a powerful effect on those so labelled. Old people are lumped together in a single category which has the negative characteristics of low social status, non-productivity, physical ill health and imminent brain failure (Norman 1984). This is extremely damaging and hinders efforts to treat the autumn of one's life as a joyful, liberating, peaceful period of psychological growth. Of course the privileged (presidents, archbishops, judges, surgeons) are not so labelled, although they often use the stereotype to refer to others. Alison Norman notes that even the Archbishop of Canterbury, a classical scholar, has described himself as playing 'geriatric tennis', a strictly meaningless term.

Ageism can be fought by direct attack, as is the case with racism and sexism, and by encouraging old people to protest against such stereotypes and publicise their creativity and discoveries. This would contribute to a new and wider vocabulary and favourable changes of attitude. Brocklehurst (1984) sees only two ways of remedying the debased geriatrics' position and status; by making the practice of geriatrics so excellent and widespread that the term becomes properly understood and respected, or by changing the name. The problem is that no other word fits as correctly. The Americans carefully avoid geriatrics and have adopted gerontology, which is the study of ageing in all living things, and should not refer only to old people, or only to diseases of old people. A gerontologist is thus a scientist and not a clinician. Some geriatric departments have switched to 'clinical gerontology', meaning health care of the elderly, but this is still imprecise. The Anglo-Saxon word 'eld' meaning elderly forms the root of words which convey wisdom as well as age, such as the old term 'alderman' (sic), an elected councillor in local government in Britain. Brocklehurst suggests using 'eld health' in the same way as paediatricians use 'child health'. He prefers, however, the strategy of making geriatrics an excellent specialty and reverting to its real meaning—the medicine of old age. This is supported by

Malcolm Johnson in Chapter 1. Then 'no longer will the adjective "geriatric" be butchered into a noun describing an old man (or old woman)' (Brocklehurst 1984, p 28, parenthesis added). By the same token, 'geriatric nursing' and 'geriatric nurse' are, strictly, inaccurate, although they are convenient terms to use, as we have seen in a number of chapters in this book (e.g. Chapter 22). Far better to describe oneself as nursing elderly people, and to teach nurses, other health workers, patients and the public the true meaning of geriatrics.

SUCCESSFUL AGEING

Merton's (1957) self-fulfilling prophecy, that what we believe will happen, applies to so much in social life. It applies in part to the success or failure of the banking system, to education (teachers' expectations of students' examination performance), to sexism and what we expect of women (see Chapter 16 by Christine Webb), and to ageing and old age. If we expect low quality we will get it. This has been supported by research, particularly in long-term settings for elderly people (Evers 1981a, b, Baker 1983) and is discussed with reference to old people with dementia by Julia Brooking in Chapter 18.

With the self-fulfilling prophecy in mind, Novak (1983) set out to study 'good ageing' by interviewing 60 active, 'successful', old people in Canada. She wanted to find the healthiest, happiest, most articulate people possible. She justifies this sample bias by arguing that the number in this group will expand and we can learn from them in order to help others. She suggested, 'We need to look at the best ageing has to offer so that we are not doomed by our own expectations to bring about the worst' (p 232).

The overriding finding from this study was that good age does not come without psychological effort. A clear series of three stages emerged which defined positive development from mid-life to old age, but this pattern was visible only for those who had successfully

moved into late life. It was true regardless of ethnic background, sex or income. All three stages were associated with a realisation that ageing should not be denied. People who deny that they are ageing because they want to stay young are less likely to prepare for ageing or to cope successfully with old age. The cost of denial is the shock that one has aged. The first stage is the *challenge*, realising that change must occur, not denying the fact of ageing and identifying new goals. Then comes the *acceptance*, accepting the challenge that alternative goals are necessary. This transition is not easy and may cause anxiety. It takes courage to age successfully. Finally, the stage of *affirmation*, when the old person can affirm that she has accepted ageing and is no longer part of the work-oriented hierarchy; she has accepted that she is taking part in a different 'game'. No longer does she strive for high status rewards but is much more concerned with family and friends. Novak maintains that affirmation is the discovery of the meaning of one's life, and, once discovered, the old person is more likely to help other people. This in itself avoids isolation and meaninglessness to one's life.

Health, social, education and voluntary services can do much to help old people age successfully, but they must first lose their traditional attitudes and assumptions. Jay (1983) observes that for generations it has been assumed that medical advances improve health. Local health initiatives organised by community groups are challenging this assumption, by demystifying medicine, by emphasising prevention rather than cure, and by educating the public towards a better understanding of the meaning of health and of ways of achieving good health. Community health councils (CHCs), established in England in 1974, were the first real attempt to introduce a line of communication for the public and to encourage community participation. They could be much more influential than they are but they are given very little power to influence the priorities for care and the allocation of funds. As Jay points out, some members of the medical profession, who may feel a threat to their own vested interest, may be hostile towards CHCs, and there has been controversy and uncertainty about their future. They should be developed as an effective consumer voice, not threatened (Batchelor 1984).

Locally-based health projects (such as self-help groups) have had a mixed reception from the medical and nursing professions, who often see them as a threat to their own work. But on the contrary, these projects have not been set up to compete with conventional services so much as to complement National Health Service provision, and to avoid illness and the need to burden the services. Effective health promotion through prevention rather than treatment has the greatest chance for significantly reducing ill health and mortality in industrialised countries, and it is encouraging to learn that many general practitioners, nurses and health visitors are working closely with community groups to this end, and are enthusiastic about what is being achieved.

Hospital and community nurses can do much to help old people to become healthy, stay healthy and look after themselves. Old people could remain passive recipients of health care information and services, or they could be encouraged to take an active part in planning and practising preventive health care. They could also be listened to more. Nurses would understand old peoples' beliefs and attitudes better so that they may help them appreciate why some of these views may be incompatible with health. Most elderly people, and unfortunately, many nurses and doctors, believe that health problems of the elderly are due to old age and must be accepted. Understanding this fallacy should be central to any preventive work. Old people and their professional and lay carers can learn that much ill health can be prevented as well as treated.

Exercise benefits everyone, even old and frail people who have chronic diseases. It will increase fitness rather than 'wear out' the body which some old people actually believe. Evidence about good and bad diet has grown enormously, and what constitutes a healthy diet today is very different from 40 years ago. Sugar, salt, butter, cream, rich meats, white bread and refined foods used to be the recognised foods of high quality in Britain rather than the unrefined, wholefood, high roughage, low fat diet advocated today (see Chapter 11 by Sue Thomas). It is extremely difficult to change the habits of a lifetime particularly when there is no obvious sign of ill health (as with high blood pressure or constipation), and when taste buds deteriorate so much that it is tempting to add even more seasonings.

It is not only the old people who need education about healthy living; friends, relatives and health care workers may also hold mistaken beliefs. Often the old person's behaviour will not change without change in attitudes and behaviour of their supporters. Education is available to old people in pre-retirement groups, Open University courses, old people's clubs and special health courses for the elderly. Nurses have a valuable opportunity to give patients health care information and advice on an individual basis in hospital and the community, based on their knowledge of the patient's previous lifestyle. They could exploit the opportunity much more than they do, by a change in their own attitudes and awareness and enhancement of their own skills, particularly skills of communication.

REFERENCES

Acheson E D 1982 The impending crisis of old age: a challenge to ingenuity. Lancet 1: 592–594

Baker D E 1983 'Care' in the geriatric ward: an account of two styles of nursing. In: Wilson-Barnett J (ed) Nursing research: ten studies in patient care. Wiley, Chichester

Ballard R 1983 Race and the census: what an 'ethnic' question would show. New Society 64: 212–214

Batchelor I 1984 Policies for a crisis? Some aspects of DHSS policies for care of the elderly. Occasional Papers No. 1, Nuffield Provincial Hospitals Trust, London

Borkman T 1982 Ageism. In: Kolker A, Ahmed P I (eds) Aging. Elsevier, New York

Brocklehurst J C 1984 What's in a name. New Age 24:28

Davies A 1982 Elderly, British and black. Voluntary Action 13: 18–19

Ernst N S, Glazer-Waldman H R (eds) 1983 The aged patient: a source book for the allied health professional. Year Book Medical Publishers, Chicago

Evers H 1981a Woman patients in long-stay geriatric wards. In: Hutter B, Williams G (eds) Controlling women: the normal and the deviant. Croom Helm, London

Evers H 1981b Tender loving care. In: Copp L A (ed) Care of the aging. Recent advances in nursing series, no. 2, Churchill Livingstone, Edinburgh

Evers H 1983 Elderly women and disadvantage: perceptions of daily life and support relationships. In: Jerrome D (ed) Ageing in modern society. Croom Helm, London

Hodgson J 1984 The age of statistics: in the USSR, US and UK. British Journal of Geriatric Nursing 3(5): 12–15

Isaacs B 1981 Ageing and the doctor. In: Hobman D (ed) The impact of ageing: strategies for care. Croom Helm, London

Jay P 1983 Health for all: a role for the community. Journal of the Royal College of Physicians 17: 2, 93–94

Kuhn M 1980 Grass-roots gray power. In: Fuller M M, Martin C A (eds) The older woman: lavender rose or gray panther. Charles C Thomas, Springfield, Illinois, ch 23

Lewis M, Butler R N 1980 Why is Women's Lib ignoring old women? In: Fuller M M, Martin C A (eds) The older woman: lavender rose or gray panther. Charles C Thomas, Springfield, Illinois, ch 22

Macdonald B, Rich C 1984 Look me in the eye: old women, aging and agism. Spinsters Ink, San Francisco

Merton R K 1957 Social theory and social structure, Revised edn. Free Press, Illinois

Norman A 1984 Word play. New Age 24:29

Novak M 1983 Discovering a good life. International Journal of Ageing and Human Development 16: 231–239

Phillipson C 1982 Capitalism and the construction of old age. Macmillan, London

Roebuck J 1983 Grandma as revolutionary: elderly women and some modern patterns of social change. International Journal of Ageing and Human Development 17: 249–266

Rossiter C, Wicks M 1982 Crisis or challenge? Family care, elderly people and social policy. Study Commission on the Family

Shegog R F A (ed) 1981 The impending crisis of old age: a challenge to ingenuity. Oxford University Press

S. J. Redfern

29

The elderly patient

In the previous chapter, the discussion focused on the elderly person living in a youth-oriented, industrialised society. In this chapter, we focus on the frail old person who requires continued support in an institutional setting or who needs shorter-term hospital care. The chapter contains two sections, one on the quality of living and the other on the quality of dying. No attempt has been made to be comprehensive in coverage but the aim has been to discuss issues, some of which have been raised in earlier chapters, and which require thought and debate by nurses. The choice of issues is based largely on those raised by students. They are profoundly concerned about what they see as the plight of old people who are 'living' and dying in our hospitals and residential Homes, where the opportunity for a fulfilling life or comfortable and peaceful death may not be available to them.

We hope that readers will find these issues sufficiently contentious to want to debate them in their own settings and, in doing so, will examine the quality of care they give to their own patients.

QUALITY OF LIVING

A great deal of research has been published on the quality of life and on nursing care in different settings for old people. In this section, we look at two issues in nursing which have not, on the whole, emerged as high quality aspects of patient care. The first is communicating with elderly patients or clients and the second is the organisation of nursing care of old people in different institutional settings. Striking an optimum balance between allowing old people the rights to which any adult is entitled and avoiding unnecessary risk is a theme which runs through the whole chapter and is perhaps the key to successful and high quality nursing. It continues in the discussion of surgery for old people. Two surgical conditions are singled out for discussion because they are so common: the aged hip and vascular problems of the lower limbs, some of which require amputation.

Communicating with elderly patients

The research published on the amount and quality of communication with elderly patients makes sobering reading. Levels of social interaction between nurses and elderly patients are low, are even lower for elderly confused patients and do not increase when more nurses are on duty (Miller 1978, Wells 1980, Godlove et al 1981, Gilbert 1984; Jill Macleod Clark in chapter 4 of this book).

Godlove et al (1981) observed 65 old people in day hospitals, hospital wards, local authority old people's Homes, and day centres in London. Although the staff were aware of the observers, the most consistent finding was that, between 10 a.m. and 4 p.m., most of the old people spent most of their time doing nothing (70% in hospital wards, 62% in old people's Homes, 54% in day hospitals, and 51% in day centres; Richard 1983). Those who attended day hospitals spent only 18% of their time on rehabilitation and treatment activities, which was less than the time spent on these activities in day centres, whose primary function is to meet social needs. Interaction through conversation or physical contact was lowest in the old people's Homes (3%) and the day centres (5%), and rather more in the hospital wards (11%) and the day hospitals (18%), although nowhere was it very substantial.

Staffing levels did not vary significantly between the settings, and the researchers observed examples of both downright cruelty on the one hand and sensitive staff on the other doing their utmost to retain some dignity and comfort for their patients. The authors suggest that nurses in training should spend time doing similar observations of nurse–patient interaction and should discuss their findings with ward and teaching staff. This could be educational for everyone.

A resident of an old people's Home has experienced such inadequate care and has had the courage to write about it (Chambers 1982). She maintains that the objectives of care are inadequate, and advocates two steps to catalyse change. Firstly, consumer participation in the way lives are organised with residents' committees taking an active and influential role. Consumer participation is discussed in more detail in the next section. A 'listening service', which would enable a resident to discuss anything with a sympathetic listener. This could help sort out problems, avoid loneliness, and enhance feelings of worth. Many residents have the skills and qualities to do this for their companions. It is a tragedy that nurses and other care staff do so little.

Organising nursing care of old people

We are constantly being told that 'old age is not an illness', but this phrase becomes ambiguous when applied to very old people. It is helpful because it encourages society to adopt positive expectations about ageing and old age and it discourages old people from sinking into a sick role. On the other hand, increasing frailty is inevitable with very old age, and so even if not a 'sickness' in the medical sense, the care required is not very different from that needed by people who are sick, dependent or disabled (e.g. the stroke or multiple sclerosis victim). Nurses have the most important role of all health care workers in getting the balance right between fulfilling the nursing needs of old people and ensuring as much independence as possible, and a sense of well-being and purpose in life. Much of the research shows that nurses fail to get the balance right and are more concerned with the risks that independence must carry, than with the rights that old people, like anyone else, have in choosing the way they live.

It is easy for nurses who look after frail, dependent and often ill old people in hospital wards to assume that very little can be done because these are inevitable consequences of old age. These nurses do not often see healthy old people as part of their work, and so they tend to generalise what they see to all old people. The outcome may be inadvertently to encourage these old people in their care to enter into vicious cycles of disability and dependency, which involve a loss of function and activity in excess of that which can be explained by the undeniable fact of ageing or by the effects of disease (Muir Gray 1984). The disability cycle starts with the loss of function resulting from disabling disease which leads to the loss of ability to perform certain actions. The joint stiffness, muscle weakness and loss of confidence which result from typical disease produce further loss of function and an inability to perform more actions. The vicious cycle of dependency makes matters worse. The increasing difficulty an old person has in performing a task means that someone else will probably do it for her. She is less likely to perform it and other activities on subsequent occasions, she will be less involved in decision making, will lose mental and physical fitness and become increasingly dependent and disabled.

When chronic disease is present, it is essential for nurses to promote and sustain exercise in order to prevent loss of fitness, strength and stamina. They should encourage old people to undertake their own personal care and also to keep exercising, such as stretching, walking, dancing, cycling or swimming. One man of 89 years emphasises how much more stable and mobile he is on a bicycle than on his feet (Clark-Kennedy 1982). The fear of accident so often takes precedence, that nurses, other health workers and relatives at home overprotect the old person and inadvertently assist the vicious cycles. Old people are resourceful and self-reliant if

allowed to be. The job of nurses and other health professionals is to work on their disabilities and handicaps so that they do not interfere with that resourcefulness and self-reliance.

The balance between rights and risks

No one has complete liberty and freedom of choice, but old people have less than most. 'There are ways in which society further restricts this narrowing range of choice by imposing on elderly people forms of care and treatment which are the fruit of social perception, social anxiety, convenience and custom rather than inescapable necessity' (Norman 1980, p 3).

This lack of choice, which has been mentioned in other chapters of this book, (e.g. Chapters 2, 7, 23) occurs in all settings. Old people are removed from their homes when they could have remained there with support; they are deprived of dignity in hospitals and old people's Homes, and are not consulted about their care and treatment. Norman (1980) highlights the fundamental need for a change in attitude by society, health and social workers, and old people themselves, away from paternalistic overprotection from risk towards the right to self-determination for each person within the limits of available resources.

Old people in institutions are treated very differently from those outside. Outside, people are permitted to rock climb and hang-glide even though the costs of rescue and disaster are high. Old people at home can live at considerable risk of accidents because of their unsafe environment. But in residential Homes fire precautions have to be so extensive that the increased fees necessary for covering the cost mean that old people cannot afford to live there, or their mobility is reduced because they cannot get through heavy fire doors with a walking-frame. They are not asked how much risk they are prepared to take. The fear of scandal, disaster and litigation takes precedence.

The problem may be even worse for

confused old people living at home. Pressure from relatives and neighbours on the police, the welfare services and the primary health care team to remove an old lady from her familiar decrepitude, neglect and squalor to a clean, efficient hospital or residential Home, can be overwhelming for her. There, her confusion, bewilderment and anxiety are likely to increase; she can no longer choose what she does; she becomes restless, disoriented, anorexic and increasingly frail, apathetic, and incontinent; and she knows no one. She is given drugs to calm her down, which increase her confusion and incontinence, and the outcome is a chest infection and death within a few days. This occurs even though she was healthy but dirty when admitted. Or, she may survive at the cost of becoming depersonalised, accepting of loving care and attention by the nurses, being totally dependent with no choice and responsibilities. Skilled nursing and medical care can keep her alive but at what cost to her quality of life? She might have preferred death.

This is an extreme case, but it does happen. It raises the difficulty of getting the balance right between respecting the rights and wishes of the old lady and those of her neighbours and relatives. It may be right to let her live in squalor and to refuse help if this does not cause danger or inconvenience to her or her neighbours, but the difficulty is knowing what level of inconvenience to the neighbours outweighs an individual's choice to stay at home. Perhaps the answer is to ensure that the health care team in the hospital or residential Home get the balance right between the risk of independence and the risk of institutionalisation.

Loss of one's home results in bereavement and produces a grief reaction similar to that occurring when losing a relative. There is plenty of evidence that the mortality rate is high during the first three months after moving to an institution, and this occurs irrespective of the condition of the old person or the nature of the institution (Norman 1980). Cognitive ability, physical status, personality factors, and preparing thoroughly for the change are powerful predictors of successful relocation. But it is those who would be the most successful in adapting who are the least likely to need to be moved, because they have their own resources and initiative. Norman also maintains that the evidence suggests more fatal accidents occur in institutions than at home (even allowing for the greater frailty of institutional residents), and so if the main objective is to avoid 'risk', then relocation in an institution may not be the answer.

Most elderly people admitted to hospital for medical treatment recover and return home. But some become longer-term patients because the relatively minor illness has caused a crisis in the system of support at home. It is often the case, except in progressive geriatric units, that a disease is given as the reason for admission rather than that the spouse cannot manage. This means that the real reason may not be the focus of attention and the old person may find it difficult to get fit enough to go home. Or the patient may be detained in hospital because other diseases, which she has lived with for years, are diagnosed. In an acute medical ward, there may not be the facilities, staff nor motivation to take time to rehabilitate her, with the result that prolonged rehabilitation in a geriatric unit is necessary before she can go home. The long period away from home may have, in Norman's (1980) terms, closed up the 'social space', and the outcome may be long-term care and a gradual move towards Muir Gray's (1984) vicious cycles of disability and dependency. Thus, although hospital admission for old people may be life saving, the dangers must be weighed against the advantages. This problem is increasingly recognised by geriatricians, especially those who do home visits before admission and find out about the patient's circumstances. The wish to keep the old person at home if possible is paramount, and if hospital admission is necessary, the aim is that it should be as short as possible.

Similar problems can occur when old people move to residential Homes. The problems may be worse because in hospital the patient is only in danger of becoming a permanent resident, whereas in a residential Home this is virtually a certainty. It is important that a full medical and social assessment is done before the decision to move into a residential Home is made, irrespective of whether the move is from home or hospital. This will ensure that the move is the right decision for the old person.

Moving to live with a child is also a loss. It may not be successful or not turn out to be permanent, and since the old person will have given up her home, the outcome may be a residential Home or long-stay hospital. If such a move is permanent, the old person's needs may not be met because of an overprotective, anxious daughter. Norman (1980) points out that much more public education is needed concerning the advantages and disadvantages of an old person moving in with her child's family, and about the potential danger of meeting the child's anxieties and needs rather than the old person's wishes. We need to move towards a system where old people either give up their homes because they want to or, if it is impossible for them or their family to cope at home, are supported by the full range of statutory and voluntary domiciliary services.

Nursing old people in hospital

In Chapter 22, Helen Evers discusses the development of geriatric medicine and nursing; in Chapter 23, Barbara Wade illustrates the lack of choice found in so many long-term settings; and in Chapter 7, Amanda Stokes-Roberts discusses what can be done to enhance well-being of patients and residents in institutions. A generally depressing picture reported in research studies concerning the organisation of nursing care emerges. Some of the issues they have raised are given further attention here. The issue of rights versus risk is particularly relevant to old people in hospital. It is not unusual to see today's hospital wards, particularly long-stay ones, retaining the traditions of the old public hospitals, with rigid lines of authority, housed in a barely disguised workhouse where the patients still carry the stigma

of weakness and social incompetence, are seen as recipients of charity and are expected to be obedient, submissive and grateful (Norman 1980). The principles of compulsion and custody continue. Patients are admitted or ordered to hospital, are detained there, and are released. This is the language of custody, not hospitality. Attitudes associated with the Poor Laws continue—relegation, obedience, batch processing and lack of choice.

Hospitals need certain rules to achieve their primary aims of healing and rehabilitation, which result inevitably in some loss of autonomy. But, in many long-stay wards, rules inhibit autonomy and work against the goal of rehabilitation. If an old person cannot retain her dignity and autonomy as an individual, she cannot be successful at establishing herself back into the community, nor can she possibly become a purposeful being in a long-stay ward.

Elderly patients in long-stay wards may be subjected to routines and deprived of more choice than that given a two-year-old. In Chapter 25 of this book, Pauline Fielding refers to the routinisation and depersonalisation of hospital patients. Hospital routines of times for rising and retiring and mealtimes are usually extremely rigid and totally different to one's routine at home. Opportunity for choice is often missing. For example, choice of menu: although a choice exists, it is so often the case that the menus are filled in by a nurse or ward clerk (Wade et al 1983). Staff in geriatric wards encourage their patients to dress in dayclothes, but so often the patients have no choice, and the dress worn last week may turn up on someone else next week. Clothing should be personal, labelled, attractive, dignified and sufficient. It should include a full complement of underwear, including suspender belts to keep stockings up. It follows that a personal clothing system requires an adequate selection, labelling, laundry, ironing, storage and repair service, which many wards do not have, even though this has been Department of Health and Social Security policy since 1972 (DHSS 1972). A number of studies have shown the successful outcome of implementing a personal clothing service (Adams 1984, for a review of the literature).

Control of money is a function most of us take for granted. It is anomalous that pensioners in Britain are required to give up earned benefit in return for long-term medical and nursing care, but the hospital providing the care gets no direct benefit (Norman 1980). Retirement pensions are reduced by £13.60 per week after an old person with no dependants has been in hospital for eight weeks, and drop to £6.80 after one year (Smith 1984). The rationale is that the sum taken covers the costs of living at home and these are now met by the National Health Service. But in reality elderly patients forego their income and economic independence and receive no benefit since they 'live' in some of the worst conditions in the health service. In some long-stay wards patients do not even get the £6.80. The administration's fear of theft overrides the old person's need for independence and dignity. Norman (1980) describes one hospital where a clerk visits every patient every two weeks to inform her how much money she owns, and to discuss what she would like to buy. It could be a personal television or radio, a present for relatives, a bottle of brandy, a regular supply of wholemeal bread, or a taxi ride round the town. Why is this not done by more hospitals? It could be a valuable role for volunteers.

As Helen Evers makes clear in Chapter 22, helping elderly patients to maintain or increase their independence has not been a high nursing priority in the past. With the development of progressive geriatric units, however, the necessity of maintaining independence is now realised although nurses have been slow to discard their protective role. Clarke (1978) describes how nurses working in a psychogeriatric ward unintentionally socialised their patients into dependency. The aims of the nurses were to keep the patients fed, clean and dry and they worked hard to achieve this. The valued nurse was one who did not 'waste time' listening, talking, writing, and encouraging independence in her patients. The valued patient was silent and submissive and allowed herself to be treated as a dependent product to be processed gratefully.

Many nurses working in geriatric wards have positive attitudes towards working with old people, but they are often patronising and emphasise ritualistic routines rather than giving individualised care to the patients (Wells 1980). Wells maintains that responsibility for the problem lies primarily with nursing education. If students are not taught to give nursing care using an individualised, problem-solving approach, and allowed to practise that way of nursing in all clinical settings, then few nurses responsible for the delivery of care will be in a position to stimulate change and improve the quality of nursing.

Caring for the old is a low status specialty in nursing and it is likely that many nurses working in geriatric wards do so out of convenience rather than a genuine desire to enhance the quality of care for old people. Much of the work is described as dull, 'basic' and unskilled and can be left to untrained nursing students and auxiliaries. 'Real' nursing comprises the high status work of 'dressings, drips and drama' (Evers 1981a) and is not found in long-stay wards. 'Basic' nursing is heavily routinised, and easily conforms to rigid hierarchical control. This acts as another constraint to individualised care and innovation.

In contrast to this view, the pioneers in nursing old people (e.g. Norton 1965) insist that it is this speciality which provides the opportunity for 'real' nursing because the emphasis is on the caring role of the nurse. Sander and Walden (1984) emphasise the challenge of nursing elderly people and the need for nurses in this field to become specialists. Evers (1981a) found that those nurses who preferred to work on geriatric wards did so because of the opportunity they had to care for the 'whole person' rather than a diseased organ, and to get to know the patients and their relatives really well. Yet despite this, care observed by Clarke (1978), Wells (1980), Evers (1981a, 1981b) and Baker (1983) was routinised and task oriented.

Evers (1981b) makes it clear that the predominantly 'warehousing' approach to patient care fails to fulfil the objectives for hospital care of the elderly explicit in various government and other policy documents (e.g. Department of Health and Social Security 1978, 1979, British Geriatrics Society and Royal College of Nursing 1975). She identified four objectives:

(a) to make full use of all diagnostic and rehabilitation resources with the aim of discharging patients from hospital as soon as possible;

(b) to promote patients' physical and psychological independence whilst in hospital;

(c) to enable patients to engage in purposeful activity whilst in hospital in order to ensure their self-esteem and an optimum quality of life;

(d) to give patients access to the multidisciplinary team who have specific expertise in the care of the elderly.

The energy found in progressive geriatric units enables perhaps all the objectives to be fulfilled for the 'acute career' patient, who follows the medical model of diagnosis–treatment–cure–discharge home. This success has been due largely to the initiative of geriatricians, supported by nurses and therapeutic staff. In long-stay wards, however, where geriatricians have not taken the lead, care often falls far short of all these objectives. As the research quoted shows, the factors which produce institutionalisation (depersonalisation, social distance, block treatment, lack of variation in daily routine) described by King and Raynes (1968) are prevalent. The 'mortification' or psychological self-extinction (Goffman 1961) of the inmates of the total institution can still be found in long-stay settings. Nurses have been slow to take up the challenge of the long-stay patient. Here is a specialty which is crying out for improvement and in which the nurse could take a key role. Where progress has been made the initiative has usually come from someone else, occupational therapists and physiotherapists (Glossop 1983), or clinical psychologists (Woods and Holden 1982), with nurses taking very little interest except perhaps in some progressive units for the elderly mentally ill (e.g. Rowden 1983).

We could speculate on the many reasons which could account for this nursing apathy, but perhaps one of the most important is their training, which is medically oriented and hospital based. Relatively little attention is given to acquiring interpersonal communication skills, to psychosocial care and social policy. Happily, undergraduate nursing students in the British universities and polytechnics are educated in the social sciences as well as the basic medical sciences, and many of these students choose to work with the elderly because of the opportunities for responsibility, autonomy and challenge that this kind of nursing offers. But the innovative nurse will find it very difficult to discuss and implement new ideas unless she or he is supported by a progressive geriatric team which is open to change. Staff in a more traditional, closed environment are likely to feel threatened by innovation, will close ranks, and either force the innovater to conform to their practices or to leave. Achieving change on one's own is close to impossible for the relatively junior ward nurse. There appear to be two options for success. Either the nurse implements her ideas through an understanding doctor, in which case the nursing staff view the idea as a medical instruction and therefore as credible; this approach cannot enhance the emerging professionalisation of nursing. Or all the nurses on the ward, the untrained, those in training, and the qualified nurses, go on a course together so that the ideas for change can be discussed by all of them and they all feel part of the decision-making process. They will be more likely to have an interest in seeing changes implemented successfully than if they had been excluded. In this case, the ward would have to be closed for a short period, and this could be timed to coincide with a period of ward redecoration.

In defence of those nurses who do attempt to innovate and improve patient care, they sometimes find that it is very difficult to give high quality care or to achieve change because the resources to provide a minimum service are not available. The nurse is in a dilemma if she (or he) cannot provide the care she knows is required. She can take the traditional course of action chosen by many nurses, that is, make the best of things and keep quiet. Or, she can voice her concerns loudly and agitate for change. Nurses are more enthusiastic about publicising examples of poor standards of care in the nursing press, and agitation like this is important. Nurses have a professional responsibility to document instances when they are forced to let patients down or when they cannot be the patient's advocate. They should shout about failing the patient rather than respond defensively.

There are, of course, examples where local initiatives have been taken successfully by nurses, particularly in small community hospitals where the environment is less clinical and can be made more homely. One example is the work at Burford Cottage Hospital in Oxfordshire, England, where nurses have taken the lead. The care is individualised, planned and evaluated, the nurses receive continuing education and support in primary nursing and introducing change, and nursing research is encouraged (Swaffield 1983).

Over the past decade in Britain the nursing process has been recommended as the method of organising nursing care, and professional and educational bodies in nursing are advocating its widespread use. But very little research has been done in Britain to evaluate the quality of patient care, although there have been workload and audit studies to assess the quantity of nursing and the relationship with staff appraisal (Miller 1984). Miller, however, has studied the quality of care. She compared two different methods of work organisation (nursing process and task allocation) in geriatric wards in terms of their effect on patients. Her first difficulty was in finding geriatric wards which really were using the nursing process. She located 10 hospitals in Britain which claimed to be using it in at least one geriatric ward, but the number dropped to five when Miller applied specific criteria: the existence of written care plans, no

fragmentation of care, continuity of care, co-ordination of care and accountability for care. She paired each nursing process ward with a 'matched' task allocation ward, and compared them on physical, psychological and social outcomes of care.

The results were different for short- and long-stay (more than one month) patients. There was no difference in patient outcome for short-stay patients, who were occupied with intensive medical and therapeutic intervention. In contrast, there were large and significant differences between the two kinds of ward for long-stay patients. Long-stay patients in the nursing process wards were much happier, much less incontinent (urinary and faecal), much less dependent and undertook much more self-care than those in the task allocation wards. It is clear that individualised, planned nursing care is essential for long-stay patients because it enhances their quality of life. Miller also counters the persistant cry that the nursing process cannot be implemented because of lack of staff. She found that there was no increase in the quantity of nursing given to patients in the nursing process wards except that nurses talked with them more. Thus it is the method of work organisation rather than staffing levels which affects outcome for long-stay patients.

These results are exciting and show the challenge and scope for change in the care of old people which nurses could initiate. We are sufficiently optimistic to believe that initiatives like those at Burford and in Miller's nursing process wards will spread. Nurses caring for old people in institutions will become less medically oriented and less apathetic. They will do much more to encourage patients to retain their self-respect and their dignity, to avoid depression and the 'learned helplessness' syndrome (Seligman 1975) and to look forward to the future.

Care of the old people in residential Homes

There is widespread evidence that the distribution of dependency and need for nursing of old people is similar in residential Homes and long-stay geriatric wards (Wade et al 1983), and Barbara Wade herself discusses this in Chapter 23 of this book. Much of the discussion in the previous section, therefore, applies to old people in residential Homes (local authority or 'Part III', voluntary and private Homes). There is also evidence (Peace 1983, Willcocks et al 1983) that residents want control over their environment, single bedrooms, self-determination in activities of daily living, and no enforced participation in communal activities. These authors argue that the needs of the individual should take precedence over group needs and living accommodation should consist of residential flatlets which are lockable and which contain full toilet/washing facilities, plenty of storage space, snack-making equipment and space for one's own furniture and for entertaining visitors. Communual rooms should be provided for meals and relaxation with television and bar facilities.

It is important to cater for different needs and to provide a variety of facilities. Norman (1984) discusses the advantages of the 'hotel' model and the 'group unit' model of living and suggests that the advantages of both should be available. Residents would have the freedom to be alone when they wished and at other times to meet other residents and participate in group activities and carrying out chores. A high quality of life and self-determination has been achieved in some residential Homes even when the physical facilities have been less than ideal.

Old people living in residential Homes are entitled, as is any other adult, to control their own activities, finances and social affairs unless restriction is required in order to provide necessary care, or to protect the lives of other residents. Some residential Homes achieve this autonomy and make a real effort to improve residents' quality of life even if it means increasing the risks taken. Others are not homely, they are rigid, routinised, institutional, and residents are not consulted or given choice. The residents' day is organised to suit the staff, independence is not encouraged, there is very little privacy, residents are required to surrender their pension books and they do not participate with daily chores (Norman 1980). The Department of Health and Social Security (1978) has urged local authorities to make improvements. It recommends that old people should have control of their pension books, should choose their own food from the menu, have flexible mealtimes, be able to come and go as they please, choose when to get up and go to bed, choose and keep their own clothes, have access to facilities for making snacks, have space for entertaining visitors and help in running the Home. These opportunities should be available for all those who wish it. Those who do not want to, or cannot take such control should be exceptions. Allowing this kind of autonomy and quality of life involves necessary risk, and this should be recognised by service staff.

Residential Homes will become homely only if all the staff are proud of and independent in their work. But 'as long as residential care of the elderly is perceived as a second-class occupation which provides 'warehousing' for 'geriatrics' and does not require professional skills or offer adequate reward, those who work in this field will pass on their sense of uselessness and rejection to residents' (Norman 1980, p 41). There is a long way to go before care of old people is seen to be a rewarding and valuable specialty. Before this happens, change must occur to the status of 'geriatrics', to societal attitudes towards elderly people, to pay and conditions of service for staff and to education of staff.

There is no doubt that some old people want dependence and no effort or responsibility. Should they be persuaded to be less passive, dependent and immobile? There is no question that individuals should be allowed to exercise choice even if that means passivity. Some people will choose dependence if they find themselves in a large-scale, anonymous old people's Home, whereas they would want to retain independence and choice if the Home were small, friendly and homely, without imposed group activities. The aim should be to keep life to as close as it was at home, or to improve it, since many old people are very inactive at home. This process of 'normalisation' implies that normal activities outside and inside the Home are continued—visiting shops, pubs, church, friends and relatives, walking in the park, voting on polling day.

An excellent idea is the 'written contract' (Norman 1980) which is agreed between resident and residential Home when the resident arrives. It should be individualised and identify clearly any necessary rules and regulations of the Home and the reasons for them. It should stipulate that the Home would never prevent individual choice unless there was a clear danger to the resident or to others, and that certain activities (bathing alone, locking doors, going to the pub alone) would not be prevented as long as the resident was able to make the choice responsibly and was aware of the risks. This kind of contract would reduce the Home's obsession with safety at all costs and the fear of litigation which dominates so much decision making. Patients in the United States are accustomed to receiving a standard statement of their rights, but this is not common practice in Britain. However, Norman (1980) refers to an initiative taken by East Sussex County Council. Since 1979, this authority has developed a standard contract for all residents in its old people's Homes. The contract makes clear that staff and management accept that some risk is inevitable, and it refers to quality of life, independence and choice, responsibility for one's own actions, privacy, consultation and participation in decision making, access to community health facilities, going out, having visitors and one's own possessions. There is a formal complaints procedure, and regular monitoring of residents' opinions. It is very encouraging to see this initative, and other authorities could follow East Sussex's lead. It is, however, sobering that such contracts are necessary, and it reflects an erosion of old people's rights.

The increased dependency of residents in old people's Homes means that many require skilled nursing care, and the community nursing services find it difficult to meet this need in addition to their existing caseloads. No one denies that nursing care should be given, but district nurses have argued that residential Homes should employ their own nurses who could ensure continuity of care. Making use of district nurses means that this care must be fragmented and much needed nursing time and skill is taken away from old people living in their own homes (Bleatham and Bowling 1983). The argument put forward against employing nurses in residential Homes is that they will become like hospitals. This underlines the recommendation that nurses need training in psychosocial care and in methods of work organisation which enable old people's physical needs to be met within a homely, non-clinical atmosphere. This should help to remove the conflict between social work values and the medical model of care so often raised by social workers (Willcocks et al 1983).

The Centre for Policy on Ageing, in London, is concerned to ensure an adequate quality and quantity of care for old people living at home as well as in residential Homes. The two services should be complementary, not alternatives for resources, and they should overlap. For example, residential Homes could provide day and weekend care, temporary care after discharge from hospital, short-stay care to relieve the family, and rehabilitation after bereavement, illness or self-neglect. There could be a more flexible use of all settings—home, residential Home, nursing Home, hospital—which encourages independence and promotes a high quality of life for old people who need support.

The case for National Health Service nursing Homes

In Chapter 22, Helen Evers discusses the wisdom of a non-medicalised nursing care facility for old people requiring long-term nursing care, and Jo Hockley (Chapter 21) mentions the potential for such units for the care of dying people. Barbara Wade, in Chapter 23, describes the study commissioned by the Department of Health and Social

Security into the development of state-run nursing Homes. In Scotland, state nursing Homes for the elderly mentally infirm, particularly, have been recommended since 1970 by the Scottish Home and Health Department (Dalley 1983), and the SHHD has monitored the success of one such unit in Glasgow (McIntosh 1983). Another unit, a state nursing Home in England, has also been extremely successful (Storrs 1982).

The 'supportive model' of organisation, described in Chapter 23, was recommended for nursing Homes, and there was virtually unanimous agreement amongst nurses in each of the settings observed that the Homes should be run by nurses. Opinions were divided concerning the other care staff. Some thought that care assistants should be sufficient, others advocated a mix of trained nurses and assistants, and still others thought that all the care staff should be trained nurses. Wade and her colleagues (1983) felt strongly that the nursing Homes would be successful only if a movement away from the medical cure-oriented approach was made, and that nurses trained in giving individualised total care were employed. The leadership style of the head of the Home would be crucial in determining the type of care given and in preventing the Homes from becoming like geriatric wards, and she or he would have to receive appropriate education for this role.

Opinion from health and social workers is divided about the likely success of the state nursing Home in terms of the residents' quality of life. Professional jealousies and territorial boundaries might prevent this new form of care from being successful because it depends on effective co-operation between these groups. Social work personnel are suspicious of medical and nursing dominance because they see the care being removed from their control and run on sick-role lines. Nurses are enthusiastic and see an opportunity for expanding their role, and most doctors are either fairly neutral or strongly against the idea because they see it as an erosion of medical control (Dalley 1983). One doctor, however, a psychiatrist (Batchelor 1984), argues strongly for nurse-run nursing Homes. He maintains that nurses have the ability and the motivation to take such responsibility, and that too much attention has been paid by the Department of Health and Social Security to warnings expressed by doctors that standards of care will fall.

Two conclusions (among others) emerged clearly from the study by Wade and her colleagues (1983). The hospital environment is inappropriate in meeting the needs of old people requiring long-term care, and staffing and therapeutic input to local authority residential Homes is inadequate to meet the needs of residents because so many are highly dependent on nursing care and surveillance. The authors recommended that long-stay geriatric wards should be phased out, except for a few kept for 'holiday admissions' to relieve caring families, and short-stay admissions for medical and psychogeriatric assessment and intervention. Alternative provision should be provided in state nursing Homes but taking account of the role of residential Homes. If there were no change made to the residential Homes, then a three-tier system would emerge:

(a) Nursing Homes run by the National Health Service with extensive nursing care and rehabilitation
(b) Private nursing Homes
(c) Residential Homes run by social service departments of local authorities which need but do not have the resources of the nursing Homes.

The health and social services in this country are run by different, inflexible bureaucracies with different local boundaries. As Wade and her colleagues maintain, the logical solution would be to develop a new form of care which would incorporate aspects of both nursing and residential Homes, and would be the responsibility of a single administrative body containing representatives of both the health and social services. This would allow nursing and therapeutic input to be directed where it was most needed, and continuity of care for old people would be achieved without them having to move when they became dependent.

There should also be the means for this joint administrative body to liaise with a third bureaucracy, the housing department which provides sheltered housing (described in Chapter 26). If the present sheltered housing schemes had 'very sheltered housing' and nursing Home-type annexes, then old people living there who came to require more care would not have to be moved. Legislation is required for the necessary flexibility to be achieved. If state nursing Homes are set up within the existing framework, then the present inequalities in the care provision for the elderly will continue.

It will take a long time before state nursing Homes are introduced across the country. In the meantime, some old people are living out their lives in misery in long-stay hospitals and residential Homes. Nurses have a responsibility and a great opportunity to take the initiative in the care of these old people, to improve their quality of life and to achieve the satisfaction of doing 'real' nursing.

Surgery for old people

A substantial proportion of the beds in surgical wards are occupied by elderly people. Vowles (1979) found in Devon, England, that 30% of surgical patients and more than 50% of all surgical emergency admissions were over 65 years. With increasing numbers of elderly people, the use of resources must be assessed together with the achievements gained in operating on so many old people. Is surgery the treatment of choice? Is it contributing to survival of the unfittest? How much 'heroic' surgery is performed on old people which fails to give them an increased quality of life? Are the patient and her family given an opportunity to take part in the decision to operate?

Selecting an arbitrary age limit for surgery is unethical and unsatisfactory. Many elderly people enjoy a greatly enhanced quality of life after surgery, which is its aim. The surgeon,

together with the whole health care team, including patient and relatives, must consider many factors in the decision to operate: the prognosis of disease, the risk of surgery, the chance of cure, the chance of palliation, the patient's will to live, her average life expectancy, the presence of other problems, her degree of disability, and the chances of complications developing (Vowles 1979). The surgeon should discuss all the alternatives to surgery with the patient and should help the patient make the final decision. If the patient makes an informed choice and rejects surgery, provided she is judged competent to make that decision, then it should be respected.

Vowles (1979) has identified questions that every surgeon should consider with old people:

Which is likely to be longer, the natural course of the disease or the patient's expectation of life?

Without surgery what will be the patient's quality of life?

What chance has the patient of surviving surgery?

Should the operation be elective and soon, or is it better to leave well alone and risk emergency surgery later?

Should the operation be radical and heroic or modified and palliative?

Assessment for surgery

Assessment should be comprehensive and done by the surgeon and the geriatrician, with support from the knowledge of nurses, health visitor and social worker where possible. Old people admitted to hospital have on average nine separate diagnoses (Vowles 1979) and so the medical and nursing assessment is more difficult than for a younger patient. Other problems may need attention before surgery can be contemplated. Another problem for the doctors is that the usual signs of a diagnosis, or problems post-operatively, may not occur in old people. For example, pain may be absent or vague and difficult to pinpoint; response to fever may be confusion and weakness rather than a raised temperature and abnormal white cell count; a thrombo-embolism may be 'silent' with no pleural pain or haemoptysis; vomiting may not be obvious but occur as quiet regurgitation and aspiration into the lungs. It may be difficult for an inexperienced doctor to recognise that the patient is very ill, and there is much the vigilant nurse can do to prevent disaster.

The quality of life after surgery

This should be at least as good as before surgery, and preferably better. As with anyone, old people value health over longevity, and palliative surgery which gives a few more high quality years to an 80-year-old may be preferable to radical surgery. The British Geriatrics Society's motto, 'Add life to years', is essential for surgeons to remember, particularly when the mortality rate of emergency surgery of old people is double that of elective surgery in this age group (Vowles 1979).

It is essential that the hospital team has knowledge of the patient's home circumstances, suitability of housing, the health of a spouse, etc. and that these are considered with reference to appropriate aftercare. It may be that a follow-up visit is done with the geriatrician or general practitioner (family doctor), and attendence at a day hospital might be an additional help in rehabilitation.

If the surgery was not successful, the question of whether it should have been done will be raised. This is difficult to answer, but Vowles (1979) refers to a study done in the Oxford region of England in which 750 patients over the age of 65 years had elective surgery. The conclusions reached were that, on the whole, patients whose operations had relieved their symptoms lived fuller lives than before the operation, and those whose symptoms were not relieved, or who developed new ones, led more restricted lives. Mortality for the whole group was 8%, usually for non-surgical reasons. The dilemma of whether or not to operate underlines the importance of assessing, preparing and knowing the patient and her family very well before surgery, and

ensuring that the patient and family are involved in making the decision.

Mortality rates

Following surgery, mortality is higher for old people compared with younger age groups and this should be taken into account in the decision to operate. Figures like those in Table 29.1 may cause the surgeon who wants to operate at all costs to think twice. However, age should not be the only criterion when assessing surgical risk. The increased mortality for both elective and emergency surgery is related to factors other than age (pneumonia, cardiac complications, malignancy-related complications). It is true, though, that old people with heart disease, diabetes or dementia are at greater risk (Mohr 1983).

On the other hand, if the surgeon decides to do as little as is necessary to solve the problem, which is often what is advocated, then the problem may recur when the patient is older and less able to withstand the assault of surgery. If the patient is carefully and properly assessed, prepared, anaesthetised and

Table 29.1 Mortality for abdominal surgery (emergency and elective) by age. Source: Ziffren and Hartford (1972) quoted by Vowles (1979)

Abdominal operation	Percentage mortality by age			
	<60	60–69	70–79	80+
Appendicectomy	0.1	3.3	2.7	16.6
Repair of inguinal hernia	0.1	0.2	1.6	3.3
Cholecystectomy	0.8	2.8	5.5	5.4
Partial gastrectomy	3.9	5.0	11.2	19.8
Exploratory laparotomy for inoperable lesion	6.9	9.0	16.6	31.6
Aortic graft	7.5	9.2	16.4	22.2
Closure of wound dehiscence	17.7	15.7	36.3	66.6
Resection/anastomosis of small intestine for obstruction	14.2	13.9	24.3	35.7
Partial colectomy	6.4	6.8	5.4	9.0
Abdominoperineal resection	0.7	4.3	7.6	11.5
Colostomy	5.6	8.1	8.3	14.2

given meticulous post-operative care, then most old people can survive any operation (Vowles 1979). Recovery depends mainly on avoiding complications which old people cannot cope with because they lack the necessary reserves. Vowles makes clear that the old person experiences more 'loss of elasticity' than the young, which is physical and psychological (e.g. she may give up the struggle) and so knowledge of her state of mind before the operation may be critical to her survival. Nurses caring for aged surgical patients must be involved in the decision to operate and have knowledge of the risk/benefit balance for each patient.

The aged hip

As populations age there is an increasing incidence of fractured femurs, and degenerative and rheumatoid arthritis (Ling 1979). These conditions are not fatal in themselves but their effects on health are severe, causing incessant pain, immobility and a reduced quality of life. The problems are likely to reach epidemic proportions over the next 20 years, and, without adequate planning and resources, many services and professionals will be stretched beyond breaking point (orthopaedic surgeons, geriatricians, nurses, physiotherapists, occupational therapists, psychiatrists, general practitioners, social workers, community services, and the patients' families).

Rheumatoid arthritis strikes 41% of people aged over 65 years, and virtually everyone (96%) over 75 years has osteoarthrosis (Ling 1979) although these figures are not confined to hip disease. Total hip replacement surgery, pioneered in Britain, has made a huge impact on the quality of life of old people because of the pain relief and restoration of function it brings. The benefits for old people of this operation are greater than for almost any other. From the cost-benefit point of view, too, these operations are economic, the cost of treatment being exceeded by the benefits in terms of return to productive work (Ling 1979) and avoiding burden on the services.

Arthritic conditions of the hip appear to be more common for men than women, but the incidence of fractured neck of femur is much higher for elderly women (Table 29.2). As with arthritis of the hip, the number of fractured femurs will rise in the next few years and the increased demand on the services will be enormous.

Emergency admission to hospital is essential for people with fractured femurs, and Ling (1979) suggests how the services might cope. The length of hospital stay could be reduced from a current average of 22.5 days to 20 days. This would require intensive physiotherapy and nursing resources for rehabilitation to be achieved. Secondly, the available treatment facilities could be increased, which would mean a large injection of funds, unlikely in the present economic climate. Thirdly, the number of fractures could be reduced by establishing reasons for and preventing old people from falling, by preventing and treating osteoporosis and osteomalacia, both of which weaken bone, and by reducing long-term drug effects which affect bone density. Osteomalacia is relatively easy to prevent and treat, with vitamin D and calcium. Osteoporosis is more difficult. Ling (1979) quotes evidence in favour of physical exercise, fluoride, calcium, low doses of synthetic human parathyroid hormone, and oestrogen therapy for women without ovaries.

Table 29.2 Incidence of fractured neck of femur by age and sex. Source: Gallanaugh et al (1976) quoted by Ling (1979)

		Femoral neck fractures per 1000 population								
Age:	<60	−64	−69	−74	−79	−84	−89	−94	≥95
Men		0.42	0.52	0.70	1.31	2.34	5.13	8.08	14.00	20.00
Women		0.43	1.08	1.58	3.54	6.30	13.03	22.93	32.76	26.15

Vascular problems and amputation

Arteriosclerosis increases with age, and is more prevalent for men than women until the menopause, when it equalises (Vowles and Halliday 1979). It occurs more frequently in tobacco smokers and those with diabetes mellitus or polycythaemia. Improved techniques of diabetic control mean that more diabetics survive into old age when complications are more common than for young diabetics. In fact, major arterial lesions are no more common for diabetics but, when they do occur, healing is slower and neuropathy and sepsis are more likely. Michael Hobday refers briefly to the care of the diabetic foot in Chapter 9.

Severe intermittent claudication, or pre-gangrene, often requires aorto-iliac or femoro-popliteal graft surgery. This is major surgery for old people, but it can improve their quality of life substantially. The chances of a graft remaining potent is higher in old than young people because the occlusive arteriosclerosis is probably no longer progressive.

Unfortunately, the life expectancy of the elderly arteriosclerotic amputee is not good. Seventy-five per cent survive one year, 33% survive five years and have a 50% chance of losing the other leg (Vowles and Halliday 1979). Motivation and psychological strength are essential for these old people. For some, an amputation is another sign of their inability to cope with life, but for others, it is a challenge and the relief of pain is what is important. Talking to other amputees is a great help together with communal rehabilitation with a specialist physiotherapist. Nurses can do a lot to continue this rehabilitation and to ensure that patients keep in touch with each other. Elderly amputees find artificial limbs difficult to manage, but in expert hands many will achieve independence. For those who cannot, full independence in a wheelchair can increase quality of life a great deal.

Concluding this section on surgery for old people, we have all seen examples where extensive 'heroic' operations have been performed which have not given the patient an increased quality of life. On the other hand, many old people are living happier, pain-free, more independent lives as a result of surgery, and age should never be allowed to become a negative criterion for surgery. Careful assessment, preparation and aftercare by a well-coordinated health care team, together with close involvement of the patient and her family in all stages of the process, is the strategy most likely to be successful.

QUALITY OF DYING

Care of people who are dying is one of the areas which requires much more attention in terms of the quality of care given. Nursing and medical training focuses almost exclusively on treating those who will get better and aiming for cure, and so it is no surprise that nurses and doctors working in general settings, are ill-equipped and uncertain how to care for the dying person. This section begins with a discussion of the patient's right to refuse treatment, and the complex issue of informed consent. Following this, the focus is on the care of dying people, and some of the lessons to be learned from hospice care are emphasised.

The patient's right to refuse treatment

Advances in medical expertise (resuscitation techniques, life-support systems, etc.) have led to increased public debate on the issue of discontinuing active treatment of a dying or comatose patient, particularly if this is known to be her wish. This is not voluntary euthanasia or assisted suicide, which is a deliberate hastening of death (see Jo Hockley, Chapter 21 of this book).

Consent to treatment is a complex issue and is discussed in some detail by Norman (1980). The Medical Defence Union stipulates that people have a right to refuse treatment, and going ahead without consent could lead to a successful claim for damages. Informed consent cannot be given without sufficient information, and yet we suspect that many elderly patients do not receive such information and so cannot give proper informed consent. There is a mass of evidence that hospital patients want more information and that what they do get is inadequate. They feel their intelligence is underrated and they dislike the exclusion from discussions about them so typical of the ward 'round'. This is even more the case for elderly patients who may be particularly reticent about asking questions and be unable to communicate effectively. On the other hand, some patients say they do not want to know very much; they want to submit themselves to the doctors' care and take no active part. Nurses can do a lot to check whether this is really what the patient wants.

Lawyers who specialise in ethics maintain that a conscious patient who refuses treatment must have that wish respected whatever her condition, provided she is sufficiently 'mature and lucid' to make that decision (Kennedy 1978 in Norman 1980). If the doctor thinks the patients is not lucid enough, then the decision can be ignored. This is a crucial issue in the care of old people. How many times have we seen a patient fed through a nasogastric tube against her will because she is refusing to eat? Many nurses disagree with the decision because they thought the patient's refusal was made lucidly, which it probably was. Yet later on, the patient has recovered her health and vigour and is now very pleased to be alive. In this case, it was right that she should have been tube fed until able to eat, but does it mean that she cannot have been in a lucid frame of mind when she refused treatment? The definition of lucidity is extremely difficult, particularly for old people who are confused or dying. Doctors are bound to vary in their definition. If our patient above, instead of eventually accepting the nasogastric tube, tries to remove it, is this refusal to co-operate equivalent to refusal to consent to treatment, or is she too confused to make a lucid decision?

The question of lucidity is even harder to answer because many patients will be taking drugs to relieve pain and distress and these may affect their mental competence. Kennedy maintains that the doctor should be the final arbiter, but can and should he or she carry that burden alone? It is much more likely that the correct decision is reached for an individual patient after discussion with all those who know the patient well, including the family and friends as well as the patient. In some cases, the doctor may be the least able to make the decision because (s)he does not know the patient well enough.

This kind of discussion would ensure that the patient's values and beliefs are taken into account in the decision making. In McCullough's (1984) terms, the patient's 'value history' would not be ignored. If the doctor either insists on treatment being given or respects the patient's wishes even if they turn out to be misguided, then in both cases the 'hidden' middle ground is ignored, that is, the material which is based on the patient's value history. It is this which should become the basis for decision making rather than merely that which the doctor thinks is right for the patient. Such knowledge would enable a decision to be made whether, for example, to treat aggressively or more palliatively, and every decision made would be an individual one. The patient, her family and the primary care team are in the best position to know the patient's value history, and the hospital consultant should make use of their knowledge. It may, however, be necessary for the health professionals to help the family to distinguish between their own wishes and the patient's values.

Making use of the value history is implicit in the goal of 'living wills' which identify the patient's wishes about terminal treatment (see Chapter 21). Similarly, value histories should be considered important in decisions concerning non-terminal treatment. It does mean, however, that someone in the health care team must get to know the patient and her family very well and preferably before she becomes ill. The general practitioner is unlikely to be able to devote enough time to this, but it could be an extremely important role for the health visitor in the first instance, and the district and hospital nurse when the old person becomes a patient. If health professionals would take this albeit complex approach to decision making, then the principle of self-determination, which is fundamental to the concept of consent would be respected. The idea of the value history is closely related to the importance of the biographical approach to the understanding of ageing, described by Malcolm Johnson in Chapter 1.

Whether or not to instigate an energetic resuscitation procedure with an elderly patient presents a moral dilemma for the nurse. It is not at all clear when or how decisions on this are made. Although most elderly patients who die move into a terminal phase of the illness and gradually deteriorate, the nurse must know how to respond in the event of a sudden collapse. Knowledge of the patient's value history, and the relationship (s)he has built with the patient over time may enable her to make the 'right' decision, but often there is some kind of policy on the ward. It is not at all clear how the decision is arrived at, but usually it reaches the nurse as an instruction and is made by the doctor without discussion with the ward team. There should be no place for a ward policy on an issue like this which requires a decision specific to an individual patient. The nurse would never be certain that the policy was the right one for an individual case. But if true consultation and co-ordination occurred, as has been advocated earlier, between all members of the health care team, then the dilemma would be unlikely to occur.

Care of dying people

Today, most people (70%) in Britain die in an institution, which is in contrast to the position a few generations ago, when home was the commonest place (Ch. 21). Now the trend seems to be reverting to home care with the development of more home management teams specialising in the care of dying patients. This trend parallels the government policy of increasing care in the community, but, since these specialist teams are the initiatives of the hospice movement, there is little evidence that they are reaching most old people who are in the terminal phase of illness. Automatically moving a terminally ill old person into hospital can do immeasurable harm, particularly when 63% of chronically ill people spend more than a year dying (Doyle 1981). Doyle informs us that studies have shown that 60% of patients have at least five symptoms when they die, and they do not tell the doctor about half of these, thinking them too trivial.

So much can be done for dying old people and they deserve the most energetic and skilled nursing care available. This is the time when they need more communication with nurses, not less, and the loneliness that many experience is overwhelmingly cruel. The poem written by the old lady of 90 just before her death, which appears in Chapter 21, bears witness to this.

Jo Hockley in Chapter 21 describes the quality of care that hospices give to dying people. So much can be learned from hospice care and using their techniques is surely the aim for all carers of dying people, irrespective of where they are. It is a painful and embarrassing reminder that hospices are necessary because of the inadequate care that most dying people receive in other settings.

> Consumers in both general and geriatric hospitals assert that they are too institutionalised, too authoritarian, too rigid in their routines, too threatening in their staff hierarchies. Patients and visitors appreciate the relaxed atmosphere of hospices, the constant availability of staff to talk to them, the intense energy and enthusiasm devoted to symptom relief and the efforts that are made to restore patient dignity. More than anything, they eulogise about the policy of honesty in hospices, the clear explanations, the lack of deceit, the respect for patients who seek genuinely to know the truth, or as much of the truth as they can at that time bear. (Doyle 1981, p 177.)

Just as there are specialist nurses in stoma care, infection control, parenteral nutrition and so on, there is a need for specialist nurses working as part of a care team for the dying to bring the principles of hospice care into general and geriatric wards, and to teach their skills to hospital staff.

Doyle (1981) identifies five prerequisites for adequate terminal care. First, there must be staff adequately trained in terminal care to advise nurses and doctors whose main aim is to cure and rehabilitate, and who therefore have inadequate experience with dying patients. Second, true non-hierarchical team-work is essential with doctors, nurses, social workers, chaplains, occupational therapists, speech therapists, physiotherapists, patients and relatives. Regular team meetings are important and should be led by the person who best knows the patient, who may not be the doctor. Third, the system of allocating nurses must be sufficiently flexible to allow changes to be made at short notice. Visitors should be allowed complete freedom of access, should be given a space for privacy and solitude, and should be allowed to partic-ipate in intimate nursing procedures if they wish. Fourth, an adequate staff support system is essential, so that any member of the team has the opportunity to discuss his or her own emotions, feelings of guilt, isolation, disappointment, failure and inadequacies. Finally, there should be an organised follow-up system for bereaved relatives which is not confined only to the first three weeks after the death. Research shows that the maximum risk periods are much later, at six weeks, three months, six months and one year. Very few bereaved people receive this kind of attention.

It is not so easy to provide the hospice approach to care of the dying in hospitals which focus on treating disease. With long-stay patients particularly, it may be difficult to identify the terminal phase of life because there may be no acute illness. Furthermore, it may be difficult for nurses to accept impending death and to keep their 'emotional distance', particularly if they have developed a close bond with the patient over a long period. The nurse may reject the doctor's judgment that the patient is dying.

There is a great need for nurses and doctors to receive training in care of the dying and to regard it as positive care, not as failure. Nurses need emotional support to help them cope with their own feelings about death, and also to be able to provide relatives of the patient with the support needed. Too often, in their own uncertainty, they insist that relatives leave the patient when nursing procedures are performed, when the relatives would prefer to help and the patient wants them to. Relatives feel they cannot protest, or if they do, they are often ignored. As Norman (1980) observes, children are vigorously defended and protected by their parents and by the National Associ-ation for the Welfare of Children in Hospital (NAWCH). There is no similar protection for old people. Organisations like Age Concern and Help the Aged have not taken up this challenge.

Care of dying people is an area in which nurses should take a key role. They are in a position to get to know the patient and her family well and to help the patient find fulfil-ment in the final period of her life. Hospices have developed because the care of dying people in institutions is inadequate. Nurses should be taught how to meet the patient's physical needs and above all, her psycho-logical needs. There is very little evidence of a co-ordinated, effective team approach to the care of the dying in most hospitals and specialist teams could be introduced to advise staff on how best to meet the patient's needs. Hospices and their home care counterparts tend to focus on people with cancer, yet it would be wrong if all patients had 'good' deaths only in a specialist setting. It would be much more effective to bring the principles of hospice care into all institutions, so that everyone who is close to death feels comfort-able, peaceful, close to relatives and friends, and prepared to die.

REFERENCES

Adams S 1984 Clothing in elderly patients in medical and geriatric wards and the relationship of clothing to self-esteem. Undergraduate Dissertation, Department of Nursing Studies, Chelsea College, University of London

Batchelor I 1984 Policies for a crisis? Some aspects of DHSS policies for the care of the elderly. Occasional Papers No. 1. Nuffield Provincial Hospitals Trust, London

Bleatham C, Bowling A 1983 If we don't shout now. Nursing Times Community Outlook 79(15): 89–90

British Geriatrics Society and Royal College of Nursing 1975 Improving geriatric care in hospital. Royal College of Nursing, London

Chambers R 1982 How to combat 'doing nothing'—two steps to catalyse change in homes for the elderly. Social Work Service 32(winter): 51–53

Clarke M 1978 Getting through the work. In: Dingwall R, McIntosh J (eds) Readings in the sociology of nursing. Churchill Livingstone, Edinburgh

Clark-Kennedy A E 1982 A bicycle is best. Geriatric Medicine 12: 74–77

Dalley G 1983 The nursing home: professional attitudes to the introduction of new forms of care provision for the elderly. In: Jerome D (ed) Ageing in a modern society. Croom Helm, London

Department of Health & Social Security 1972 Minimum standards in geriatric hospitals and departments. HMSO, London

Department of Health and Social Security 1978 A happier old age. HMSO, London

Department of Health and Social Security 1979 The way forward. HMSO, London

Doyle D 1981 Terminal care of the elderly. In: Kinnaird J, Brotherston J, Williamson J (eds) The provision of care for the elderly. Churchill Livingstone, Edinburgh

Evers H 1981a Women patients in long-stay geriatric wards. In: Hutter B, Williams G (eds) Controlling women: the normal and the deviant. Croom Helm, London

Evers H 1981b Tender loving care. In: Copp L A (ed) Care of the ageing. Recent advances in nursing series, Churchill Livingstone, Edinburgh

Gilbert M 1984 Challenging stereotypes. Nursing Mirror 158(16): 42–43

Glossop E S 1983 Improving quality of life: a case study of a geriatric unit. In: Denham M J (ed) Care of the long stay elderly patient. Croom Helm, London

Godlove C, Richard L, Rodwell G 1981. Time for action: an observation study of elderly people in four different care environments. Social Services Monograph: Research in Practice. Joint Unit for Social Services Research, University of Sheffield

Goffman E 1961 Asylums. Doubleday, New York

King R D, Raynes N V 1968 An occupational measure of inmate management in residential institutions. Social Science and Medicine 2: 41–53

Ling R S M 1979 Problems of the aged hip. In: Vowles K D J (ed) Surgical problems in the aged. Wright, Bristol

McCullough L B 1984 Medical care for elderly patients with diminished competence: an ethical analysis. Journal of the American Geriatrics Society 32(2): 150–153

McIntosh J B 1983 Experimental care for the elderly. Occasional papers. Nursing Times 79(25): 56–57

Miller A F 1978 Evaluation of the care provided for patients with dementia in six hospital wards. Unpublished MSc thesis, University of Manchester

Miller A F 1984 Nursing process and patient care. Nursing Times Occasional Paper. 80(13): 56–58

Mohr D N 1983 Estimation of surgical risk in the elderly: a correlative review. Journal of the Medical Geriatrics Society 31: 99–102

Muir-Gray J A 1984 The prevention of disability and handicap. Nursing Mirror 158(22): 29–30

Norman A J 1980 Rights and risk. National Council for the Care of Old People (now Centre for Policy on Ageing), London

Norman A J 1984 Bricks and mortals: design and lifestyle in old people's homes. Centre for Policy on Ageing Reports No. 4. CPA, London

Norton D 1965 Nursing in Geriatrics. Gerontologia Clinica 7: 59–60

Peace S 1983 Residential life of the elderly in the UK: a consumer viewpoint. Ageing International 10(2): 8–12

Richard L 1983 Time for action. Nursing Mirror 156(13): 17–19

Rowden R 1983 A sense of harmony. Nursing Times 79(37): 9–11

Sander R, Walden E 1984 So much to learn. Nursing Times 80(32): 50–51

Seligman M E P 1975 Helplessness: on depression, development and death. Freeman, San Francisco

Smith R 1984 Rights guide to non-means-tested social security benefits, 6th edn. Child Poverty Action Group, London

Storrs A 1982 What is care? British Journal of Geriatric Nursing 1(4): 12–14

Swaffield L 1983 A model for the future? Burford. Nursing Times 79(2): 13–16

Vowles K D J 1979 Surgery for the aged. In: Vowles K D J (ed) Surgical problems in the aged. Wright, Bristol

Vowles K D J, Halliday C E 1979 Vascular problems and the aged amputee. In: Vowles K D J (ed) Surgical problems in the aged. Wright, Bristol

Wade B, Sawyer L, Bell J 1983 Dependency with dignity. Occasional Papers on Social Administration no. 68. Bedford Square Press, London

Wells T 1980 Problems in geriatric nursing care. Churchill Livingstone, Edinburgh

Willocks D, Peace S, Kellaher L 1983 A profile of residential life: a discussion of key issues arising out of consumer research in one hundred old-age homes. In: Jerrome D (ed) Ageing in modern society. Croom Helm, London

Woods R T, Holden U P 1982 Reality orientation. In: Isaacs B (ed) Recent advances in geriatric medicine Churchill Livingstone, Edinburgh

S. J. Redfern

30

The nurse's role and provision of health care for old people

In this final chapter we move from focusing on the elderly patient, which is the subject of Chapter 29, to the nurse's role in the care of old people, and the provision of health care. In the third section, we have highlighted some aspects of nursing care which are areas of nursing responsibility and which need research by nurses working independently or as members of multidisciplinary research teams. The list of areas is short and selective. Readers will have many more ideas which are equally in need of investigation.

THE NURSE'S ROLE IN THE CARE OF OLD PEOPLE

Independent nurse practitioner

'If prevention and health is *everybody's* business, does this necessitate any realignment of position between doctors, patients, nurses, therapists, and other paramedical workers?' (Austin 1979, p 145, emphasis in original.)

In the last Chapter, it is abundantly clear that, although exciting initiatives have been taken by nurses, a lot more could be done to improve the quality of living and of dying of old people. Nursing has, it seems, on the one hand, encouraged the development of specialist nurses who advise their colleagues and patients on specific areas of nursing (stoma therapists, infection control nurses, incontinence advisers, breast cancer specialists etc.). Yet, on the other hand, they have given away the fundamental 'basic' nursing care to unqualified students and auxiliaries. The hospital nurse caring for old people is perhaps the nurse who has, to the greatest extent, allowed others to take over nursing care. The geriatrician takes an energetic approach to diagnosis, treatment, rehabilitation, cure and discharge home and requires the specialist skills of the physiotherapist, occupational therapist, speech therapist, dietician and social worker to achieve his or her aim of optimum health for the patient and discharge home. The nurse, however, is everybody's assistant. She (or he) carries out medical instructions and ensures treatments are given, and she prepares the patient for therapy by the specialist, or delegates someone else to do this. She, typically, does not co-ordinate or continue the work of non-nurse specialists. Her principal role seems to be as a facilitator for others; she reacts to their instructions rather than taking the initative herself.

There is tremendous scope for nurses caring for old people in geriatric, psychiatric and community settings to extend the traditional role of doctor's handmaiden more in line with that of the independent, autonomous health care practitioner. This would require nurses to develop a sufficient knowledge base which would enable them to use their clinical judgment alongside but independent of medical expertise. In certain circumstances, as when nursing patients who are acutely ill, then nurses would, of course, defer to doctors when carrying out medical treatments. But the nurse would continue to work towards maintaining and improving the patient's health after completion of the acute treatment, and preferably before illness occurs. As Austin (1979) observes, nursing would become continual rather than episodic and need not be related to a medically oriented setting. Community nurses, especially health visitors, argue that they are giving continual, preventive care as independent practitioners. This is true, but with the exception of those specialising with the elderly, most generic health visitors see child health as their main responsibility (Fitton 1984b; Robertson 1984), and do not see working with old people as so rewarding (see Chapter 27).

Austin (1979) argues for the development of a nurse practitioner who is better suited to the practice of *health* care than the disease-oriented doctor. The impact of bureaucracy and professional territoriality, many believe, has not encouraged health care but has instead promoted a sickness service. The health and well-being of society is more likely to be dependent on factors such as a clean environment, good housing, adequate nutrition, a satisfactory minimum income, physical exercise, stress-alleviating interpersonal relationships and job satisfaction than on medical factors. Austin maintains that the welcome growth of preventive medicine has not been an active effort by the medical profession to promote health, and she sees the need for four changes if the promotion of health is to become a reality: more democratic forms of control, humane organisation and management, realistic resource allocation, and changes in the relationships between professionals, and between professionals and their clients or patients.

The health promotion oriented independent nurse practitioner is not uncommon in parts of the United States and Canada and has been a normal feature of developing countries, with their 'barefoot doctors', although these latter practitioners are not usually nurses. The 'geriatric nurse practitioner' in the United States is an independent practitioner, teacher and consultant to hospital and community nurses, and has assumed a role caring for the health of old people which doctors in that country do not want. The demise of the North American nurse practitioner has been forecast by some members of the medical profession (Spitzer in Nursing Mirror 1984) because doctors maintain that they can cope with the workload which they see as theirs. But whether this will include the geriatric nurse practitioner as well as those working in areas traditionally regarded as the territory of doctors remains to be seen.

In Britain, the independent nurse practitioner is a rarity, but has been successful in the community setting of general practice (Stilwell 1984). Nurse practitioners are unlikely to develop in this country until nurses are both willing and able to accept accountability as well as being allowed autonomy in their work. The present standard nurse training does not equip them for this, nor is continuing education mandatory for all nurses, which means that their knowledge is not necessarily kept up-to-date. The signs are, however, that progress is being made. The growth of degree-level nurse education in universities and polytechnics is giving a small proportion of nurses a comprehensive grounding in the nursing sciences. Research in nursing is increasing, and it is much more common than in the past to find nurses with research degrees working in clinical practice. One example is Pauline Fielding, the author of Chapter 25, who has a doctor of philosophy degree and is a sister in charge of a geriatric unit in London.

The Department of Health and Social Security (1981) and the professional body, the Royal College of Nursing (1981), have been active in advocating the need for a professional career structure in clinical nursing. Promotion would be dependent on acquisition of general and specialist post-basic qualifications, and peer review, as well as on experience. These developments will provide nurses with the skills, knowledge and attitudes necessary to take on the independent practitioner role. The nurse practitioner would be primarily concerned with nursing practice, but must have a thorough grasp of the literature, research and theory development in the field, and be skilled at relating this knowledge to practice.

It is easier to envisage the successful development of the independent nurse practitioner in the primary care field of community nursing which is less dominated by medicine than hospital nursing. Much as I and other contributors to this book (e.g. Helen Evers, Chapter 22) would like to see a breakdown in the hospital/community boundary with the properly educated professional nurse caring for old people in health and illness irrespective of location, this would not be possible within the present hospital structure in Britain.

The time is ripe for community nurses to take the initiative and develop their role within the current climate of public opinion which is critical of conventional medicine. The development of public awareness for the need for nutrition and exercise for health, the self-help movement, and the rise of alternative therapies have created an ideal environment for nurses to take the lead. Yet community nurses, particularly district nurses, are 'lagging behind the public in utilising and building on innovative approaches and demystifying professional care' (Turton 1984, p 41).

The nurse who has most contact with old people in the community is the district nurse, and the research evidence suggests that the care district nurses provide is inadequate, especially with respect to health education, counselling and rehabilitation (Turton 1983, 1984; Fiona Ross in Chapter 26 of this book). They spend most of their time on physical nursing procedures. District nurses see themselves as giving skilled care to people identified as sick, and this does not include preventive care which is regarded as the province of the health visitor, although Fiona Ross (Chapter 26) maintains this is part of the district nurse's role. But, as noted above, health visitors generally restrict their preventive role to child care. As with hospital nurses, this fragmentation of care is compounded by the handing over of 'skilled' aspects of nursing care to non-nurse specialists (physiotherapists, occupational therapists, social workers, etc.), and of 'basic' nursing to untrained nursing auxiliaries, care assistants and home helps. Thus both district and hospital nurses have abdicated their role as providers of comprehensive patient care.

Turton (1984) maintains that nursing management and education are responsible for the lack of district nurse initiative. Management 'appears to value obedience and conformity to current practice rather than independence and initiative' (p 40). The conventional hospital-based, treatment-of-disease oriented nurse training does not prepare district nurses to be flexible and responsive to social and technological change, to be leaders and co-ordinators of care at patient, family, team, local and national levels, and to be the patient's advocate. Turton is critical of the present criteria used for selecting students into nurse training, which value conformity and competence in convergent thinking (seeking single solutions to problems) rather than the non-conformist creativity of the divergent thinker. She describes an educational model based on holistic medicine which could be used as the basis for the district nurse training curriculum:

> Emphasis would be placed on understanding the factors that make the individual vulnerable to disease—the complex interplay of body, mind and spirit, and/or a recognition and deployment of the skills of the "pharmacopoeia of people" available to aid the patient and his carer. The role of the district nurse as a health educator in its broadest sense is equally important—not as a didactic teacher, but as a facilitator, enabling patients and carers to co-operate actively in sharing information and maximising their self-healing potential in a more egalitarian relationship with the health professionals' (p 42).

If district nurse training were to develop along these lines, then the argument for a single community nurse for the elderly, rather than the present fragmentation between the district nurse and health visitor, may gain support. In spite of their preference for children, health visitors see their unique skills as essential in the care of old people (Fitton 1984a, 1984b, and Chapter 27 of this book by Alison While). But, since district nursing focuses almost entirely on old people (see Chapter 26 by Fiona Ross) and since most health visitors' priority is with children and their families, then combining district nurse and health visitor training into a curriculum for educating a generalist community nurse for the elderly would surely be a wise move. Such a move has its supporters (e.g. Batchelor 1984), and Nuttall (1984) has predicted this will occur within five years.

Community psychiatric nurses who have a major role with the elderly mentally ill have taken the initiative to become active and valuable members of the primary care team. Although there are few teams in Britain whose prime focus is on mentally ill old people (see Chapter 24), the organisation of care adopted by them could be extended into other areas of community care. The team is a cohesive one, consisting of community psychiatric nurse, psychogeriatrician, social worker and clinical psychologist. One member takes the role of key worker depending on the client's needs, and co-ordinates the services required to enable the old person and the family to cope at home. The key worker is the first point of contact for client, family, neighbour and other health care workers, which ensures proper co-ordination of services and avoids the fragmented care so typical of non-psychiatric community and hospital nursing. These community psychiatric nurses have developed an independent practitioner role, which could be extended to the care of other old people.

Nurse education

There is plenty of evidence in the literature that basic and post-basic education of nurses in Britain and in other countries is inadequate (Cox 1983, World Health Organisation 1983, Hall 1984a). Concern is so great in England that the Royal College of Nursing set up a Commission on Nursing Education in April 1984 to examine the whole field of nurse education and training and to make recommendations.

If we look at the definition of nursing given by the World Health Organisation, it is clear that nursing is seen in terms of health promotion as well as caring for the sick and dying:

> *Nursing* is a fundamental human activity and in its organised form a discrete health discipline. Its primary responsibility is to assist individuals and groups (families/communities) to optimise function throughout the lifespan as well as to care during acute and protracted illness and disability. It also makes social contributions maintaining, promoting and protecting health, caring for the

sick and providing rehabilitation. It is concerned with the psychosomatic and psychosocial aspects of life as these affect health, illness and dying (WHO 1983, p 31, emphasis in original).

If health for all is to be achieved by the year 2000, then nursing education and practice must move away from the present emphasis on hospital-based disease-oriented care. The World Health Organisation stipulates that basic curricular for nurse education should include theories of human development and ageing, self-care, health promotion and community health, as well as the development of disease, disability and social dysfunction, and specific treatments and rehabilitation.

A vision of the nurse of the future, provided by Hall (1984) underlines the need for change in basic nurse education. She outlines 12 features of this future nurse:
— She would focus on health rather than ill health and recognise her role as a health educator.
— She would operate as a member of a true team, recognising her own unique role and that of the other professionals.
— She would work with individuals and their families in attaining and promoting health.
— She would have a comprehensive knowledge base and be able to initiate and direct her own subsequent learning.
— She would be competent in relevant nursing skills including those of communication.
— She would be analytical and critical without being defensive, and be able to conceptualise.
— She would be able to apply and adapt general principles to particular situations.
— She would make use of research.
— She would recognise both the art and science of nursing.
— She would understand the need for continuing education to maintain her competence, and the value of higher education for new and extended roles.
— She would accept the responsibility of professional accountability and understand its implications.
— She would be committed to a standard of professional conduct based on ethical principles.

Hall firmly believes that nursing students should cease to be part of the National Health Service labour force and that the proportion of nurses educated to degree level should increase. If newly qualified nurses possessed the qualities outlined by Hall, then those who specialised in the care of old people would be in an ideal position to develop their knowledge and skills through further education and research, and to take the lead in improving the standards of health care for the elderly. Many people, including Hall, recommend that nurse teachers should be graduates and there should be an increase in joint appointments between teaching and research, between research and practice, and between teaching and practice. The arguments for joint teaching–practice posts are appealing because teaching would occur in clinical areas. But in the present structure in the United Kingdom, teachers could not take a full-time clinical load and carry responsibility for student and postbasic teaching and research. This role would be easier for the independent nurse practitioner or clinical nurse specialist, who would not carry full-time clinical responsibility.

THE PROVISION OF HEALTH CARE FOR OLD PEOPLE

Present provision

Health for all people in the world by the year 2000 was the goal adopted by the World Health Organisation at its conference on primary health care held in Alma Ata in Russia in 1978. The development of primary health care services was seen as the principal means of achieving this goal. Yet there is little evidence, especially in western society, that politicians, doctors, nurses, social workers and ancillary workers are working together towards primary health care and away from high technology hospital care (O'Neill 1983). In his book, which was supported by the

World Health Organisation, O'Neill warns that there is more likely to be a health crisis for all by the year 2000, unless radical and co-ordinated measures are taken by the public, the health and social service professions, industry and governments.

The Department of Health and Social Security has admirable long-term aims for the National Health Service. These are to increase service provision for the elderly, the mentally ill and the mentally handicapped, to move the priority from hospital to community-based care, and to redistribute resources from richer to poorer regions. However, there is little evidence that these aims are being achieved, except perhaps the last. Expenditure on community health services has not been substantially increased (Hall 1984b), which means that the bulk of the care of old people still falls on the family, mainly on its women members.

The present organisation of health care for old people in this country is hampered by a division of responsibility and lack of co-ordination between authorities, a point raised in other Chapters of this book (Chapters 22, 23, 24, 26 and 29). The Department of Health and Social Security is responsible for the state pension scheme and age-related financial help; the local authorities (i.e. local government) for personal social services and old people's residential Homes; the National Health Service for hospital and domiciliary health services; and the Department of the Environment and district housing authorities for sheltered housing. Furthermore, the General Medical Council is responsible for the content of medical education, and the national boards for nurse training. In Britain there is no co-ordinated central policy for social services and health care and no forum for developing a policy except at parliamentary Cabinet level. A proposal for co-ordination was put forward in 1975, but this disappeared into oblivion (Acheson 1982).

Pensions

The provision of pensions and benefits to the elderly is disjointed, illogical, inequitable, and discriminates against those of modest means and those in long-term National Health Service care. The system discourages initiative and freedom of choice, is too complex to understand and is wasteful to run (Acheson 1982). Means testing occurs for old people moving into local authority residential Homes (Part III), and in long-stay wards patients surrender most of their state pension and so they have no control over this income.

Community care

Some 90% of old people in Britain live in their own homes (Tinker 1984). Relocation, particularly into old people's Homes, nursing Homes and long-stay hospitals has been related to an increase in morbidity and mortality, and so old people should be moved only as a last resort and with their agreement. Wardens of sheltered housing have an increasingly difficult job because the proportion of very frail old people has increased, and they often need 24-hour cover. Alarm and communication systems help but only if the old person can reach them when required and understand how to use them. Each district should have a comprehensive housing policy which co-ordinates the needs of the elderly for sheltered housing, places in old peoples' Homes and the requirements of the demented and disturbed (Acheson 1982).

In the community, many maintain that the general practitioner (family doctor) has the central role, but apart from the few with a special interest in old people, most general practitioners give an inadequate service, are not interested in the elderly, do not have knowledge of geriatrics, and do not want this role (Bosanquet 1978). Neither do the Family Practitioner Committees, who have had responsibility for developing primary care services since 1974, adequately moniter the general practitioner service (Batchelor 1984). Some doctors are enthusiastic, and have set up screening programmes, or visit all those at risk with the help of a health visitor or district nurse, but this is unusual. The district nursing service is one of the strengths of the National Health Service, and should receive a much greater slice of the budget in order to meet a mandate to cater for the needs of old people living in the community.

Hospital care

The powerful medical profession continues to regard the 'elderly problem' as a threat to their services to other groups, as potential 'bed blockers', and as preventing them from treating 'interesting cases' (Bosanquet 1978). Bonsanquet observes that the attitudes of the medical profession are similar today compared with 20 years ago, in spite of virtually similar circulars, about the need to develop more extensive services for the elderly, issued by the DHSS at regular intervals during that period. However, as Helen Evers points out in Chapter 22, progress has been made since the 1940s by only a small band of very active, visionary geriatricians who set up the progressive geriatric departments that we have today. But hostility, prejudice, a lack of understanding and the lack of a wish to change amongst most of the medical profession has meant that the development of geriatric medicine as a recognised and respected specialty has been slow. Its future remains precarious. Although the debate continues as to whether geriatrics should be strengthened as an age-related service, or integrated with general medicine or abandoned altogether (see Chapter 22), most writers favour an age-related service (Bosanquet 1978, Grimley Evans 1981, Isaacs 1981). This course is supported even though recruitment of suitable doctors and nurses will continue to be difficult. The progressive units have no difficulty in attracting staff, and so what is known to be successful should be developed rather than abandoned.

There are more than 300 consultant geriatricians in Britain, which amounts to one for 20 000 of the population over 65 years (Isaacs 1981). Many would think this ratio is impressive but it is too low to meet the growing needs of old people. Most of these geriatricians do not have the facilities enjoyed by

progressive geriatric units and cannot achieve the aims of swift admission, diagnosis, rehabilitation and a supported return home to the patient's preferred place of residence. Failure to achieve this results in further deterioration in the patient's health, the development of complications, and greater dependency. Without the facilities of a district general hospital, a full service cannot be provided, and an accumulative effect occurs in which high calibre doctors and nurses are not attracted to the specialty, or if they are they soon lose heart, leave and may not be replaced.

Much less progress has been made in the care of the elderly mentally infirm in spite of continuous advice and pressure from the DHSS to set up psychogeriatric units as part of the geriatric service. The advice has, generally, not been taken, and many health authorities have no psychogeriatric service, which means that these old people are cared for by the geriatrician and his or her colleagues. The problems experienced by the geriatric service are even worse for the psychogeriatric service, with its very small number of psychogeriatricians who, with community and hospital psychiatric nurses, psychologists, occupational therapists and social workers, have improved the care for these old people and their families.

Many doctors and nurses find communicating with old people difficult, their multiple medical and nursing problems daunting and their often unconventional presentation of disease perplexing. Many non-specialist doctors, according to Isaacs (1981), handle elderly patients in one of three ways. First is 'fractionation', where the doctor who finds that forming a relationship with the whole patient is so difficult that (s)he resorts to relating to parts only, e.g. the diseased heart, lungs or kidney. This (s)he treats successfully and sends home with its owner. With 'abrogation', the doctor blames the patient for putting him or her into a difficult position because it is impossible to classify her into a disease category. The doctor abrogates responsibility by referring the patient to the geriatrician, with a note to say that the patient has been fully investigated, nothing definite has been found, and health at such a great age is impossible, and so would the geriatrician provide continuing care. The third method is 'defamation', where patients are described as 'bed blockers', and wards are 'cluttered' with unresponsive elderly patients. Isaacs observes that doctors display their exasperation by using various forms of restraint, such as cot sides, restraining chairs, catheters and sedation. These reflect the frustration of doctors rather than meeting the needs of the patients.

These means of encounter are relevant to nurses also, who on the whole, have adopted doctors' approaches to patients. Consider the general medical ward nurse who says the ward has changed from being interesting and acute to boring, heavy and 'geriatric'. Many nurses working in actual geriatric wards also hold these views and do not have the skills necessary to engage in mutually beneficial encounters with the patient. The skill of the geriatrician and the specialist nurse is in being able to develop effective encounters with the old person and her family, and to do this in successful collaboration with the whole health care team. In acute medicine and nursing, each worker may be able to play his or her part reasonably successfully with little reference to the others. With the care of old people, each member of the team must recognise the work of the others and modify his or her approach accordingly. The nurse's role in co-ordinating the efforts of the team members into a 24-hour programme is unique to nursing and fundamental to the quality of care.

Recommendations for the future

A recent report by a working group set up by the Office of Health Economics (Teeling Smith 1984) underlines the failure of the 1946 National Health Service Act to cater for people with chronic disease, or to encourage care in the community, or to promote positive health. There is little doubt that care provision for old people in this country will not improve without closer liaison between the health,

social services, and housing authorities. The present sporadic and disconnected services must be co-ordinated under a joint planning arrangement. A co-ordinated policy at central and local government level is required in order for regional and district health authorities to integrate their services successfully with local authorities and voluntary organisations (Shegog 1981, Batchelor 1984). Acheson (1982) has identified a central policy which will fulfil two major principles: the policy of 'least removal' so that old people are relocated once only if at all, and the recognition that individual wishes vary, and choice and privacy are paramount for most potential clients. The central policy requires a Minister for co-ordination of all services for the elderly (a point made by Michael Green in Chapter 13), and these services should be centrally co-ordinated by an interdepartmental committee. Responsibility for special housing for old people should be moved from the Department of the Environment to the Department of Health and Social Security to facilitate effective co-ordination. More suitable accommodation should be provided, with sheltered housing schemes linked to old people's Homes. Batchelor (1984) argues for much greater devolution of responsibility and accountability to local level, with less use made of inappropriate, centrally defined norms and standards.

Acheson (1982) also emphasises the need for a review of the pension and subsides system to one which is more equitable, less complex, promotes independence and enables old people to control their finances. Furthermore, each health authority should have a physician responsible for co-ordinating health services for the very frail elderly, in the hospital, community and mental health service. Acheson is convinced that it is within society's powers to maximise quality of life and minimise dependency of old people. If society fails, this would not be through a lack of resources, but through an inability to take a broad view in co-ordinating effort, and in allowing those with vested minority interests to continue to hold too much power and preserve their territoriality.

In their own homes, old people often find

it difficult to retain their independence and to summon help in an emergency. They need effective alarm systems, a general practitioner and primary care team whose priority is with preventive care, and increased access to volunteer help.

There is evidence of improvement in local authority residential Homes towards preserving individuality and privacy with more private bedrooms and toilets (Shegog 1981). The National Health Service nursing Homes should be homely, unregimented and not run like hospitals.

The large number of old people with dementia and depression (see Chapters 18 and 19) implies the need for priority support for them and their families. Shegog (1981) stipulates that each health authority should have an integrated service for the elderly mentally infirm which contains inpatient beds, day hospitals, a specialist day centre with residential accommodation, and intensive family support. There should be a certain amount of controlled sharing of facilities with other old and handicapped people. There has been substantial resistance to the integration of services for the elderly and elderly mentally frail, critics maintaining that the interests and needs of the demented may be swamped by the needs of the numerically dominant physically handicapped elderly. What is perhaps a more important reason is that psychiatrists object to integration with geriatric medicine, because they see themselves as having a separate identity. This insistence on clearly demarcated boundaries does nothing to meet the needs of old people. It is extremely confusing for general practitioners or relatives who may be unsure whom to contact before a definite diagnosis is made. Shegog and his colleagues recommend a joint assessment and review between specialists in geriatric medicine and psychiatry and from nursing, paramedical, social services and housing authorities.

The general recommendation for hospital care is for true and effective teamwork and joint planning, with no resistance resulting from demarcation lines between professions

and departments (Shegog 1981, Batchelor 1984). Closure of long-stay wards would release funds for small jointly run nursing units, which would provide more suitable care at less cost. As discussed earlier, the central government must act to enable funds from different sources to be used jointly by the health and local authorities. An efficient geriatric service is possible without exorbitant resources, and the increase in the very elderly and their health needs makes this the group most in need of more resources until the end of the century. If we ignore them, they will not simply go away. 'The threat of a national scandal grows yearly, and enlightened self-interest, if no nobler motive, should persuade health service administrators to grasp some urgent nettles' (Grimley Evans 1981, p 146).

Given a mixed economy in this country, more use could be made of voluntary (charity) and commercial nursing Homes. As Shegog (1981) observes, some are excellent and luxurious and are run more flexibly and cheaply than state Homes. But the abundant opportunities for abuse will continue to exist until all these Homes are included in the newly instigated health service and local government inspection system. If this inspectorate were effective, then placing more old people in the independent private sector would leave a reserve capacity in the public (state) sector for the future increase in numbers.

Nursing education was discussed earlier in this chapter. Education of medical students about the elderly is still grossly inadequate. Bosanquet (1978) observes that medical teaching on ageing and the elderly often occupies two weeks of a five-month medicine course, compared with six months devoted to surgery and five months to paediatrics. Yet most of our graduates become general practitioners and are confronted far more with illness of old people than with surgery. The powerful advocates of clinical freedom are responsible for a gross misfit between medical education and practice and the needs of the community, and the Department of Health and Social Security has no influence on the content of the medical school curriculum.

Education is required at all levels of the service and also for the public so that they are better informed about preventive health, self-care and alternative therapies. Heller (1978) predicts that people will take more responsibility for their own health and will influence decision making through increasingly powerful patient committees and community health councils. He sees the basic health care unit as the primary care team controlled by the community it serves. It would have a wider membership than at present and would include general practitioners, district nurses, health visitors, social and community workers, and those concerned with legal and welfare rights and income maintenance. The primary care team would have well-defined links with medical, institutional, community and domiciliary facilities, and would encourage well-supported family and self-care to replace professional input where possible. The principal functions of the primary care team would be crisis intervention for medical and social stress, health education to prevent crises, and changing those factors which lead to poor health (environmental, occupational, class, sexist and ageist factors).

Some local initiatives

On a national level the care provision of old people is fragmented, uncoordinated and often inadequate, but there have been a number of local initiatives described by Shegog (1981) and others which could be duplicated elsewhere.

Age Concern's Wigston day centre and volunteer scheme. The national charity, Age Concern, provides a 'drop-in' service and lunch club at Wigston in the north of England. A Neighbourhood Help officer recruits and organises a band of volunteer street wardens who support old people at risk without families. They make visits, do shopping, collect pensions, help with financial problems, provide meals when carers are on holiday, and provide a 'welcome home' service for those discharged from hospital (bed airing, fire

lighting, food stocking). The street wardens are helped by casual volunteers.

The day centre has a dining room, workshop and shop, and is planning a television room and hairdressing and chiropody service. It has a paid part-time manager and a part-time cook, and voluntary helpers.

The Glaven District Caring scheme in Norfolk was set up to bring home help, nursing, meals, and other services to 12 villages in remote rural areas. It is based in a warden supervised group housing scheme close to the general practitioner's surgery. A day centre and day hospital were added, which provide bathing facilities, physiotherapy, occupational therapy and lunch club. Meals-on-wheels and home helps are provided, and nursing covers old people's needs in the centre and at home. The co-ordinator is salaried, but most of the helpers are volunteers, many being nurses.

Kent Community Care project was the initiative of the director of social services for Kent. Social workers mobilise help for the elderly at risk, so avoiding the need for hospital or residential care. The social workers have a budget to buy in services, and helpers are paid a small sum. This scheme was evaluated against a control group and fewer old people who took part in the scheme moved to institutional care compared with members of the control group.

The Stockport model was developed in response to the decision that domiciliary rather than residential services should be strengthened. It has three elements. Social services officers were appointed who are responsible for co-ordinating all care for each client in their area. A radio alarm and mobile warden service operates round the clock every day, and there are 1600 mainly elderly clients in the system. High dependency sheltered housing and a residential Home are run jointly by the health and social service authorities. Care assistants provide help in both schemes, and district nurses, general practitioner, physiotherapist and occupational therapist visit the residential Home, which is run by an officer-in-charge. This is a good example of a jointly administered and funded scheme in which admissions are controlled by the area social services officer in consultation with the officer-in-charge and the geriatrician.

Cottage Homes were set up originally in Mill Hill, London, to provide for the dependent elderly and infirm of the Linen and Woollen drapers' trade (King's Fund Centre 1979). The scheme has now spread to Derby and Glasgow and consists of cottages, flats with bathrooms, bed-sitting rooms, rest Home rooms and nursing wing beds. This is a flexible, voluntary scheme in which each resident has her own possessions and own personal space. It is similar to the much admired Danish nursing Home system (see below).

Care of old people in different industrial countries

A useful overview of the care of old people in industrialised countries is provided by Nuberg (1981). Most industrial countries provide health care for old people through the same general system which serves all age groups, be it a national health service, national insurance programme, private insurance, voluntary sick funds or public welfare programme. The United States is an exception with Medicare, a form of national health insurance only available to the elderly.

As a specialty, geriatric medicine has developed in only a few countries such as Britain and the USSR, although Sweden has a long-term care specialty. The United States National Institute on Ageing is against establishing geriatrics as a separate specialty, preferring all physicians to be trained in the biology of human ageing and geriatric medicine.

Preventive health

Most countries have some kind of preventive health measures, although often they fail to reach the elderly population. Sweden's government requires its local authorities to inform its citizens about their rights and its

postmen check on old people. Scotland makes good use of health visitors, and in some parts everyone over 70 years is visited by a health visitor.

In the USSR, physicians refer old people to 'groups of health' where they can get health and hygiene education, learn first-aid and are encouraged to exercise. In the USA, self-help groups are available for stabilising and improving health, and providing exercise and relaxation for old people.

Social services

Many countries have services like home helps, escorts, laundry, meals-on-wheels, senior centres and transport, but the provision tends to be piecemeal. Some of these are required by law in only Britain and Sweden. In France, each service area must provide at least three of the following: pre-retirement training, home helps, home nursing, day centres, health education, telephones, hot meals, referral services or organised physical exercise.

Housing

In all industrialised countries, old people are more likely than other age groups to live in substandard housing. Often, in the United Kingdom, they live in houses which have become too large for them, and they have paid off the mortgage but they cannot keep up with the running costs and repairs. The charity Help the Aged in Britain has an imaginative 'gifted housing' scheme in which elderly owners of large houses donate them to Help the Aged who convert them into flats for rent to other old people. In exchange the donors live there rent-free for the rest of their lives, and have no repair costs to meet. They also acquire company if they want it, and emergency assistance if needed.

In Denmark, specially equipped apartments for the disabled are built into new housing developments, so that disabled people remain integrated in their communities. Denmark's long-term care policy places a high priority on privacy, and the approach has been to replace residential Homes with combined sheltered housing and nursing wings (Millard 1983). Everyone has a single room with connecting toilet and shower, and they chose their own furniture and furnishings. The room is seen as the resident's territory and staff knock before entering. Denmark's long-term care is of high quality, but they have not developed an energetic short-term programme incorporating diagnosis, treatment, rehabilitation and discharge, as is the case in Britain. In contrast, the British system has concentrated on short-term geriatric medicine to the detriment of long-term care.

In the United States and Germany private enterprise builds retirement communities, with recreational facilities, which are attractive for those who can afford them although only a few have comprehensive social and health services. The concept of these 'continuing care communities' is largely unfamiliar in Britain, but they aim to meet the housing, personal and health care needs of old people on one site (Hearnden 1983). They resemble an estate or small village with small flats or bungalows and communal buildings for meals, activities and services. The most comprehensive complexes provide sheltered housing, domiciliary services such as home help, and long-term nursing care in the flats or in high dependency units. Thus housing and lifetime care is provided in return for an entrance fee and regular service and maintenance charges. The attitudes towards these communities tend to polarise. Enthusiasts say they are ideal for retired people because they provide care, company and activities for like-minded old people. Critics say they are undesirable ghettoes for the affluent (Hearnden 1983).

Hearnden examined the viability of continuing care communities in Britain run on independent non-profit making lines. He concluded that they could be financially and socially viable but they would not be cheap. Each community would need 300–400 residents each paying realistic service charges (£200–£500 monthly) in addition to an entrance fee of £20 000–£35 000. He estimates that perhaps one in four elderly householders could afford it after selling their houses. Options for reasonably well off people even in this country are very inadequate, and where they exist, they are much more expensive than this. Therefore, a continuing care community would be a reasonable buy for those who would choose its way of life, although it would be anathema to others. It would seem a good idea to maximise choice in this way as long as the provision for the less affluent is not jeopardised.

Apart from these retirement communities, long-term care institutions in the United States range from residential Homes for the elderly, private and state nursing Homes, psychiatric hospitals and chronic care hospitals. They may be profit or non-profit making but the average charges are beyond the means of most old people (House 1983). The facilities operate under the Medicare and Medicaid programmes. Medicare is a health insurance programme for the elderly and Medicaid is a welfare programme for the poor. They were designed to meet the medical needs of these high risk groups. Extended care, intermediate care and skilled nursing facilities are provided under the Medicare/Medicaid system and all have to fulfil certain standards of care in order to qualify for reimbursement of funds. Thus all long-term facilities are inspected on a regular basis. Some provide high quality care but many appear inadequate (House 1983). Strictly speaking, the licences of those not up to standard should be withdrawn, but it is difficult to do this because the need for nursing Home beds is acute in most areas. Therefore, in practice, licences are revoked only if flagrant abuse has occurred over several years.

A progressive and comprehensive policy on the care of old people has not been developed in the United States, and there is general agreement that the very sick and medically complex patient gets less than ideal care (House 1983). Staff tend to be scarce and doctors are absent, and potent tranquillisers frequently are used as restraints in consequence. Regimentation of the environment and the patient's day is very apparent and arranged to suit the staff. House observes that recruitment, retention and training of staff are great problems and responsibility for direct care tends to fall on untrained nurse aides. The few registered nurses are usually occupied on administrative duties.

Pressure groups

Pressure groups which lobby for self-determination are particularly well developed in the United States (American Association of Retired Persons, National Council of Senior Citizens, Gray Panthers). Sweden's pensioner groups have obtained legislation to provide income security and health and social services to the elderly (Nuberg 1981). The Federal Republic of Germany, the Netherlands and France all have legislation requiring retirement and nursing Homes to have elected councils of residents to advise their administrators. In some Homes residents serve on the board of directors and so they have considerable power. Pressure groups are less well developed in the United Kingdom than the United States but they are likely to increase, and future generations of old people are less likely than present-day elderly to acquiesce when offered inadequate services (see Chapter 1).

Conclusion

Although a continuum of care is the policy in many countries, services in most are piecemeal and variable. Services are generally underdeveloped in the USA and the Federal Republic of Germany, and the United Kingdom has a fairly extensive service but a lack of co-ordination between the health and social services. Poland has overcome this by giving the health ministry control of all services, but this has resulted in a medically dominated service.

In Canada, the province of Manitoba has got closer to an optimum balance. All services are administered by the Department of Health and Community Services which provides a complete continuum from home services to different levels of institutional care. Individuals are assessed by a diagnostic team and assigned to the most appropriate level of care. Services are administered centrally but implemented with local discretion, and so community resources, volunteers, etc. can be employed (Nuberg 1981). It is not clear what opportunity there is for individual choice in this system. It seems that no country has got the balance quite right for the care of its elderly people.

RESEARCH INTO NURSING ELDERLY PEOPLE

Research into the care of old people has become a more popular field of nursing research over recent years. Some 20% of the papers presented at the annual research conference in 1984, organised jointly by the Workgroup of European Nurse Researchers and the Royal College of Nursing, related to the elderly. In this final section are listed a number of areas in the nursing care of old people which need more research. The choice is based on topics raised in earlier chapters of this book, and on my own awareness of research needs gained from my teaching and research experience.

Quality of care of old people

As discussed in Chapter 29, very little research into evaluating the quality of patient care in terms of patient outcomes has been attempted in the United Kingdom. Miller's (1984) work is a notable exception. More work which compares methods of work organisation is required. Helen Evers (Chapter 22) and Pauline Fielding (Chapter 25) point to the need for more research to compare the effects of different kinds of wards (e.g. acute medical, orthopaedic, geriatric, psychogeriatric) and of multipurpose wards on patients' recovery and well-being. It has been found, for example, that long-stay patients in medical wards fare less well than those in geriatric wards (Fielding 1982).

Communicating with old people

The research literature mentioned in chapters 4 and 29 shows clearly that nurses spend very little time communicating either verbally or in non-verbal ways with elderly patients in hospital wards. There is a pressing need for nurses to develop effective communication skills, and Jill Macleod Clark (Chapter 4) identifies four areas relating to communication which tend to be unmet in care of the institutionalised elderly: the need for social contact and interaction; explanation and confirmation; advice, education and support; and comfort and reassurance. Communication is an area in which nurses, above all, should be specialists.

Loneliness

Loneliness is a topic which is frequently referred to in the literature, but which is relatively under-researched (Wenger 1983). It presents measurement difficulties because people are often reluctant to admit to loneliness, and the fear of loneliness may be the real problem rather than actual loneliness. Information on the nature and extent of loneliness is required, particularly of old people living in institutions and alone at home. Relief of extreme isolation and loneliness may be crucial for mental health.

Related to loneliness is the extent to which old people want to and do engage in different activities and interests (see Chapter 7). Research is needed on the effect of various activities, such as music, art and exercise therapy, and cooking, and of discussions on the well-being of old people. As Morva Fordham suggests in Chapter 15, activities and stimulation might reduce daytime sleeping from boredom and might improve night-time sleep. She also suggests that loneliness might be reduced and the quality of sleep improved if elderly patients were settled down for the night by their relatives. Also, the relationship of personal possessions and pets on the well-being of old people in long-stay institutions needs to be better understood. The opportunity for peace and solitude is rare in institutional life. How common is this problem for old people?

Noise

Uncontrolled and intrusive noise is unbearable, and has been used for brainwashing and torture in political contexts. Noise increases the communication problems of old people (see Chapter 4) and reduces the quality of sleep (see Chapter 15). Incessant noise from television and radio is very common in wards and dayrooms, and if combined with patients' cries and amplified by hearing aids, it can be intolerable (Norman 1980). Long-term elderly patients in hospital wards put noise amongst their most serious dislikes (Raphael and Mandeville 1979). We need information on the prevalence of noise from various sources (including nurses at night) and the effects on patients' quality of life and of sleep.

Falls

One of the 'giants of geriatrics', it is not clear what the factors are which unequivocally predispose old people to falls (see Chapter 8). This is a complex research area which Bernard Isaacs and his team at Birmingham University in the United Kingdom have been studying for some years. Nurses could collaborate in research programmes which study the relationship of various interventions to the incidence of falls.

Dementia

Another 'giant' which has at last attracted medical research funds. The growing problem of old people makes this a priority research area, and there is a need for nurses to collaborate in research into the management of old people with dementia.

Incontinence

Incontinence is a third 'giant' which is a research priority and is the subject of a research programme led by John Brocklehurst at Manchester University. Many topics spring to mind appropriate to nursing research (see Chapter 12). For example:

— The management of patient toileting by nurses in hospital wards, and the extent to which toileting regimes match individual micturition patterns.
— The effect of bed/chair protection on incontinence levels.
— Whether incontinence is reduced in a reality oriented, purposeful environment.
— The frequency with which urinary catheters are inserted for incontinence before other methods have been tried.
— The frequency with which appropriate catheter equipment is used (leg drainage bags, bag holders which are hidden from view, etc.) which preserves the patient's dignity.
— The reasons for and prevalence of bladder washouts for catheterised patients; what solution is used for irrigation, and the frequency with which safe closed irrigation is used.

Constipation

The prevention and management of constipation is an area of nursing responsibility which is often not handled well, particularly in long-stay settings. The evidence suggests that the prevalence of constipation in old people in hospital is high (e.g. Wright 1974). Chris Norton in Chapter 12 emphasises the need for a comprehensive nursing assessment of bowel function, and makes clear that recording a 'Yes' or 'No' answer is inadequate. Nurses need information on faecal amount, consistency, ease of passage, the use of laxatives, and so on. Also, in the management of constipation, we need more knowledge about the effect of different treatments and preventive regimes, such as exercise and diet; and on the use of laxatives by old people today.

Self-medication

There are immense problems of drug compliance by elderly people (see Chapter 20). There are many reasons for this, but lack of comprehension by patients is an important one on which nurses have influence. As Jill David (Chapter 20) suggests, suitable patients should be taught to administer their own drugs well before discharge from hospital, so that difficulties can be revealed and removed.

Single records

Communication between hospital and community workers, in both directions, is often poor (see Chapter 26), and research is needed on the feasibility of producing a single set of patients' notes which can accompany the patient wherever she goes, be it hospital, home, or nursing Home.

Risk-taking

Nurses and managers of hospitals and residential Homes are understandably concerned about the risk of litigation following accidents to patients. The outcome is that a detailed formal procedure is instigated when accidents occur even when the patient has come to no harm. The result is often that old people can be over-protected and prevented from doing anything that carries the slightest risk, such as boiling a kettle, and this reduces the likelihood that they will have independence and choice (see Chapters 23 and 29). More information is needed on the frequency of accidents, of allowing reasonable risk, and on the psychological damage to the patient who is restrained mechanically (cot sides, geriatric chair) and chemically (sedatives, tranquillisers). What is the frequency of accident form completion, and is there a relationship between number of accident forms and over-protection of elderly patients/clients?

Research wards

A few health authorities are introducing

3</

research wards into their hospitals where clinical nursing research can be carried out on a continuing basis. These are an excellent idea because they can effectively bridge the gap between research and practice, research can lose its ivory tower image, nurses and students can be exposed to research in the course of their work and get experience of conducting studies, and patients and staff are readily accessible for participation in studies, although the usual requirements concerning ethical approval and informed consent would have to be followed.

SUMMARY AND CONCLUSIONS

In this chapter we have looked briefly at the role of the nurse caring for old people, particularly at the feasibility of developing a nurse practitioner role. The need for improvement in this and other industrial countries makes the climate right for nurses to take the initative in promoting change and improvements in care. This is not easy for most nurses. They are not given a sufficiently comprehensive education, nor are they accustomed to initiating change. The style of working, at least in hospital nursing, is such that they are expected to be fully exposed on the job for the whole of their working time. Traditionally, nurses do not choose to, nor are they given time to, absent themselves for reading, thinking and writing. Other hospital workers (doctors, therapists, teachers) are visitors to the ward and can work more independently. They are in an easier position when wanting to introduce changes in their care.

The second section in this chapter moves away from a solely nursing orientation, and aims to provide an overview of health care provision. It is essential that nurses caring for old people understand the complexity of health care in this country and widen their skills so that they can operate as equal and contributing members of the health care team and can add their voices to debates on the care of old people. The emphasis in this book is on the organisation of health care for old people in Britain, although this chapter contains a brief look at some of the care provision in other industrialised countries.

The aim of the final section on nursing research needs has not been to present a comprehensive review of available research, but to suggest areas which would benefit from more research. If these thoughts stimulate readers to examine their own practices, to learn more about different aspects of nursing old people which interest them, and to investigate nursing questions for themselves, then the quality of nursing care can only improve and with it the quality of life for old people.

REFERENCES

Acheson E D 1982 The impending crisis of old age: a challenge to ingenuity. Lancet 1: 592–594
Austin R 1979 Practising health care: the nurse practitioner. In: Atkinson P, Dingwall R, Murcott A (eds) Prospects for the national health. Croom Helm, London
Batchelor I 1984 Policies for a crisis? Some aspects of DHSS policies for care of the elderly. Occasional Papers No 1, Nuffield Provincial Hospitals Trust, Oxford
Bosanquet N 1978 A future for old age. Towards a new society series. Temple Smith, London
Cox C 1983 Mightier than an army. Nursing Mirror 156:15 Nurse Education Conference Report, vi–vii
Department of Health and Social Security 1981 Professional development in clinical nursing—the 1980s. DHSS, London
Fielding P 1982 An examination of student nurse attitudes towards old people in hospital. Unpublished PhD Thesis, University of Southampton
Fitton J M 1984a Health visiting the elderly: nurse managers' views—1. Nursing Times Occasional Paper. 80(10): 59–61
Fitton J M 1984b Health visiting the elderly: nurse managers' views—2. Nursing Times Occasional Paper. 80(11): 67–69
Grimley Evans J 1981 Hospital care for the elderly. In: Shegog R F A (ed) The impending crisis of old age: a challenge to ingenuity. Oxford University Press for Nuffield Provincial Hospitals Trust, Oxford
Hall C 1984a A springboard to the future. Nursing Mirror 158(4): 39–41
Hall C 1984b A time for vision. Nursing Mirror 158(3): 32–35
Hearnden D 1983 Continuing care communities: a viable option in Britain? Centre for Policy on Ageing Report no. 3, CPA, London
Heller T 1978 Restructuring the health service. Croom Helm, London

House G 1983 Institutionalised elderly. In: Ernst N S, Glaser-Waldman H R (eds) The aged patient: a source book for the allied health professional. Year Book Medical Publishers, Chicago

Isaacs B 1981 Ageing and the doctor. In: Hobman D (ed) The impact of ageing: strategies for care. Croom Helm, London

Millard P H 1983 Long-term care in Europe: a review. In: Denham M J (ed) Care of the long-stay patient. Croom Helm, London

Miller A F 1984 Nursing process and patient care. Nursing Times Occasional Paper. 80(13): 56–58

Norman A 1980 Rights and risk. National Corporation for the Care of Old People (now Centre for Policy on Ageing), London

Nuberg C 1981 Programmes and services for the elderly in industrialised countries. In: Hobman D (ed) The Impact of Ageing: strategies for care. Croom Helm, London

Nursing Mirror 1984 The nurse practitioner. (Editorial.) Nursing Mirror 158(1):21

Nuttall P 1984 Shape of things to come? Nursing Times 80(1): 8–10

O'Neill P D 1983 Health crisis 2000. Heinemann, London

Raphael W, Mandeville J 1979 Old people in hospital. King Edward's Hospital Fund for London, London

Robertson C 1984 Old people in the community. 1. Health visitors and preventive care. Nursing Times 80(34): 29–31

Royal College of Nursing 1981 A structure for nursing. RCN, London

Shegog R F A (ed) 1981 The impending crisis of old age: a challenge to ingenuity. Oxford University Press for National Provincial Hospitals Trust, Oxford

Stilwell B 1984 The nurse in practice. Nursing Mirror 158(21):17

Tinker A 1984 Health and housing. Nursing Times 80(18): 57–59

Teeling Smith G 1984 A new NHS Act for 1996. Office of Health Economics, London

Turton P 1983 Health education and the district nurse. Nursing Times Community Outlook 79(32): 222–229

Turton P 1984 Nurses working in the community. Nursing Times 80(22): 40–42

Wenger C 1983 Loneliness: a problem of measurement. In: Jerrome D (ed) Ageing in modern society, Croom Helm, London

World Health Organisation 1983 Medicosocial work and nursing: the changing needs. EURO Reports and Studies 79. WHO Regional Office for Europe, Copenhagen

Wright L 1974 Bowel function in hospital patients. Study of Nursing Care Series 1 no. 4, Royal College of Nursing, London

Index